CURRENT TOPICS IN PUBLIC HEALTH

Edited by **Alfonso J. Rodriguez-Morales**

Current Topics in Public Health
http://dx.doi.org/10.5772/56648
Edited by Alfonso J. Rodriguez-Morales

Contributors

Michael Adedigba, Isaiah Oke, Regina Arobieke, Nkechi Chuks Nwachukwu, Orji Frank Anayo, Ositadinma Chinyere Ugbogu, Yasutaka Chiba, Etsuji Suzuki, Erika Rodriguez-Wulff, Leonardo Sosa Valencia, Juan Sepúlveda-Arias, Adalucy Alvarez-Aldana, Cristian Díaz-Vélez, Víctor Soto-Cáceres, Eric Ricardo Peña-Sánchez, Moisés Alexander Apolaya-Segura, Edén Galán-Rodas, Adrian Bolivar-Mejia, Boris Eduardo Vesga Angarita, Charles Ntungwen Fokunang, Alfonso J. Rodriguez-Morales, Diana M. Castañeda-Hernández, Niyi Awofeso, Naser Al Jaser, Peter Papoh Ndibewu, Prince Ngobeni, Mosiur Rahman, Abdur R Mia, Syed Emdadul Haque, Nowsheen Sharmin Purabi, Sar Choudhury, Maria De Lourdes Pereira, Irvathur Krishnananda Pai, Fernando Garcia E Costa, Spencer Moore, Emma Bassett, Jason Turner, Simone Singh, Connie Evashwick, Steven Eastaugh, Klara Slezakova, Simone Morais, Maria Carmo Pereira, Claudia Marin-Kelso, Susan Kinnear, Zobaidul Kabir, Julie Mann, Lisa Bricknell, Emanuela Barbini, Paolo Barbini, Pietro Manzi, Balwinder Singh, Ajay Parsaik, John Berry, Matthew R Hipsey, Justin Brookes, Jalila Jbilou, Réjean Landry, Salaheddine El Adlouni, Nabil Amara, Erasto Mbugi, Carmen Luisa Betancur Pulgarín, Salim Mattar, Nelson Alvis, Marco Gonzalez

Published by InTech
Janeza Trdine 9, 51000 Rijeka, Croatia

Publishing Process Manager Sandra Bakic
Technical Editor InTech DTP team
Cover InTech Design team

Additional hard copies can be obtained from orders@intechopen.com

Current Topics in Public Health, Edited by Alfonso J. Rodriguez-Morales
p. cm.
ISBN 978-953-51-1121-4

For EU product safety concerns:
IN TECH d.o.o., Prolaz Marije Krucifikse Kozulić 3, 51000 Rijeka, Croatia,
info@intechopen.com or visit our website at intechopen.com.

Meet the editor

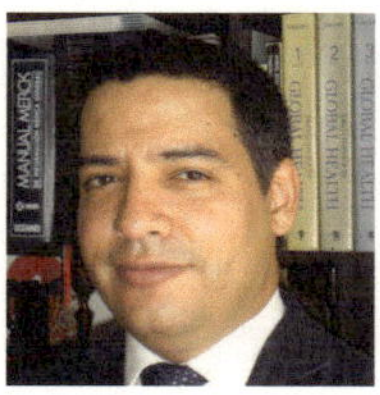

Prof. Alfonso J. Rodriguez-Morales - Medical Doctor (MD), Universidad Central de Venezuela, Caracas, Venezuela, in 2003; Master of Sciences in Protozoology (MSc), Universidad de Los Andes, Trujillo, Venezuela, 2004-2005; Diploma in Tropical Medicine & Hygiene (DT-M&H), Universidad Peruana Cayetano Heredia, Lima, Peru and University of Alabama at Birmingham, USA, 2009. He is fellow of the Royal Society for Tropical Medicine & Hygiene (FRSTMH), UK, 1998. Fellow of the Faculty of Travel Medicine (FFTM) of the Royal College of Physicians and Surgeons of Glasgow (RCPSG), UK, 2010. Candidate to Doctor in Parasitology (PhD), Universidad Central de Venezuela, 2005-2008. Editor, Journal of Infection in Developing Countries. Chair, Comission of Scientific Publications and Teaching of the Latin American Society for Travel Medicine. Editorial Board, Travel Medicine and Infectious Diseases. Guest Editor, Special Issue "Immunology of Zoonotic Infections", Clinical and Developmental Immunology. Member of the Advisory Board, Peruvian Journal of Experimental Medicine and Public Health. Associated Editor, Journal of the Colombian Association of Infectious Diseases. Assistant Editor, Journal of the Faculty of Health Sciences, Universidad Tecnológica de Pereira, Pereira, Risaralda, Colombia. Former Member of the Venezuelan Society of Public Health. Full Member of the Colombian Association of Infectious Diseases. Author of 118 articles published in international journals. Editor of the book Current Topics in Tropical Medicine (ISBN 978-953-51-0274-8).

Contents

Preface

Public health is a major health discipline in the world. Defined as the science and art of preventing diseases, prolonging life and promoting health through the organized efforts and informed choices of the society, organizations (public and private), communities and individuals, this discipline has been renewed by the incorporation of multiple actors, professions, knowledge areas, as well as being impacted and promoted by multiple technologies, particularly information ones. As a changing field of knowledge, public health requires evidence-based information and regular updates, even more in the context of a world in epidemiological transition. Health impacts of climate change are currently in the quest of the Millennium Development Goals, and most of them are related to the activities of public health. "Current Topics in Public Health" presents updated information on multiple topics related to actual areas of interest in this growing and exciting medical science, with the conception and philosophy that we are working to improve the health of the population, rather than treating diseases of individual patients; taking decisions about collective health care that are based on the best available, current, valid and relevant evidence; and finally within the context of available resources. Public health should be a complex science helping in the decision, actions and changes in the health of the world. In a globalized society this is emphasized not just in a particular nation but in the whole world.

Public health topics can diverge from basic aspects of this discipline to multiple applications in very specialized related fields. With these conceptions in mind, this book includes different topics on public health of current international interest, trying to update the most significant research in many of them as well as to offer a multinational perspective on different aspects. This book has been organized in 8 major sections: I) Methods in Public Health; II) Healthcare Systems; III) Evidence-based Public Health; IV) Communicable Diseases in Public Health; V) Non-Communicable Diseases in Public Health; VI) Environmental Public Health; VII) Pharmacoepidemiology and Pharmacosurveillance in Public Health; and VIII) Research, Ethics, Social and Teaching Issues in Public Health.

Section I includes topics covering from epidemiological and statistical analyses up to the implications of new technologies in public health research. Section II includes topics covering experiences from different countries in healthcare systems research. Section III includes topics on philosophy of evidence-based medicine applied to public health, clinical epidemiology and evidence assessment in public health. Section IV includes topics on the epidemiology of infectious diseases, human immunodeficiency virus (HIV), human papiloma virus (HPV), tuberculosis, and viral haemorrhagic fevers. Section V includes topics on the burden of chronic diseases of global relevance such as cancer and cardiovascular diseases. Section VI includes topics related to different environmental issues of relevance for the public health. Section VII includes a topic on antibiotic pharmacosurveillance. And finally, section VIII includes chapters about issues on research, as well on social epidemiology and related fields, ethical issues and on the teaching in public health.

Following the same philosophy as we had on the previous book, "Current Topics in Tropical Medicine" (Rodriguez-Morales AJ, 2012), this books does not intend to be an exhaustive compilation and this first edition has included not just multiple different topics but also a wide geographical participation from many countries. Its online availability allows it to reach a wide audience in the world. This book has been endorsed by the Council of the Faculty of Health Sciences of the Universidad Tecnológica de Pereira, Pereira, Colombia (Meeting No. 014, July 17, 2012). Continuing on the series of "Current Topic" books, now, we are planning to develop "Current Topics in Infectious Diseases", so if you are interested in participate in this endeavor as an author of one or more chapter, please contact us.

I would like to give especial thanks to InTech, and particularly to Ana Nikolic, Dragana Manestar and Sandra Bakic, for the opportunity to edit this interesting and important book, as well for their constant support. I want to dedicate this book to my family and particularly to my lovely wife, Diana, my strongest support; she provides everything in my life; and also to my friends and my undergraduate and postgraduate students of health sciences in Venezuela, Colombia and around Latin America.

We hope our readers will enjoy this publication as much as I did reading the chapters of "Current Topics in Public Health".

Alfonso J. Rodriguez-Morales
Infection and Immunity Research Group and Department of Community Medicine,
Faculty of Health Sciences, Universidad Tecnológica de Pereira, Pereira,
Risaralda, Colombia

Office of Scientific Research,
Cooperativa de Entidades de Salud de Risaralda (COODESURIS),
Pereira, Colombia

Instituto José Witremundo Torrealba, Universidad de Los Andes,
Trujillo, Venezuela

Section 1

Methods in Public Health

Chapter 1

Academic' Policy Briefings: What Determines Health Researchers' Involvement in Public Health Policy Informing?

Jalila Jbilou, Réjean Landry,
Salah-Eddine El Adlouni and Nabil Amara

Additional information is available at the end of the chapter

http://dx.doi.org/10.5772/53536

1. Introduction

Over the last decade there has been widespread interest in the Organization for Economic Co-operation and Development (OECD) countries in ensuring that the best available evidence underpins policymaking process and the ways in which health services are organized and delivered (Lavis, Rottingen et al. 2012). The rational underlining this paradigm is of two perspectives: an economic one that supports a return of investment from public funded research and a social one that supports a better care and better health outcomes for individuals and the entire population. In Canada, this is reflected in the structure of the federal and provincials' health systems (introduction of research and development units to support policy and decision making) and the specific programs of funding agencies (grants for systematic reviews projects, for knowledge dissemination activities, for collaborative and applied research, and the investment in CADRE program) (CIHR 2007).

The emergence of the evidence based paradigm and the actual policy discourse of the knowledge economy offer an ideal platform for collaborative research. Considering particularities of academia and public health professionals one can imagine that new challenges have to be addressed by academics (Limb 2012): 1) how to produce operational outputs and 2) How to transfer them effectively to public health policy makers? In the healthcare sector, knowledge and scientific evidence flow are now considered critical for health system development and for population health status (Ettelt and Mays 2011). For public health sector, the remaining question is: how to effectively integrate evidence on modifiable risk factors and cost-effectiveness of population-based interventions designed to reduce these risks in public health programs and policies development? Governments around the world had developed public capital ventures to support applied and fundamental research to improve the impact of publicly funded research, seen as a public good, and increase the return on investment for a much more cost-effective health system, a better population health status and the reduction of health inequalities (Orton, Lloyd-Williams, et al. 2011; Waters 2011). In short, this perspective puts universities as key actors to drive societies towards the knowledge economy. For public health sector, universities produce evidence, expertise and knowledge through various traditional channels of information i.e. human resources training (graduate and post-graduate), applied research, translational research and academic consulting. Recently, universities have been encouraged to develop links with governmental institutions in a series of new modes of partnership: collaborative research, participative action research, evaluative research, experts groups on specific topics and academic policy informing (policy briefs). *"Policy briefs are a relatively new approach to packaging research evidence for policymakers."* (Lavis, Permanand et al. 2009).

However, during the last two decades, the health sector has been under tremendous pressure in responding to the ongoing global political situation, economic constraints, ecologic changes and social and demographic challenges. Thinking new ways to support decision making, in such rapidly changing context, calls for proactive strategies and timely actions. Evidence-based public health policy informing through academic policy briefings provision is different from evidence based medicine, in which gold standards evidence, is mainly systematic reviews, meta-analysis and randomized controlled trials. Public health policy process is complex, involves series of actors (institutions and individuals) and decision levels (micro, meso and macro level) and requires evidence from different research domains policy sciences, economics, epidemiology, community health or healthcare management that may offer sometimes conflicting information.

Literature on public health policy making process and impact of evidence and research findings on this process is not optimal and calls for rethinking knowledge transfer strategies in this domain, especially through the perspective of health academics. Indeed, traditionally health and medical academics role was exclusively centred on teaching and leading research on clinical practices, patients' behaviour and healthcare management with a major focus on evidence based decision making in clinical practices. Less attention had been paid to public health policy informing and evidence-based public health. Therefore, public health policy informing requires not only the production of useful knowledge, which relates to the needs of public health, but also to ensure its transfer to policy makers in timely, easy and ready to use format. According to authors (Carroll, Cooke et al. 2006; Jetha, Robinson et al. 2008; Lavis, Moynihan et al. 2008), informing public health policymaking through academic policy briefings (APB) is an effective strategy to improve healthy policies formulation and to consolidate the strategic interface between academics and the governmental organizations. Canada has promoted knowledge brokers and health policy analysts as key actors (or intermediaries) to close the university-government gap. However, these new roles are still to develop and to better clarify for an optimal effectiveness. Public health policies as an evidence informed policy making process has implication for researchers, who should be striving to be

http://dx.doi.org/10.5772/53536

more involved with policy making and studying the implications of policies on public health care interventions and programs (De Palma 2002; Hanney and Block 2009; Lomas and Brown 2009). Major researches had been done to better understand what determine decision makers' utilization of research results and evidence. However, we still not know much on what makes health and medical academics perform knowledge translation activities, especially in terms of APB. Indeed, implementing academic policy informing as a new role for health and medical academics will need strategic approaches to support its performance and maintenance as a routine strategy to foster public health knowledge translation into health policies. Thus, in this paper, we propose to explore determinants of health and medical academics involvement in preparing and presenting APB to public health policy makers, as part of their contribution to the knowledge translation process.

2. Overview of the existing literature

One of the greatest challenges facing evidence informed policymaking is not necessarily the accessibility to evidence but actually getting it used while the process is under a series of internal and external pressures such as stakeholders influences (lobbying and administrative bureaucracy), economic factors (cost containing, efficiency and systems performance), and professionals (corporative pressure and clinical autonomy) (Moore 2006; Bowen, Erickson, et al. 2009). More recently, with the spreading of the evidence informing policy paradigm, universities and academics are seen as an additional major pressure (Clancy et al. 2012). The Canadian health care system, like those in OECD countries, confronts continued pressures (cost constraints; systems performance and services quality challenges; population health demographics and epidemiology). Public health researchers can influence policy making in different ways. Providing valuable information to policy makers is a challenging process for researchers. It implies not only the demonstration of lab or pilot effectiveness but also their transferability at large, their flexibility to contextualization, the clarification of needed resources and the anticipation of impacts on the system and the population. Such type of information requires clear understanding of policy formulation process, public health programs development and management, health professionals' constraints and population and social values and expectations. Involving health researchers in policy makers' informing through APB calls for rethinking academics' social role and a major shift from "Neutral technicians" to "Issue Advocate" (Sabatier and Jenkins-Smith 1999). Knowledge transfer literature shows that APB should be thought of as a set of rules and institutional arrangements designed to encourage transparent and balanced use of evidence and research results in health policy making (Cookson 2005). In a dynamic world where contingencies and crisis are constant the evidence and research results are to inform rather to shape the process. Thus, researchers have to engage in better highlighting information that is relevant for decision and policymaking (Lavis, Davies et al. 2005). But a range of barriers to knowledge and/or evidence utilization in health policy making process still exist such as the system bureaucratization, the decision-making centralization, the conflict of evidences/values/culture, the nature of evidence and knowledge (qualitative research…), policymakers attributes (lack of research culture, competencies, skills and resources) and the persistent asymmetry of information between researchers and policy makers (Hanney, Gonzalez-Block et al. 2003, Thacker et al. 2005). Nutley and al. (2003) summarise the four key requirements that are necessary for improving evidence use in policy and one of them is the effective *dissemination* of evidence to where it is most needed and the development of effective means of providing wide access to knowledge. Politicians utilize evidence depending on related benefits and risks that they are ready to take during decision-making process (Walshe and Rundall 2001). A large literature exists on policy makers' determinants and especially on the procedural components of their utilization of evidence (e.g. information systems, capacity building, structural organization, organizational factors, utilization types….) (Dobrow, Goel et al. 2004; Mitton and Donaldson 2004; Ouimet, Landry et al. 2006; Jbilou, Amara et al. 2007; Lavis et al. 2012). But less is known on health researchers' contribution in this process. It will go beyond rehearsing the challenges, and question some of our basic assumptions about how health researchers could help to achieve a more equitable and a more efficient health policymaking? The answer to this question is closely dependant on the answer to: What factors challenge or help health academics performing Academic Policy Briefings (APB)?

3. Conceptual framework

The move to more informed policy making has been a recent and much-advocated feature of public policy, especially in health and social care. An essential element of this approach is to make available synthesis of evidence in an accessible format. APB the most studied formats, had been explored under policy analysts' perspective but never under health academics' perspective. A range of issues limit research results use in policy making process. Two broad areas of issues: the format in which the results are presented and the forum for whom the results are designated. The format issues include the manner, the time and the philosophy in which research reports are presented. The forum issues involve undertaking a clear response to specific problems or concerns, so as to guide decision and action. I did an extended review of the literature to clarify the concept of APB performance by health academics. There is a wide consensus on the fact that APB should be better approached as a personal behavior. Literature presents APB as a dual phenomenon based on two conceptual components: 1) the structural component that depends closely on both organizational and individual characteristics and 2) the relational component that depends on networks and links. Thus, we extracted from the literature a range of factors that have a confirmed or potential effect on APB performance by academic researchers (Figure 1): Relational capital (governmental health organizations), domain of research (health policy, health services, population health) and orientation of research (applied or basic research), self perceptions (efficacy, credibility, barriers to research utilization), personal area of interests (systematic review, clinical guidelines), Existence of a clear strategy of research dissemination, availability of electronic channel for information flow (such as Internet, weekly published newsletters, electronic Websites), participation in expert groups and committees (consultancy), radicalness of research results and individual characteristics (gender, education, university position, diversification of workplace).

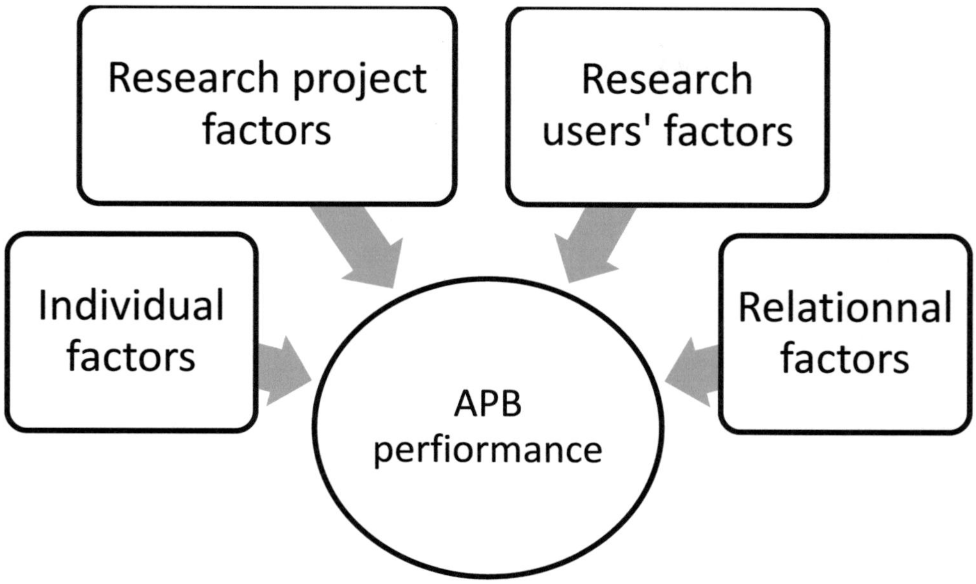

Figure 1. Operational framework

This paper considers the role of health academics as actors in social and health development, and the implications for approaches to knowledge, through knowledge transfer and exchange (KT&E) activities. It will determine the major factors that explain why health academics write and transmit APB to policy makers and derive incentives and strategies to put in place to support them perform this KT&E activity that consolidate the Triple Helix interface between universities and governments.

4. Methodology and data

4.1. Population under study

The project titled "Factors that incite researchers in the health sciences to engage in KT activities leading to the utilization of their results in Canadian health care system." Ad concerned a representative sample (health research domains and Canadian provinces) of researchers from all Canadian medical schools and faculties (medicine, nursing, pharmacy, community medicine, healthcare management and policy). Names and addresses of researchers were collected from provincial registries of health researchers and from the websites of all the 16 Canadian medical schools with no regard to their status as faculty members or other categories of researchers, since provincial registries do not specify this information. We selected a stratified random sample of 3814 health researchers from the 5712 that have been identified, with stratification designed to ensure a regional distribution in line with the distribution of the Canadian population and the distribution of Canadian medical school revenues for biomedical and health care research. Among the 3814 individuals in the original sample, 2207 were deemed ineligible. The reasons for their ineligibility are the following: the language used was different from English or French (n=11), part of an over-sample in a single province that had been requested by a financing partner (n=120), impossible to reach either an individual or voice mail after more than 25 calls (n=707), and other reasons (n=1369) such as not a faculty member, not conducting research anymore, on sabbatical vacation or in an administrative post, moved, retired, or incorrect or discontinued telephone numbers. From the 1607 faculty members eligible to be included in the final sample, 10 asked to be interviewed later but were never reached again, 23 ended the call before the questionnaire had been completed, and 596 refused to participate (after a recall). The survey generated 978 adequate responses to the questionnaires for a net response rate of 60.86%. The regional distribution of respondents is very close to what was originally targeted in the sampling strategy.

4.2. Instrument for data collection

Based on an extended review of the literature and on a previous questionnaire developed by authors to explore knowledge transfer activities among social sciences researchers (Landry and Amara 2001), we built a comprehensive questionnaire to map knowledge translation activities and their predictors. The questionnaire was assessed by an advisory committee comprised of health researchers, clinicians, health system managers and policymakers. They reviewed its preliminary drafts in regard of its feasibility (length), its appropriateness (concordance with academic professional context) and its intelligibility (clarity of questions). The questionnaire includes close-ended questions and was administered by telephone by a survey firm that uses computer-assisted telephone interviewing (CATI) technology, which allows for simultaneous data entry and data coding.

4.3. Data analysis

A range of issues limit the research results used in the policymaking process (Gregrich, 2003). There are two broad areas of issues: those linked to the format and those related to the forum. The format issues include the manner, the time and the philosophy in which research reports are presented. The forum issues involve undertaking a clear response to specific problems or concerns, so as to guide decision and action (Gregrich, 2003). Based on those two assumptions, we built a question to measure PMI. We considered that involvement in PMI is accomplished when both actions are completed: preparing and presenting targeted reports on specific health topics. The question that measures the PMI is *the following: 'Do you prepare and present targeted reports on specific health topics to policy makers?'* The answers were: Yes =1 or No=0.

The analysis plan is based on the estimation of an econometric model through a Logistic regression model applied to identify predictors of APB among public health academics.

$$APB = \beta 0 + \beta 1\ INFOCHAN + \beta 2\ LnUNSIZ + \beta 3\ STRATKET + \beta 4\ RELCADM + \beta 5\ HOSP\&UNIV + \beta 6\ PERCRED + \beta 7\ PEREFFIK + \beta 8\ EXPERPRO + \beta 9\ RESPECIA + \beta 10\ MOSDEG + \beta 11\ PROFES + \beta 12\ GENDER + \beta 13\ USRECAP + \beta 14\ APPLYRES + \beta 15\ INNOVAT + \varepsilon$$

Where,

βi (i= 0…….15) are the coefficients to estimate.

5. Results

5.1. Descriptive statistics

Of the 978 respondents who participated in the survey, the average number of researchers that had undergone APB is 35%. Among the 978 respondents, 91.6% had a PhD/MSc and 8.4% had only a professional degree such as medical doctor, nurse or pharmacist. However, 78.5% of the respondents were men. Among the respondents, 85.6% carry their work at university, 60.6% at a teaching hospital and 8.0% in other type of organizations. The population repartition of the study by fields of activity reveals that 44.3% declare working in fundamental health sciences, 43.8 % in clinical sciences and 12.0% in public health or population health sciences (Health policy research, health services research, health promotion research).

Only 35% of the respondents consider that they perform APB. While 72% of them declared that they are active in applied research and 14% active in political sciences research. The sample is made of 78.5% of men, 83.6% hold a PhD, 25.7% hold a clinical certification (MD, Nurse, pharmacist…) and 46.1% are professors or assistant professors.

5.2. Logistic regression model estimation

The econometric model used here to estimate the predictors of APB performance among health academics show that there are seven facilitators and two barriers. Having a clear and well defined strategy for KT&E is a predictor of APB. The KT&E strategy as measured in this work relate on 4 activities: to define the intended users or beneficiaries of the project's results, the description of dissemination goals and strategies, the researcher personal follow-up with users to assess how useful project information is and the personal follow-up with users to assess how easily project information could be applied. Such an approach is drawn on the participatory action research perspective.

The results presented here show that effective collaboration between academics and governments institutions is based on the relational aspects (relational capital with government has a positive impact on APB) but also on structural aspects (KT&E formal strategy). More, health academics' research profile is important in terms of APB performance. For example, being active researcher in political sciences, combination of research settings (at the hospital and at the university) and developing innovative research are predictors of APB. The perceived credibility has also a positive impact on APB. The past professional experience, as health administrators, has also a positive and significant impact on APB. However, the results show that being active in applied research and the availability of electronic channels of research information flow are inhibitors of APB performance by health academics.

Independent variables		
	Coeff. β	*EXP β*
Organizational factors		
Availability of electronic channels of information flow [INFOCHAN]	-.630$^{(***)}$	.533
Size of research unit [LnUNSIZ]	.1389$^{(NS)}$	1.148
Formal Strategy for KE&T [STRATKET]	.467$^{(***)}$	1.596
Individual factors		
Relational capital with Government [RELCADM]	.961$^{(***)}$	2.614
Combination of research settings [HOSP&UNIV]	.410$^{(*)}$	1.507
Perceived credibility [PERCRED]	.865$^{(**)}$	2.374
Perceived efficacy on policy decision making [PEREFFIK]	.169$^{(NS)}$	1.184
Administrative Experiential Assets [EXPERPRO]	.019$^{(*)}$	1.019
Health Policy Research [RESPECIA]	1.340$^{(**)}$	3.818
Cognitive Assets [MOSDEG]	.012$^{(NS)}$	1.012
Academic position [PROFES]	-.174$^{(NS)}$	.841
Gender [GENDER]	.118$^{(NS)}$	1.125
Research users' factors		
Users' receptive capacity [USRECAP]	.093$^{(NS)}$	1.097
Research project factors		
Applied research projects [APPLYRES]	-.445$^{(*)}$	.641
Innovativeness of research [INNOVAT]	.260$^{(*)}$	1.297
Constant	-5.031$^{(***)}$	.007
Total number of cases:	606	
Chi-square (d.f.):	171.626 (15)	
Nagelkerke R^2 (Pseudo R Square):	.351	
Percentage of correct prediction	77.9%	

Table 1. Econometric model estimation

6. Conclusion and implications

With this contribution, we take a first step toward closing the gap in the literature concerning APB, with a special emphasis on the role of medical schools. The overarching hypothesis in this study, therefore, is: academic policy briefing development is a function of its endowments in financial, relational and intellectual capital with the two first being provided by the university and the others by the researcher. We test this hypothesis on a pan Canadian sample of researchers affiliated to medical schools.

http://dx.doi.org/10.5772/53536

Strong relationships between academics and policymakers appear to increase the prospects for research use (Lavis, Moynihan et al. 2008). Many research projects have been undertaken to address the factors that increase the prospects for research use by public policymakers and encourage partnerships between researchers and policymakers that allow for their interaction around the tasks of asking and answering relevant policy questions (Lavis 2006). Much less progress has been made understanding what factors impact on academics involvement in the triple helix model and especially in its non commercial part as for developing academic policy briefings (APB). We still need to address APB performance determinants among public health academics to improve the evidence informed policy making process. An important proportion of public health research is related to social and welfare care dimensions and topics and has no impact on patenting or copyright which may inhibit its dissemination to policymakers and may rely exclusively on researchers' involvement in research push activities, such as APB performance.

The results presented here show that APB performance is an individual behavior that is under specific professional orientation, organizational structural factors and personal motivation rather than individual social and demographic characteristics such as gender, most advanced education degree or academic position. Indeed, public health academics seem to be of traditional culture since they still relate on personnel relational capital (the relational capital with governmental institutions through face-to-face meetings and collaborative research) rather than electronic interface (through websites and electronic newsletters) to disseminate their research results. Moreover, organizational factors are of major relevance to support APB performance among public health academics. Having a formal strategy of knowledge exchange and transfer is an important factor for facilitating evidence flow from academic department to policymakers' offices. Universities have to support and stimulate administrative involvement of public health researchers. This type of activities may raise more awareness about stakes of policy decision making context and helps academics understand the contingencies of administrative decision process and the relevance of developing APB to improve the follow of research results to support this process. Moreover, researchers how carried out their research in different research settings, at the university and at the clinical settings, performed APB more than those having a single setting of research, at the university. This result lets us suggest that public health researchers need to be exposed to different realities and contingencies to better perform APB. Bilateral collaboration between university and government institutions had been developed extensively these last two decades and resulted, unfortunately, in innovations that lacked a context to be put to use. Health sector had beneficed largely from these collaborations with little accountability since intellectual property and its translation into policies, services products and process had been called the "death valley". The emergence of public health entrepreneurs called for more accountability and more knowledge translation among public health researchers. Thus, developing effective multi-sectors networks is a critical activity to improve and innovate in teaching and training for strategic knowledge transfer competencies among public health researchers.

In terms of research related factors, being involved in health policy research and developing innovative research are major factors of APB performance. However, those involved in applied research were less likely to perform APB. These results let us suggest that more efforts have to be invested to support applied research academics and show them how to develop and how to disseminate APB to improve utilization of their research results. Finally, we found out that the perceived credibility has a positive impact on APB performance. In fact, the more the researcher believes that his research is useful and is used to support policymaking the more he gets involved in APB development and dissemination to targeted audiences.

In knowledge transfer literature, less attention had been paid to the existing differences between academics, political analyst and knowledge brokers in terms of roles, legitimacy and inputs in developing policy briefings. Indeed, policy briefings had traditionally been prepared by policy analysts. The evidence based paradigm has raised new concerns about who would analyze and synthesize research results. In Canada, *"a knowledge broker (KB) is a popular knowledge translation and exchange (KT&E) strategy emerging in Canada to promote interaction between researchers and end users, as well as to develop capacity for evidence-informed decision making."* (Dobbins, Robeson et al. 2009) However, APB by health academics is a new concept (Carroll, Cooke et al. 2006). Health and health research is complex and diversified; thus, it is hard to propose a standard approach for research push. APB is an individual behavior that needs a cultural change among health academics. To improve the performance of APB among health academics the university has to make intrinsic efforts. For example, a new system of awards has to be developed to value and support KT&E activities. In terms of capacity building, health academics have to be supported to build an effective KT&E strategy (Pope, Mays et al. 2006). Since, it is not only important to disseminate but also to evaluate the usefulness, the utility and the impact of the APB (Field et al. 2012; Kurko et al. 2012; Lavis, Rottingen, et al. 2012). There is also a major challenge for low and middle income countries where there is a need for implementing effective structured policymaking processes, establishing functional KT&E platforms and leveraging policymakers and researchers' engagement in KT&E activities (Collender et al. 2012; El-Jardali et al. 2012; Uneke, Ezeoha, et al. 2012). We explored the perspective of researchers from medical schools through a cross-sectional survey, which allowed us to control for faculties and schools idiosyncrasies and for time. However this approach necessarily limits the generalizability of these results cross other university departments. Future research should attempt to test the model predicting APB across a larger number of departments, especially those who carry public health research, to enhance the external validity of the presented model. We speculate that disciplinary specificities in terms of predictors will be identified.

Acknowledgements

Authors would like to thank the Canadian Institute for Health Research (CIHR) for the financial support provided to PrRéjean Landry, director of the CIHR Chair on knowledge transfer and innovation (Université Laval). Dr. Jalila Jbilou contribution was supported by the CIHR Team in Familial Risks of Breast Cancer Grant (CRN-8752-1) and the Ministry of Economic Development, Innovation and Export Trade of Quebec – Supporting grant (PSR-SIIRI-701).

http://dx.doi.org/10.5772/53536

Author details

Jalila Jbilou[1,2,3*], Réjean Landry[4], Salah-Eddine El Adlouni[3] and Nabil Amara[4]

*Address all correspondence to: jalila.jbilou@umoncton.ca

1 Centre de formation médicale du Nouveau Brunswick-Université de Sherbrooke (QC), Canada

2 Réseau de santé Vitalité (NB), Canada

3 Université de Moncton (NB), Canada

4 Université Laval (QC), Canada

References

[1] Bowen, S, Erickson, T, et al. (2009). More Than "Using Research": The Real Challenges in Promoting Evidence-Informed Decision-Making." Healthc Policy , 4(3), 87-102.

[2] Collender, G, Gabrysch, S, et al. (2012). Reducing maternal mortality: better monitoring, indicators and benchmarks needed to improve emergency obstetric care. Research summary for policymakers." Trop Med Int Health.

[3] Carroll, C, Cooke, J, et al. (2006). Bridging the gap: the development of knowledge briefings at the health and social care interface." Health Soc Care Community , 14(6), 491-8.

[4] Clancy, C. M, Glied, S. A, & Lurie, N. (2012). From Research to Health Policy Impact". Health Services Research, doi:j.1475-6773.2011.01374.x, 47, 337-343.

[5] Cookson, R. (2005). Evidence-based policy making in health care: what it is and what it isn't." J Health Serv Res Policy , 10(2), 118-21.

[6] Dobbins, M, Robeson, P, et al. (2009). A description of a knowledge broker role implemented as part of a randomized controlled trial evaluating three knowledge translation strategies." Implement Sci 4: 23.

[7] Dobrow, M. J, Goel, V, et al. (2004). Evidence-based health policy: context and utilisation." Soc Sci Med , 58(1), 207-17.

[8] El-Jardali, F, Ataya, N, et al. (2012). A multi-faceted approach to promote knowledge translation platforms in eastern Mediterranean countries: climate for evidence-informed policy." Health Res Policy Syst 10(1): 15.

[9] Ettelt, S, & Mays, N. (2011). Health services research in Europe and its use for informing policy." J Health Serv Res Policy 16 Suppl , 2, 48-60.

[10] Field, P, Gauld, R, et al. (2012). Evidence-informed health policy- the crucial role of advocacy." Int J Clin Pract , 66(4), 337-41.

[11] Hanney, S. R, Gonzalez-block, M. A, et al. (2003). The utilisation of health research in policy-making: concepts, examples and methods of assessment." Health Res Policy Syst 1(1): 2.

[12] Hanney, S. R, & Gonzalez-block, M. A. (2009). Evidence-informed health policy: are we beginning to get there at last?" Health Res Policy Syst 7:30

[13] Jbilou, J, Amara, N, et al. (2007). Research-based-decision-making in Canadian health organizations: a behavioural approach." J Med Syst , 31(3), 185-96.

[14] Jetha, N, Robinson, K, et al. (2008). Supporting knowledge into action: The Canadian Best Practices Initiative for Health Promotion and Chronic Disease Prevention." Can J Public Health 99(5): I, 1-8.

[15] Lavis, J, Davies, H, et al. (2005). Towards systematic reviews that inform health care management and policy-making." J Health Serv Res Policy 10 Suppl , 1, 35-48.

[16] Lavis, J. N. (2006). Research, public policymaking, and knowledge-translation processes: Canadian efforts to build bridges." J Contin Educ Health Prof , 26(1), 37-45.

[17] Lavis, J. N, Moynihan, R, et al. (2008). Evidence-informed health policy Case descriptions of organizations that support the use of research evidence." Implement Sci 3: 56., 4.

[18] Lavis, J. N, Permanand, G, et al. (2009). SUPPORT Tools for evidence-informed health Policymaking (STP) 13: Preparing and using policy briefs to support evidence-informed policymaking." Health Res Policy Syst 7 Suppl 1: S13.

[19] Lavis, J. N, Rottingen, J. A, et al. (2012). Guidance for evidence-informed policies about health systems: linking guidance development to policy development." PLoS Med 9(3): e1001186.

[20] Limb, M. (2012). Evidence is still not informing policy on obesity, conference hears." BMJ 344: e1023.

[21] Lomas, J, & Brown, A. D. (2009). Research and advice giving: a functional view of evidence-informed policy advice in a Canadian Ministry of Health." Milbank Q , 87(4), 903-26.

[22] Kurko, T, Silvast, A, et al. (2012). Is pharmaceutical policy evidence-informed? A case of the deregulation process of nicotine replacement therapy products in Finland." Health Policy 105(2-3): 246-55.

[23] Mitton, C, & Donaldson, C. (2004). Health care priority setting: principles, practice and challenges." Cost Eff Resour Alloc 2(1): 3.

[24] Moore, R. A. (2006). Evidence-based policy-making." Clin Chem Lab Med , 44(6), 678-82.

[25] Niedzwiedzka, B. M. (2003). Barriers to evidence-based decision making among Polish healthcare managers." Health Serv Manage Res , 16(2), 106-15.

[26] Ouimet, M, Landry, R, et al. (2006). What factors induce health care decision-makers to use clinical guidelines? Evidence from provincial health ministries, regional health authorities and hospitals in Canada." Soc Sci Med , 62(4), 964-76.

[27] Orton, L, Lloyd-williams, F, et al. (2011). The use of research evidence in public health decision making processes: systematic review." PLoS One 6(7): e21704.

[28] Peirson, L, Ciliska, D, et al. (2012). Building capacity for evidence informed decision making in public health: a case study of organizational change." BMC Public Health 12: 137.

[29] Pope, C, Mays, N, et al. (2006). Informing policy making and management in healthcare: the place for synthesis." Healthc Policy , 1(2), 43-8.

[30] Sabatier, P. A, & Jenkins-smith, H. C. (1999). Theories of the Policy Process., Boulder: Westview Press.

[31] Thacker, S. B, Ikeda, R. M, et al. (2005). The evidence base for public health informing policy at the Centers for Disease Control and Prevention." Am J Prev Med , 29(3), 227-33.

[32] Uneke, C. J, Ezeoha, A. E, et al. (2012). Promotion of evidence-informed health policymaking in Nigeria: Bridging the gap between researchers and policymakers." Glob Public Health.

[33] Waters, E. (2011). Evidence of new innovations: investing in evidence synthesis, generation and translation ensures public health innovations improve population health." Perspect Public Health 131(3): 103.

[34] Walshe, K, & Rundall, T. G. (2001). Evidence-based management: from theory to practice in health care." Milbank Q IV-V., 79(3), 429-57.

[35] Hurst, S. A, Borisch, B, et al. (2011). Public health: how much evidence is needed to support our policies?" J Public Health Policy , 32(1), 135-41.

[36] Katikireddi, S. V, Higgins, M, et al. (2011). How evidence based is English public health policy?" BMJ 343: d7310.

[37] Larsen, M, Gulis, G, et al. (2011). Use of evidence in local public health work in Denmark." Int J Public Health , 57(3), 477-83.

[38] Macdonald, I. A, & Atkinson, R. (2011). Public health initiatives in obesity prevention: the need for evidence-based policy." Int J Obes (Lond) 35(4): 463.

[39] Waters, E, Hall, B. J, et al. (2011). Essential components of public health evidence reviews: capturing intervention complexity, implementation, economics and equity." J Public Health (Oxf) , 33(3), 462-5.

Chapter 2

Bayesian Approach in Medicine and Health Management

Emanuela Barbini, Pietro Manzi and Paolo Barbini

Additional information is available at the end of the chapter

http://dx.doi.org/10.5772/52402

1. Introduction

Statistical decision theory deals with scenarios where decisions have to be made under a state of uncertainty, and its goal is to provide a rational framework for dealing with such situations. These scenarios are typical in most of the problems of medical decision-making.

The Bayesian procedure is a particular way of formulating and dealing with these type of problems. It has great promise in putting health-related decision making on a more rational basis, thus making the assumptions more obvious, and making the decisions easier to explain and defend [1]. This approach can be used to support the decision-making process in many application fields, as, for example, diagnosis and prognosis [2], risk assessment [3] and health technology assessment [4]. A wide-ranging collection of applications of Bayesian statistics in the biomedical field can be found in thematic books [5-7].

Bayes's theorem appeared in a posthumous publication by Thomas Bayes [8]. It gives a simple and uncontroversial result in probability theory, but its practical application has been the subject of considerable controversy for more than two centuries and, only recently, a more balanced and pragmatic perspective has emerged. In summary, the Bayesian approach offers a method of formalizing a priori beliefs and of combining them with the available observations, with the goal of allowing a rational derivation of optimal decision criteria.

This chapter is an introduction to the modern world of Bayes procedures for professionals with a minimal background in biostatistics. In particular, we analyze the main theoretical aspects of the Bayesian approach and we review current thinking on the value of this approach as a decision-support system in medicine and health management. It is hoped that this discussion stimulates reflection on the subject and elicits new ideas and inspiration for people involved in problems of public health.

2. The Bayes decision rule

Statistical decision-making can be seen as a process of inferring, from past observations, predictions that then can be used to perform an action. A typical problem is to determine to which class a given sample belongs. The estimation of the class membership can provide a key support to decision making.

The first step of the process is the formalization of the underlying unknown reality (class membership). This is done by considering that this unknown reality can be represented by an entity (ω) taking values on a state space (Ω). Often, ω is a single unknown numerical quantity. In other problems, it may be an ordered set of numerical parameters (a vector) or the elements of Ω may not be of numerical nature. In the present chapter, we assume that ω is a single quantity.

An observation and/or measurement process allow us to obtain a set of numbers which make up the observation vector ($\mathbf{x}$). This observation vector is assumed to be a random vector whose conditional density function depends on ω. In formal probabilistic terms, this dependence is expressed by the class-conditional probability function $p(\mathbf{x}|\omega)$. The observations $\mathbf{x}$ are also called features and the feature vector is the input to the decision rule by which the sample is assigned to one of the given class.

The Bayesian approach to decision theory brings into play another element: *a priori* knowledge which concerns ω, in the form of a probability function $P(\omega)$. This probability is usually referred to as the prior.

When the prior probabilities and the class-conditional probability functions are known it is possible to derive a formal decision rule, which allows us to decide to which class a given sample ($\mathbf{x}$) belongs. For simplicity of discussion we will treat the two-class problem. The generalization to more than two classes is immediate.

Let $\mathbf{x}$ be the observation vector and let be ω_1 and ω_2 the two classes to which $\mathbf{x}$ may belong. A decision rule based on probabilities can be written as follows [9]

$$\begin{aligned} P(\omega_1 \mid \mathbf{x}) \geq P(\omega_2 \mid \mathbf{x}) \quad &\Rightarrow \quad \mathbf{x} \in \omega_1 \\ P(\omega_1 \mid \mathbf{x}) < P(\omega_2 \mid \mathbf{x}) \quad &\Rightarrow \quad \mathbf{x} \in \omega_2 \end{aligned} \tag{1}$$

where $P(\omega_i|\mathbf{x})$ is the conditional probability of ω_i given $\mathbf{x}$ (i=1,2), that is the probability of ω_i if $\mathbf{x}$ has occurred. This conditional probability is also known as the *a posteriori* probability of ω_i given $\mathbf{x}$.

Bayes's theorem allows us to write the *a posteriori* probabilities of ω_1 and ω_2 as a function of the *a priori* probabilities ($P(\omega_1)$ and $P(\omega_2)$) and the class-conditional probability functions ($p(\mathbf{x}|\omega_1)$ and $p(\mathbf{x}|\omega_2)$), giving

http://dx.doi.org/10.5772/52402

$$P(\omega_i \mid \mathbf{x}) = \frac{P(\omega_i) \times p(\mathbf{x} \mid \omega_i)}{p(\mathbf{x})} \qquad i = 1,2 \tag{2}$$

where p(**x**) is the probability density function of **x**.

In the case of two mutually exclusive classes, p(**x**) can be expressed as

$$p(\mathbf{x}) = p(\mathbf{x} \cap \omega_1) + p(\mathbf{x} \cap \omega_2) = P(\omega_1) \times p(\mathbf{x} \mid \omega_1) + P(\omega_2) \times p(\mathbf{x} \mid \omega_2) \tag{3}$$

Therefore, the posterior probabilities in equation 2, which determine the decision rule in equation 1, can be calculated on the basis of the prior and class-conditional probabilities. This confirms that the Bayesian approach, combining *a priori* beliefs with available observations, updates the knowledge in the light of experience.

Combining equation 1 with equation 2, the previous decision rule based on probabilities can be rewritten as follows

$$\begin{array}{lll} P(\omega_1) \times p(\mathbf{x} \mid \omega_1) \geq P(\omega_2) \times p(\mathbf{x} \mid \omega_2) & \Rightarrow & \mathbf{x} \in \omega_1 \\ P(\omega_1) \times p(\mathbf{x} \mid \omega_1) < P(\omega_2) \times p(\mathbf{x} \mid \omega_2) & \Rightarrow & \mathbf{x} \in \omega_2 \end{array} \tag{4}$$

or, equivalently,

$$\begin{array}{lll} l(\mathbf{x}) = \dfrac{p(\mathbf{x} \mid \omega_1)}{p(\mathbf{x} \mid \omega_2)} \geq \dfrac{P(\omega_2)}{P(\omega_1)} & \Rightarrow & \mathbf{x} \in \omega_1 \\ l(\mathbf{x}) = \dfrac{p(\mathbf{x} \mid \omega_1)}{p(\mathbf{x} \mid \omega_2)} < \dfrac{P(\omega_2)}{P(\omega_1)} & \Rightarrow & \mathbf{x} \in \omega_2 \end{array} \tag{5}$$

The term l(**x**) is called the likelihood ratio and the ratio $P(\omega_2)/P(\omega_1)$ is the threshold value of the likelihood ratio for the decision.

Equation 5 corresponds to the Bayes's decision rule for minimum error and defines the decision boundary between the two classes. In particular, when $p(\mathbf{x} \mid \omega_1)$ and $p(\mathbf{x} \mid \omega_2)$ are Gaussian with mean vectors $\boldsymbol{\mu}_1$ and $\boldsymbol{\mu}_2$, respectively, and covariance matrices $\boldsymbol{\Sigma}_1 = \boldsymbol{\Sigma}_2$, the decision boundary is linear. Analogously, when $p(\mathbf{x} \mid \omega_1)$ and $p(\mathbf{x} \mid \omega_2)$ are Gaussian with mean vectors $\boldsymbol{\mu}_1$ and $\boldsymbol{\mu}_2$, respectively, and covariance matrices $\boldsymbol{\Sigma}_1 \neq \boldsymbol{\Sigma}_2$, the decision boundary is quadratic. Finally, when $p(\mathbf{x} \mid \omega_1)$ and/or $p(\mathbf{x} \mid \omega_2)$ are not Gaussian, the shape of the decision boundary cannot be defined a priori. Figures 1 and 2 show two-dimensional examples for Gaussian class-conditional probability functions when $\boldsymbol{\Sigma}_1 = \boldsymbol{\Sigma}_2$ and $\boldsymbol{\Sigma}_1 \neq \boldsymbol{\Sigma}_2$, respectively.

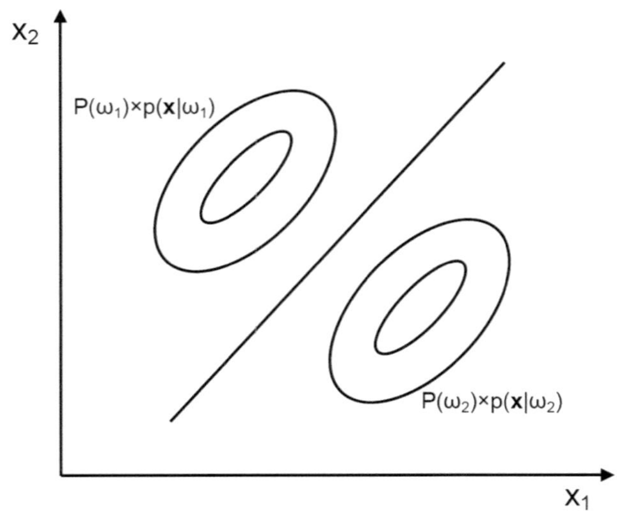

Figure 1. Decision boundary for Gaussian class-conditional probability functions when $\Sigma_1 = \Sigma_2$. Ellipses depict contour lines.

The decision rule of equation 1 implies that we should choose the class whose posterior probability is largest. Bearing in mind that the sum of $P(\omega_1|\mathbf{x})$ and $P(\omega_2|\mathbf{x})$ is equal to 1, this means setting the posterior class-conditional probability threshold (P_t) equal to 0.5, that is, **x** is assigned to class ω_i if $P(\omega_i|\mathbf{x})$ is greater than 0.5. However, the decision rule may be formulated using somewhat different reasoning. Often, in medical applications, the decision rule must account for the cost of a wrong decision. In this case, a cost can be assigned to each correct and wrong decision and P_t is chosen to obtain the minimum risk decision rule. From a purely mathematical point of view, the selection of costs is equivalent to a change in prior probabilities.

The discrimination capacity of a classification model assesses model performance in assigning correctly a sample to a class. Many criteria exist for evaluating discrimination capacity. A common way for the two-class problem is to evaluate sensitivity (SE) and specificity (SP). SE can be interpreted as the fraction of cases from ω_1 (for example, diseased patients or high-risk subjects) which are correctly classified, while SP gives the fraction of correctly classified cases from ω_2 [10]. Generally, SE and SP depend on the chosen probability threshold P_t to which the posterior probability is compared.

A receiver operating characteristic (ROC) curve is a graphic representation of the relationship between the true-positive fraction (TPF=SE) and false-positive fraction (FPF=1-SP) obtained for all possible choices of P_t.

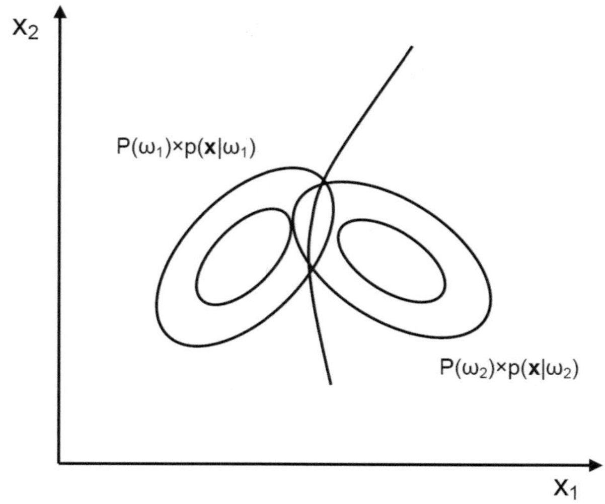

Figure 2. Decision boundary for Gaussian class-conditional probability functions when $\Sigma_1 \neq \Sigma_2$. Ellipses depict contour lines.

In medical applications the area under the ROC curve (AUC) is the most commonly used global index of discrimination capacity, although alternative indices can be used [11]. The AUC can be interpreted as the chance that a case randomly selected from ω_1 will be correctly distinguished from a randomly selected case from ω_2. An AUC value equal to 1 implies perfect forecasts, while an AUC of 0.5 reflects random forecasts.

3. Estimation of class-conditional probability functions

The Bayesian decision rule provides an optimal solution to the classification problem when the underlying probabilistic structure is known. Actually, this occurs very rarely. When the probabilistic structure is not known, the most common approach to solve the problem is to estimate it from a set of available experimental data. This set of samples is called training set. Thus the class-conditional probability functions are estimated from the training set and the Bayes's rule is implemented using the estimated functions. It should however be emphasized that the Bayesian decision rule obtained in this way does not maintain its optimality characteristics.

If we can assume that the class-conditional probability functions have a well-defined structure which can be characterized by a finite number of parameters, we can derive the Bayesian decision rule using the parameter estimates. In this case the problem is the estimation of the set of parameters and this corresponds to a parametric approach. Unfortunately, in some cases we cannot assume a parametric form for the class-conditional probability functions and in order to apply the Bayesian decision rule, we have to somehow estimate these functions, using an unstructured (nonparametric) approach. The nonparametric approach is complex and its description is not an objective of our discussion. The reader interested in this topic can find an exhaustive treatment of the problem in the specific literature [12].

Generalization is an issue of crucial importance for decision models which were designed on a training set. It is defined as the capacity of the model to maintain the same performance on data not used for training, but belonging to the same population. It is therefore estimated by testing model performance on a different set of available experimental data (testing data). The model generalizes well when the decision errors in testing and training data sets do not differ significantly. From this point of view, the optimal model is the simplest possible model designed on training data which shows the highest possible performance on any other equally representative set of testing data. Excessively complex models tend to overfit, which means they show an error on the training data significantly lower than on the testing data. Overfit is a sort of data storage precluding the learning of decision rules. It must be avoided since it causes loss of generalization.

Later in this chapter we will focus on various Bayesian models, frequently utilised in medicine and in health management, using the parametric approach to define the decision rule. After a brief description of each model, we will show an applicative example bringing out the main strengths and weaknesses of the various models.

4. The Bayes linear classifier

In many cases the class-conditional probability functions are assumed to be Gaussian, that is

$$p(\mathbf{x}|\omega_i) = \frac{1}{(2\Pi)^{q/2}} |\boldsymbol{\Sigma}_i|^{-1/2} \exp\left\{-\frac{1}{2}(\mathbf{x}-\boldsymbol{\mu}_i)^T \boldsymbol{\Sigma}_i^{-1} (\mathbf{x}-\boldsymbol{\mu}_i)\right\} \tag{6}$$

where $\boldsymbol{\mu}_i$ is the mean of class ω_i, $\boldsymbol{\Sigma}_i$ the covariance matrix, q the dimension of the observation vector (i.e. the number of features used). $|\boldsymbol{\Sigma}_i|$ indicates the determinant of $\boldsymbol{\Sigma}_i$ and superscript T indicates matrix transposition.

In this condition the problem to be solved is the estimation of $\boldsymbol{\mu}_i$ and $\boldsymbol{\Sigma}_i$. Therefore, the number of parameters to be estimated to identify $p(\mathbf{x}|\omega_i)$ is equal to $q(q+3)/2$, which corresponds to q parameters of the mean vector and $q(q+1)/2$ parameters of the covariance matrix. The greater the number q of features, the greater the number of parameters to be estimated to define the normal class-conditional probability function. Of course, given a set of training data, the accuracy of model parameter estimates rapidly worsens as q increases, leading to a significant loss in generalization capacity.

A simplifying hypothesis that is often made is to assume that the two classes have identical covariance matrices (homoscedasticity), which, as said above, leads to obtain a linear decision boundary. In fact, in this case the decision rule in equation 5 can be rewritten as

$$(\boldsymbol{\mu}_2 - \boldsymbol{\mu}_1)^T \boldsymbol{\Sigma}^{-1}\mathbf{x} + \frac{1}{2}(\boldsymbol{\mu}_1^T \boldsymbol{\Sigma}^{-1}\boldsymbol{\mu}_1 - \boldsymbol{\mu}_2^T \boldsymbol{\Sigma}^{-1}\boldsymbol{\mu}_2) \le \ln\frac{P(\omega_1)}{P(\omega_2)} \quad \Rightarrow \quad \mathbf{x} \in \omega_1$$
$$(\boldsymbol{\mu}_2 - \boldsymbol{\mu}_1)^T \boldsymbol{\Sigma}^{-1}\mathbf{x} + \frac{1}{2}(\boldsymbol{\mu}_1^T \boldsymbol{\Sigma}^{-1}\boldsymbol{\mu}_1 - \boldsymbol{\mu}_2^T \boldsymbol{\Sigma}^{-1}\boldsymbol{\mu}_2) > \ln\frac{P(\omega_1)}{P(\omega_2)} \quad \Rightarrow \quad \mathbf{x} \in \omega_2 \tag{7}$$

which identifies the following linear boundary

$$(\boldsymbol{\mu}_2 - \boldsymbol{\mu}_1)^T \boldsymbol{\Sigma}^{-1}\mathbf{x} + \frac{1}{2}(\boldsymbol{\mu}_1^T \boldsymbol{\Sigma}^{-1}\boldsymbol{\mu}_1 - \boldsymbol{\mu}_2^T \boldsymbol{\Sigma}^{-1}\boldsymbol{\mu}_2) = \ln\frac{P(\omega_1)}{P(\omega_2)} \tag{8}$$

where $\boldsymbol{\Sigma} = \boldsymbol{\Sigma}_1 = \boldsymbol{\Sigma}_2$.

Under this hypothesis, the total number of parameters to be estimated to define the decision rule for a two-class problem becomes q(q+5)/2.

The Bayes linear classifier is a simple approach, but, in the Bayes sense, it is optimal only for normal distributions with equal covariance matrices of the classes. However, in many cases, the simplicity and robustness of the linear model compensate the loss of performance occasioned by non-normality or non-homoscedasticity.

This type of model has been used for estimating morbidity probability after heart surgery [13]. The classifier was developed and tested analysing data acquired in a set of 1090 patients who underwent coronary artery bypass grafting and were admitted to the intensive care unit (ICU) of the University Hospital of Siena (Italy) over a period of three years (2002–2004). A collection of 78 preoperative, intraoperative and postoperative variables were considered as likely risk predictors, that could be associated with morbidity development in the ICU. A dichotomous (binary) variable was chosen as ICU outcome (morbidity). Data was ranked chronologically on the basis of patient hospital discharge and organized in a database. The database was divided into two sets of equal size (545 cases each): a training set consisting of patients in odd positions in the original ranked database and a testing set consisting of the other patients, that is, those in even positions in the original database. To ensure that alternate allocation of cases did not introduce systematic sampling errors, training and testing data was compared using statistical significance tests. Before developing the formal decision-model, a feature selection was performed, which reduced the variables from 78 to 8, thus the number of parameters estimated from the training set to identify the two class-conditional probability functions was equal to 52.

Discrimination capacity was quantified by AUC estimated on bootstrap data. For testing data, the 95% confidence interval (CI) of AUC was also calculated. Generalization was evaluated as the percentage difference in AUC between training and testing data. The AUC values were equal to 0.815 and 0.778 for training and testing sets, respectively, while CI for testing data was equal to [0.722-0.831]. The percentage difference in AUC between training and testing data was 4.5%.

5. The Bayes quadratic classifier

When the class-conditional probability functions are assumed to be Gaussian, but the two classes have not identical covariance matrices, a Bayes quadratic classifier should be employed. In this case, the decision rule in equation 5 can be expressed as a quadratic function of the observation vector **x** as

$$
\begin{aligned}
&\frac{1}{2}(\mathbf{x}-\boldsymbol{\mu}_1)^T\boldsymbol{\Sigma}_1^{-1}(\mathbf{x}-\boldsymbol{\mu}_1)-\frac{1}{2}(\mathbf{x}-\boldsymbol{\mu}_2)^T\boldsymbol{\Sigma}_2^{-1}(\mathbf{x}-\boldsymbol{\mu}_2)+\frac{1}{2}\ln\frac{|\boldsymbol{\Sigma}_1|}{|\boldsymbol{\Sigma}_2|}\le\ln\frac{P(\omega_1)}{P(\omega_2)} \quad \Rightarrow \quad \mathbf{x}\in\omega_1\\
&\frac{1}{2}(\mathbf{x}-\boldsymbol{\mu}_1)^T\boldsymbol{\Sigma}_1^{-1}(\mathbf{x}-\boldsymbol{\mu}_1)-\frac{1}{2}(\mathbf{x}-\boldsymbol{\mu}_2)^T\boldsymbol{\Sigma}_2^{-1}(\mathbf{x}-\boldsymbol{\mu}_2)+\frac{1}{2}\ln\frac{|\boldsymbol{\Sigma}_1|}{|\boldsymbol{\Sigma}_2|}>\ln\frac{P(\omega_1)}{P(\omega_2)} \quad \Rightarrow \quad \mathbf{x}\in\omega_2
\end{aligned}
\tag{9}
$$

which identifies a non linear (quadratic) boundary. The Bayes quadratic classifier in equation 9 requires the estimation of q(q+3) parameters from the training set.

Also this type of model has been used for estimating the probability of morbidity after heart surgery in the same set of 1090 patients who underwent coronary artery bypass in the University Hospital of Siena over the period 2002–2004 [13]. The quadratic model was developed and tested using the same training and testing sets which were employed to define the linear model above-discussed. In this case the procedure of feature selection reduced the variables from 78 to only 3 features, thus the number of parameters to be estimated from the training set was equal to 18. For the quadratic model the AUC values were equal to 0.780 and 0.785 for training and testing sets, respectively, while the 95% confidence interval of AUC, calculated in the testing set, was equal to [0.738-0.832].

The above results indicated that both linear and quadratic Bayesian classifiers had acceptable discrimination capacities on test data, because their AUC was always greater that 0.7 and less than 0.8 [14]. However, the quadratic model showed a greater power of generalization, because the AUC values calculated in the training and testing sets were nearly identical. This may be due to two causes:

1. the quadratic model, which releases the assumption of identical covariance matrices, is better suited to the actual probabilistic structure of the problem,
2. the number of parameters to be estimated from the training set for the quadratic model is smaller than that of the linear model (18 vs. 52), thanks to the smaller number of features needed to define the model.

6. The naïve Bayes approach

Even if the Gaussian assumption is correct, when the number of features necessary to define the decision rule is high, the previous linear and quadratic Bayesian models can lead to unsatisfactory results, due to the large number of parameters that must be estimated from the training data to identify the class-conditional probability functions. In these cases one way to try to solve the problem is to use a naïve Bayes approach.

The naïve Bayes approach assumes that the features are all conditionally independent of one another within each class [15]. Consequently, given a q-dimensional observation vector $\mathbf{x} = (x_1, x_2, \ldots, x_q)$ and two classes ω_1 and ω_2, the *a posteriori* probabilities of equation 2 can be rewritten as

$$P(\omega_i \mid \mathbf{x}) = \frac{P(\omega_i) \prod_{j=1}^{q} p(x_j \mid \omega_i)}{p(\mathbf{x})} \qquad i = 1,2 \tag{10}$$

where $p(x_j \mid \omega_i)$ is the class-conditional probability of feature x_j (j=1,2,….,q) conditioned on ω_i.

This assumption dramatically simplifies the problem of estimation from training data. In fact one-dimensional class-conditional distributions can be estimated for each feature individually, reducing a multidimensional task to a number of one-dimensional tasks. Despite its simplicity, the naïve Bayes classifier can often outperform more sophisticated classification methods and shows good average performance in terms of classification accuracy, even when the assumption of independence does not hold [16-18]. Actually, the naïve Bayes classifier estimates the parameters required for accurate classification using less training data than many other classifiers. This makes it particularly effective for datasets containing many features.

A naïve Bayes classifier is generally easy to understand and its induction is extremely fast if all features are discrete. In particular, for each class ω_i, a discrete feature x_j with K values $(d_{1j}, d_{2j}, \ldots, d_{Kj})$ can be simply characterized by the K-dimensional vector $[P(d_{1j} \mid \omega_i), P(d_{2j} \mid \omega_i), \ldots, P(d_{Kj} \mid \omega_i)]$ describing the class-conditional probability of this variable. In these conditions the class-conditional probability functions in equation 10 can be estimated by frequency counts from the training set.

A similar scheme may also be used when the feature set contains discrete and/or continuous variables. In this case, each continuous feature x_j can be discretized by grouping the observations of the whole training set into M groups of equal size (quantile intervals), denoted Q_{1j}, $Q_{2j}, \ldots, Q_{Mj}$. Thus, the continuous feature x_j is also characterized by class-conditional probability vectors $[P(Q_{1j} \mid \omega_i), P(Q_{2j} \mid \omega_i), \ldots, P(Q_{Mj} \mid \omega_i)]$ where $P(Q_{hj} \mid \omega_i)$ (h = 1,2,….,M) is the probability that x_j lies in the quantile interval Q_{hj} conditioned on ω_i [i = 1,2].

Recently, a naïve Bayes classifier was used to develop a locally-customized model for planning transfusion requirements in cardiac surgery [19]. The procedure allows transfusion planning to be designed and customized to a specific clinical setting on the basis of local available evidence. The size of the sample used in the study was 3182 patients.

The available patient sample was divided into two classes:

a. class of *negative* patients: patients who received no red blood cells in the intensive care unit after cardiac surgery (1107 patients),

b. class of *positive* patients: patients who received at least one pack of red blood cells (2075 patients).

Firstly, eleven dichotomous variables and six continuous variables were chosen as a set of likely independent predictors for planning transfusion quantities on the basis of qualitative evidence and previous knowledge. Univariate statistical analysis was then performed for each potential predictor in order to assess statistical differences between the classes of patients. Two dichotomous variables did not show statistically significant differences between classes and were eliminated from classifier design. Therefore fifteen variables giving statistical differences between the classes were used as features to design the naïve Bayes classifier.

Before developing the naïve Bayes classifier, the six continuous features were rendered discrete by dividing each into ten intervals of equal frequency. This was done by identifying the deciles for the whole sample of patients.

In order to evaluate the performance of this decision model, a confusion matrix was generated by the leave-one-out method, according to which each case in the training set is analysed by a classifier trained using the rest of the cases (Table 1). The overall classification accuracy was 73.7% and its corresponding 99% confidence interval was [71.7%, 75.7%].

The results shown in Table 1 reveal that although the naïve Bayes classifier cannot exactly distinguish negative from positive patients, it correctly classified about three-quarters of cases with a SE of 71.2% and a SP of 78.4%. Thus it seems to provide useful additional information for recognizing patients with transfusion requirements.

		Predicted class		**Correct classification percentage**
		Positive	Negative	
Actual class	Positive	1478	597	71.2% (SE)
	Negative	239	868	78.4% (SP)
Overall correct-classification percentage: 73.7%				
99% confidence interval: [71.7%, 75.7%]				

Table 1. Confusion matrix and correct-classification percentages obtained by the leave-one-out method. SE = Sensitivity, SP = Specificity

7. Naïve Bayes classifiers and scoring systems

Part of the difficulty of medicine is to turn qualitative judgments into quantitative assessments. To face this problem, physicians have often proposed scoring systems with the intent to summarize a set of items by means of a quantitative score. While scoring systems should never be used in place of a physician's judgment, they are undoubtedly very simple and attractive tools to analyse data and to use as decision-support systems.

The idea of using scoring systems in public health issues goes back many years ago. For example, in 1911, Hill suggested an elementary score system for determining the real relative importance of the different infectious diseases [20].

At first the methodology used to develop scoring systems was rather empirical, but over time the design of such systems has made use of more reliable quantitative techniques. Although different methodologies can be used, a naïve Bayes approach can represent a straightforward way to develop trustworthy scoring systems. In fact, in the presence of discrete (qualitative or quantitative) variables and discretized continuous variables, equation 10 can be rewritten as

$$P(\omega_i \mid \mathbf{x}) = \frac{P(\omega_i)\prod_{j=1}^{q1} P(d_{xj} \mid \omega_i)\prod_{j=1}^{q2} P(Q_{xj} \mid \omega_i)}{P(\mathbf{x})} \qquad i = 1,2 \tag{11}$$

where q1 and q2 are the number of discrete and continuous features, respectively, (q1 + q2 = q), d_{xj} is the value of the j-th discrete variable and Q_{xj} the quantile interval containing the j-th continuous variable.

The decision rule of equation 1 becomes

$$\begin{aligned} &\frac{P(\omega_1)}{P(\omega_2)}\prod_{j=1}^{q1}\frac{P(d_{xj} \mid \omega_1)}{P(d_{xj} \mid \omega_2)}\prod_{j=1}^{q2}\frac{P(Q_{xj} \mid \omega_1)}{P(Q_{xj} \mid \omega_2)} \geq 1 \quad \Rightarrow \quad \mathbf{x} \in \omega_1 \\ &\frac{P(\omega_1)}{P(\omega_2)}\prod_{j=1}^{q1}\frac{P(d_{xj} \mid \omega_1)}{P(d_{xj} \mid \omega_2)}\prod_{j=1}^{q2}\frac{P(Q_{xj} \mid \omega_1)}{P(Q_{xj} \mid \omega_2)} < 1 \quad \Rightarrow \quad \mathbf{x} \in \omega_2 \end{aligned} \tag{12}$$

Writing equation 12 in logarithmic form, the decision rule is

$$\begin{aligned} &S = \sum_{j=1}^{q1}\ln\frac{P(d_{xj} \mid \omega_1)}{P(d_{xj} \mid \omega_2)} + \sum_{j=1}^{q2}\ln\frac{P(Q_{xj} \mid \omega_1)}{P(Q_{xj} \mid \omega_2)} \geq \ln\frac{P(\omega_2)}{P(\omega_1)} \quad \Rightarrow \quad \mathbf{x} \in \omega_1 \\ &S = \sum_{j=1}^{q1}\ln\frac{P(d_{xj} \mid \omega_1)}{P(d_{xj} \mid \omega_2)} + \sum_{j=1}^{q2}\ln\frac{P(Q_{xj} \mid \omega_1)}{P(Q_{xj} \mid \omega_2)} < \ln\frac{P(\omega_2)}{P(\omega_1)} \quad \Rightarrow \quad \mathbf{x} \in \omega_2 \end{aligned} \tag{13}$$

We can note that S is a sum of q addends

$$S = \sum_{j=1}^{q} w_{xj} \tag{14}$$

where w_{xj} (j = 1,2,…,q) can be regarded as terms separately weighing the information given by each feature x_j. These weights are log-likelihood ratios, which can be determined from the training set. S is the total score: if S is less than ln $[P(\omega_2)/P(\omega_1)]$, the observation vector **x** is classified in ω_2, otherwise **x** is classified in ω_1. ln $[P(\omega_2)/P(\omega_1)]$ is the threshold value, independent of **x**, which is equal to 0 when $P(\omega_1) = P(\omega_2)$.

In conclusion, the decision rule in equation 13 defines a scoring system corresponding to a naïve Bayes classifier.

8. Bayesian networks

The simplicity and surprisingly high accuracy of the naïve Bayes classifier have led to its wide use, and to many attempts to extend it. In particular, naïve Bayes is a special case of a Bayesian network.

Bayesian networks are a flexible tool particularly suited to problem-solving [21]. They are graphic probability models of knowledge that lend themselves to modelling in situations of uncertainty. For example, a Bayesian network could represent the probabilistic relationships between diseases and symptoms. Thus, given symptoms, the Bayesian network can be used to compute the probabilities of the presence of different diseases.

A Bayesian network is a directed acyclic graph, in which nodes represent random variables and arcs represent conditional dependencies between variables. Each nodes is associated with a probability table. The probability of a node can be calculated when the values of its incoming nodes are known. To describe a Bayesian network we need to specify the graph structure and the values of each probability table based on data.

The example in figure 3 shows a simple Bayesian network in which the various nodes are represented as circles and the corresponding variables are dichotomous and therefore discrete. The arc between nodes A and C with arrow in direction A to C, indicates that A has an influence on C (A is parent of C). The lack of an arc between two nodes indicates their conditional independence: for example, nodes C and D are independent of each other.

Each node has quantitative probability information. Nodes with parents (nodes C and D in figure 3) are characterised by a conditional probability table that defines the effects of the parents on the node, whereas nodes without parents (nodes A and B) are associated with a probability *a priori*. Thus P(A) is the probability of event A and $x_{\bar{A}B}$ is the probability of event C if event B occurs but not event A. Once the topology of the Bayesian network has been determined, the conditional probability distribution of all variables and their parents must be specified.

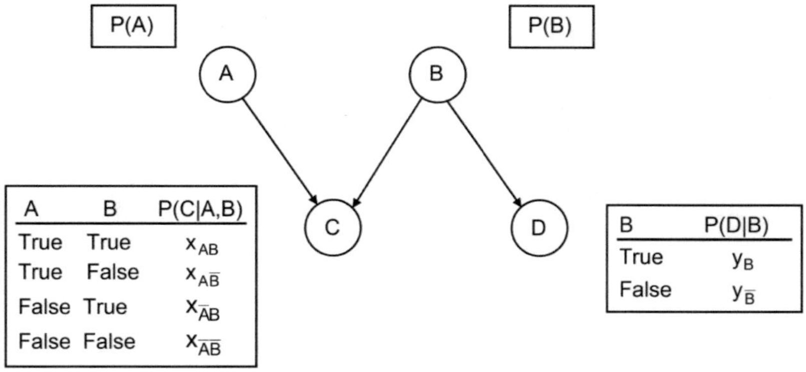

Figure 3. Simple example of Bayesian network with four nodes, two of which (nodes C and D) have parents.

The procedures required to develop and use models based on Bayesian networks may be not simple, but there is a number of commercial software packages. Information about various software packages available for Bayesian networks is provided by Murphy [22].

Learning the structure of a Bayesian network from data can be a critical point. An alternative approach can be to combine statements about the structure of Bayesian network from multiple experts into a single structure that more closely captures the dependencies in the domain. This structure is then refined, and its parameters estimated, using standard Bayesian network learning algorithms.

Bayesian networks can be applied to study major public health problems [23-25]. For illustrative purposes, we will start with a brief description of a fairly complex Bayesian network that has been proposed as a model of heart disease by researchers at the University of South Carolina [26]. Although, as the authors point out, the model is merely a prototype, it lends itself well to being used to explain the operation of a Bayesian network. The Bayesian network structure is shown in figure 4.

The structure proposed shows that the heart disease has five parents (adverse medicine, high blood pressure, atherosclerosis, family history and serum selenium). Two of these (adverse medicine and family history) have no parents, while the remaining three (high blood pressure, atherosclerosis and serum selenium) are, in turn, nodes with parents. In particular, atherosclerosis has four parents, three of which (high serum triglycerides, high serum LDL cholesterol and cholesterol/HDL) are influenced by the type of diet. Absence of moderate exercise directly influences the atherosclerosis. The structure in figure 4 also shows that heart disease influences four variables (ECG, angina pectoris, myocardial infarction and heart beat rate).

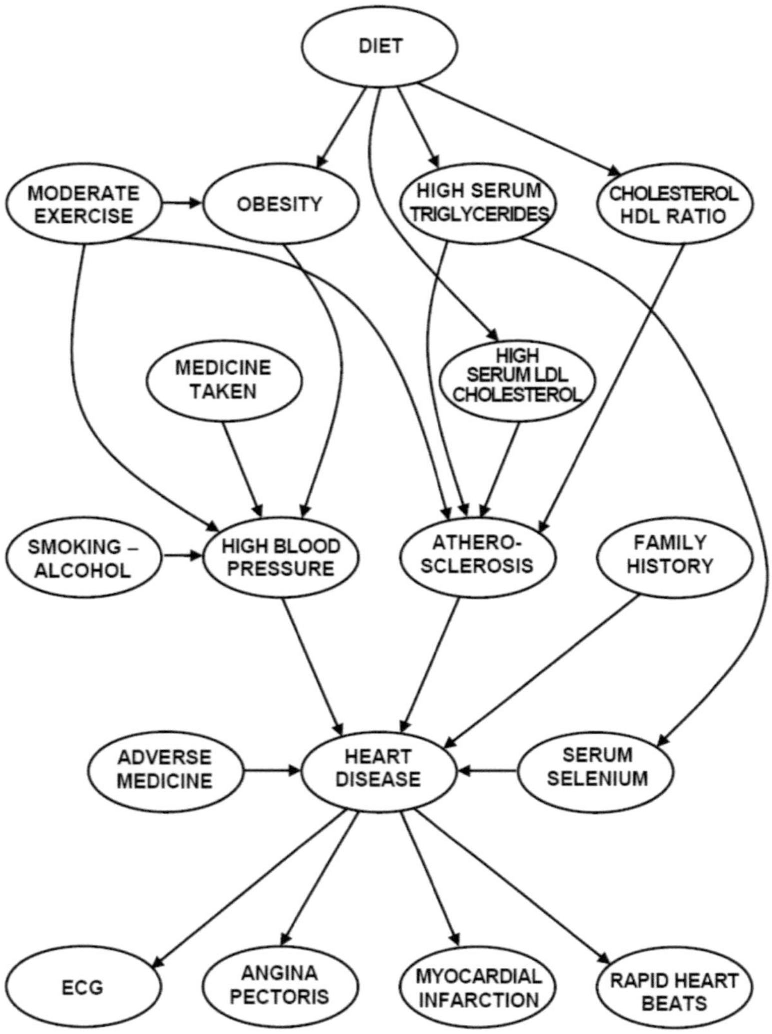

Figure 4. Bayesian network structure of the model of heart disease.

The above analysis indicates that the Bayesian network structure alone can be seen as a kind of mental map, i.e. as a diagram in which concepts are presented in graphic form. Of course, the diagram provides only qualitative information, but, by associating each node with a probability table, it is possible to obtain precise quantitative information on the whole system operation. For example, on the basis of their data, the authors found that the conditional probability of atherosclerosis is equal to 0.84 when moderate exercise is absent and serum triglycerides, serum LDL cholesterol and cholesterol HDL ratio are high [26]. The conditional probability of atherosclerosis drops to 0.20 when moderate exercise is present and serum triglycerides, serum LDL cholesterol and cholesterol HDL ratio are low [26].

Actually heart disease is a very complex system and the network shown above, despite its eighteen nodes, is a very simplified model that does not take into account important factors. For example, there is a significant chance that some inhibitor prevents atherosclerosis when serum triglycerides are high. Therefore the network in figure 4 is a useful example for explaining the operation of a Bayesian network, but does not lend itself to assess the actual strength of this approach.

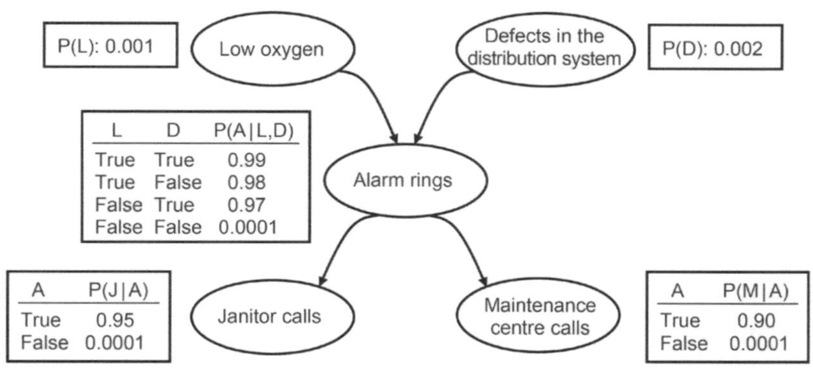

Figure 5. Bayesian network representing the medical gas plant control system. Events L, D, A, J and M represent low oxygen, defects in the distribution system, alarm rings, janitor calls and maintenance centre calls.

The strength of the approach is well illustrated by the Bayesian network which has been developed at the University Hospital of Siena (Italy) for assessing the performance of a control system of the medical gas plant (figure 5). The network takes into consideration a medical gas system connected to an alarm. The alarm rings when the pressure of oxygen falls below safety level in the main tank, but it may also ring for defects in the distribution system, such as a leaking pipe.

The alarm rings in two places, the janitor's lodge and the maintenance centre, which are responsible for calling the crisis unit. Both these places may commit errors in activating the crisis unit. For example, the janitor may not hear the alarm because he is busy giving information to users, or the maintenance centre may not hear it because of boiler noise. The network is a representation of a real situation where uncertainty exists. In other words, the network does not directly model the fact that the janitor is busy giving information to users or that the maintenance centre is noisy. These factors (and an infinite number of others) are summarised by the uncertainty associated with the links between the nodes "alarm rings" and "janitor calls" and between "alarm rings" and "maintenance centre calls". The probability tables therefore enable an enormous set of circumstances to be summarised by an approximate model of a much more complex situation.

Once the Bayesian network and the probability tables have been specified, it is possible to evaluate the effective reliability of the hospital system in monitoring the medical gas plant, allowing answers to be given to questions about its actual functioning. For example, important questions to be answered can be:

a. What is the probability that the crisis unit is called by at least one of the two places where the alarm rings when the oxygen in the tank is insufficient or when the distribution system is damaged?

b. What is the probability that the oxygen system has neither of these problems when the crisis unit is called by the janitor (false alarm by janitor)?

c. What is the probability that the oxygen is insufficient or the oxygen system damaged when the janitor calls the crisis unit?

When the calculations are done, it emerges that the probability that the crisis unit be called when oxygen is low is 97.5%. Similarly, the probability that the janitor or the maintenance centre call the crisis unit for damage to the system is 96.5%. Actually in this example the alarm system is not infallible, because when the problem is low oxygen pressure in the tank there is a 98% probability of the alarm ringing and that probability falls to 97% when the problem is a defect in the distribution system (see table in figure 5). Consequently the above results suggest that the protocol in place to call the crisis unit (janitor plus maintenance centre) is efficient.

However, when the performance of the protocol is further evaluated, some criticalities emerge. The model makes it possible to determine that once the janitor has called the crisis unit, there is a 6.5% probability of sufficient oxygen and no damage to the oxygen distribution system, which is no longer negligible. This important discovery is not immediately obvious from the design of the system and the reliability of the various components (alarm, janitor and maintenance centre) taken separately. The result is actually due to the fact that the absolute probabilities of low oxygen and system damage are very small (0.001 and 0.002, respectively), because these events occur very rarely. Assuming a very rare event, even if the probability that the janitor calls in the absence of alarm ring is almost zero (0.0001), the network points out that a call from the janitor does not mean certainty or almost certainty of a problem in the system. In other words, there is a non negligible probability (about 6.5%) of there being neither low oxygen nor damages when the janitor calls. This weakness is inherent to the system but does not have particularly serious consequences, because the only effect is that in some cases the crisis unit alerted by the janitor will not find any problem in the plant. Since this would rarely happen, its cost is very low.

The answer to the third question shows that once the janitor has called the crisis unit, the probability that oxygen is low in the main tank is about 31.5% and that the distribution system is damaged about 62%. This difference is due to the fact that while both events are rare, system damage has twice the probability a priori of low oxygen (0.002 vs. 0.001).

http://dx.doi.org/10.5772/52402

In summary, the response of the Bayesian network to the above questions indicates that in the case of problems, the protocol provides a very efficient response, practically equivalent to that of a pure alarm device, but a call from the janitor may sometimes be a false alarm.

9. Conclusion

The Bayesian approach is a way of formulating and dealing with problems where decisions have to be made under a state of uncertainty. This situation is very frequent in problems of medical decision-making.

Although Bayes's theorem was published in 1763, the use of Bayesian techniques to develop decision-support systems in medicine and health management is recent. The design of a reliable Bayesian model often requires the use of complex algorithms and its development may involve not trivial calculations. This presented a barrier to the use of the Bayesian approach until the development of numerical methods and powerful computers during the late 20th century.

The advantages of the Bayesian approach are that it offers intuitive and meaningful inferences, that it gives the ability to tackle complex problems and that it allows the incorporation of prior information in addition to the data. In particular, the simple and intuitive nature of the Bayes's theorem as a mechanism for synthesising information and updating personal beliefs is an attractive feature, which has facilitated its spread in the medical field.

In conclusion, although the Bayesian approach is not the only way to tackle the problem of decision making under uncertainty, it is undoubtedly a very useful tool to be used in medicine and health management, because it allows the professional to make decisions on rational bases, thus making the choices easier to explain and defend.

Acknowledgements

This work was partly financed by the University of Siena, Italy.

Author details

Emanuela Barbini[1], Pietro Manzi[1] and Paolo Barbini[2,3*]

*Address all correspondence to: paolo.barbini@unisi.it

1 Health-Care Management, University Hospital of Siena, Italy

2 Department of Surgery and Bioengineering, University of Siena, Italy

3 Biomedical Engineering Unit, University Hospital of Siena, Italy

References

[1] Kadane, J. B. (2005). Bayesian methods for health-related decision making. *Statistics in Medicine*, 24(4), 563-567.

[2] Sheppard, J. W., & Kaufman, M. A. (2005). A Bayesian approach to diagnosis and prognosis using built-in test. *IEEE Transactions on Instrumentation and Measurement*, 54(3), 1003-1018.

[3] Barbini, E., Cevenini, G., Scolletta, S., Biagioli, B., Giomarelli, P., & Barbini, P. (2007). A comparative analysis of predictive models of morbidity in intensive care unit after cardiac surgery- Part I: model planning. BMC Medical Informatics and Decision Making 7:35 10.1186/1472-6947-7-35 published online 22 November 2007

[4] Spiegelhalter, D. J., Myles, J. P., Jones, D. R., & Abrams, K. R. (2000). Bayesian methods in health technology assessment: a review. *Health Technology Assessment*, 4(38), 1-130.

[5] Berry, D. A., & Stangl, D. K. (1996). Bayesian biostatistics. *New York: Marcel Dekker, Inc.*

[6] Broemeling, L. D. (2007). Bayesian biostatistics and diagnostic medicine. *Boca Raton, FL: Chapman & Hall/CRC.*

[7] Moyé, L. A. (2008). Elementary Bayesian biostatistics. *Boca Raton, FL: Chapman & Hall/ CRC.*

[8] Bayes, T. An essay towards solving a problem in the doctrine of chances. By the late Rev. Mr. Bayes, F. R. S. communicated by Mr. Price, in a letter to John Canton, A. M. F. R. S. (1763), *Philosophical Transactions, Giving Some Account of the Present Undertakings, Studies and Labours of the Ingenious in Many Considerable Parts of the World*, 53, 370-418.

[9] Duda, R. O., Hart, P. E., & Stork, D. G. (2001). Pattern classification. *New York: John Wiley & Sons, Inc.*

[10] Friedman, G. D. (2004). Primer of epidemiology. *New York: The McGraw-Hill Companies, Inc.*

[11] Lasko, T. A., Bhagwat, J. G., Zou, K. H., & Ohno-Machado, L. (2005). The use of receiver operating characteristic curves in biomedical informatics. *Journal of Biomedical Informatics*, 38(5), 404-415.

[12] Fukunaga, K. (1990). Introduction to statistical pattern recognition. *San Diego, CA: Academic Press.*

[13] Cevenini, G., Barbini, E., Scolletta, S., Biagioli, B., Giomarelli, P., & Barbini, P. (2007). A comparative analysis of predictive models of morbidity in intensive care unit after cardiac surgery- Part II: an illustrative example. BMC Medical Informatics and Decision Making 7:36 10.1186/1472-6947-7-36 published online 22 November 2007

[14] Hosmer, D. W., & Lemeshow, S. (2000). Applied logistic regression. *New York: John Wiley & Sons, Inc.*

[15] Mitchell, T. M. (1997). Machine Learning. *New York: The McGraw-Hill Companies, Inc.*

[16] Domingos, P., & Pazzani, M. (1997). On the optimality of the simple Bayesian classifier under zero-one loss. *Machine Learning*, 29(2-3), 103-130.

[17] Lavrac, N., Zupan, B., Kononenko, I., Kukar, M., & Keravnou, E. T. (1998). Intelligent data analysis for medical diagnosis: using machine learning and temporal abstraction. *AI Communications*, 11(3-4), 191-218.

[18] Demichelis, F., Magni, P., Piergiorgi, P., Rubin, M. A., & Bellazzi, R. (2006). A hierarchical naïve Bayes model for handling sample heterogeneity in classification problems: an application to tissue microarrays. BMC Bioinformatics 7:514 10.1186/1471-2105-7-514 published online 24 November 2006

[19] Cevenini, G., Barbini, E., Massai, M. R., & Barbini, P. (2011). A naïve Bayes classifier for planning transfusion requirements in heart surgery. *Journal of Evaluation in Clinical Practice.*, Article first published online: 23 Aug, 10.1111/j.1365-2753.2011.01762.x.

[20] Hill, H. W. (1911). A "score system" for determining the real relative importance of the different infectious diseases. *Journal of the American Public Health Association*, 1(1), 7-9.

[21] Russell, S., & Norvig, P. (2010). Artificial intelligence: a modern approach. *Upper Saddle River, NJ: Pearson Education.*

[22] Murphy, K. (2012). Software packages for graphical models/Bayesian networks. http://www.cs.ubc.ca/~murphyk/Software/bnsoft.html, update 14 June.

[23] Burnside, E. S., Rubin, D. L., Fine, J. P., Shachter, R. D., Sisney, G. A., & Leung, W. K. (2006). Bayesian network to predict breast cancer risk of mammographic microcalcifications and reduce number of benign biopsy results: initial experience. *Radiology*, 240(3), 666-673.

[24] Li, J., Shi, J., & Satz, D. (2008). Modeling and analysis of disease and risk factors through learning Bayesian networks from observational data. *Quality and Reliability Engineering International*, 24(3), 291-302.

[25] Mnatsakanyan, Z. R., Burkom, H. S., Coberly, J. S., & Lombardo, J. S. (2009). Bayesian information fusion networks for biosurveillance applications. *Journal of the American Medical Informatics Association*, 16(6), 855-863.

[26] Ghosh, J. K., & Valtorta, M. (2000). Building a Bayesian network model of heart disease. *Proceedings of the 38th annual on Southeast regional conference, ACM-SE00 ACM-SE 2000- 38th Annual ACM Southeast Regional Conference, 7-8 April 2000, Clemson, South Carolina, USA. New York, NY, USA: ACM*, 2000, 239-240, 10.1145/1127716.1127770.

Chapter 3

Causal Inference with Intermediates: Simple Methods for Principal Strata Effects and Natural Direct Effects

Yasutaka Chiba and Etsuji Suzuki

Additional information is available at the end of the chapter

http://dx.doi.org/10.5772/53193

1. Introduction

A central problem in natural science is identifying general laws of cause and effect. Medical science is devoted to revealing causal relationships in humans [1]. The framework for causal inference applied in epidemiology can contribute substantially to clearly specifying and testing causal hypotheses. In some situations, conditioning on an intermediate, which may be between the cause (exposure) and effect (outcome), is of concern for biomedical researchers and public health practitioners [2-4]. In particular, there is a conflict in the perinatal epidemiology literature between the desire to obtain birth-weight-specific associations [5-7] and increasing awareness that conditioning on this variable can give rise to severe biases [8-11]. The difficulty arises because birth weight may be on a pathway from the exposure of interest to the perinatal outcome. For example, if the exposure is maternal smoking and the outcome is infant mortality, maternal smoking may partly affect infant mortality through its effects on fetal growth or on the timing of delivery, thereby potentially through the intermediate, birth weight. In an analysis conditioned on an intermediate, without controlling for the common causes of the intermediate and the outcome, biased results and paradoxical findings can emerge [2-4,12].

It has been reported that maternal smoking appears to have a protective effect against infant mortality among infants with low birth weight [13-15]. This perplexing association is often referred to as the *birth-weight paradox*. This relationship is exemplified by data from cohort-linked birth certificate and infant mortality files for 1997 from the National Center for Health Statistics (NCHS), which are complete files for all US births in 1997 with a 1-year follow-up for infant mortality. Table 1 gives infant mortality statistics stratified by smoking and low-birth weight [16]. In this table, only singletons are included, smoking status is dichotomized (any smoking during pregnancy versus none), and low birth weight is defined as a birth weight of less than 2,500 g. In the whole population, the crude risk difference was 9.9 – 5.9 = 4.0 (95%

confidence interval [CI]: 3.7, 4.4) per 1,000 live births. However, when we stratified the analysis by birth weight (a potential intermediate between maternal smoking and infant mortality), the risk difference was 4.9 – 2.4 = 2.5 (95% CI: 2.3, 2.7) per 1,000 live births in the subpopulation with birth weight ≥ 2,500 g, whereas it was 51.5 – 64.1 = –12.6 (95% CI: –15.0, –10.1) per 1,000 live births in the subpopulation with birth weight < 2,500 g, seemingly illustrating the birth-weight paradox.

		Infant mortality		
		Live birth	**Infant death**	**Deaths per 1,000**
Birth weight	Smoker	353,335	1,729	4.9
≥ 2,500 g[a]	Non-smoker	2,453,633	5,838	2.4
Birth weight	Smoker	40,383	2,192	51.5
< 2,500 g[b]	Non-smoker	137,154	9,387	64.1
Overall[c]	Smoker	393,830	3,950	9.9
	Non-smoker	2,591,452	15,384	5.9
Total		3,749,676	23,693	6.3

[a]Missing information on 40,747 women.

[b]Missing information on 727,384 women.

[c]Missing information on 768,753 women.

Table 1. Infant mortality (number of deaths per 1,000 live births) among women with singleton pregnancies in the 1997 cohort-linked birth certificate infant mortality files from the National Center for Health Statistics, by birth weight and smoking status

The apparent protective effect of maternal smoking among low-birth-weight infants is an artifact of conditioning on an intermediate without adequate control for intermediate-outcome confounding [8]. In the birth-weight paradox, in addition to maternal smoking, birth defects can be a cause of both low birth weight and infant mortality (Figure 1), but birth defects were not considered in the analysis. For mothers who are smokers and have low-birth-weight infants, the low birth weight could either be a consequence of smoking or a birth defect. For mothers who are non-smokers and have low-birth-weight infants, the low birth weight cannot be a consequence of smoking, and some other cause must be operating [8]. Thus, a comparison of smoking and non-smoking mothers without controlling for birth defects will artificially bias the comparison. For this group of low-birth-weight infants, no smoking and low birth weight occurring together is more likely to be associated with the presence of a birth defect. This form of bias is sometimes referred to as collider-stratification bias [17-20] because, on the path $A \rightarrow M \leftarrow U \rightarrow Y$, two arrows collide at node M. The intermediate variable does not need to have an effect on the outcome for such bias to occur (*i.e.*, the dashed arrow from M to Y in Figure 1 is absent); all that is necessary is for the exposure to affect the intermediate and for there to be an unmeasured common cause of the intermediate and the outcome. Unfortunately, intermediate-outcome confounding cannot be eliminated even when the exposure is randomized.

http://dx.doi.org/10.5772/53193

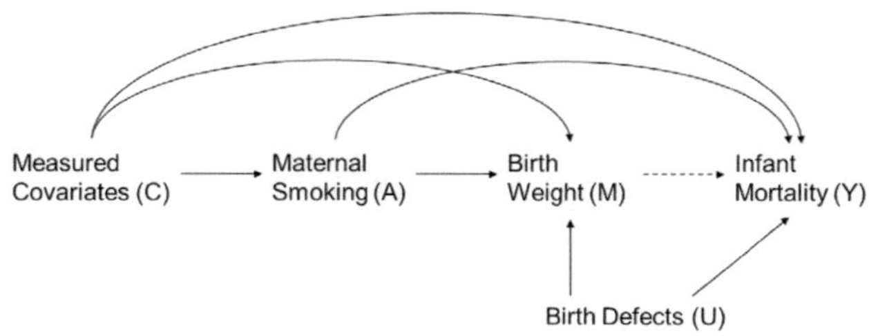

Figure 1. Diagram illustrating the relationships among an exposure (smoking status: *A*), an intermediate (birth weight: *M*), an outcome (infant mortality: *Y*), and both measured (*C*) and unmeasured (*U*) confounders

A considerable volume of literature highlights the hazards of conditioning on an intermediate [9,10,21], but the only solution offered to date is to abandon conditioning on the intermediate altogether. Simply not conditioning on an intermediate will often be the correct way to proceed with an analysis. When the total effect of the exposure on the outcome is of interest, there is no reason to condition on an intermediate. In general, conditioning on an intermediate will be a concern only when other types of effect, such as the direct effect of the exposure on the outcome (not acting through the intermediate), are considered.

In this chapter, we discuss two analytical approaches to help draw inferences when the effect of interest may be obtained by conditioning on an intermediate. The two approaches include (i) the principal stratification approach to assess the *principal strata effect* (PSE), which is a causal effect conditioned on the subpopulation of individuals for whom the intermediate would occur irrespective of exposure status, and (ii) the intervention-based approach to assess the *natural direct effect* (NDE), which is a causal effect capturing what would be realized if the exposure were to occur and its effect on the intermediate were somehow blocked. Each approach has a different interpretation and different methods for the inference. When sensitivity analysis techniques are used for the inference, a range of estimates, rather than a single estimate, will be obtained. As will be discussed later, the two approaches estimate different causal effects, and the resulting estimates would not be expected to be the same. We illustrate each by applying it to the NCHS data in Table 1, causing the birth-weight paradox to evaporate. The approaches are applicable to a variety of similar settings in all areas of epidemiological research.

This chapter is organized as follows. Section 2 introduces the notation used throughout the chapter. Section 3 defines the PSE and presents a simple method for sensitivity analysis. The method is illustrated using the NCHS data. In a similar manner, the NDE is discussed in Section 4. In Section 5, the relationship between these two causal effects is briefly discussed, although this may be somewhat theoretical. Finally, Section 6 offers some concluding remarks.

2. Notation and concepts

We let A denote the exposure of interest (*i.e.*, maternal smoking status), with $A = 1$ for a smoking mother and $A = 0$ for a non-smoking mother. M is the intermediate (*i.e.*, birth weight), with $M = 1$ for a low birth weight (< 2,500 g) and $M = 0$ for a higher birth weight (≥ 2,500 g). Y is the outcome of interest (*i.e.*, infant mortality), with $Y = 1$ for an infant death and $Y = 0$ for a live birth. We let C denote a set of baseline characteristics measured prior to or concurrent with the exposure, and U denote a set of unmeasured confounders between the intermediate (M) and the outcome (Y) (*e.g.*, birth defects). The relationship among the variables is depicted in Figure 1. We assume that no confounder exists between A and M or between A and Y (in Figure 1, a direct arrow from C to A is removed), although this assumption is not practical in the current setting[1]. Nevertheless, even in cases in which confounders exist between these variables, theories presented in this chapter hold conditional on the confounders (C).

Using the above notation, a comparison of the infant mortality risks between smoking and non-smoking mothers with infants of low birth weight can be described as follows:

$$E[Y \mid A=1, M=1]-E[Y \mid A=0, M=1],$$

where $E[Y \mid A = 1, M = 1]$ is estimated by the sample mean of Y (*i.e.*, infant mortality risk) among smoking mothers whose infants had a low birth weight (51.5/1,000) and $E[Y \mid A = 0, M = 1]$ is estimated by the sample mean of Y among non-smoking mothers whose infants had a low birth weight (64.1/1,000). Although simple, this comparison is not a fair comparison because it compares outcomes for different populations, rather than for the same population with respect to the effect of maternal smoking status on infant mortality. In the second population with $(A, M) = (0, 1)$, even if mothers are smokers, the infants may still have a low birth weight. However, in the first population with $(A, M) = (1, 1)$, if the mothers are non-smokers, some infants may not have a low birth weight. The subpopulation in which infants may have a low birth weight from smoking mothers but not from non-smoking mothers is included in the sample mean when examining smoking mothers whose infants have a low birth weight, but would not be included in the sample mean when examining non-smoking mothers whose infants have a low birth weight. To fairly compare the effect of maternal smoking status in the same population, we need an alternative to the measure described above.

Response type	Potential outcomes		Description
	Y(1)	Y(0)	
1	1	1	Always birth death
2	1	0	Birth death only with maternal smoking
3	0	1	Birth death only with maternal non-smoking
4	0	0	Never birth death

Table 2. Response types for outcome Y (*i.e.*, infant mortality) and corresponding potential outcomes

To illustrate the ideas, we use the concept of potential (or counterfactual) outcomes [22,23]. We let $Y(a)$ denote the potential outcome for each individual if, possibly contrary to fact, the exposure were set to level a. When A is binary, the two possible potential outcomes for each individual are $Y(1)$ and $Y(0)$, which respectively correspond to the outcomes that would have happened to the individual with and without maternal smoking. Note that for each individual,

1 Unfortunately we do not have access to the full NCHS dataset and can only use the published data [16]. Therefore, we cannot implement any analyses in which the confounders are taken into account.

only $Y(1)$ or $Y(0)$ can be observed, depending on the actual exposure status. As a result, individuals can be classified into four different response types, as enumerated in Table 2. Based on these potential outcomes, we can describe the population risk of Y in the presence of A as E[$Y(1)$] and that in the absence of A as E[$Y(0)$]. Thus, a causal risk difference in the whole population is given by

$$\mathrm{E}[Y(1)] - \mathrm{E}[Y(0)].$$

In other words, the above measure quantifies the total effect of A on Y. Under the assumption that no confounder exists between A and Y, one can infer a causal effect of A on Y by simply comparing the observed sample mean of Y among smoking mothers (*i.e.*, $\mathrm{E}[Y \mid A = 1]$) and the observed sample mean of Y among non-smoking mothers (*i.e.*, $\mathrm{E}[Y \mid A = 0]$). Thus, the causal risk difference can be estimated by calculating an associational risk difference as follows:

$$\mathrm{E}[Y \mid A=1] - \mathrm{E}[Y \mid A=0].$$

In the NCHS data, this measure is calculated as 9.9 – 5.9 = 4.0 per 1,000 live births.

Likewise, we let $M(a)$ denote the potential intermediate for each individual if, possibly contrary to fact, the exposure were set to level a. Thus, there are two possible potential intermediates, $M(1)$ and $M(0)$, resulting in four different response types (Table 3). The concept of PSE is closely related to these response types, as discussed in the following section.

	Potential intermediates		
Response type	**M(1)**	**M(0)**	**Description**
1	1	1	Always low birth weight
2	1	0	Low birth weight only with maternal smoking
3	0	1	Low birth weight only with maternal non-smoking
4	0	0	Never low birth weight

Table 3. Response types for intermediate *M* (*i.e.*, birth weight) and corresponding potential intermediates

Finally, we let $Y(a,m)$ denote the potential outcome for each individual if A were set to a and M were set to m. In this setting, there would be four potential outcomes for each individual, resulting in 4 × 4 = 16 possible response types [24,25]. Using the concept of these potential outcomes, PSE and NDE will be defined in Sections 3 and 4.

3. Principal stratification approach

As an alternative to the crude measure, we introduce the principal stratification approach. We define the PSE in Section 3.1 and present a simple method for the sensitivity analysis under the assumption in Section 3.2. In Section 3.3, the method is illustrated using the NCHS data. In Section 3.4, we present a sensitivity analysis formula by relaxing the assumption used in

Section 3.2, although the form may not be simple. The derivations of the equations and inequalities presented in this section are given in Appendix 1.

3.1. Principal strata effect

One approach to making a fair comparison involves assessing the effect of the exposure on the outcome among the subpopulation for which the intermediate would be present irrespective of the exposure status. For example, we might be interested in the effect among the subpopulation for which infants would have a low birth weight irrespective of maternal smoking status. This subpopulation for which the intermediate will occur irrespective of the exposure is sometimes referred to as a principal stratum [26]. More generally, a principal stratum is a subpopulation defined by the joint potential intermediates ($M(0)$, $M(1)$). If exposure A and intermediate M are binary, there are four possible principal strata:

i. Those for which the intermediate will occur irrespective of exposure status: always low birth weight (response type 1 in Table 3);

ii. Those for which the intermediate will occur with exposure but not without exposure: low birth weight only with maternal smoking (response type 2 in Table 3);

iii. Those for which the intermediate will occur without exposure but not with exposure: low birth weight only with maternal non-smoking or defiers (response type 3 in Table 3); and

iv. Those for which the intermediate will not occur irrespective of exposure status: never low birth weight (response type 4 in Table 3).

If we are interested in whether maternal smoking has a protective effect among low-birth-weight infants, one potentially relevant question within the context of principal stratification is whether maternal smoking has a protective effect among the subpopulation in which infants would have a low birth weight irrespective of maternal smoking status ($M(0) = 1$, $M(1) = 1$). This effect is referred to as a PSE or a principal stratum direct effect, and is formalized as follows [27,28]:

$$\text{PSE} \equiv \text{E}[Y(1) - Y(0) \mid M(0) = 1,\ M(1) = 1].$$

This measure quantifies the total effect of A on Y among the subpopulation defined by the response type of M. The advantage of using the principal stratification approach is that it essentially avoids the problem of conditioning directly on the intermediate. Instead, we condition on the principal stratum, which is essentially an underlying characteristic of the individual. It is like conditioning on a baseline covariate [16]. However, a disadvantage of this approach is that we do not know who is in each principal stratum. For example, we do not know which infants will have a low birth weight irrespective of maternal smoking status. Because we cannot identify the individuals who fall into each principal stratum, we cannot estimate the PSE directly from the observed data. However, the PSE can be estimated from the data by making a number of assumptions [28-30]. Because the PSE cannot be identified when unmeasured confounders exist between the intermediate and the outcome, as shown in Figure

1, some researchers have used sensitivity analysis techniques to assess the magnitude of the PSE [27,31,32].

3.2. Sensitivity analysis method

To derive a simple sensitivity analysis formula, we require the following assumption, which is sometimes referred to as a monotonicity assumption [33]:

Assumption 1. $M(0) \leq M(1)$ for all individuals.

This assumption implies that there are no individuals for whom the intermediate would occur without exposure but not with exposure (*i.e.*, no defiers exist), because $M(1) = 0$ and $M(0) = 1$ cannot hold simultaneously under this assumption. In the context of the smoking-birth weight example, this implies that there is no infant who would have a low birth weight if their mother was a non-smoker, but would not have a low birth weight if their mother was a smoker. When this is the case, the PSE can be expressed as the difference between the crude risk difference and a sensitivity parameter, under Assumption 1 [32]:

$$\text{PSE} = \text{E}[Y \mid A = 1, M = 1] - \text{E}[Y \mid A = 0, M = 1] - \alpha, \quad (1)$$

where the sensitivity parameter α is given by

$\alpha = \text{E}[Y(1) \mid A = 1, M = 1] - \text{E}[Y(1) \mid A = 0, M = 1]$.

The interpretation of this sensitivity parameter is the difference in infant mortality risks under maternal smoking for two subpopulations: the subpopulation with smoking mothers whose infants had a low birth weight, and the subpopulation with non-smoking mothers whose infants had a low birth weight. The parameter is not identified from the observed data.

The sensitivity analysis can be easily conducted. The sensitivity parameter α is set by the investigator according to what is considered plausible. The parameter can be varied over a range of plausible values to examine how conclusions vary according to different parameter values. The confidence interval of the true PSE for a fixed value of α can be obtained simply by subtracting α from the upper and lower confidence limits of the crude risk difference. Therefore, we can graphically display the result of the sensitivity analysis, where the horizontal axis represents the sensitivity parameter and the vertical axis represents the true PSE.

As it may be troublesome to determine the range of α values to examine in some situations, we present a range of values that α can take under some plausible assumptions. These assumptions are straightforward extensions of those developed to assess the total effect of an exposure on the outcome [34-37]. The first assumption, sometimes referred to as the assumption of monotone treatment selection [35-37], is formalized as follows in the current setting:

Assumption 2. $\text{E}[Y(1) \mid A = 1, M = m] \leq \text{E}[Y(1) \mid A = 0, M = m]$ for all m.

This assumption will hold if the subpopulation with $(A, M) = (0, m)$ is less healthy than the subpopulation with $(A, M) = (1, m)$ when the larger value of Y is more harmful. In the context of the smoking-birth weight example, Assumption 2 with $m = 1$ implies that the subpopulation with $(A, M) = (0, 1)$, which consists of low-birth-weight infants with non-smoking mothers, would be a less healthy population than the subpopulation with $(A, M) = (1, 1)$, which consists of low-birth-weight infants with smoking mothers. Assumption 2 with $m = 0$ implies that the subpopulation with $(A, M) = (0, 0)$, which consists of those who do not have a low birth weight with non-smoking mothers, would be a less healthy population than the subpopulation with $(A, M) = (1, 0)$, which consists of those who do not have a low birth weight with smoking mothers.

Assumption 2 with $m = 1$ seems arguably plausible, because in the subpopulation with $(A, M) = (0, 1)$, even if mothers were smokers, infants would have a low birth weight and the mortality risk in this subpopulation would likely be higher than that in the subpopulation with $(A, M) = (1, 1)$. However, Assumption 2 with $m = 0$ may seem less plausible to some investigators. Nevertheless, Assumption 2 with $m = 0$ is still reasonable because under Assumption 1, Assumption 2 with $m = 0$ is equivalent to assuming:

$$E[Y(1) \mid M(0)=0, M(1)=0] \leq E[Y(1) \mid M(0)=0, M(1)=1],$$

which implies that the infant mortality risk in the subpopulation consisting of those who would never have a low-birth-weight infant is not more than that in the subpopulation consisting of those who would have a low-birth-weight infant only with a smoking mother. Under the scenario in which the mother is a smoker, this would indeed be the case. Thus, Assumption 2 with $m = 0$ is also arguably reasonable. We note that under Assumption 1, Assumption 2 with $m = 1$ is equivalent to assuming:

$$E[Y(1) \mid M(0)=0, M(1)=1] \leq E[Y(1) \mid M(0)=1, M(1)=1],$$

which implies that the infant mortality risk in the subpopulation consisting of those who would have a low-birth-weight infant only with a smoking mother is not more than that in the subpopulation consisting of those who would always have a low-birth-weight infant.

When Assumption 2 holds in addition to Assumption 1, the range of α becomes [32]:

$$\frac{(p_1 - p_0)\{E[Y \mid A=1, M=0] - E[Y \mid A=1, M=1]\}}{p_0} \leq \alpha \leq 0,$$

where $p_a = \Pr(M = 1 \mid A = a)$.

The second assumption is sometimes referred to as the assumption of monotone treatment response [34,36,37] and is formalized as follows in the current setting[2]:

Assumption 3. $E[Y(0) \mid A=a, M=m] \leq E[Y(1) \mid A=a, M=m]$ for all a and m.

In the context of the smoking-birth weight example, this assumption implies that in the subpopulation with $(A, M) = (a, m)$, the infant mortality risk is higher if the mother was a smoker than if the mother was a non-smoker, which seems reasonable. When, in addition to Assumption 1, Assumption 3 holds, the range of α becomes:

2 The assumption of monotone treatment response was originally given as an assumption for all individuals; *i.e.*, $Y(0) \leq Y(1)$ for all individuals [34]. Therefore, Assumption 3 is a somewhat weaker assumption than the original one.

http://dx.doi.org/10.5772/53193

$$\left\{\begin{matrix}(1-p_0)\mathrm{E}[Y \mid A=0,\ M=0] \\ -(1-p_1)\mathrm{E}[Y \mid A=1,\ M=0] \\ -(p_1-p_0)\mathrm{E}[Y \mid A=1,\ M=1]\end{matrix}\right\} \Bigg/ p_0 \le \alpha \le \mathrm{E}[Y \mid A=1,\ M=1] - \mathrm{E}[Y \mid A=0,\ M=1].$$

When it is considered that, in addition to Assumption 1, both Assumptions 2 and 3 hold, we can use a narrower range derived under these two assumptions.

3.3. Illustration

We now apply the principal stratification approach to the NCHS data shown in Table 1. As noted in Section 1, the crude difference in the mortality risk of low-birth-weight infants between smoking and non-smoking mothers was –12.6 (95% CI: –15.0, –10.1) per 1,000 live births, suggesting that maternal smoking has a protective effect against infant mortality for low-birth-weight infants.

To calculate the PSE defined in Section 3.1, we adjust this crude estimate by the sensitivity parameter α. We set the range of α per 1,000 live births to $-22.1 \le \alpha \le -12.6$ because the ranges were calculated as $-22.1 \le \alpha \le 0$ under Assumption 2 and $-84.0 \le \alpha \le -12.6$ under Assumption 3. Figure 2 shows the result of the sensitivity analysis over this range of α, for which the lower and upper limits of the PSE per 1,000 live births were 0.0 (95% CI: –2.4, 2.4) and 9.6 (95% CI: 7.1, 12.0), respectively.

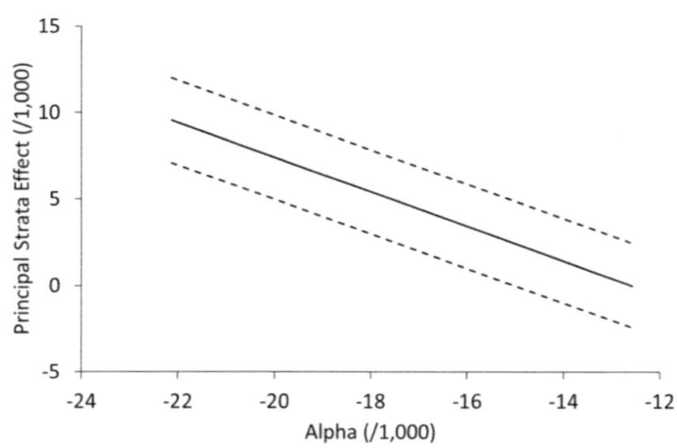

Figure 2. Sensitivity analysis of the principal strata effect (per 1,000 live births); the solid line indicates the principal strata effect and broken lines indicate 95% confidence intervals

The result of this sensitivity analysis for the PSE suggests that maternal smoking has a harmful effect on the subpopulation of infants who would have a low birth weight irrespective of maternal smoking, although the lower limit of the 95% confidence interval for the PSE was still smaller than 0 when α per 1,000 live births was larger than –15.0. Therefore, we can say that the birth-weight paradox was resolved in terms of the PSE.

3.4. Sensitivity analysis without the monotonicity assumption

The monotonicity assumption (Assumption 1) is a strict assumption because the inequality ($M(0) \leq M(1)$) must hold for all individuals. If just one defier exists, this assumption does not hold. Therefore, we introduce a sensitivity analysis for the PSE without the monotonicity assumption. This sensitivity analysis formula requires the following three sensitivity parameters, instead of α:

$$\beta_1 = \mathrm{E}[Y(1) \mid M(0)=1, M(1)=1] - \mathrm{E}[Y(1) \mid M(0)=0, M(1)=1],$$

$$\beta_2 = \mathrm{E}[Y(0) \mid M(0)=1, M(1)=1] - \mathrm{E}[Y(0) \mid M(0)=1, M(1)=0],$$

$$\beta_3 = \Pr(M(0)=1, M(1)=0).$$

In the context of the smoking-birth weight example, the parameter β_1 is the difference in the infant mortality risk under maternal smoking between the subpopulation consisting of those who would always have a low birth weight and the subpopulation consisting of those who would have a low birth weight only with a smoking mother. As discussed in Section 3.2, β_1 will take a positive value. β_2 is the difference in the infant mortality risk under maternal non-smoking between the subpopulation consisting of those who would always have a low birth weight and the subpopulation consisting of those who would have a low birth weight only with a non-smoking mother (defier). β_2 will also take a positive value. β_3 indicates the proportion of defiers. In this context, even if the value of β_3 is not zero, it will be very small.

Using these three sensitivity parameters, the PSE can be expressed as follows [38]:

$$\mathrm{PSE} = \mathrm{E}[Y \mid A=1, M=1] - \mathrm{E}[Y \mid A=0, M=1] + \frac{p_1 - p_0 + \beta_3}{p_1}\beta_1 - \frac{\beta_3}{p_0}\beta_2. \quad (2)$$

It will be more difficult to determine the values or ranges of these three sensitivity parameters (β_1, β_2, and β_3) compared with those of only one sensitivity parameter (α). Furthermore, it will be difficult to display the result of the sensitivity analysis. For example, in the NCHS data, if we set (β_1, β_2, β_3) = (30.0, 2.0, 0.1) per 1,000 live births, the PSE is 1.7 per 1,000 live births. A larger value of β_1 makes the PSE larger. Conversely, a larger value of β_2 makes the PSE smaller.

4. Intervention-based approach

As another alternative to the crude measure, we introduce the intervention-based approach. In Section 4.1, we define two types of direct effects, the controlled direct effect (CDE) and the NDE, both of which are based on interventions on the intermediate [2,39]. We mainly focus our discussion on the NDE. A simple method for the sensitivity analysis is presented in Section 4.2 and is illustrated in Section 4.3 using the NCHS data. The derivations of equations and inequalities presented in this section are given in Appendix 2.

http://dx.doi.org/10.5772/53193

4.1. Controlled and natural direct effects

The CDE captures the effect of exposure A on outcome Y by intervening to fix intermediate M to m. Using the notation $Y(a,m)$, the CDE is defined as

$$\mathrm{CDE}(m) \equiv \mathrm{E}[Y(1, m)] - \mathrm{E}[Y(0, m)],$$

Contrary to the PSE, the CDE is a causal effect concerning the whole population. In the context of the smoking-birth weight example, the CDE with $m = 1$ captures the effect of maternal smoking on infant mortality if all infants were intervened to have a low birth weight; the CDE with $m = 0$ captures the effect of maternal smoking on infant mortality if all infants were intervened to not have a low birth weight. However, interventions on birth weight seem inconceivable.

The NDE differs from the CDE in that the intermediate M is set to the level $M(0)$, which would have naturally been under the exposure level of $A = 0$. Therefore, to describe the NDE, we need to integrate information about $M(a)$ and $Y(a,m)$. This yields the compound potential outcome $Y(a,M(a^*))$. In this case, individuals can be classified into 4 × 16 = 64 combined response types, each of which has a corresponding pattern of compound potential outcomes [24]. Using the compound potential outcome, the NDE is defined as[3]

$$\mathrm{NDE} \equiv \mathrm{E}[Y(1, M(0))] - \mathrm{E}[Y(0, M(0))],$$

which compares the effect of an exposure on the outcome if the intermediate were set to what it would have been when exposure A was set to 0. In the context of the smoking-birth weight example, the NDE compares what would have happened to an infant if the mother had been a smoker versus a non-smoker and if the infant had the birth weight status that would have occurred due to maternal non-smoking. Corresponding to the NDE is a natural indirect effect (NIE). The NIE is defined as

$$\mathrm{NIE} \equiv \mathrm{E}[Y(1, M(1))] - \mathrm{E}[Y(1, M(0))],$$

which compares the effect of the intermediate at levels $M(1)$ and $M(0)$ on the outcome when exposure A is set to 1. The NIE can be interpreted as a causal effect when intervention is made to block a direct link between the exposure and the outcome (an arrow between A and Y in Figure 1), rather than to block a variable itself [39]. Therefore, the NIE is an indirect component of the total effect, acting through the intermediate. Note that the total effect decomposes into the NDE and NIE, *i.e.*, $\mathrm{E}[Y(1)] - \mathrm{E}[Y(0)] = \mathrm{NDE} + \mathrm{NIE}$. This decomposition holds at not only the population level but also the individual level; when we define the individual natural direct and indirect effects by $\mathrm{NDE}(\omega) \equiv Y(1,M(0)) - Y(0,M(0))$ and $\mathrm{NIE}(\omega) \equiv Y(1,M(1)) - Y(1,M(0))$, respectively, for each individual ω,

$$\begin{aligned} Y(1) - Y(0) &= Y(1, M(1)) - Y(0, M(0)) \\ &= \{Y(1, M(1)) - Y(1, M(0))\} + \{Y(1, M(0)) - Y(0, M(0))\} \\ &= \mathrm{NIE}(\omega) + \mathrm{NDE}(\omega). \end{aligned}$$

3 We can also define the NDE under the exposure level of $A = 1$ as $\mathrm{NDE} \equiv \mathrm{E}[Y(1,M(1))] - \mathrm{E}[Y(0,M(1))]$. The NIE corresponding to this NDE is equal to $\mathrm{E}[Y(0,M(1))] - \mathrm{E}[Y(0,M(0))]$.

This decomposition may help in understanding the meaning of the NDE, *i.e.*, the NDE is a direct component of the total effect and does not act through the intermediate.

If there is no interaction between the effects of exposure A and intermediate M on outcome Y in the sense that $E[Y(1,m)] - E[Y(0,m)]$ does not vary with m, the CDE and NDE coincide. The difference between a total effect and a CDE cannot generally be interpreted as an indirect effect and thus cannot be used to assess mediation. This is because when there is an interaction between the effects of exposure A and intermediate M on outcome Y, the CDEs may differ from the total effect even when A is not a cause of M. When there is an interaction between A and M, the CDEs will differ with different values of m, and thus one of the CDEs will differ from a total effect. Therefore, in general, CDEs cannot be used for decomposition of a total effect into direct and indirect effects. We note that the CDE will often be of greater interest in policy [39], and the NDE will often be of greater interest in the evaluation of etiology [39-41].

Similar to the CDE, the NDE is also a causal effect concerning the whole population, and it can be estimated from the data under certain assumptions [42,43]. However, neither the CDE nor the NDE can be identified when an unmeasured confounder exists between the intermediate and the outcome, as in Figure 1. Therefore, sensitivity analysis techniques have been discussed to assess their magnitudes [4,44-48]. In the next subsection, a simple sensitivity analysis method for the NDE is presented. Methods for the CDE are found elsewhere [4,44,47].

4.2. Sensitivity analysis method for the natural direct effect

Although the monotonicity assumption (Assumption 1) was necessary to derive a simple sensitivity analysis formula for the PSE, this assumption is not required to derive one for the NDE.

For each possible value of intermediate M (= 0, 1), we consider the following sensitivity parameter:

$$\gamma_m = E[Y(1, m) \mid A=1, M=m] - E[Y(1, m) \mid A=0, M=m].$$

The sensitivity parameter $\gamma_1 = E[Y(1,1) \mid A = 1, M = 1] - E[Y(1,1) \mid A = 0, M = 1]$ is a contrast of infant mortality risks for two subpopulations. In a manner similar to the sensitivity parameter α for the PSE, the first subpopulation with $(A, M) = (1, 1)$ consists of smoking mothers whose infants had a low birth weight, and the second subpopulation with $(A, M) = (0, 1)$ comprises non-smoking mothers whose infants had a low birth weight. We then consider whether the infants in these two subpopulations would have lived or died if we had intervened to fix mothers to be smokers and infants to have a low birth weight; *i.e.*, we consider $Y(1,1)$. The contrast between the infant mortality risks in these two subpopulations under this particular intervention is our sensitivity parameter, γ_1. This parameter differs from α for the PSE in that it considers two interventions, which fix A to 1 and M to 1, whereas α considers one intervention, which fixes A to 1. As described above, it is not realistic to consider an intervention to fix the birth weight of an infant. This is a disadvantage of using the sensitivity parameter γ_1 in the smoking-birth weight context. Analogously, the other sensitivity parameter, $\gamma_0 = E[Y(1,0) \mid A = 1, M = 0] - E[Y(1,0) \mid A = 0, M = 0]$, can be interpreted. The parameters are not identified from the observed data.

We now consider a weighted mean of the sensitivity parameters γ_1 and γ_0, where the respective weights are the probabilities of infants with low birth weights and not from non-smoking mothers, *i.e.*, $\Pr(M=1 \mid A=0)$ and $\Pr(M=0 \mid A=0)$:

$$\Gamma = \sum_{m=0}^{1} \gamma_m \Pr(M=m \mid A=0). \tag{3}$$

After calculating the crude risk differences $E[Y \mid A=1, M=m] - E[Y \mid A=0, M=m]$ and probabilities $\Pr(M=m \mid A=0)$ for $m=0, 1$, the NDE can be expressed as the difference between the weighted means of the two crude risk differences and Γ, *i.e.*,

$$\text{NDE} = \sum_{m=0}^{1} \{E[Y \mid A=1, M=m] - E[Y \mid A=0, M=m]\} \Pr(M=m \mid A=0) - \Gamma. \tag{4}$$

The variance of the first term in equation (4) is calculated by the delta method, $\text{var}(\hat{s}\hat{t}) = \text{var}(\hat{s})\text{var}(\hat{t}) + s^2\text{var}(\hat{t}) + t^2\text{var}(\hat{s})$, where s and t are replaced by the estimates $\hat{s}$ and $\hat{t}$. In a manner similar to the sensitivity analysis for the PSE, the sensitivity analysis for the NDE can be conducted easily. The sensitivity parameters γ_0 and γ_1 are set by the investigator according to what is considered plausible. The parameters can be varied over a range of plausible values to examine how the conclusions change according to the different parameter values. However, to obtain the confidence interval of the true NDE for the fixed values of γ_m, we must calculate not only the variance of the first term in equation (4) but also the variance of Γ, because Γ depends on the probabilities $\Pr(M=m \mid A=0)$, which must be estimated from the observed data. However, if γ_m were constant across the strata of m, Γ would no longer depend on $\Pr(M=m \mid A=0)$, and thus we could simply subtract Γ from both limits of the confidence interval for the first term in equation (4) to obtain the confidence interval for the true NDE. Similarly, for a data set large enough that the estimates of $\Pr(M=m \mid A=0)$ were very precise, the approximate confidence interval for the true NDE could be obtained by subtracting Γ from both limits of the confidence interval for the first term in equation (4).

We can determine the upper limits of γ_m by using the following assumptions, which are similar to Assumptions 2 and 3 for the PSE:

Assumption 2*. $E[Y(1, m) \mid A=1, M=m] \le E[Y(1, m) \mid A=0, M=m]$ for all m.

Assumption 3*. $E[Y(0, m) \mid A=a, M=m] \le E[Y(1, m) \mid A=a, M=m]$ for all a and m.

The upper limit of γ_1 is $\gamma_1 \le 0$ under Assumption 2* with $m=1$ or $\gamma_1 \le E[Y \mid A=1, M=1] - E[Y \mid A=0, M=1]$ under Assumption 3* with $a=0$ and $m=1$. These upper limits are equal to those of $\alpha = E[Y(1) \mid A=1, M=1] - E[Y(1) \mid A=0, M=1]$ for the sensitivity analysis of the PSE in Section 3.2. Unfortunately, the lower limit of γ_1 cannot be derived under these assumptions, even when Assumption 1 is added, because we are considering interventions on not only exposure A but also intermediate M (see Appendix 2). Furthermore, it is somewhat difficult to interpret these assumptions because of intervention on the intermediate M. The upper limit of γ_0 is $\gamma_0 \leq 0$ under Assumption 2* with $m = 0$ or $\gamma_0 \leq \mathrm{E}[Y \mid A = 1, M = 0] - \mathrm{E}[Y \mid A = 0, M = 0]$ under Assumption 3* with $a = 0$ and $m = 0$. From these upper limits of γ_m, the upper limit of Γ is calculated using equation (3).

Assumptions 2* and 3* (2 and 3) relate to monotone treatment selection and monotone treatment response regarding the exposure, respectively. We can also make these types of assumptions about the intermediate [49]:

Assumption 4. $\mathrm{E}[Y(a, m) \mid A=a, M = 0] \leq \mathrm{E}[Y(a, m) \mid A=a, M = 1]$ for all a and m.

Assumption 5. $\mathrm{E}[Y(a, 0) \mid A=a^*, M=m] \leq \mathrm{E}[Y(a, 1) \mid A=a^*, M=m]$ for all $a, a^*,$ and m.

In the context of the smoking-birth weight example, Assumption 4 implies that infants with a low birth weight, representing the subpopulation with $(A, M) = (a, 1)$, would be a less healthy than infants who did not have a low birth weight, representing the subpopulation with $(A, M) = (a, 0)$, where maternal smoking status is common among these two subpopulations. Assumption 5 implies that in the subpopulation with $(A, M) = (a^*, m)$, the infant mortality risk would be higher if infants had a low birth weight than if infants did not have a low birth weight. As this would indeed be the case, Assumptions 4 and 5 seem arguably reasonable. Under these assumptions, although ranges of γ_m cannot be derived, the range of Γ can be derived as follows:

$$-(1-p_0)\{\mathrm{E}[Y \mid A=1, M=1]-\mathrm{E}[Y \mid A=1, M=0]\} \leq \Gamma \leq p_0\{\mathrm{E}[Y \mid A=1, M=1]-\mathrm{E}[Y \mid A=1, M=0]\}.$$

While Assumptions 2* and 3* can lead to only the upper limit, Assumptions 4 and 5 can lead to both limits. Furthermore, when Assumption 1 is added, under Assumptions 1 and 5, the lower limit of Γ is improved to:

$$\Gamma \geq -(p_1-p_0)\{\mathrm{E}[Y \mid A=1, M=1]-\mathrm{E}[Y \mid A=1, M=0]\}.$$

However, neither the lower nor the upper limit can be derived under only one of the Assumptions 4 and 5.

4.3. Illustration

We now apply this intervention-based approach to the NCHS data shown in Table 1. To calculate the NDE defined by equation (4), we determine a range of values for Γ. Under Assumptions 2* and 3*, the respective upper limits of γ_0 and γ_1 per 1,000 live births were calculated as $\gamma_0 \leq 0$ and $\gamma_1 \leq -12.6$. By substituting these upper limits into equation (3), we obtained $\Gamma \leq -0.7$ per 1,000 live births. Under Assumptions 4 and 5, the range of Γ per 1,000 live births was calculated as $-44.0 \leq \Gamma \leq 2.6$. Under Assumptions 1 and 5, the lower limit was improved to $\Gamma \geq -2.4$ per 1,000 live births. Therefore, we set the range of Γ per 1,000 live births as $-2.4 \leq \Gamma \leq -0.7$. Because the sample size was large, we obtain the approximate confidence interval for the true NDE by subtracting Γ from both limits of the confidence interval for the first term in equation (4). The result of the sensitivity analysis over this range of Γ is shown in Figure 3. With this range of Γ, the lower and upper limits of the NDE per 1,000 live births were 2.4 (95% CI: 2.0, 2.7) and 4.0 (95% CI: 3.7, 4.4), respectively.

http://dx.doi.org/10.5772/53193

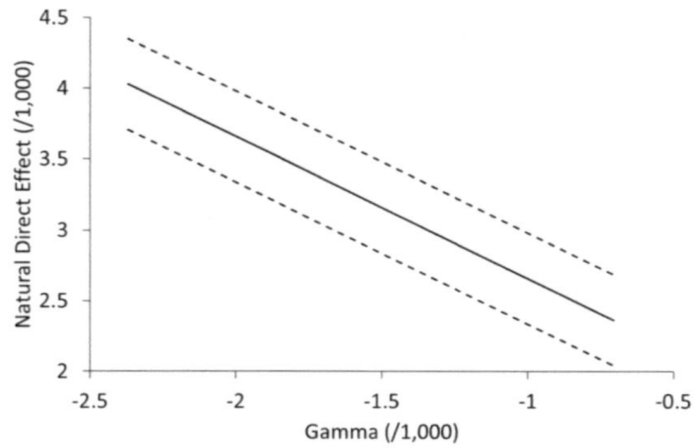

Figure 3. Sensitivity analysis of the natural direct effect (per 1,000 live births); the solid line indicates the natural direct effect and broken lines indicate 95% confidence intervals

The result of this sensitivity analysis for the NDE suggests that maternal smoking has a directly harmful effect on infant mortality. Thus, the birth-weight paradox is also resolved in terms of the NDE.

5. Relationship between the principal strata effect and the natural direct effect

We briefly discuss the relationship between the PSE and NDE. Again, we note that the individual NDE is defined as $\mathrm{NDE}(\omega) \equiv Y(1,M(0)) - Y(0,M(0))$. It can then be shown that, when there is no natural direct effect for any individual, there is no principal strata effect [50], *i.e.*,

Theorem 1. If $\mathrm{NDE}(\omega) = 0$ for all ω, then $\mathrm{PSE} = 0$.

To prove this theorem, we consider a probability of $Y(1) - Y(0) = 0$ conditional on $\{M(0) = 1, M(1) = 1\}$, *i.e.*, $\Pr(Y(1) - Y(0) = 0 \mid M(0) = 1, M(1) = 1)$. This indicates a probability that the PSE is equal to 0. We prove Theorem 1 by showing that this probability is equal to 1 under the assumption that $\mathrm{NDE}(\omega) = 0$ for all ω. The proof is as follows:

$$
\begin{aligned}
&\Pr(Y(1)-Y(0)=0 \mid M(0)=1, M(1)=1)\\
&=\Pr(Y(1, M(1))-Y(1, M(0))+\mathrm{NDE}(\omega)=0 \mid M(0)=1, M(1)=1)\\
&=\Pr(Y(1, M(1))-Y(1, M(0))=0 \mid M(0)=1, M(1)=1)\\
&=\Pr(Y(1, 1)-Y(1, 1)=0 \mid M(0)=1, M(1)=1)\\
&=\Pr(0=0 \mid M(0)=1, M(1)=1)\\
&=1,
\end{aligned}
$$

where the first equation is from the decomposition of the total effect to the NDE and NIE, the second is by $\mathrm{NDE}(\omega) = 0$, and the third is because $Y(1,M(a))$ is equal to $Y(1,1)$ conditional on $M(a) = 1$. This completes the proof.

The converse of this theorem does not hold: the absence of a PSE does not imply the absence of a NDE. Nevertheless, from the contraposition of this theorem, when there is a PSE, there must be some individuals for whom there is a NDE. The results of the sensitivity analyses in Sections 3.3 and 4.3 showed that the true PSE was not smaller than 0 and that the true NDE was larger than 2.3. The results do not contradict the contraposition of Theorem 1.

6. Conclusion

In this chapter, we described two approaches related to calculating the effect of an exposure on an outcome that is conditional on potential intermediates or one that does not act through the intermediate. Here, we made an impractical assumption in the observational studies that no confounder exists between the exposure and the outcome or between the exposure and the intermediate. Nevertheless, the methodologies described here also hold conditional on confounders if no unmeasured confounder exists between these variables. We considered a risk difference as the effect measure, but the methodologies can be extended to other effect measures.

Each approach has a unique interpretation and its own strengths and weaknesses. In the principal stratification approach, one conditions on the subpopulation for which the intermediate would occur irrespective of exposure. An advantage of this approach is that the subpopulation is a particularly high-risk group in which the intermediate will necessarily occur. A disadvantage is that we do not know who is in the subpopulation such that the intermediate will occur irrespective of the exposure. In the intervention-based approach, the NDE appears to capture the effect of an exposure on the outcome if the intermediate was set to what it would be when the exposure is set to 0. An advantage of this approach is that it can be used to decompose the total effect into direct and indirect components. A disadvantage is that it is difficult to understand the meaning of the NDE from the form. In addition, it is difficult to interpret the sensitivity parameter for the sensitivity analysis, although this may be avoided by applying a parametric model [46].

In many studies, the total effect of the exposure on the outcome in the whole population may be of central interest, and then none of the approaches described here are required. The approaches described here are of relevance only when the investigators are interested in the direct effect of the exposure not acting through the intermediate or the effect of the exposure on the outcome for certain groups at high risk for the intermediate. In some birth weight settings, the exposure or intervention under study may occur after birth in some cases [6]. In these cases, birth weight becomes a pre-exposure baseline variable, and the approaches described here are not needed. These settings should be distinguished from those similar to the birth-weight paradox. When the approaches described here are of relevance, both the PSE and NDE may be in a consistent direction in some situations, as seen in Sections 3.3 and 4.3. However, it is important to note that the two approaches need not give effect estimates in the same direction. Having effect estimates in different directions with the two approaches is not necessarily an indication that one of the estimates is in the wrong direction. The two approaches estimate two different effects (effects for two different populations), and these may in fact be in different directions. Before these approaches are applied, it is important to be clear about the scientific or policy question.

The approaches described in this chapter are applicable to a number of similar settings in all areas of epidemiological research. As the existing literature has made clear, conditioning on an intermediate can be problematic and can give rise to severe biases. In many contexts, conditioning on an intermediate is not necessary and is best avoided. Nevertheless, there are cases in which conditioning on an intermediate is of scientific or policy interest. We have shown that alternative approaches can be used to draw inferences in such settings. Although these methodological tools are imperfect and need to be interpreted carefully, they can be useful in examining conditional and direct effects.

Appendix

Appendices 1 and 2 outline the derivations of the equations and inequalities presented in Sections 3 and 4, respectively. As noted in Section 2, we assume that no confounder exists between A and M or between A and Y. This assumption leads to the independency assumption that $M(a)$, $Y(a)$, and $Y(a,m)$ are independent of A. In addition, we require two assumptions. The first is the no-interference assumption that one individual's outcome does not depend on the exposure status of other individuals. The second is the consistency assumption that when $A = a$, the potential outcomes $Y(a)$ and $M(a)$ are equal to the observed outcomes Y and M, respectively. Likewise, we assume that when $A = a$ and $M = m$, the potential outcome $Y(a,m)$ is equal to Y. For simplicity, we use the notations $E_{ij}(a) = \mathrm{E}[Y(a) \mid M(0) = i, M(1) = j]$ and $\pi_{ij} \equiv \Pr(M(0) = i, M(1) = j)$.

Appendix 1: Derivations of equations and inequalities in Section 3

Derivation of equation (1)

Using α, PSE can be expressed as follows:

$$\begin{aligned}\mathrm{PSE} &\equiv E_{11}(1)-E_{11}(0)\\ &=\mathrm{E}[Y(1)\mid M(0)=1]-\mathrm{E}[Y(0)\mid M(0)=1]\\ &=\mathrm{E}[Y(1)\mid A=0,\ M=1]-\mathrm{E}[Y(0)\mid A=0,\ M=1]\\ &=\{\mathrm{E}[Y(1)\mid A=1,\ M=1]-\alpha\}-\mathrm{E}[Y(0)\mid A=0,\ M=1]\\ &=\mathrm{E}[Y\mid A=1,\ M=1]-\mathrm{E}[Y\mid A=0,\ M=1]-\alpha,\end{aligned}$$

where the second equation is by Assumption 1, the third is by the independency and consistency assumptions, the fourth is by using $\alpha = \mathrm{E}[Y(1) \mid A = 1, M = 1] - \mathrm{E}[Y(1) \mid A = 0, M = 1]$, and the last is again by the consistency assumption.

Proof that Assumption 2 is equivalent to assuming that $E_{01}(1) \le E_{11}(1)$ and $E_{00}(1) \le E_{01}(1)$

The relationship between π_{ij} and $p_a = \Pr(M = 1 \mid A = a)$ is

$$\pi_{11}+\pi_{01}=p_1,\ \pi_{10}+\pi_{0_0}=1-p_1,\ \pi_{11}+\pi_{1_0}=p_0,\ \text{and}\,\pi_{0_1}+\pi_{00}=1-p_0 \qquad \text{(A1)}$$

because $\Pr(M(a) = m) = \Pr(M(a) = m \mid A = a) = \Pr(M = m \mid A = a)$ by the independency and consistency assumptions. Furthermore, because $E[Y(a) \mid A = 1, M = 1] = E[Y(a) \mid M(1) = 1]$ by the independency assumption, this conditional expectation can be expressed as

$$E[Y(a) \mid A=1, M=1] = \frac{\pi_{11}E_{11}(a) + \pi_{01}E_{01}(a)}{\pi_{11} + \pi_{01}}. \tag{A2}$$

Similarly,

$$E[Y(a) \mid A=0, M=1] = \frac{\pi_{11}E_{11}(a) + \pi_{10}E_{10}(a)}{\pi_{11} + \pi_{10}}, \tag{A3}$$

$$E[Y(a) \mid A=1, M=0] = \frac{\pi_{10}E_{10}(a) + \pi_{00}E_{00}(a)}{\pi_{10} + \pi_{00}}, \tag{A4}$$

$$E[Y(a) \mid A=0, M=0] = \frac{\pi_{01}E_{01}(a) + \pi_{00}E_{00}(a)}{\pi_{01} + \pi_{00}}. \tag{A5}$$

As $\pi_{10} = 0$ (no defier exists) under Assumption 1, (A1) reduces to

$$\pi_{11} = p_0,\ \pi_{00} = 1 - p_1,\ \text{and}\ \pi_{01} = p_1 - p_0,$$

where it is assumed that $\pi_{01} > 0$ (*i.e.*, $p_1 > p_0$). Using $\alpha = E[Y(1) \mid A = 1, M = 1] - E[Y(1) \mid A = 0, M = 1]$ and $\alpha' = E[Y(1) \mid A = 1, M = 0] - E[Y(1) \mid A = 0, M = 0]$, (A2)–(A5) with $a = 1$ can be expressed respectively as

$$E[Y \mid A=1, M=1] = \frac{p_0E_{11}(1) + (p_1 - p_0)E_{01}(1)}{p_1}, \tag{A6}$$

$$E[Y \mid A=1, M=1] - \alpha = E_{11}(1), \tag{A7}$$

$$E[Y \mid A=1, M=0] = E_{00}(1), \tag{A8}$$

$$E[Y \mid A=1, M=0] - \alpha' = \frac{(p_1 - p_0)E_{01}(1) + (1 - p_1)E_{00}(1)}{1 - p_0}. \tag{A9}$$

The differences between (A6) and (A7) and between (A8) and (A9) lead to, respectively

$$\alpha = \frac{p_1 - p_0}{p_1}\left\{E_{01}(1) - E_{11}(1)\right\},$$

$$\alpha' = \frac{p_1 - p_0}{1 - p_0}\left\{E_{00}(1) - E_{01}(1)\right\}.$$

Assumption 2 with $m = 1$ is equivalent to $\alpha \le 0$, and that with $m = 0$ is equivalent to $\alpha' \le 0$. Thus, Assumption 2 is equal to assuming that $E_{01}(1) \le E_{11}(1)$ with $m = 1$ and $E_{00}(1) \le E_{01}(1)$ with $m = 0$, because $p_1 > p_0$ by assumption.

Derivations of ranges of α under Assumptions 2 and 3

Substituting (A7) into (A6) gives

$$E_{01}(1) = E[Y \mid A=1, M=1] + \frac{p_0}{p_1 - p_0}\alpha, \tag{A10}$$

and substituting (A8) into (A9) leads to

$$E_{01}(1) = E[Y \mid A=1, M=0] - \frac{1 - p_0}{p_1 - p_0}\alpha'. \tag{A11}$$

Given that these two equations are equal, some algebra yields

$$p_0\alpha + (1-p_0)\alpha' = -(p_1 - p_0)\{\mathrm{E}[Y \mid A=1, M=1] - \mathrm{E}[Y \mid A=1, M=0]\}. \tag{A12}$$

Then, a range of α under Assumption 2 is derived by $\alpha \leq 0$ and by substituting $\alpha' \leq 0$ into (A12).

Under Assumption 3,

$$\begin{aligned}\alpha &= \mathrm{E}[Y(1) \mid A=1, M=1] - \mathrm{E}[Y(1) \mid A=0, M=1]\\ &\leq \mathrm{E}[Y(1) \mid A=1, M=1] - \mathrm{E}[Y(0) \mid A=0, M=1]\\ &= \mathrm{E}[Y \mid A=1, M=1] - \mathrm{E}[Y \mid A=0, M=1],\end{aligned}$$

and similarly $\alpha' \leq \mathrm{E}[Y \mid A=1, M=0] - \mathrm{E}[Y \mid A=0, M=0]$. Thus, a range of α under Assumption 3 is derived by $\alpha \leq \mathrm{E}[Y \mid A=1, M=1] - \mathrm{E}[Y \mid A=0, M=1]$ and by substituting $\alpha' \leq \mathrm{E}[Y \mid A=1, M=0] - \mathrm{E}[Y \mid A=0, M=0]$ into (A12).

Derivation of equation (2)

Using $\beta_1 = E_{11}(1) - E_{01}(1)$, $\beta_2 = E_{11}(0) - E_{10}(0)$ and $\beta_3 = \pi_{10}$, (A2) with $a = 1$ can be expressed as

$$\begin{aligned}\mathrm{E}[Y \mid A=1, M=1] &= \frac{(\pi_{11}+\pi_{01})E_{11}(1) - \pi_{01}\{E_{11}(1) - E_{01}(1)\}}{\pi_{11}+\pi_{01}}\\ &= E_{11}(1) - \frac{p_1 - (p_0 - \pi_{10})}{p_1}\left\{E_{11}(1) - E_{01}(1)\right\}\\ &= E_{11}(1) - \frac{p_1 - p_0 + \beta_3}{p_1}\beta_1,\end{aligned}$$

and (A3) with $a = 0$ can be expressed similarly as

$$\begin{aligned}\mathrm{E}[Y \mid A=0, M=1] &= \frac{(\pi_{11}+\pi_{10})E_{11}(0) - \pi_{10}\{E_{11}(0) - E_{10}(0)\}}{\pi_{11}+\pi_{01}}\\ &= E_{11}(0) - \frac{\pi_{10}}{p_0}\left\{E_{11}(0) - E_{10}(0)\right\}\\ &= E_{11}(0) - \frac{\beta_3}{p_0}\beta_2.\end{aligned}$$

The difference between these two equations leads to equation (2).

Appendix 2: Derivations of equations and inequalities in Section 4

Derivation of equation (4)

Using γ_m and Γ, $\mathrm{E}[Y(1,M(0))]$ can be expressed as follows:

$$\begin{aligned}\mathrm{E}[Y(1, M(0))] &= \mathrm{E}[Y(1, M(0)) \mid A=0]\\ &= \sum_m \mathrm{E}[Y(1, M(0)) \mid A=0, M(0)=m]\Pr(M(0)=m \mid A=0)\\ &= \sum_m \mathrm{E}[Y(1, m) \mid A=0, M=m]\Pr(M=m \mid A=0)\\ &= \sum_m \{\mathrm{E}[Y(1, m) \mid A=1, M=m] - \gamma_m\}\Pr(M=m \mid A=0)\\ &= \sum_m \mathrm{E}[Y \mid A=1, M=m]\Pr(M=m \mid A=0) - \Gamma,\end{aligned}$$

where the first equation is by the independency assumption, the third is by the consistency assumption, and the fourth is by $\gamma_m = \mathrm{E}[Y(1,m) \mid A=1, M=m] - \mathrm{E}[Y(1,m) \mid A=0, M=m]$. The simpler calculation expresses $\mathrm{E}[Y(0,M(0))]$ as

$$\begin{aligned}E[Y(0, M(0))] &= E[Y(0)] \\ &= E[Y \mid A=0] \\ &= \sum_m E[Y \mid A=0, M=m]\Pr(M=m \mid A=0).\end{aligned}$$

The difference between these two equations leads to equation (4).

The reason that the lower limit of γ_m cannot be derived under Assumptions 2* and 3*

A range of α can be derived because (A10) and (A11) are equal. In the setting in which γ_m is used instead of α and α', under Assumption 1, the following equations are derived, instead of (A10) and (A11):

$$E_{01}(1, 1) = E[Y \mid A=1, M=1] + \frac{p_0}{p_1 - p_0}\gamma_1, \quad \text{(A13)}$$

$$E_{01}(1, 0) = E[Y \mid A=1, M=0] - \frac{1-p_0}{p_1 - p_0}\gamma_0, \quad \text{(A14)}$$

where $E_{ij}(a,m) = E[Y(a,m) \mid M(0) = i, M(1) = j]$. Because these two equations are not equal, the lower limit of γ_0 (γ_1) cannot be derived using the upper limit of γ_1 (γ_0) under Assumptions 2* and 3*, even under Assumption 1.

Derivations of ranges of Γ under Assumptions 4 and 5 and Assumptions 1 and 5

By the consistency assumption, $E[Y(1,m) \mid A = 1, M = m] = E[Y \mid A = 1, M = m]$. Using Assumptions 4 and 5, the following inequality can be derived:

$$\begin{aligned}\sum_m E[Y(1, m) \mid A=0, M=m]\Pr(M=m \mid A=0) &\le \sum_m E[Y(1, 1) \mid A=0, M=m]\Pr(M=m \mid A=0) \\ &= E[Y(1, 1) \mid A=0] \\ &= E[Y(1, 1) \mid A=1] \\ &= \sum_m E[Y(1, 1) \mid A=1, M=m]\Pr(M=m \mid A=1) \\ &\le \sum_m E[Y(1, 1) \mid A=1, M=1]\Pr(M=m \mid A=1) \\ &= E[Y \mid A=1, M=1],\end{aligned}$$

where the first inequality is by Assumption 5 with $a = 1$ and $a^* = 0$, the third equation is by the independency assumption, and the fifth inequality is by Assumption 4 with $a = 1$ and $m = 1$. Substituting the above equation and inequality into equation (3) leads to

$$\begin{aligned}\Gamma &\ge \sum_m E[Y \mid A=1, M=m]\Pr(M=m \mid A=0) - E[Y \mid A=1, M=1] \\ &= -\{E[Y \mid A=1, M=1] - E[Y \mid A=1, M=0]\}\Pr(M=0 \mid A=0).\end{aligned}$$

A similar calculation gives the upper limit.

Equations (A13) and (A14) hold under Assumption 1 and $E_{01}(1,0) \le E_{01}(1,1)$ holds under Assumption 5 with $a = 1$, $a^* = 0$ and $m = 1$. Substituting (A13) and (A14) into this inequality leads to

$$-(p_1 - p_0)\{E[Y \mid A=1, M=1] - E[Y \mid A=1, M=0]\} \le p_0\gamma_1 + (1 - p_0)\gamma_0 = \Gamma.$$

Acknowledgements

This work was supported partially by Grant-in-Aid for Scientific Research (No. 23700344) from the Ministry of Education, Culture, Sports, Science, and Technology of Japan.

http://dx.doi.org/10.5772/53193

Author details

Yasutaka Chiba[1*] and Etsuji Suzuki[2]

1 Division of Biostatistics, Clinical Research Center, Kinki University School of Medicine, Japan

2 Department of Epidemiology, Graduate School of Medicine, Dentistry and Pharmaceutical Sciences, Okayama University, Japan

References

[1] Greenland S, Morgenstern H. Confounding in health research. *Annual Review of Public Health* 2001; 22(1) 189-212.

[2] Robins JM, Greenland S. Identifiability and exchangeability for direct and indirect effects. *Epidemiology* 1992; 3(2) 143-155.

[3] Cole SR, Hernán MA. Fallibility in estimating direct effects. *International Journal of Epidemiology* 2002; 31(1) 163-165.

[4] VanderWeele T.J. Bias formulas for sensitivity analysis for direct and indirect effects. *Epidemiology* 2010; 21(4) 540-551.

[5] Kiely JL. Some conceptual problems in multivariable analyses of perinatal mortality. *Paediatric and Perinatal Epidemiology* 1991; 5(4) 243-257

[6] Kiely JL, Kleinman JC. Birth-weight-adjusted infant mortality in evaluations of perinatal care: towards a useful summary measure. *Statistics in Medicine* 1993; 12(3-4) 377-392.

[7] Kramer MS. Biology vs. methodology in investigating causal pathways for infant mortality. *Paediatric and Perinatal Epidemiology* 2009; 23(5) 414-416.

[8] Hernández-Díaz S, Schisterman EF, Hernán MA. The birth-weight "paradox" uncovered? *American Journal of Epidemiology* 2006; 164(11) 1115-1120.

[9] Schisterman EF, Whitcomb BW, Mumford SL, Platt RW. Z-scores and the birth-weight paradox. *Paediatric and Perinatal Epidemiology* 2009; 23(5) 403-413.

[10] Whitcomb BW, Schisterman EF, Perkins NJ, Platt RW. Quantification of collider-stratification bias and the birthweight paradox. *Paediatric and Perinatal Epidemiology* 2009; 23(5) 394-402.

[11] Wilcox AJ, Weinberg CR, Basso O. On the pitfalls of adjusting for gestational age at birth. *American Journal of Epidemiology* 2011; 174(9) 1062-1068.

[12] Judd CM, Kenny DA. Process analysis: estimating mediation in treatment evaluations. *Evaluation Review* 1981; 5(5) 602-619.

[13] Yerushalmy J. The relationship of parents' cigarette smoking to outcome of pregnancy –implications as to the problem of inferring causation from observed associations. *American Journal of Epidemiology* 1971; 93(6) 443-456.

[14] Wilcox AJ. Birthweight and perinatal mortality: the effect of maternal smoking. *American Journal of Epidemiology* 1993; 137(10) 1098-1104.

[15] Platt RW, Joseph KS, Ananth CV, Grondines J, Abrahamowicz M, Kramer MS. A proportional hazards model with time-dependent covariates and time-varying effects for analysis of fetal and infant death. *American Journal of Epidemiology* 2004; 160(4) 199-206.

[16] VanderWeele TJ, Mumford SL, Schisterman EF. Conditioning on intermediates in perinatal epidemiology. *Epidemiology* 2012; 23(1) 1-9.

[17] Hernán MA, Hernández-Díaz S, Robins JM. A structural approach to selection bias. *Epidemiology* 2004; 15(5) 615-625.

[18] VanderWeele TJ, Robins JM. Directed acyclic graphs, sufficient causes and the properties of conditioning on a common effect. *American Journal of Epidemiology* 2007; 166(9) 1096-1104.

[19] Glymour MM, Greenland S. Causal diagrams. In: Rothman KJ, Greenland S, Lash TL (eds.) *Modern Epidemiology* 3rd ed. Philadelphia: Lippincott Williams and Wilkins; 2008. p183-209.

[20] Cole SR, Platt RW, Schisterman EF. Illustrating bias due to conditioning on a collider. *International Journal of Epidemiology* 2010; 39(2) 417-420.

[21] Basso O, Wilcox AJ. Intersecting birth weight-specific mortality curves: solving the riddle. *American Journal of Epidemiology* 2009; 169(7) 787-797.

[22] Little RJ, Rubin DB. Causal effects in clinical and epidemiological studies via potential outcomes: concepts and analytical approaches. *Annual Review of Public Health* 2000; 21(1) 121-145.

[23] Hernán MA. A definition of causal effect for epidemiological studies. *Journal of Epidemiology and Community Health* 2004; 58(4) 265-271.

[24] Suzuki E, Yamamoto E, Tsuda T. Identification of operating mediation and mechanism in the sufficient-component cause framework. *European Journal of Epidemiology* 2011; 26(5) 347-357.

[25] Hafeman DM, VanderWeele TJ. Alternative assumptions for the identification of direct and indirect effects. *Epidemiology* 2011; 22(6) 753-764.

[26] Frangakis CE, Rubin DB. Principal stratification in causal inference. *Biometrics* 2002; 58(1) 21-29.

[27] Egleston BL, Cropsey KL, Lazev AB, Heckman CJ. A tutorial on principal stratification-based sensitivity analysis: application to smoking cessation studies. *Clinical Trials* 2010; 7(3) 286-298.

[28] Chiba Y, Taguri M, Uemura Y. On the identification of the survivor average causal effect. *Journal of Biometrics and Biostatistics*, 2011; 2(5) e104.

[29] Hayden D, Pauler DK, Schoenfeld D. An estimator for treatment comparisons amongst survivors in randomized trials. *Biometrics* 2005; 61(1) 305-310.

[30] Chiba Y. Marginal structural models for estimating principal stratum direct effects under the monotonicity assumption. *Biometrical Journal* 2011; 53(6) 1025-1034.

[31] Sjölander A, Humphreys K, Vansteelandt S, Bellocco R, Palmgren J. Sensitivity analysis for principal stratum direct effects, with an application to a study of physical activity and coronary heart disease. *Biometrics* 2009; 65(2) 514 -520.

[32] Chiba Y. Bias analysis for the principal stratum direct effect in the presence of confounded intermediate variables. *Journal of Biometrics and Biostatistics* 2010; 1(1) 101.

[33] Angrist JD, Imbens GW, Rubin DB. Identification of causal effects using instrumental variables (with discussion). *Journal of the American Statistical Association*, 1996; 91(434) 444-472.

[34] Manski CF. Monotone treatment response. *Econometrica* 1997; 65(6) 1311-1334.

[35] Manski CF, Pepper JV. Monotone instrumental variables: with an application to the returns to schooling. *Econometrica* 2000; 68(4) 997-1010.

[36] Manski CF. *Partial identification of probability distributions*. New York: Springer-Verlag; 2003.

[37] Chiba Y. Causal inference in randomized trials with noncompliance. In: Śmigórski K (ed.) *Health Management – Different Approaches and Solutions*. Rijeka: Intech; 2011. p315-336.

[38] Chiba Y, VanderWeele TJ. A simple method for principal strata effects when the outcome has been truncated due to death. *American Journal of Epidemiology* 2011; 173(7) 745-751.

[39] Pearl J. Direct and indirect effects. In: Breese J, Koller D (eds.) *Proceedings of the Seventeenth Conference on Uncertainty in Artificial Intelligence*, 2-5 August 2001. San Francisco: Morgan Kaufmann; 2001. p411-420.

[40] Joffe M, Small D, Hsu CY. Defining and estimating intervention effects for groups that will develop an auxiliary outcome. *Statistical Science* 2007; 22(1) 74-97.

[41] Hafeman DM, Schwartz S. Opening the black box: a motivation for the assessment of mediation. *International Journal of Epidemiology* 2009; 38(4) 838-845.

[42] Petersen ML, Sinisi SE, van der Laan MJ. Estimation of direct causal effects. *Epidemiology* 2006; 17(3) 276-284.

[43] VanderWeele TJ. Marginal structural models for the estimation of direct and indirect effects. *Epidemiology* 2009; 20(1) 18-26.

[44] Kaufman S, Kaufman JS, MacLehose RF, Greenland S, Poole C. Improved estimation of controlled direct effects in the presence of unmeasured confounding of intermediate variables. *Statistics in Medicine* 2005; 24(11) 1683-1702.

[45] Imai K, Keele L, Yamamoto T. Identification, inference and sensitivity analysis for causal mediation effects. *Statistical Science* 2010; 25(1) 51-71.

[46] VanderWeele TJ, Vansteelandt S. Odds ratios for mediation analysis with a dichotomous outcome. *American Journal of Epidemiology* 2010; 172(12) 1339-1348.

[47] Chiba Y. Monte-Carlo sensitivity analysis for controlled direct effects using marginal structural models in the presence of confounded mediators. *Communications in Statistics – Theory and Methods* 2012; 41(10) 1739-1749.

[48] Tchetgen Tchetgen EJ, Shpitser I. Semiparametric theory for causal mediation analysis: efficiency bounds, multiple robustness, and sensitivity analysis. *Annals of Statistics* (in press).

[49] Chiba Y. Bounds on controlled direct effects under monotonic assumptions about mediators and confounders. *Biometrical Journal* 2010; 52(5) 628-637.

[50] VanderWeele TJ. Simple relations between principal stratification and direct and indirect effects. *Statistics and Probability Letters* 2008; 78(17) 2957-2962.

Chapter 4

Use of Analytical Methods and *In-silico* Techniques in Public Health Research

Peter Papoh Ndibewu and Prince Ngobeni

Additional information is available at the end of the chapter

http://dx.doi.org/10.5772/54006

1. Introduction

In this chapter, we briefly summarize the concept of analytical methodologies used for detecting, measuring, and/or monitoring in public health research. Additionally, this chapter describes *in silico* ADME, ADMET and ADME/Tox approaches or models relevant to analytical methodologies for public health researchers or practitioners.

Recently, adopted technologies to cope with this type of scientific demand in terms of drug development and testing are the applications of *in silico* techniques used in pharmaceutical companies in the process of drug discovery (Ndibewu et al., 2012; Vallero, 2012; Lipinski et al., 1997; Leeson & Springthorpe, 2007). Two fast growing examples involve the use of cheminformatics (also known as chemoinformtaics) and chemical informatics which is the use of computer and informational techniques, applied to a range of problems in the field of chemistry (Langdon et al., 2011; Brown, 2011). These *in silico* techniques are employed in pharmaceutical companies in the process of drug discovery (Lipinski, 2004). These methods can also be used in chemical and allied industries in various other forms (Pradeep, 2009). Combined with the accuracy of data obtained with validated analytical methods, this encompasses the mixing of those information resources necessary to transform data into information and information into knowledge for the intended purpose of making better decisions faster in the area of drug lead identification and optimization. The outcome is clearly the efficiency in public health research and the beneficiary is mankind. In the section that follows, we briefly summarize *in silico* pharmacokinetics, widely designated as ADME approaches or models relevant to analytical methodologies for public health researchers or practitioners (Yamashita & Hashida, 2004). Pharmacokinetics is the study of the time course of a drug within the body and incorporates the processes of absorption, distribution, metabolism and excretion (ADME) (Van de Waterbeemd & Gifford, 2003). The extent of distribution will depend on the structural and physicochemical properties of the compound (Fig. 1).

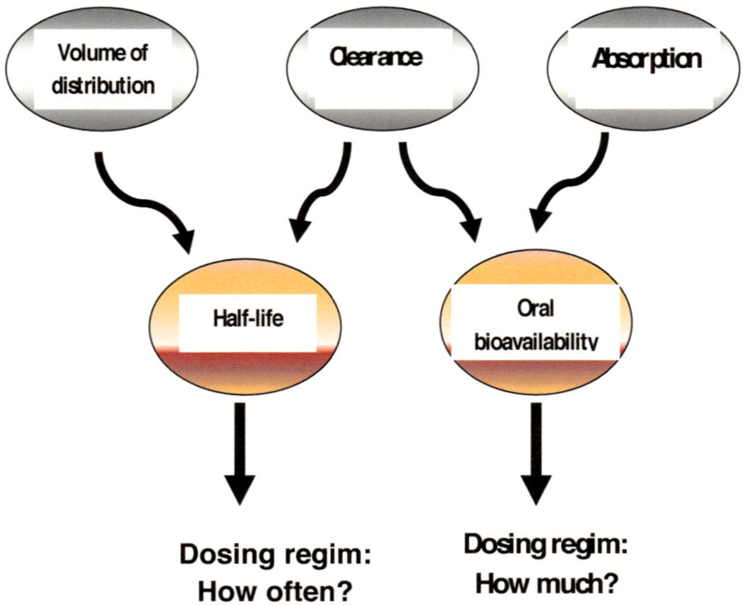

Figure 1. ADME flow chart showing volume of distribution (V_d): is a theoretical concept connecting administered dose with actual initial concentration (C_o) present in circulation, $V_d = Dose/C_o$; Unbound volume, $V_{du} = Vd/f_u$, where f_u is the fraction of unbound; Clearance (Cl) of the drug from the body mainly takes place via the liver and the kidney; Bioavailability is given by area under the curve (AUC) = F x Dose/Cl; Half-life ($t_{1/2}$) is the time taken for a drug concentration in plasma to reduce by 50% (is function of the clearance and volume of distribution, and determines how often a drug needs to be administered ($t_{1/2} = 0.693V_d/Cl$) (Van de Waterbeemd & Gifford, 2003).

Figure 2 shows a simple ADME decision-making flow sheet which will incorporate predictors for volume of distribution, oral bioavailability, half-life ($t_{1/2}$), distribution\protein binding module including percentage plasma protein binding values (*%PPB*) and drug affinity constant to human serum albumin represented by log K^a_{HSA} constants. The adaptability of this simple form has continuously refine existing models by building on larger and higher-quality data sets crucial to the success of the *in silico* approaches as grouped by Van de Waterbeem and Gifford (2003) in the form of problem areas for which predictive models could be helpful (Fig. 2). And during these past few years, the range of models have further expanded to include, for example, models for various transporters, metabolism by non-P450 enzymes, plasma protein binding, and so (Lu et al., 2003; Ekins et al., 2001).

Figures 2a and 2b outline the parameters in the prediction of a safe drug given in acceptable dose, which it is ultimately hoped will be reliably obtainable from molecular structure and appropriate descriptors using a suite of predictive models. This expression had earlier been made clear by Japertas and coworkers (2011).

http://dx.doi.org/10.5772/54006

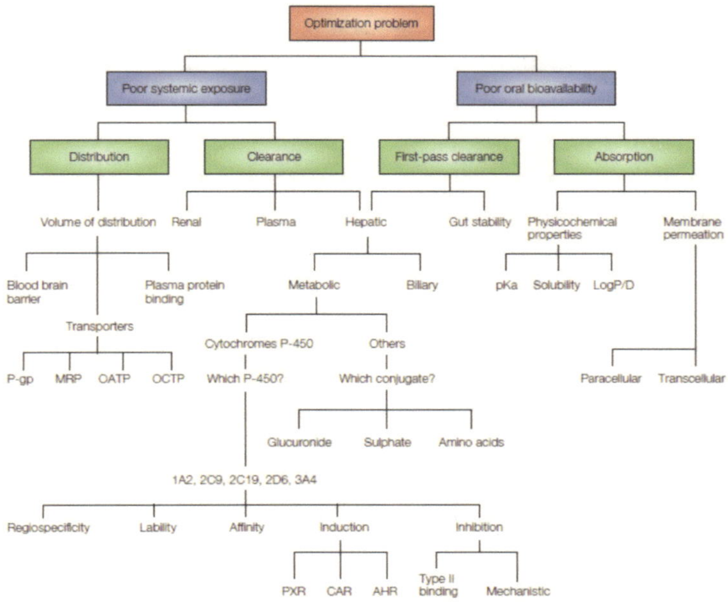

(a)

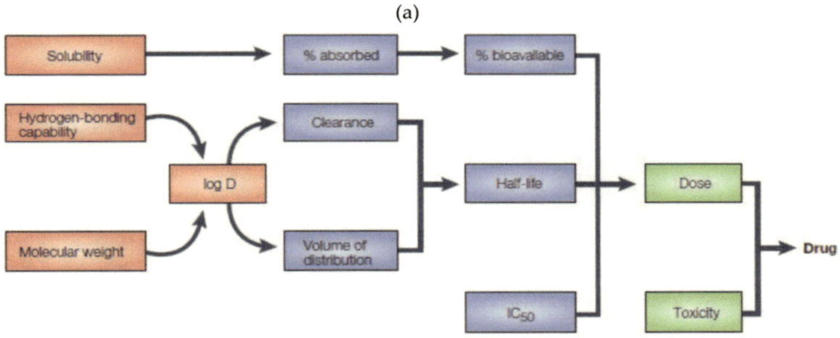

(b)

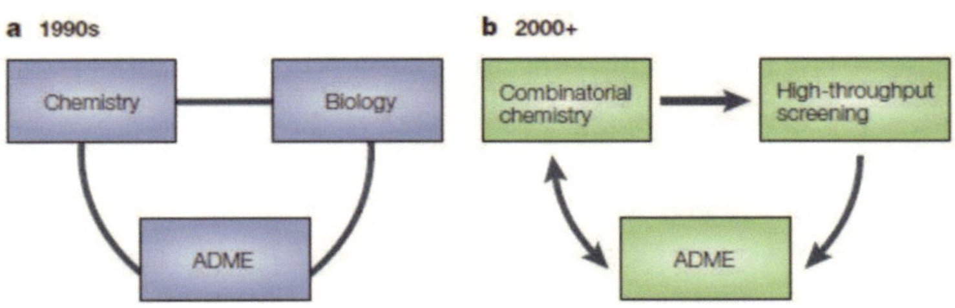

(c)

Figure 2. a. An analysis of the crucial ADME processes for which predictive models are available or are being developed (Carlson & Segall, 2002). b. Prediction paradigm ranging from models for simple physicochemical properties (H-bonding capacity, Molecular mass, Solubility and lipophilicity (log*D*)) to models for ADME properties (% drug absorbed & bioavailability, clearance, volume of distribution and half-life ($t_{1/2}$)) to complex endpoints (binding (IC_{50}), to molecular target of new drug and its required dose and toxicity potential (Waterbeemd & Gifford, 2003). c. The evolution of drug discovery and the changing role of ADME studies I (Waterbeemd & Gifford, 2003)

In figure 2c (Waterbeemd & Gifford, 2003), the form *a* depicting the classical project-collaboration approach between chemistry, biology and drug metabolism (ADMES) groups in the 1990s is shown to *b* which is a much more automated world at the start of this millennium in which combinatorial chemistry (*CombiChem*), high throughput screening and ADME studies are linked together in a streamlined fashion.

It should be noted that all three activities shown in figure 3 can even be carried out by separate companies of research units or even researchers in health departments or for health interest. A good example is the Medical Research Council (MRC) of South Africa which supports unit health research projects towards a nationally planned and prioritized health sectors. Furthermore, the wide introduction of *in silico* and high-speed in vivo methods could redefine the traditional meaning of ADME to Automated Decision-Making Engine. To reflect, one sees that considerable effort has equally been devoted into the development of *in silico* models for the prediction of oral absorption (Veber et al., 2002; Agoram et al., 2001; Parrott & Lavé, 2002; Yu et al., 2000). This range from the simplest models based on a single descriptor, such as log P or log *D*, or polar surface area, which is a descriptor of hydrogen-bonding potential to combo or meta- or QSAR models.

2. Analytical methods in health research

As analytical methods become increasingly sophisticated and capable for the detection of each component in a sample (Barnes & Dourson, 1988), including biological systems (Kote-Jarai et al. 2011), it is critical to separate and quantify them. Methods such as mass spectrometry (MS) and high performance chromatography (HPLC) routinely ensure these in many laboratories around the world (Thorp et al., 2011). HPLC instrumentations provide crucial analytical data (Beitler, 1995) used to calculate or predict drug's affinity constants ($log\ K_a^{HSA}$) (Packard et al., 1996; Endo et al., 1982). For nearly half a century, analytical and testing methods as opposed to empirical approaches have played a key role in the identification of key diseases causative toxins (Barnes & Dourson, 1988; Bathija, 2003) and drug-like compounds to cure them (Kote-Jarai et al., 2011; Moore & Carpenter, 1999).

In this process, as tons of data are being produced with the analytical chemists struggling to make sense out of the bunch, the health researcher and health practitioners are faced with a constant task to make better and faster decisions in the area of disease treatment and prevention based on laboratory results. In the midst of all this, there is the requirement not only to produce efficient drugs, in enough quantities, to cure diseases but their development at the pace at which pandemics are spreading around the globe is also required, for example, cancer and HIV & AIDS.

As far as the identification of data needs is crucial in clinical laboratories, the quest for methods to determine biomarkers of exposure and effect of diseases in the public health is also growing fast. Hence, analysis of metabolites of drugs in humans or animals can provide a biomarker of exposure that is sensitive to low levels of exposure and correlates well with exposure concentrations. Methods for determining biomarkers of exposure in humans are needed to determine background levels in the population and levels at which biological effects occur. For example, Abdel-Rahman et al. (1980a & 1980b) developed a method to quantitatively and qualitatively measure the metabolites of chlorine dioxide (e.g., ClO_2^-, and ClO^-) in biological fluids. These biomarkers may be used to indirectly measure chlorine dioxide exposure.

In the absence of sensitive and reliable methods for determining diseases vector-borne metabolites and biomarkers of exposure, mechanistic models of tissue distribution of drug compounds have been used (Rowley et al., 1997) to assess levels at which biological effects occur in the population and mitigate disease occurrence. Poulin et al. (Poulin & Theil, 2002; Poulin & Krishna, 1995) developed tissue composition-based equations for calculating tissue-plasma partition coefficients ($P_{t:p}$).

The following expressions are used (equations 1 and 2) (Yamashita & Hashida, 2004):

$$P_{t:p\,nonadipose} = \frac{P_{o:w}(V_{nlp} + 0.3V_{php}) + (V_{wt} + 0.7V_{pht})}{P_{o:w}(V_{nlp} + 0.3V_{php}) + (V_{wp} + 0.7V_{php})} x \frac{f_{Up}}{f_{Ut}} \tag{1}$$

$$P_{t:p\,adipose} = \frac{D^*_{vo:w}(V_{nlt} + 0.3V_{pht}) + (V_{wt} + 0.7V_{pht})}{D^*_{vo:w}(V_{nlp} + 0.3V_{php}) + (V_{wp} + 0.7V_{php})} x \frac{f_{Up}}{1} \tag{2}$$

$P_{o:w}$ is the n-octanol:buffer partition coefficient of non-ionized species at pH 7.4.

$D^*_{vo:w}$ is the olive oil:buffer partition coefficient of both the nonionized and ionized species at pH 7.4, V is the fractional tissue volume content of neutral lipids (*nl*), phospholipids (*ph*), and water (*w*), t is the tissue, p is the plasma and f_u is the unbound fraction.

These equations are based on the assumption that each tissue and plasma is a mixture of lipids, water and plasma proteins in which the drug can be homogeneously distributed.

The first term of these equations is based on the drug Lipophilicity-hydrophilicity balance of tissues and plasma due to their lipid and water contents, while the second term of the equation considers the binding to common proteins present in plasma and plasma interstitial space.

3. Use of *In-silico* techniques and chemical informatics in health research

Even though disease mapping has been done for over a hundred years, historically, the focus in health research has been on person and conventional medicinal chemistry targeting specific disease treatment with little regard for the implications of *de novo* molecular design costs. Also, the need for high throughput screening in drug discovery research for public health interest has surfaced as a top priority in the last decade (Norris et al., 2000; Green et al, 1974).

However, the testing of much lead drug-like candidates often fails because of unsatisfactory ADME properties (Zmuidinavicius et al., 2003). In handling this challenge, ADME studies employing *in silico* techniques to improve the rate of success in the more costly downstream stages of drug development before clinical trials has gain tremendous interest in public health research methodologies. In this light, *in silico* ADME studies use various models developed for predicting ADME properties of compounds from their chemical structures and integrating them to simulate the kinetics at the organ or body levels Carlson & Segall, 2002; Podlogar et al., 2001; Ekins et al., 2001). Data-based approaches such as quantitative structure-activity relationship (QSAR) (Zhaou et al., 2001, Yoshida & Topliss, 2000), similarity searches, 3D-QSAR (Jones et al., 1996) and structure-based methods such as ligand-protein docking and pharmacophore modeling are amongst approaches currently used. In addition, several methods of integrating ADME properties to predict pharmacokinetics at the organ or body level have been studied (Agatonovic-Kustrin, 2001; Van de Waterbeemd, 2001; Ho et al., 2000; Jacoby et al., 2009; Lave et al., 1999). All these effort is to reduce the risk of late-stage attrition of drug development and to optimize screening and testing by looking at only the promising compounds. Recently, researchers have equally develop keen interest in *de novo* molecular design (Good et al., 1995; Clark et al., 1995), predictive modeling, graph theory, molecular similarity and diversity, virtual ligand docking, scaffold hopping (Langdon et al., 2010), multi-objective optimization Nicolaou et al., 2007), molecular descriptors, bioisosteric replacement, machine learning and evolutionary algorithms (Gillet, 2008).

In the last decade, a wide variety of descriptors used in QSAR studies have been developed (Khan et al., 2009; Miners et al., 2006). A subset of these descriptors is potentially useful for predicting ADME properties. Many QSAR studies on BBB permeation of drugs have been published recently. In the big junk of these works (Wichmann et al., 2007; Zhao et al., 2007; Cuadrado et al., 2007; Katritzky et al., 2006; Garg & Verma, 2006; Hemmateenejad et al., 2006; Narayanan & Gunturi, 2005) experimental data are represented as log*BB* constants or as qualitative (binary) index subdividing all compounds into 'CNS positive' and "CNS negative" classes according to presence or lack of central nervous system (CNS) activity. Table 1 summarizes the most notable QSAR models (log*PS*) representing blood/brain partitioning coefficients at equilibrium conditions (log*BB*)(Goodwin & Clark, 2005; Abbott, 2004) showing that typical data sets involved only 20-30 compounds.

Log*PS* is based on *in vivo* kinetic permeability measurements using intravenous administration (Oldendorf, 1971), brain uptake index (Bickel, 2005; Oldendorf, 1971) and *in situ* perfusion in rat or mouse (Bickel, 2005; Dagenais et al., 2000; Takasato et al., 1984;). Where, P (cm s^{-1}) is observed permeability across BBB, whereas S (cm^2/g) is surface area of brain capillary endothelium which equals to ~ 100 – 130 cm^2 in rats (Abraham, 2004; Bodor & Buchwald, 1999). PS product can be calculated from Kety-Renkin-Crone equation of capillary transport (K_{in} = F. (1- $e^{-PS/F}$)), and by its physical meaning, PS is equal to the unidirectional influx rate constant (K_{in}) corrected for cerebral blood flow (F). Earlier attempts of log*PS* prediction were largely restricted by the lack of high quality data. A subset of statistical techniques can deal with larger sets of molecular descriptors aimed at finding relationships or patterns in data

http://dx.doi.org/10.5772/54006

sets. For examples, multiple linear regressions (MLR) and partial least square (PLS) (Norinder & Österberg, 2001).

References	Descriptors	*N*	R^2	RMSE
Levin[19]	Log(P.MW$^{-1/2}$)	22	0.83	-
Abraham and coworkers[10,24]	Solvation parameters (A, B, E, S, V_x)	18	0.95	0.48
		30	0.87	0.52
Bodor and Buchwald[11]	Log*P*(log*D*)	58	0.90	0.62
Liu et al.[5]	Log*D*, PSA, vsa base	23	0.74	0.50
Luco and Marchevsky[25] (review of earlier studies)	Log*P*, different *MW* functions	7-37	0.80-0.96	-
This literature	Log*P*, HD, HA, V_x, ion fractions (p*Ka* function)	125[a]	0.84	0.48
		53[b]	0.82	0.49

[a]Training set; [b]Validation set.

Table 1. Summary of QSAR Models for Predicting LogPS (Lanevskij et al., 2008)

These illustrations show how *in silico* chemistry or cheminformatics and high-throughput screening have increased the possibility of finding new lead compounds at much shorter time periods than conventional medicinal chemistry. With judicious selection of lead compounds and constant monitoring of physical properties (especially Lipophilicity (equation 1) or other major physchem parameter) during optimization, medicinal chemists have an opportunity to help alleviate the appalling attrition rates, estimated at 93–96% (Norris et al., 2000) in clinical drug development (Bhal et al.,. This means that physicochemical properties in small-molecule drug discovery are completely under the control of medicinal chemists and can easily be calculated before chemical synthesis. It is, however, important to emphasize here that when interpreting results from prediction models, that the predictions are only as good as the dataset used to create the model. So when we calculate a prediction, if the training set does not contain chemical structures that are similar to the particular compound in question, the predicted result may not be reliable, regardless of the actual result of the prediction.

From various literature sources (Bhal, 2007; Sazonovas et al., 2010), it is reported that ADME and toxicity prediction models can be a valuable part of many different research workflows, including virtual screening, metabolite identification, impurity analysis and chemical safety, reliability index (*RI*) value (0 – 1) in addition to the predicted probability result (Japertas et al., 2010) which is an indicator of how well spatial chemical space around a particular compound is represented within the training set of the model (Fig. 3)

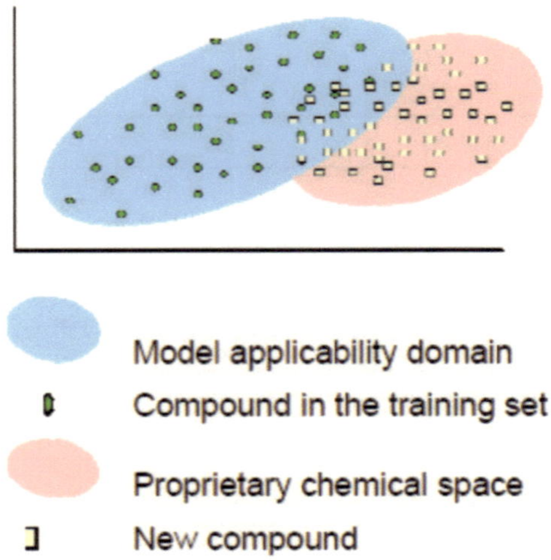

Figure 3. Model applicability domain versus proprietary chemical space, predicted using ACD/Log*D* Suite (Bhal & Coworkers, 2007)

The development of *in silico* technologies or chemical informatics over the last 20 years has, thus, provided a more powerful and rapid ability to examine clinical decision-making and answers to critical public research health issues based on scientifically validated models from an un biased an empirical question based on a minimally biased appraisal of all the relevant empirical studies. This, in turn, has fostered the discussion of policy of drug discovery relevant to health issues as well as health services and planning, in conjunction with the use of clinical investigations and disease surveillance. Such reviews aim to improve ethically relevant decisions in public healthcare research or policy. With this in mind, identification of a lead compound or biochemical starting point for a drug discovery program has been highlighted recently as a critically important activity, reflected by lead generation strategies being widely implemented in the pharmaceutical industry (Jupertas, 2007).

For a more robust process, calculated quantitative parameters will provide further information though slightly different from the core predictive pharmacokinetic data. These parameters show great inter relation. Such parameters include the drug's affinity constants ($log\ K_a^{HSA}$) to human serum albumin (the major carrier protein in plasma). Experimental data come from direct chromatographic determination of binding strength to that particular protein. These parameters are usually calculated as follows (Bhal et al. 2007):

$$\log K_a^{HSA} = \log\left(\frac{[LA]}{[L[A]]}\right). \tag{3}$$

Where [LA] is the concentration of ligand bound to albumin, [L] is that of free ligand, and [A] is the concentration of free albumin which, estimated at ~ 0.6 *mM* in human plasma.

http://dx.doi.org/10.5772/54006

%PPB values represent the overall fraction of drug bound in human plasma, i.e. accounts for interactions with different proteins: albumin, α-1-acid glycoprotein, liproteins, SHBG, transortion, etc. In vitro measurements of the extent of plasma protein binding usually involve equilibrium dialysis, ultrafiltration or ultracentrifugation methods. The supplementary distribution/V_d module calculates apparent volume of distribution of drugs in human body expressed in litres per *Kg* body weight (*L/Kg*). This expression is given as: $\%PPB = (1\text{-}f_u)\ x\ 100\%$, Where f_u is a fraction of free (unbound) drug in plasma (0 -1). Note that predictive models for %PPB and $\log_a^{HSA}$ are derived using GALAS (Global, Adjusted Locally According to Similarity) modeling methodology consisting of global (baseline) statistical model (based on *PLS* with multiple bootstrapping, using a predefined set of fragmental descriptors), and local correction to baseline prediction (based on the analysis of model performance for similar compounds from the training set = self-training library). Because of the percentage (*%PPB*) scale platform of the overall protein binding in plasma, values are linearized prior to modeling and converted to apparent serum affinity constants, $\log K_{app,}$ the main parameter used in modeling. With this, final prediction can be converted back to *%PPB* using the following expression (Bhal et al., 2007):

$$\%PPB = \frac{\log K_{app}}{1 + \log K_{app}} x100\% \tag{4}$$

To illustrate the performance of *%PPB* and $\log_a^{HSA}$ models, validation set compounds within Model Applicability Domain (MAD) ($RI \geq 0.3$) is taken from Bhal et al. (2012) and shown in figures 4. In equation (y), the local part of the model provides the basis for estimating reliability of prediction by means of calculated Reliability Index (*RI*) values that range from 0 – 1. 0 means unreliable prediction and 1 fully reliable or ideal prediction. The *RI* values can also be used for interpreting prediction results, for example in setting the cut-off point ($RI = 0.3$), meaning that if compound falls outside of the MAD, the respective prediction should be totally discarded from further analysis irrespective of *%PPB* and log_a^{HSA}.

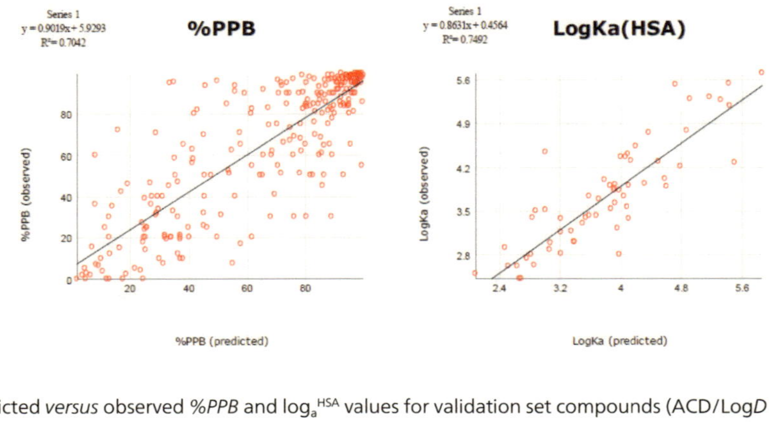

Figure 4. Predicted *versus* observed *%PPB* and $\log_a^{HSA}$ values for validation set compounds (ACD/Log*D* Suite).

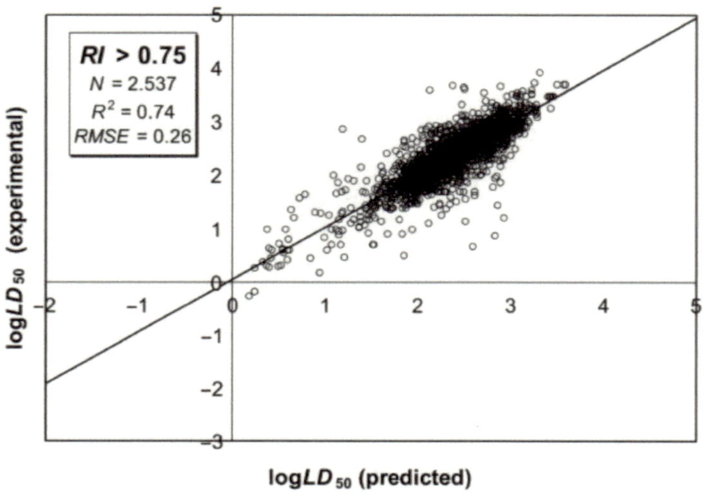

Figure 5. Predicted *versus* experimental values of *logLD*$_{50}$ (with a very high *RI > 0.75*) *%PPB* and $\log_a^{HSA}$ values for validation set compounds (Bhal et al., 2012).

In figures 5 and 6, both models produce highly accurate results, while even better statistical characteristics are observed if only predictions of moderate and high reliability index are considered.

In order to understand the behavior of drug compounds in the real world, Bhal et al. (2012) has used ACD/Predictors such as log*P*, log*D*, solubility, and pKa to evaluate and predict the likely behavior of 5-Methoxy-2-(1-piperidin-4-ylpropyl)pyridine (Fig. 7), a compound prior to its synthesis. Lipophilicity is represented by the descriptors log*P* (also known as K_{ow} or P_{ow}) and log*D*, and is used, for example, to help predict *in-vivo* permeability of active compounds in drug discovery and the behavior of compounds in many other areas of health related research. The partition coefficient, P, is a measure of the differential solubility of a compound in two immiscible solvents and the most commonly used commonly used solvent system is octanol-1-ol/water.

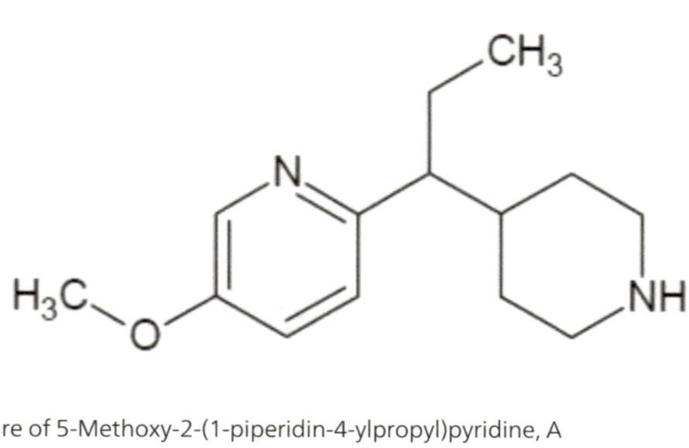

Figure 6. Chemical structure of 5-Methoxy-2-(1-piperidin-4-ylpropyl)pyridine, A

http://dx.doi.org/10.5772/54006

The *P* descriptor is a lipophilicity descriptor for neutral compounds, or where the compounds exist in a single form.

$$Partition\ coefficient,\ p=\frac{[Compound]_{octanol}}{[Compund]_{water}}$$ and Log*P* = $\log_{10}$(Partition Coefficient)

Log*P* = 1 can be explained as a ratio of 10 :1 organic:aqueous phase.

For ionizable solutes, the compounds may exist as a variety of different species in each phase at a given pH. D, typically used in the logarithmic for (lo*D*) representing the distribution coefficient which is the appropriate descriptor for ionizable compounds since it is a measure of the pH-dependent differential solubility of all species in the octanol/water system (Levin, 1980).

$$Distribution\ coefficient,\ D=\frac{\sum[Microspecies]_{octanol}}{\sum[Microspecies]_{water}}.$$

Bhal (2012) used methylamine to illustrate the difference between these two descriptors as follows: $MeNH_3^+ \rightleftharpoons MeNH_2 + H^+$, meaning that,

$P_{MeN\,H_2}=\frac{[MeN\,H_2]_{octanol}}{[MeN\,H_2]_{water}}$ and/or $P_{MeN\,H_3^+}=\frac{[MeN\,H_3^+]_{octanol}}{[MeN\,H_3^+]_{water}}$.. So, keeping the definition of D above in mind, we can write the expression of D as: $D=\frac{[MeN\,H_2]_{octanol}+[MeN\,H_3^+]_{octanol}}{[MeN\,H_{water}]+[MeN\,H_3^+]_{water}}.$

To accurately predict a compound's lipophilicity based on predicted molecular physical properties, it was imperative that the author applied the correct descriptor in an appropriate manner. In this context, log*D* instead is used in lieu of log*P* as the use of the latter to address lipophilicity concerns by drug research and manufacturing companies in the past (around 1980's and 90's) had resulted in incorrect conclusions for ionizable compounds. A good example would be to reproduce data generated by the previous author employing ACD/Log*D* in his application to discuss the significance of applying log*D* instead of log*P* using drug discovery as an example where lipophilicity is correlated with *in vivo* permeability. Using the sample molecule in figure 6 (5-Methoxy-2-(1-piperidin-4-ylpropyl)pyridine), data presented in table were calculated.

pKa	Ionization centre
4.8	Pyridine
10.9	Piperidine

Table 2. pKa values of 5-Methoxy-2-(1-piperidin-4-ylpropyl)pyridine (Bhal et al., 2012)

The pH dependence of log*D* for this sample molecule (5-Methoxy-2-(1-piperidin-4-ylpropyl)pyridine) is shown in figure 7 showing a plot of log*D* versus pH, while figure 8 displays the changing ionic forms of molecule A.

Looking at the plot in figure 8, and according to Bhal el al. (2012), we can confirm that ionization of the compound greatly affects octanol-water partitioning and that lipophilicity cannot be simplified to a constant. This is very so as lipophilicity of the compound is low below pH 12 when the majority of the compound exists in an ionized form. This would definitively be contradictory, of course, if log*P* was examined alone (Predicted log*P* is 2.7 ± 0.3 by author for comparison sake).

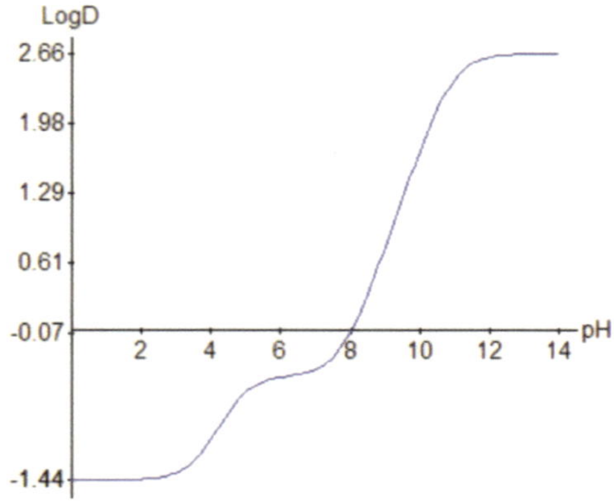

Figure 7. The logD curve of 5-Methoxy-2-(1-piperidin-4-ylpropyl)pyridine (ACD/LoD Suite), Bhal et al., 2012)

The author concludes that the negative values of log*D* (-1.44 to 0) in the physiologically relevant pH range (pH 1–8) lead us to conclude that this compound would be more susceptible to higher aqueous solubility and of lower lipophilicity in the body. As a result we would expect membrane permeability to be poor. Also, it is true as seen from graph in figure 8 the neutral form of molecule A is almost non-existent at physiologically relevant pH (1–8). This neutral form possibly dominates at ~pH 13. Conclusively, compound A is highly associated with the lipid phase (>30 fold affinity for octanol over water), and thus will likely permeate biological membranes spontaneously.

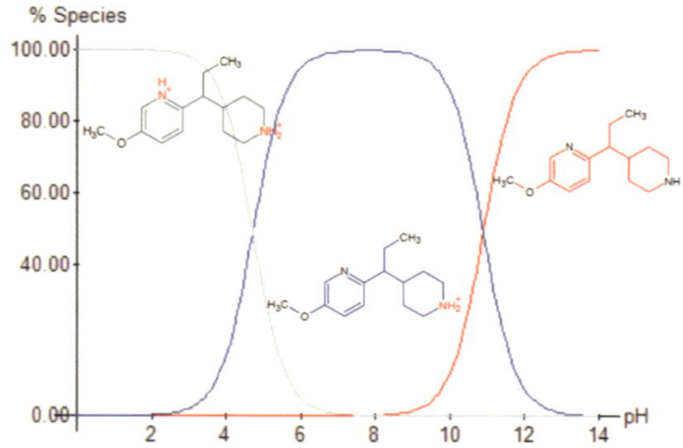

Figure 8. A graph illustrating the changing ionic forms of 5-Methoxy-2-(1-piperidin-4-ylpropyl)pyridine with pH (Bhal et al., 2012)

Figure 9 shows a schematic representation of the changing pH environments that an orally administered compound is likely to encounter in the gastrointestinal (GI) tract. From figure 9, we can observe that there is, thus, no constant pH in the body and it is therefore essential that we consider an appropriate pH when predicting the *in vivo* behavior of a drug candidate.

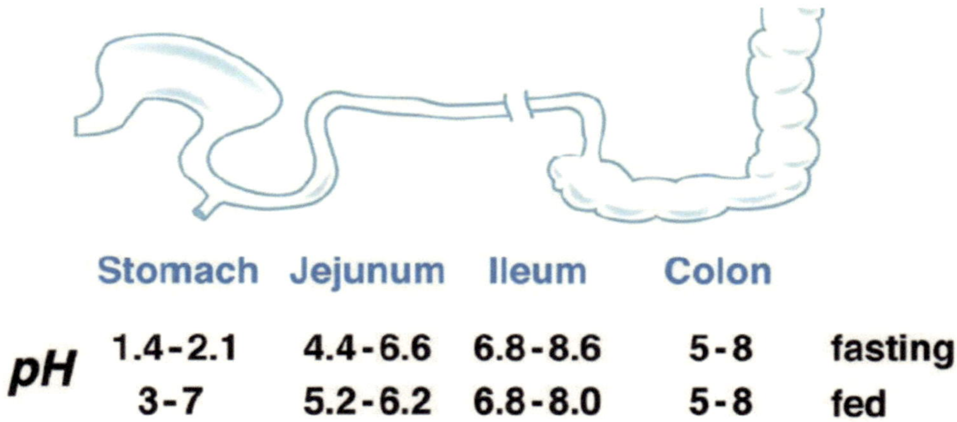

Figure 9. The pH environment of the human gastrointestinal tract (Bhal et al., 2012)

4. Implications of analytical methods and *in-silico* techniques in public health

The outcomes from a global network on the development of standardized analytical methods for the public and environmental health directly impacts on the quality of health of mankind worldwide. High quality data necessitates the development of harmonized study approaches and adequate reporting of data (Bouwmeester et al., 2011).

Priority public health scale can only be based on well-characterized dose-response relations derived from a systematic study of the bio-kinetics and bio-interactions of drugs or drug-like molecules at both organism and (sub)-cellular levels using validated analytical methods and pharmacokinetic studies. The ADME (absorption, distribution, metabolism and excretion) and toxicity effects is crucial to declare a particular molecule safe for the treatment of a particular disease and often clinical trials to arrive at a conclusive release of a new drug very costly, sometimes in the range of millions of dollars covering the cost of fundamental research through clinical trials or testing to manufacturing. Multiple content databases, data mining and predictive modeling algorithms, visualization tools, and high-throughput data-analysis solutions are being integrated to form systems-ADME/Tox (Ekins et al., 2005). More so, Ekins and co-authors (2005) reported that the functional interpretation and relevance of complex multidimensional data to the phenotype observed in humans is the focus of current research in toxicology.

In fact, increased effort is needed to develop and validate analytical methods to determine ADMET effects in complex matrices such as the human body. This implies the use of validated analytical methods and *in-silico* chemistry to reduce time and cost at developmental stage. In addition, this would allow for systematic study of sets of drug-like molecules' reactivities with specific aim to generate a data set which would allow the establishment of dose-response relations. This approach is commonly referred to as quantitative structure-activity relationship (QSAR) and has a practical implication in the process of *in-silico* algorithms optimizations. A more general but direct implications of analytical methods and *in-silico* techniques in public health is that international cooperation and worldwide standardization of terminology, reference materials, models and protocols are needed to make progress in establishing lists of essential globally acceptable drug formulation methods, clinical trials, quality control and assurance. In this way, traditional pharmacopeia and those exploiting natural biodiversity can benefit from proven methods at the grassroots' levels, especially in developing countries.

Metabolomics, metabonomics, proteomics, pharmacogenomics and toxicogenomics, are groups of latest experimental approaches that are combined with high-throughput molecular screening of targets to provide a view of the complete biological system that is modulated by a compound with direct or indirect implications of analytical methods and *in-silico* techniques development for application in the public health sector (Ekins et al., 2005). In conclusion, it is widely recognized in industry-orientated research and development of APIs (active pharmaceutical ingredients) that predicting or determining the ADME/Tox properties of molecules would help to prevent failure of many of the compounds targeted before they reach the clinic. Many authors (Bhal et al., 2012; O'Donnell et al., 2012; Ndibewu et al., 2012; Thorp, 2011; Ekins et al., 2005) agree that this has, undoubtedly, been as a result of considerable research into developing better *in-silico, in vitro* and *in vivo* methods and models.

5. General conclusion

Driven by the changes in the working paradigm in the pharmaceutical and biotechnology, and now in environmentally health-related research, *in-silico* approaches will inevitable find their place. Some insilicoids have even mentioned that this approach will save the world. This is, probably, owing to the gains recorded in terms of cost reduction and efficiency for early stage drug discovery research to the point of manufacturing of some important drugs or vaccines to which the future of mankind mercilessly rely like terminal illnesses such as cancer or HIV-AIDS. All these diseases are unquestionable public health pandemonium requiring quick systematically robust holistic research approaches to halt their effects on human evolution.

Conclusively, ADMET data is tackled in three ways, namely: first, a variety of *in vitro* assays are further automated through the use of robust laboratory integrated system (LIM); secondly, *in silico* models are used to assist in the selection of both appropriate assays, as well as in the selection of subsets of compounds to go through these screens. And thirdly, predictive models have are then developed that might ultimately become sophisticated enough to replace *in vitro* assays and/or *in vivo* experiments. So, the need for ADMET information should start with the design of new compounds. Finally, this information shall influence the decision to proceed with synthesis either via traditional medicinal chemistry or combinatorial chemistry strategies. Although, it but obvious that at this point computational approaches are the most appropriate option to get this information, we should never, however, forget that predictions can be imperfect if flawed with errors. So, optimization should be the way forward once a lead compound is obtained and further optimized using more robust mechanistic models towards clinical trials before final manufacturing and authorization for absorption as a public health drug.

6. Recommendations

Since most models are rule-based and may use descriptors that are not easily understood by the chemist or not easily translated into better molecular structures, it is important to constantly train models of datasets. A combo approach, combining first generation (basic predictive descriptors) and second generation (meta-models) computational ADMET technologies would be the best way to go.

To then get value for your money, it is clearly demonstrated that ADME predictive tools is imperative, nowadays, in the health research programs in order to cut costs and propose reliable lead drug-like compounds. It is though highly desirable and recommendable to add in-house data in the prediction models whenever available. Sensitive and reliable high throughput instrumentations are a prerequisite in generating in-house analytical data necessary for efficient and useful predictive processes. Training data sets in models would be an added advantage for a wide range of investigations in health related research.

Acknowledgements

The author would like to acknowledge the application scientists at the Advanced Chemistry Development Inc., (Toronto, Canada), in particular, Dr Sanji Bhal for providing some of the illustrative predictive examples. Many thanks go to the reviewers for their helpful suggestions and revision of this chapter. Finally, the authors are grateful to Dr GPP Kamatou of the Department of Pharmaceutical Sciences of the Tshwane University of Technology, Pretoria, South Africa, for reading through the proof of the chapter and hereby acknowledge his positive criticism.

Author details

Peter Papoh Ndibewu* and Prince Ngobeni

*Address all correspondence to: ndibewup@tut.ac.za

Tshwane University of Technology, Faculty of Science – Arcadia Campus, Department of Chemistry, Pretoria, South Africa

References

[1] Abbott, N. J. Prediction of blood–brain barrier permeation in drug discovery from in vivo, in vitro and *in silico* models. Drug Discov Today Technol. 1,407–416 (2004).

[2] Abdel-Rahman, M. S, Couri, D., Jones, J. D. Chlorine dioxide metabolism in rat. J Environ Pathol Toxicol 3:421-430 (1980b).

[3] Abdel-Rahman, M. S., Couri, D., Bull. R. J. Kinetics of ClO_2 and effects of ClO_2, ClO_2^-, and ClO_3 in drinking water on blood glutathione and hemolysis in rat and chicken. J Environ Pathol Toxicol 3,431-449 (1980a).

[4] Abraham, M. H. The factors that influence permeation across the blood-brain barrier. Eur J. Med. Chem. 39, 235–240 (2004).

[5] ACD/Log*D* Suite. www.acdlabs.com/logdsuite/ Advanced Chemistry Development, Inc., Toronto, ON, Canada. 24 April, (2007).

[6] Agatonovic-Kustrin, S., Beresford, R. & Yusof, A. P. M.Theoretically-derived molecular descriptors important in human intestinal absorption. *J. Pharm. Biomed. Anal.* 25, 227–237 (2001).

[7] Agoram, B., Woltosz, W. S. & Bolger, M. B. Predicting the impact of physiological and biochemical processes on oral drug bioavailability. *Adv. Drug Del. Rev.* 90, S41–S67 (2001).

[8] Barnes, D. G, Dourson, M. Reference dose (RfD): Description and use in health risk assessments. Regul. Toxicol. Pharmacol. 8, 471-486 (1988).

[9] Bathija, A. T. Health Risk to Fetuses, infants and children from stage 1 disinfectants and disinfectant by-products (D/DBPs). Toxicologist. 72(S-1):28 (2003).

[10] Beitler, M. K, Chin, H. B. Improved determination of chlorite and chlorate in rinse water from carrots and green beans by liquid chromatography and amperometric and conductivity detection. J. AOAC Int. 78(3),878-883 (1995).

[11] Bhal, S. K. Lipophilicity Descriptors: Understanding When to Use Log*P* & Log*D*.

[12] Bickel, U. How to measure drug transport across the blood-brain barrier. NeuroRx, 2, 15–26 (2005).

[13] Bodor, N., Buchwald, P. 1999. Recent advances in the brain targeting of neuropharmaceuticals by chemical delivery systems. Adv. Drug. Deliv. Rev. 36,229–254 (1999).

[14] Brown, N. Algorithms for Chemoinformatics. *Wiley Interdisciplinary Reviews: Computational Molecular Science.* 1(5), 716-726 (2011).

[15] Carlson, T. J. & Segall, M. D. Predictive, computational models of ADME properties. *Curr. Drug Disc.* 3, 34–36 (2002).

[16] Clark, D. E., Frenkel, D., Levy, S. A., Li, J., Murray, C. W., Robson, B., Waszkowycz, B., David R. Westhead, D. R. PRO LIGAND: An approach to de novo molecular design. 1. Application to the design of organic molecules. Journal of Computer-Aided Molecular Design. 9(1) 13-32 (1995).

[17] Cuadrado, M. U. Ruiz, I. L., Gomez-Nieto, M. A. QSAR models based on isomorphic and nonisomorphic data fusion for predicting the blood brain barrier permeability. J. Comput. Chem. 28, 1252–1260 (2007).

[18] Dagenais, C., Rousselle, C., Pollack, G. M., Scherrmann, J. M. Development of an in situ mouse brain perfusion model and its application to mdr1a P-glycoprotein-deficient mice. J. Cereb. Blood Flow Metab. 20, 381–386 (2000).

[19] Ekins, S., Nikolsky, Y., Nikolskaya, T. Techniques: Application of systems biology to absorption, distribution, metabolism, excretion and toxicity. Trends in Pharmacological Sciences. 26(4), 202-209 (2005).

[20] Ekins, S., Waller, C. L., Swaan, P. W., Cruciani, G., Wrighton, S. A. & Wikel, J. H. Progress in predicting human ADME parameters *in silico*. *J. Pharmacol. Toxicol. Methods* 44, 251–272 (2001).

[21] Endo, S., Hayashi, H., Wada, A. Affinity chromatography without immobilized ligands: a new method for studying macromolecular interactions using high-performance liquid chromatography. Anal. Biochem. 124,372-379 (1982).

[22] Garg, P. Verma, J. *In silico* prediction of blood brain barrier permeability: An Artificial Neural Network model. J. Chem. Inf. Model. 46, 289–297 (2006).

[23] Gillet, V. J. (2008) De Novo Molecular Design, in Evolutionary Algorithms in Molecular Design (ed D. E. Clark), Wiley-VCH Verlag.

[24] Good, A. C., Ewing, T. J. A., Gschwend, D. A., Kuntz, I. R. New molecular shape descriptors: Application in database screening. *Journal of Computer-Aided Molecular Design*, 9(1), 1-12 (1995).

[25] Goodwin, J. T., Clark, D. E. *In silico* predictions of blood-brain barrier penetration: Considerations to "Keep in Mind". J. Pharmacol. Exp. Ther. 315,477–483 (2005).

[26] Green, J. P., Johnson, C., Kang, S. Application of Quantum Chemistry to Drugs and Their Interactions. Annual Review of Pharmacology. 14 (4) 319-342 (1974).

[27] Han Van de Waterbeemd, H., Gifford, E. ADMET *IN SILICO* MODELLING:TOWARDS PREDICTION PARADISE? www.nature.com/reviews/drugdisc 192 2(3) 192 -204 (2003).

[28] Hans Bouwmeester, H., Lynch, I., Marvin, H. J. P., Dawson, K. A., Berges, M., Braguer, D., Byrne, H. J., Casey, A., Chambers, G., Clift, M. J. D., Elia, G., Fernades, T. F., Fjellsbø, L. B., Hatto, P., Juillerat, L., Klein, C., Kreyling, W. G., Nickel, C., Riediker, M., Stone, V. Minimal analytical characterization of engineered nanomaterials needed for hazard assessment in biological matrices. Nanotoxicology, 5(1), 1-11(2011).

[29] Hemmateenejad, B., Miri, R., Safarpour, M. A., Mehdipour, A. R. 2006. Accurate prediction of the bloodbrain partitioning of a large set of solutes using ab initio calculations and genetic neural network modeling. J. Comput. Chem. 27,1125–1135 (2006).

[30] Ho, N. F. H., Raub, T. J., Burton, P. S., Barsuhn, C. L., Adson, A., Audus, K. L. & Borchardt, R. T. Quantitative approaches to delineate passive transport mechanisms in cell culture monolayers. *Drugs Pharm. Sci.* 102 (Transport Processes in Pharmaceutical Systems), 219–316 (2000).

[31] Jacoby, E., Boettcher, A., Mayr, L. M., Brown, N., Jenkins, J. L., Kallen, J., Engeloch, C., Schopfer, U., Furet, P., Masuya, K., Lisztwan, J. Knowledge-Based Virtual Screening: Application to the MDM4/p53 Protein-Protein Interaction. In: Jacoby, E. (ed.), *Chemogenomics, Methods in Molecular Biology, vol.* 575. Humana Press, 2009.

[32] Japertas, P. Fragmentiniu˛ ir statistiniu˛ metodu˛ naudojimas biologiškai aktyviu˛ junginiu˛ strukturos-aktyvumo sa˛ryšio tyrimuose. Ph.D. thesis, Vilniaus universitetas, Vilnius (2007).

[33] Japertas, P., Dapkunas, J. Sazonovas, A. Probabilistic Model for the Prediction of the Human Liver Microsomal Metabolism Regioselectivity. QSAR, 18th Euro QSAR. Sep 19, (2010).

[34] Japertas, P., Dapkunas, J. Sazonovas, A. Trainable In-Silico Screening Filter for Various Human Cytochrome P450 Isoforms Inhibition Liability. QSAR, 18th Euro QSAR. Sep 19, (2010).

[35] Japertas, P., Kubilius, R., Sazonovas, A., Lanevskij, K. ACD/Labs, Inc., A.Mickeviciaus g. 29, LT-08117 Vilnius, Lithuania *In Silico* Techniques in Lead Optimization ACD/Labs, Inc., A.Mickeviciaus g. 29, LT-08117 Vilnius, Lithuania, ACS Fall, August 29, (2011).

[36] Jones, J. P., He, M., Trager, W. F., Rettie, A. E. 3-dimensional QSAR for inhibitors of cytochrome P4502C9. *Drug. Metab. Dispo.*, 24, 1-6(1996).

http://dx.doi.org/10.5772/54006

[37] Katritzky, A. R., Kuanar, M., Slavov, S., Dobchev, D. A., Fara, D. C., Karelson, M., Acree, W. E., Jr., Solov'ev, V. P., Varnek, A. Correlation of blood-brain penetration using structural descriptors. Bioorg. Med. Chem. 14,4888–4917 (2006).

[38] Khan, Mahmud, T.H. Sylte, Ingebrigt. Multivariate Linear Regression Models Based on ADME Descriptors and Predictions of ADMET Profile for Structurally Diverse Thermolysin Inhibitors. Letters in Drug Design & Discovery. 6(6) 428-436(9) (2009).

[39] Kote-Jarai, Z.; Amin Al Olama, A.; Leongamornlert, D.; Tymrakiewicz, m.; Saunders, E.; Guy, M.; Giles, G. G.; Severi, G.; Southey, M.; Hopper, J. L.; Sit, K. C.; Harris, J. M.; Batra, J.; Spurdle, A. B.; Clements, J. A.; Hamdy, F.; Neal, D.; Donovan, J.; Muir, K.; Pharoah, P. D. P.; Chanock, S. J.; Brown, N.; Benlloch, S.; Castro, E.; Mahmud, N.; O'Brien, L.; Hall, A.; Sawyer, E.; Wilkinson, R.; Easton, D. F.; Eeles, R. A. Identification of a novel prostate cancer susceptibility variant in the *KLK3* gene transcript. *Hum. Genet.* 129*(6)*, 687-694(2011).

[40] Lanevskij, K., Japertas, P., Didziapetris, R., Petrauskas, A. Drug Discovery Interface. Ionization-Specific Prediction of Blood–Brain Permeability. *Wiley InterScience* (www.interscience.wiley.com). 4 (3) (2008).

[41] Langdon, S. R., Ertl, P., Brown, N. Bioisosteric Replacement and Scaffold Hopping in Lead Generation and Optimization. *Mol. Inf.* 29(5), 366-385 (2010).

[42] Langdon, S. R.; Brown, N.; Blagg, J. Scaffold Diversity of Exemplified Medicinal Chemistry Space. *J. Chem. Inf. Model.* 51(9), 2174-2185 (2011).

[43] Lave, T., Coassolo, P., Reigner, B. Prediction of hepatic metabolic clearance based on interspecies allometric scaling techniques and in vitro-in vivo correlations. *Clin. Pharmacokinet.*, 36, 211-231 (1999).

[44] Leeson, P. D., Springthorpe, B. The influence of drug-like concepts on decision-making in medicinal chemistry. Natuure reviews, *drug discovery*, 6, (9), 881-890 (2007).

[45] Levin, V. A. Relationship of octanol/water partition coefficient and molecular weight to rat brain capillary permeability. J. Med. Chem. 23, 682–684 (1980).

[46] Lipinski, C. A. Lead- and drug-like compounds: the rule of five revolution. *Drug Discov. Today Technol.* 1, 337–341 (2004).

[47] Lipinski, C. A., Lombardo, F., Dominy, B. W. & Feeney, P. J. Experimental and computational approaches to estimate solubility and permeability in drug discovery and development settings. *Adv. Drug Del. Rev.* 23, 3–25 (1997).

[48] Lu, A. Y. H.,Wang, R.W., and Lin, J. H. Cytochrome P450 in vitro reaction phenotyping: a re-evaluation of approaches used for P450 isoform identification. Drug Metab Dispos 31, 345–350 (2003).

[49] Miners, J. O., Knights, K. M., Houston, J. B., Mackenzie, P.I. *In vitro-in vivo* correlation for drugs and other compounds eliminated by glucuronidation in humans: pitfalls and promises. *Biochem. Pharmacol.* 71(11), 1531-9 (2006).

[50] Moore, D. A., Carpenter, T. A. Spatial Analytical Methods and Geographic Information Systems: Use in Health Research and Epidemiology Epidemiologic Reviews 21, (2), 143-161 (1999).

[51] Narayanan, R., Gunturi, S. B. *In silico* ADME modelling: Prediction models for blood-brain barrier permeation using a systematic variable selection method. Bioorg. Med. Chem. 13,3017–3028 (2005).

[52] Ndibewu, P. P., LL Sibali, L. L., Sieliechi, J. Mnisi, L. R. Application of *in-silico* Chemistry in understanding health risk and bioaccumulation Mechanism of POPs. *ENVIRONMIN2012*, Loskop Dam, Forever Resorts, Middleburg, South Africa. 11 – 15 March (2012)

[53] Nicolaou, C. A., Brown, N., Pattichis, C. K. Molecular Optimization Using Multi-Objective Methods. *Curr. Opin. Drug. Discov. Devel.* 10(3), 316-324 (2007).

[54] Norinder, U. & Österberg, T. Theoretical calculation and prediction of drug transport processes using simple parameters and partial least squares projections to latent structures (PLS) statistics. The use of electrotopological state indices. *J. Pharm. Sci.* 90, 1076–1085 (2001).

[55] Norris, D. A., Leesman, G. D., Sinko, P. J. & Grass, G. M. Development of predictive pharmacokinetic simulation models for drug discovery. *J. Contr. Rel.* 65, 55–62 (2000).

[56] O'Donnell, III, J. J., O'Donnell, J. T., Juettner, V. M. Clinical Pharmacology for the Primary Care Physician. DM, 10,558-610 (2012).

[57] Oldendorf, W. H. Brain uptake of radiolabeled amino acids, amines and hexoses after arterial injection. Am. J. Physiol. 221, 1629–1639 (1971).

[58] Packard, B. Z., Toptygin, D. D., Komoriya, A., Brand, L. Profluorescent protease substrates: Intramolecular dimmers described by the exciton model. Proc. Natl. Acad. Sci. 93,11640-11645 (1996).

[59] Parrott, N. & Lavé, T. Prediction of intestinal absorption: comparative assessment of GastroPlus and iDEA. *Eur. J.Pharm. Sci.* 17, 51–61 (2002).

[60] Podlogar, B. L., Muegge, I. & Brice, L. J. Computational methods to estimate drug development parameters. *Curr. Opin. Drug Disc. Dev.* 4, 102–109 (2001).

[61] Poulin, P., Krishnan, K. A biologically-based algorithm for predicting human tissue: blood partition coefficients of organic chemicals. *Hum. Exp. Toxicol.*, 14,273-280 (1995).

[62] Poulin, P., Theil, F. P. Prediction of pharmacokinetics prior to *in vivo* studies. 1. Mechanism-based prediction of volume of distribution. *J. Pharm. Sc.,* 91,129-156 (2002).

[63] Pradeep, S. Bioinformatics Infrastructure FacilityNorth-East Institute of Science & Technology. http://www.scribd.com/salampradeep/d/14651445-Chemical-Informatics. http://biotech-job.blogspot.com/ (2009). [Accessed 01 June 2012].

[64] Rowley, M., Kulagowski, J. J., Watt, A.P., Rathbone, D., Stevenson, G. I., Carling. R. W., Baker, R., Marshall. G. R., Kemp, J. A., Foster, A. C, Grimwood, S., Hargreaves, R., Hurley, C., Saywell, K. L., Tricklebank, M. D., Leeson, P. D. Effect of plasma protein binding on in vivo activity and brain penetration of glycine/NMDA receptor antagonists. J Med. Chem. 40, 4053–4068 (1997).

[65] Sazonovas, A., Japertas, P., and Didziapetris, R. Estimation of reliability of predictions and model applicability domain evaluation in the analysis of acute toxicity (LD50). SAR QSAR *Environ Res*. 21, 127–148 (2010).

[66] Takasato, Y., Rapoport, S. I., Smith, Q. R. An in situ brain perfusion technique to study cerebrovascular transport in the rat. Am. J. Physiol. 247, H484–H493 (1984).

[67] Thorp, D. Powerful Analytical Chemistry Software Solutions for CROs Through ACD/Labs Subscription Service Advanced Chemistry Development, Inc. Toronto, ON, Canada, www.acdlabs.com. Feb 23, (2011).

[68] Vallero, D. A. Ethical Decisions in Emergent Science, Engineering and Technologies, In: Emerging informatics – Innovative Concepts and Applications. Edited by Miah, S. J. InTech Publisher, Janeza Trdine 9, 51000 Rijeka, Croatia, 4, 21 (2012).

[69] Van de Waterbeemd, H. Quantitative structure-absorption relationships. In: *Pharmacokinetic Optimization in Drug Research: Biological, Physicochemical and Computational Strategies*, Testa, B., Van de Waterbeemd, H., Folkers, G. & Guy, R. (Eds), Verlag HCA, Zurich (2001), pp. 499–511.

[70] Veber, D. F., Johnson, S. R., Cheng, H. Y., Smith, B. R., Ward, K. W. & Kopple, K. D. Molecular properties that influence the oral bioavailability of drug candidates. *J. Med. Chem*. 45, 2615–2623 (2002).

[71] Wichmann, K., Diedenhofen, M., Klamt, A. Prediction of blood-brain partitioning and human serum albumin binding based on COSMO-RS sigma-moments. J. Chem. Inf. Model. 47, 228–233 (2007).

[72] Yamashita, F., Hashida, M. Insilico Approaches for predicting ADME properties of drugs. *Drug Metab. Pharmacokin*. 19(15), 327-338 (2004).

[73] Yoshida, F., Topliss, J. G. QSAR models for drug human oral bioavailability. *J. Med. Chem*. 43, 2575-2585 (2000).

[74] Yu, L. X., Gatlin, L. & Amidon, G. L. Predicting oral drug absorption in humans. *Drugs Pharm. Sci.* (Transport Processes in Pharmaceutical Systems), 102, 377–409 (2000).

[75] Zhao, Y. H., Abraham, M. H., Ibrahim, A., Fish, P. V., Cole, S., Lewis, M. L., de Groot, M. J., Reynolds, D. P. Predicting penetration across the blood-brain barrier from simple descriptors and fragmentation schemes. J. Chem. Inf. Model. 47,170–175 (2007).

[76] Zhao, Y. H., Le, J., Abraham, M. H., Hersey, A., Eddershaw, P. J., Luscombe, C. N., Boutina, D., Beck, G., Sherborne, B., Cooper, I. & Platts, J. A. Evaluation of human intestinal absorption data and subsequent derivation of a quantitative structure-activity relationship (QSAR) with the Abraham descriptors. *J. Pharm. Sci.* 90, 749–784 (2001).

[77] Zmuidinavicius, D., Japertas, P., Petrauskas, A., Didziapetris, R. Progress in Toxinformatics: the Challenge of Predicting Acute Toxicity. *Curr. Top. Med. Chem.* 9(1), 2003.

Chapter 5

From Creativity to Artificial Neural Networks: Problem-Solving Methodologies in Hospitals

Pietro Manzi and Paolo Barbini

Additional information is available at the end of the chapter

http://dx.doi.org/10.5772/52582

1. Introduction

Health services, viewed systemically, are organizations and complex systems. Their management calls for managerial techniques and instruments that meet expectations raised by professional awareness of complexity and a systemic approach. Systemic approaches are methods for understanding and managing complex health systems in an effective way [1, 2].

The professional nature of health organizations calls for flexible management and continuous adaptation, leading to a real understanding of complexity through a view of organizations as open systems capable of learning within a network of systems [3]. Occupational psychology and company management need to adapt to the world of health systems and hospitals, aware that they are not exhaustive in the analysis or proposition of solutions, because only health service professionals can achieve the perfect synthesis between clinical aspects and organization, ethics and technique that is still so necessary.

The approaches described in the present chapter may be flanked by powerful methods of probability calculation and statistical inference. The aim of the chapter is to provide practical indications and describe the main methods that professionals can apply in the difficult art of health management. The perspective springs from experience in Italian hospitals.

2. Traditional problem-solving techniques

Problem-solving may be defined as an ability that enables any problem to be tackled in any sector, and usually involves systematic changes in point of view. It has various phases:

- Problem finding: realise the discomfort;

- Problem setting: describe, define and frame the question in precise terms, transforming discomfort into a well-defined problem;
- Problem analysis: break the main problem down into secondary problems;
- Problem solving: eliminate the causes and answer the questions raised by the problem;
- Decision making: decide how to act on the basis of the answers obtained;
- Decision taking: act.

Let us look at the definition of problem. A problem is:

- a difficult situation requiring a way out;
- a situation that needs to be tackled by methods that make it possible to avoid obstacles and eventually obtain a result;
- a real-life situation requiring an effective response that is not immediately clear or available;
- a situation requiring some sort of discovery, which may be creative, intuitive, inventive, rational or structural, where attention is directed to procedural activities in order to solve it.

The problem may belong to different categories: concrete, abstract, familiar, unfamiliar, hypothetical or real. We are all accustomed to such situations in daily life, probably without ever realising these details [4].

Problems may be posed by oneself or others; in self-posed problems the solver is the same as the person who posed the problem; in problems posed by others the solver tackles a problem created by third parties. The process of problem-solving is normally systematic, sequential, practical and begins when the problem is realised. Various methods of problem-solving are used in organizations. A well-known approach is summarised in Table 1.

Focus	List problems Select problem Verify and define problem	Describe problem in writing
Analyse	Decide what needs to be known Gather reference data Determine relevant factors	Reference values List critical factors
Solve	Generate alternative solutions Select a solution Develop implementation plan	Choice of solution Implementation plan
Implement	Work for the expected result Implement plan Monitor impact	Organisational commitment Implemented plan Outcome assessment

Table 1. Scheme of a problem-solving process

http://dx.doi.org/10.5772/52582

3. Motivation of personnel

Problem-solving can benefit from motivational analysis of personnel. Motivation can be defined as behaviour that directs energy towards a goal. For hospital problem-solving, motivational analysis can help coordinate efforts. To achieve these aims, occupational activity can be planned in a motivating way. There are various ways of doing this. Organisation and/or general activity should be planned with the following principles in mind:

- *combine tasks* — elementary tasks should be grouped to form a more complex task that can be assigned to a group formed *ad hoc*;
- *organise natural work units* — do not break up activities that have internal completeness;
- *establish relationships with internal and external clients* — this enables workers to perceive the utility of what they are doing and obtain feedback on their performance;
- *attribute personal responsibility* — individuals must feel directly responsible and have a sense of ownership of the results of their work;
- *increase discretionary power* — it is important to give individuals decisional power and control of resources;
- *open various feedback channels* — feedback may be intrinsic to the task or come from others, directly (by face-to-face meetings) or indirectly (by quality reporting).

Other ways of motivating personnel are management by objectives, organisational fairness and participation [5].

Management by Objectives (MB0) implies clear definition of objectives for each organisational member, combined with careful monitoring and systematic assessment, with participation of the employee in each phase of this process. This formula, proposed by Drucker [6], is widely applied and can be linked to compensation over and above fixed retribution by varying pay according to the extent to which objectives are achieved. The following steps, among others, can help to implement this policy properly:

- shared identification of objectives in a meeting of chiefs and collaborators, when how to measure achievement of objectives is also defined;
- specification of expected results in measurable terms, such as "consignment within 24 hours" or "7.5% annual increase in sales";
- assignment of temporal goals for achieving an objective;
- monitoring at regular intervals (e.g. monthly), followed by feedback enabling individuals to modify their manner of working.

Significantly, there are two main classes of objectives: contribution and competence objectives. The former are related to collaborator performance and may regard the results (e.g. 5% reduction in rejects or waste) or quality (e.g. 10% increase in customer satisfaction). The latter regard acquisition of knowledge and skills necessary for reaching contribution objectives. These skills are part of the model defined by the organisation (e.g. attention to clients, team work, innovation, time management) but not all of them are equally important for a given worker. In brief, growth objectives must not be fixed for all skills, but only for those truly significant for an individual at a given time, in relation to task.

The theory of Adams [7] favoured development of a line of research and intervention regarding organisational fairness. It aimed to promote perception of equity in the workplace, where on-site studies suggest that sense of fairness may have three main components:

a. *distributive fairness,* regarding the equity with which rewards (e.g. economic incentives or promotion) are assigned; what individuals see as the relationship between rewards and performance (result, commitment, skills, etc.);

b. *procedural fairness,* regarding the process by which such rewards are assigned; in this case what individuals see not as the result of distribution but the *rules* used for distribution (e.g. their coherence in time and between individuals, the quality of the information available on which to base evaluation, the absence of voluntary or involuntary errors by decision-makers, etc.);

c. *fairness of interactions,* regarding the quality of the relationship between management and collaborators; what the parties view as reflecting honesty, respect, courtesy, empathy, etc.

The meta-analyses of Cohen-Charash & Spector [8] and Colquitt et al. [9] show that working performance is positively associated with distributive and procedural fairness, but the latter enables better prediction of results. Moreover, the three forms of fairness are correlated positively with motivation and negatively with intention to leave the organisation and with employee turn-over.

The perception of procedural fairness is positively influenced by the possibility of taking part in the assessment process [10]. Distributive and procedural fairness are also promoted by allowing employees to appeal against decisions that regard them [11]. The above studies show that a further motivational lever concerns participation. Fifty years ago, McGregor [12] invited a whole generation of managers and organisers to revise their concept of individuals at work and change from an authoritarian to a participatory style of management. He sustained that humans are not to be considered intrinsically lazy and needful of direction and control, but that they seek growth and responsibility and are willing to work for organisational goals. Since McGregor, the concept of participation has developed and is currently considered an indispensable support for motivation. In concrete terms, there are different areas of activity in which it is possible to increase participation:

- transformation of general into specific objectives;
- decision-making;
- identification, analysis and solving of problems;
- definition of values and policies;
- implementation and monitoring of changes;

http://dx.doi.org/10.5772/52582

- control of resources (instruments, budget, consultants).

Among the advantages of a participatory management style, scientific studies showed improvement in performance and productivity, better quality and attention to clients, creation of a cooperative atmosphere and a consequent reduction in internal competition and more probability of emergence of hidden talents [13].

4. Information management

Since management of a system assumes knowledge of that system, the solution of hospital problems requires detailed knowledge of hospitals. This not only concerns structural and functional knowledge that can be obtained from official data, but also knowledge of the dynamics of internal relationships, for which it is necessary to use interviews or the technique of systematic communication. Internal dynamics elude standardized modes of acquiring information, being a partly individual, partly shared form of knowledge belonging to the emotional constitution of healthcare personnel. Since internal dynamics have to do with the deepest part of personnel motivation, they normally elude conventional interviews, which are limited to communicating ways of working or technical approaches to healthcare, and call for induced communication techniques. The manager detects uncertainty, nervousness or outright difficulty in the person being interviewed. He uses these emotions to induce the person to communicate things that are difficult to admit. These situations of emotional difficulty are found in all hospital units, even the best ones, and represent a failure of one or more staff members that the person in charge usually has difficulty in admitting. Knowledge of situations of emotional difficulty allows the manager to intervene in internal dynamics, reassuring where the dynamics generate anxiety, and intervening drastically where there is danger of uncontrolled situations with risks for patients.

The interview technique is the most common and is generally used for the heads of units or directors. The technique of systematic communication, on the other hand, is used for all personnel, without distinction of rank. It is normally more laborious and expensive, but may provide indirect information or feedback and a key to ward dynamics.

Induction of communication is a delicate art, calling for tact, astuteness and discretion on the part of the manager. The person being interviewed must have complete trust in the confidentiality of the communication and must perceive that sincerity will be rewarded through a preferential relationship with top management, even if a degree of weakness is revealed. A lever often used in induction of communication is narcissism. Many heads aspire to respect in the hospital environment and are willing to give up something to obtain consensus or an apparently dominant position over other colleagues.

Another technique of hospital management is based on acquiring unconventional information. The manager acquires information, not directly linked to hospital activity, from sources outside the hospital. This information may, for example, regard external professional activity, activities unrelated to healthcare, political orientation or the private sphere of the healthcare worker. Although unbecoming and often a source of gossip, the working environment produces much information of this type, which may come to the attention of managers without their solicitation.

A considerable source of information on hospitals comes from the press, which may amplify information not obtained through the normal channels of communication but from health personnel, despite existing prohibitions. Cases of malpractice are a typical example, but the press may also pick up news from staff wishing to air situations of internal uneasiness. Such cases of instrumental use cannot be disciplined, however they increase knowledge of internal dynamics.

These are ways in which managers pursue the aim of information asymmetry to gain advantage with respect to directors, who come to be in a position of psychological inferiority. The manager who "knows more" plays his information more astutely, only showing his "aces" when necessary and waiting for his adversary to make a mistake. These are questions of power, as management of information is in many cases closely linked to the management of power.

In conclusion, in the framework of hospital problem-solving, managers make wise use of the conventional and non conventional information they obtain, increasing information asymmetry in order to direct personnel behaviour towards better organisational performance.

5. Operative management techniques

The solution of certain hospital management problems can be attempted by five basic methods:

1. framing of responsibilities;
2. raising the level of conflict resolution;
3. delay techniques;
4. responsibility shift;
5. management through competition.

The first is a consolidated management technique regarding the definition of *who does what*. Framing of responsibilities is actually defined by the statute of the hospital in organisation and function charts. Using these charts, certain problems can be solved simply by correct distribution of responsibilities between directors (Figure 1).

The second method consists in realising that conflict exists between employees belonging to non-decisive levels of management (e.g. between nurses and auxiliaries) and in investing the next levels up with the question (in the example, the ward sister, clinic director and director of health professions). If this does not work, higher levels are invested with responsibility. Raising the level of conflict resolution normally puts an end to the conflict by easing emotivity and direct interest.

http://dx.doi.org/10.5772/52582

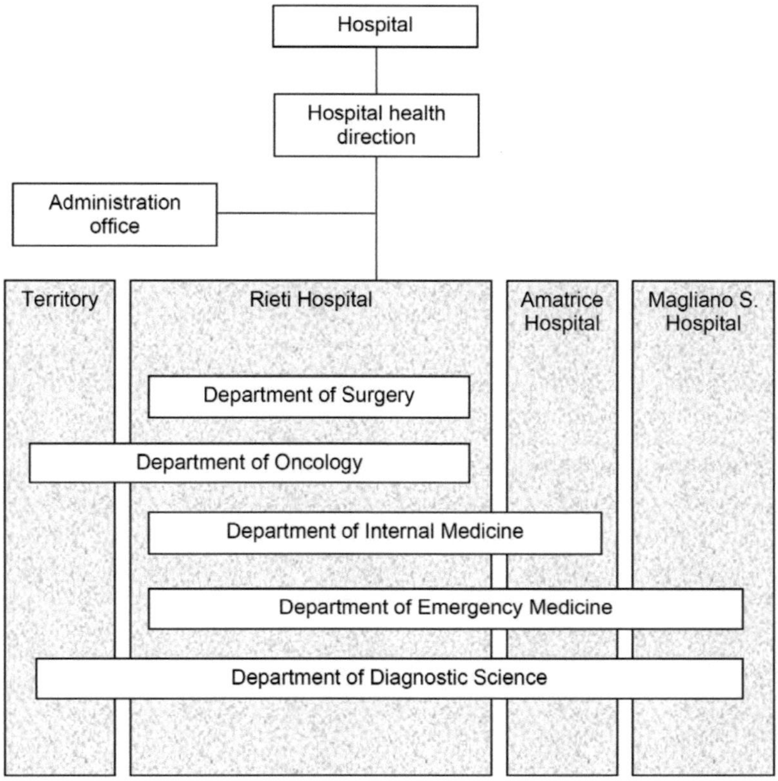

Figure 1. Function chart of Departments of Rieti-Amatrice Hospital – Italy (by kind permission of ASL Rieti).

The third method is applied when a request is patently out of proportion with the material resources or time available to provide an adequate response. Delay techniques may consist in requiring complicated forms to be filled in, asking for a detailed report or phone contact with an office known to be poorly staffed or slow to act, and so forth. The bureaucratic elephant will ensure that the request disappears into the administrative machinery.

The fourth method exploits the uncertainty or complexity of certain organisational arrangements and consists in referring the question to a third office for an opinion, verification, technical advice or further laboratory control to transfer the applicant's attention from the core problem to an unlikely external authority. Third parties are involved by sending them copies, in which something is requested of them, knowing that only a meticulous reader will discern the deception.

The fifth method (management by competition) is based on the principle of narcissism. When a problem is not tackled by a healthcare worker, it is suggested that the sector be handed over to another whose skill is well known and who would be happy to take over. Usually narcissism comes to the rescue, making the director change his mind and become more amenable to compromise.

6. Creative or heuristic methods

An innovative method of problem-solving known as "creative" was recently proposed. Its features include learning different ways of creative thinking, eliminating preformed schemes and stereotypes and taking a richer approach to problems. Creative problem-solving is particularly useful in project design phase, when the objective is to correctly identify problems and solutions using instruments that reinforce creativity by encouraging original and innovative ideas. The concept of creativity was defined appropriately by Poincaré when he stated that creativity is joining existing elements by useful new connections and that invention consists not in building useless combinations but only useful ones, which are a tiny minority. The conclusion is that a new result has value, if any, when by establishing a link between known elements, hitherto scattered and apparently unrelated, it immediately creates order where disorder seemed to reign.

This type of approach exploits heuristic methods without a mathematical foundation. The solution is identified iteratively, seeking to optimise one or more objective functions within an allowed region. Ideas are typically generated by brainstorming. The aim is to focus on the problem and then let various original solutions emerge deliberately, without any preconceived order. Discussion and exchange of opinions enable an iterative approach that leads to a solution regarded as optimal.

The processes of the creative method are:

- establish priorities;
- seek alternatives;
- formulate hypotheses;
- generate new ideas.

Creative methods can exploit mind mapping, a powerful technique of graphic representation of knowledge that provides a universal key to the potential of the mind. A mind map is a diagram in which concepts are presented in graphic form: the main idea is in the centre and more detailed information is added piece by piece (Figure 2). Mind maps express radiating thoughts and are therefore a natural function of the human mind [14].

Mind mapping is based on the results of research into:

- the possibility of the human mind to associate concepts and information in a non linear manner;
- the functional differentiation of the two lobes of the brain:

– the left lobe processes information in a linear, logical, analytical, quantitative, rational and verbal way and is stimulated by written and verbal representations;

– the right lobe works in a non linear, holistic, intuitive, imaginary and non verbal way and is stimulated by hierarchical, spatial, symbolic and coloured representations.

http://dx.doi.org/10.5772/52582

Research has led to the identification of a method that enables information and ideas to be represented through logical-rational and imaginary-creative functions. Mind maps differ from other methods of representation of knowledge because they emphasise:

- the hierarchical-associative structure of information;
- the use of elements of high perceptive impact, such as colours and images, that stimulate the creativity of the producer and capture the attention of readers.

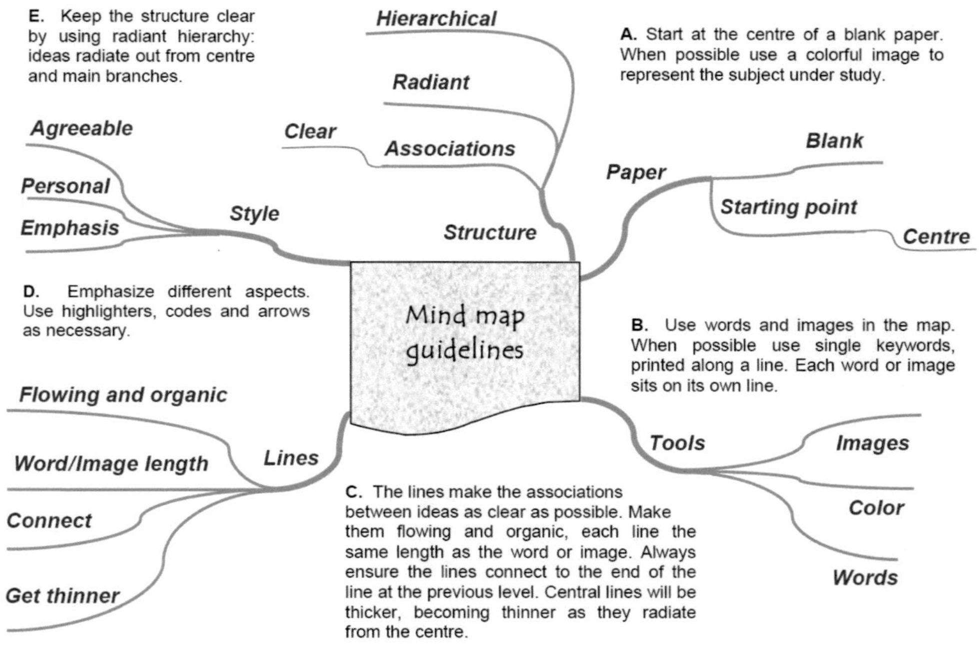

Figure 2. Mind map guidelines.

The paradigm of linear representation envisages a static beginning and end to a logical process, preventing the effective creation of associations, whereas mind maps offer a dynamic approach and envisage a centre but not an end. A graphic representation with these characteristics is very effective:

- as a support for creativity because it stimulates ideas and associations not yet elaborated (in a mind map, every branch can in turn be the centre of another more detailed mind map);
- as a support for representation, because it enables an overall vision, helping work on existing thoughts and ideas as well as on everything still to be developed from them;

- in the communication of thoughts, because it makes conceptual links graphically explicit and facilitates creation of mental associations.

For example, mind maps can be used:

- in the personal sphere to elicit ideas and then to fix and elaborate them;
- in group work to represent the information and ideas of different people on the same map, facilitating exchange and accelerating the transition from elaboration to performance;
- in the management of distributed knowledge to represent information using standards and representational devices that favour an objectivised interpretation and view.

General fields in which maps can be applied include:

- creativity: to generate ideas autonomously or in groups by brainstorming;
- analysis: to represent, evaluate and compare various options in the act of problem-solving and decision-making;
- communication: to convey information in a simple intuitive manner, emphasising logical links and facilitating dialectic and exchange;
- organisation: to structure activities, allocate resources, assign times and gather necessary information;
- documentation: to lay out documents and plan document structure.

7. Pragmatic methods

A typical example of the pragmatic approach is lean thinking. The aim is to make a little go a long way by reducing waste. The problems are studied in action and the solutions must be simple. The term *lean* indicates a process close to maximum efficiency, a process of optimisation with continuous endeavour to reduce waste and unproductive activity. The word was first used in this sense in the 1990s, but the concept is exemplified by the Toyota production system invented by Taiichi Ohno after World War II. The lean approach consists in analysing processes, mapping activities connected with processes, and identifying productive activities and their flows. Activities that add value are distinguished from those that cause a loss of value.

Application of this approach in the health services is not completely intuitive. The parallel with industry may seem bold, but the activity of a health unit is actually based on processes and pathways often similar to those of industrial production. Applied to health systems in the last 7-8 years, the model is based on recognition of the fact that all activities form production lines [15]. Activities have an ideal pathway that is rarely recognised and followed. The aim is to try to achieve an optimal pace without unnecessary interruptions and unexpected obstacles. All components of a given line of activity are brought together to decide the best pathway with the best timing and the appropriate resources. For example:

- several meetings are held to involve everyone. The components, unaccustomed to sharing their small and big problems, produce a quantity of problems, mainly organisational, that are ordered by priority and solved (capacity for teamwork is necessary);
- the organisational methods sustaining this principle include value stream maps and rapid improvement events that can be applied in specific areas known as production cells.

The techniques, clearly described and easy to learn, must be agreed on and adopted by operative personnel, becoming part of a mechanism of change (improvement) by progressive involvement plans. The aim for all is to reduce space, distance, effort, stocks and service time.

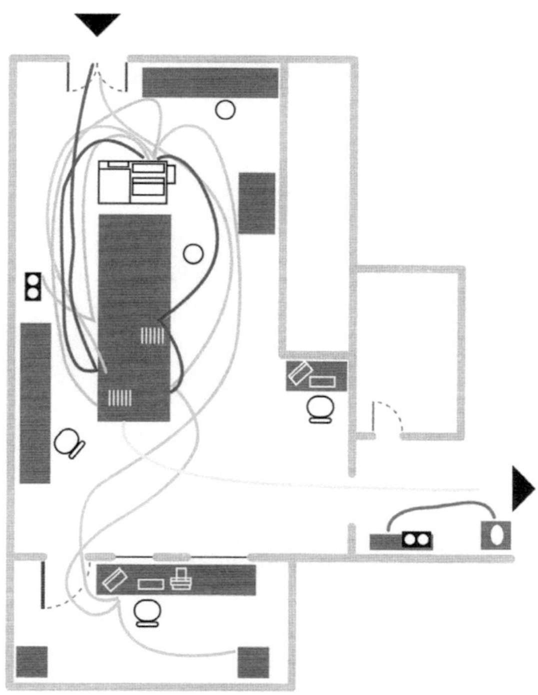

Figure 3. Example of spaghetti chart.

A graphic tool that can help in applying lean thinking is the spaghetti chart, which represents the movements of an element (patient, personnel, biological samples, etc.) in the value stream of the organisation. The tangled form of the chart may resemble a plate of spaghetti. Spaghetti charts can be used to analyse all the movements of personnel, biological samples, patients or anything else that is moved in a specific area (Figure 3). Goals take time and must be planned by the general management, without the support of which only minor progress is possible. However, once underway, the immediate results are incredible. Supply improves in the points where maps were used. The improvement becomes visible and elicits amazement that the solution was never thought of before. The challenge is met by those understanding the concept of flow and the need to maintain the wave of action. The need for territorial assistance pathways from the hospital is another necessary but not sufficient tool. Without the concept of flow, value to improve and waste to reduce, continually and obsessively, little progress is made. If a scheme is applied but not carried through, the mechanism stops. On the other hand, if it is fuelled by realisation of the true requisites, the hospital pulses with the synchronous activities of planned flows. This is possible because besides the concept of flow, not as influx of clients in part of the organisation (clinics, emergency, outpatients, operating theatres, with problems of variations in demand) but as flexible supply of services, it is fundamental to recognise the concept of waste in internal activities, estimated to be around 80-90% in current hospital activity lines [16]. The actions performed in activity lines can be improved in terms of organisation, logistics and efficiency. The concept of speed and volume of activity is not what counts, but rather the right flexibility for the volume of activity necessary and useful for patients.

8. Mathematical methods

Mathematical methods can be applied to problem-solving in two main ways: Bayesian networks and artificial neural networks, that can also be used as complementary tools.

8.1. Bayesian networks

A Bayesian network (also called belief network) is a probabilistic graphical model able to represent the dependence between random variables and to give a concise specification of the joint probability distribution [17]. This type of model is a powerful tool which can be particularly suited to describe dependencies among variables and to support the decision-making process in situations of uncertainty [18].

For explanatory purposes, an illustrative example of a simple Bayesian network model is shown in Figure 4. The network is composed of five nodes and four arrows. Each node represents a random variable (work, environment, age, disease and symptoms) and arrows represent conditional dependencies between variables. The figure points out that a disease is dependent on age, work and environment and that symptoms are dependent on the disease. According to this model, the probability of a disease is conditioned on three variables (age, work and environment), while that of symptoms depends only on the disease. $P(W)$, $P(E)$ and $P(A)$ represent the absolute probabilities of work, environment and age, respectively. $P(D|W,E,A)$ is the conditional probability of disease and $P(S|D)$ is the conditional probability of symptoms.

http://dx.doi.org/10.5772/52582

In summary, the example shows that a Bayesian network is a graph in which the following holds:

1. A set of random variables makes up the nodes of the network.
2. A set of directed links or arrows connects pairs of nodes. The intuitive meaning of an arrow from node X to node Y is that X has a direct influence on Y (X is called a parent of Y, and Y is a child of X). The lack of an arrow between two nodes indicates their conditional independence.
3. Each node has a conditional probability table that quantifies the effects that the parents have on the node. The parents of a node are all those nodes that have arrows pointing to it.
4. The graph has no directed cycles (hence is a directed, acyclic graph, or DAG).

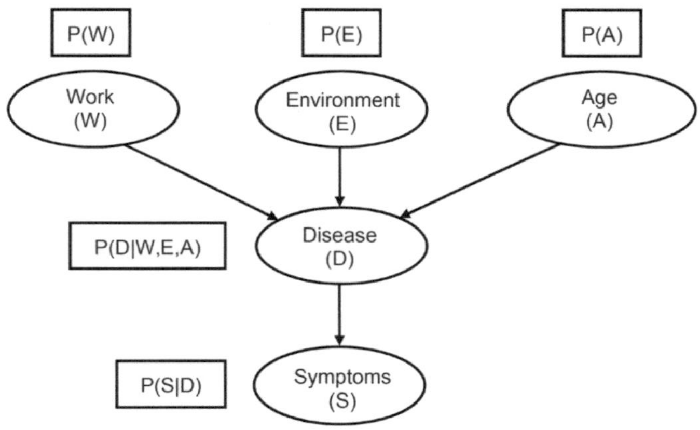

Figure 4. Illustrative example of Bayesian network. P(W), P(E) and P(A) represent the absolute probabilities of work, environment and age, respectively. P(D|W,E,A) is the conditional probability of disease and P(S|D) is the conditional probability of symptoms.

Learning the topology of a Bayesian network from data can be a difficult problem, as its associated search space is super-exponentially large. However, in a lot of cases, it can be easy for a domain expert to decide what direct conditional dependence relationships hold in the domain - much easier, in fact, than actually specifying the probabilities themselves. Once the topology of the belief network is specified, we need only specify conditional probabilities for the nodes that participate in direct dependencies, and use those to compute any other probability values.

Manual construction of a network involves various development stages. For each of these stages, knowledge is acquired from experts in the domain of application, the relevant medical literature is studied, and available patient data are analysed. As developing a Bayesian network is a creative process, the various stages are iterated in a cyclic fashion where each stage may, on each iteration, induce further refinement of the network under construction.

Bayesian networks can be used for data classification, identification of causal relationships and output prediction. They allow a domain expert to model uncertain relationships between a variable of interest with unknown values and clinical findings/observations (known variables) and are particularly useful for medical diagnosis [19-21]. Attractive features of Bayesian networks include encoding dependencies among all variables, thereby addressing problems with incomplete data; informing causal relationships, thereby increasing understanding about a problem domain and predicting consequences of treatment; combining prior knowledge (which often comes in causal form) and available data; and user friendliness of graphical representations.

From the above we can realize that Bayesian networks seem to be suitable tools in hospital context, because they are intuitive, even to the novice, and allow for incorporating qualitative knowledge and statistical information which is often easily available in medicine. Moreover, they can be used not only for clinical purposes, but for many other problems associated with the management of health, e.g. for health economic evaluations [22-23].

A special case of Bayesian network is the well-known naïve Bayes classifier. It is an ancient form of Bayesian network that continues to have particular success in various fields of application by virtue of its simplicity and good performance. Naïve Bayes models are often used in medicine for pattern recognition and to aid clinical decisions [24].

A more detailed discussion on Bayesian networks is available in the present book in the chapter entitled "Bayesian Approach in Medicine and Health Management".

8.2. Neural networks

Artificial neural networks (ANN) are powerful tools that can be used to manage knowledge and solve problems [25]. They are information processing systems that reproduce by computer the function of a very simplified biological neural network, composed of a certain number of interconnected neurons. Intelligent behaviour springs from appropriate interactions between interconnected units. Figure 5 shows an example of stratified feed-forward ANN architecture.

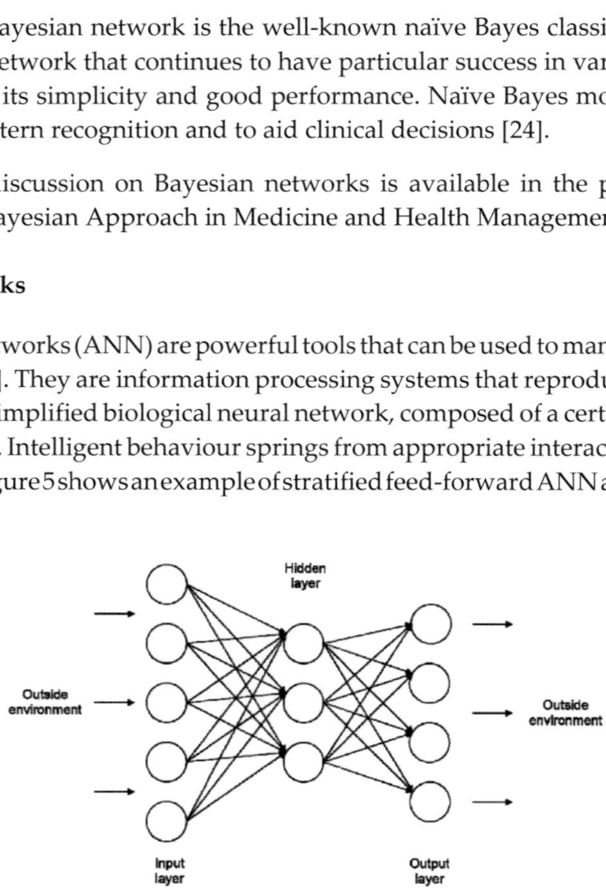

Figure 5. Example of stratified feed-forward artificial neural network architecture. The ANN architecture consists of three layers of neurons. The neurons in a layer only project onto those in the subsequent layer.

The architecture of the artificial neural network shown in Figure 5 is said to be stratified because it consists of a number of layers of neurons. It is feed-forward because the connections only project forward, that is, the flow of information moves in one direction from input to output. The neurons in a layer only project onto those in the subsequent layer. There are no connections between neurons in the same layer or between non-adjacent layers.

In a stratified feed-forward network all connections between neurons can be described quantitatively using a number of tables (matrices) equal to the number of pairs of adjacent layers. The ordered elements of each matrix represent the weights of the connections between corresponding pairs of neurons in adjacent layers.

To design an artificial neural network it is first of all necessary to carefully identify the inputs and outputs to the system in order to define the context correctly and completely. Not much can be said about the topology of the network to use, because there are no theoretical criteria that enable the ideal type of network (feed-forward or feed-back) or the optimal number of layers, neurons and connections to be identified a priori. In general, ANN topology is chosen empirically in relation to the problem to solve.

Perhaps the greatest difficulty in using ANNs for problem-solving is the difference between this type of approach and a conventional algorithmic approach. Conventional approaches use a specific algorithm and the computer is programmed to follow a set of instructions that reflect the algorithm that will solve the problem. On the other hand, ANNs use a pattern-recognition approach to the problem, exploiting the information contained in available data (data driven) rather than an algorithmic perspective. In other words, once ANN structure has been chosen, the network is trained to solve a problem using a training set of examples. Examples must be chosen with care so as not to waste time or train the network in the wrong way. Thus the performance of ANNs depend greatly on the training set: the more the set represents the problem and is complete, the better its performance and capacity to provide appropriate responses to inputs not analysed during training (generalisation power).

The ANN and conventional algorithmic approaches are not actually contradictory but complementary. In some situations one or the other is preferable, in others the two can be combined. Although ANNs have proven successful, they are not suitable for all types of problem. Current consensus on ANNs is that they do not work miracles, but if used intelligently can give surprising results. They undoubtedly have certain strengths with respect to the human brain, such as good performance even in situations where human judgment may be penalised by fatigue, lack of motivation and poor memory. A certain weak point lies in the fact that human decisions are often based on perceptions and are modified in the course of time by life's experiences that mature the person and cannot be reproduced by artificial learning.

A conclusive consideration is possible comparing Figures 4 and 5. Similarities can be observed between the structures of Bayesian networks and artificial neural networks. Despite these analogies and often similar performance, it should be borne in mind that the parameters for designing Bayesian networks are conditional probability relationships between two random variables, characteristic of the problem (network nodes), whereas those of ANNs do not have this meaning.

9. Conclusions

Hospital problem-solving is the daily bread of hospital managers and doctors with managerial roles, especially those in hospital medical management, who are the main specialists in this subject. Irrespective of clinical provenance, doctors involved in medical management acquire experience in problem-solving, usually self-taught since the subject is often neglected in specialisation schools.

As we have seen, problem-solving calls for a scientific multidisciplinary approach with psychological adaptation of method to context. The ability to interpret the system as a whole and to knowledgeably mix various management techniques are not for everyone and even the best versed colleagues need time and practice.

The author hopes that this chapter will promote reflection on the topic, suggesting fields to investigate in more detail and eliciting recognition by doctors working in hospital organisation.

Acknowledgment

This work was partly financed by the University of Siena, Italy.

Author details

Pietro Manzi[1] and Paolo Barbini[2,3*]

*Address all correspondence to: paolo.barbini@unisi.it

1 Hospital Health-Care Management, University Hospital of Siena, Siena, Italy

2 Department of Surgery and Bioengineering, University of Siena, Siena, Italy

3 Biomedical Engineering Unit,University Hospital of Siena, Siena, Italy

References

[1] Bar-Yam Y. Improving the effectiveness of healthcare and public health: A multiscale complex systems analysis. American Journal of Public Health 2006;96(3) 459-466.

[2] Resnicow K., Page SE. Embracing chaos and complexity: A quantum change for Public Health. American Journal of Public Health 2008;98(8) 1382-1389.

[3] Begun JW, Zimmerman B, Dooley K. Health care organizations as complex adaptive systems. In: Mick SM, Wyttenbach M. (eds.) Advances in health care organization theory. San Francisco, CA: Jossey-Bass; 2003. p253-288.

[4] Robertson SI. Problem solving. Hove, England: Psychology Press; 2001.

[5] Arnold J. Work psychology: understanding human behaviour in the workplace. Harlow, England: Pearson Education; 2005.

[6] Drucker PF. The practice of management. New York: Harper & Row; 1954.

[7] Adams JS. Inequity in social exchange. In: Berkowitz L. (ed.) Advances in experimental social psychology. New York: Academic Press; 1965. p267-299.

[8] Cohen-Charash Y, Spector PE. The role of justice in organizations: A meta-analysis.Organizational Behavior and Human Decision Processes 2001; 86(2) 278-321.

[9] Colquitt JA, Conlon DE, Wesson MJ, Porter COLH, Ng KY. Justice at the millennium: A meta-analytic review of 25 years of organizational justice research. Journal of Applied Psychology 2001;86(3) 425-445.

[10] Avery DR, Quiñones MA. Disentangling the effects of voice: the incremental roles of opportunity, behavior, and instrumentality in predicting procedural fairness. Journal of Applied Psychology 2002;87(1) 81-86.

[11] Tepper BJ, Lockhart D, Hoobler J. Justice, citizenship, and role definition effects. Journal of Applied Psychology 2001;86(4) 789-796.

[12] McGregor D. The human side of enterprise. New York: McGraw-Hill; 1960.

[13] Hodson R. Dignity in the workplace under participative management: Alienation and freedom revisited. American Sociological Review 1996;61(5) 719-738.

[14] Buzan T, Buzan B. The mind map book. Harlow, England: BBC Active; 2006.

[15] Graban M. Lean hospitals: Improving quality, patient safety, and employee satisfaction. New York: CRC Press; 2009.

[16] Joosten T, Bongers I, Janssen R. Application of lean thinking to health care: Issues and observations. International Journal for Quality in Health Care 2009;21(5) 341-347.

[17] Russell S, Norvig P. Artificial intelligence: a modern approach. Upper Saddle River, NJ: Pearson Education; 2010.

[18] Lucas PJF, van der Gaag LC, Abu-Hanna A. Bayesian networks in biomedicine and health-care. Artificial Intelligence in Medicine 2004;30(3) 201-214.

[19] Burnside ES, Rubin DL, Fine JP, Shachter RD, Sisney GA, Leung WK. Bayesian network to predict breast cancer risk of mammographic microcalcifications and reduce number of benign biopsy results: initial experience. Radiology 2006;240(3) 666-673.

[20] Li J, Shi J, Satz D. Modeling and analysis of disease and risk factors through learning Bayesian networks from observational data. Quality and Reliability Engineering International 2008;24 (3) 291-302.

[21] Mnatsakanyan ZR, Burkom HS, Coberly JS, Lombardo JS. Bayesian information fusion networks for biosurveillance applications. Journal of the American Medical Informatics Association 2009;16 (6) 855-863.

[22] Chacón M, Maureira B. Causal networks for modeling health technology utilization in intensive care units. In: Sanfeliu A, Martínez Trinidad JF, Carrasco Ochoa JA. (eds.), Progress in pattern recognition, image analysis and applications. Berlin: Springer; 2004, p645-653.

[23] Le QA, Doctor JN. Probabilistic mapping of descriptive health status responses onto health state utilities using Bayesian networks: an empirical analysis converting SF-12 into EQ-5D utility index in a national US sample. Medical Care 2011;49(5) 451-460.

[24] Cevenini G, Barbini E, Massai MR, Barbini P. A naïve Bayes classifier for planning transfusion requirements in heart surgery.j Journal of Evaluation in Clinical Practice. Article first published online: 23 Aug 2011, doi:10.1111/j.1365-2753.2011.01762.x.

[25] Haykin S. Neural networks and learning machines. New York: Prentice Hall/Pearson; 2009.

Section 2

Healthcare Systems

Chapter 6

Knowledge Management in Canadian Healthcare Organizations: How Do Knowledge Brokers Perform?

Réjean Landry, Jalila Jbilou, Nabil Amara and Salaheddine El Adlouni

Additional information is available at the end of the chapter

http://dx.doi.org/10.5772/54802

1. Introduction

Under the Canada's health Act, the health sector is administered and operated on a non-profit basis by the public authority. The sustainability of Canada's public health-care system depends in large part on its ability to implement strategies to improve its performance in terms of social, economic, organizational and professional. Knowledge-brokering is an emerging function in the healthcare systems worldwide. Championed as a cornerstone role for knowledge translation by the Canadian Health Services Research Foundation, the implications of understanding this function and those who undertake it are important for improving knowledge management in the healthcare sector where there is a spread of the evidence informed/based decision making (EI/BDM) movement. Knowledge brokering is defined, by the Canadian Health Services Research Foundation, through a set of basic skills that are *the ability to bring people together and facilitate their interaction; the ability to find academic research and other evidence to shape decisions; the ability to assess evidence, interpret it and adapt it to circumstance; a knowledge of marketing, communication and Canadian healthcare; and the ability to identify emerging management and policy issues which research could help to resolve*. Its mandate is to support in the organization, management and delivery of health services and its main strategy for doing so is to link decision makers and researchers to ensure effective knowledge transfer.

In an era of knowledge society and knowledge economy, the amount of information has reached unimaginable proportions. Hence, in biomedical research, one has about 15000 journals that publish approximately two million articles every year. Web search engines are not always the most accurate and appropriate way to extract the relevant information because they typically generate a large amount of unsorted information. Some innovative approaches were developed to optimize information identification and knowledge management through Strategic foresight. However, we rarely find *"ready to go"* solutions to complex problems in published documents (articles or reports). Thus, managers have to address the problem by becoming more proactive in managing how knowledge is accessed, integrated and translated into new or improved products, services or practices (Jbilou and al. 2007). Nevertheless, this knowledge translation process is complex and a major gap still exist, the so-called knowledge-to-action gaps in healthcare sector (Gagnon 2011). One of the options to close this gap between science and practice is related to the concept of boundary practices, developed by Wenger (2000) and the effective system of "bridging" across those boundaries involve organizations, groups and/or individuals acting as 'knowledge brokers'. In healthcare sector, knowledge brokering has become a popular knowledge management strategy to promote interaction/collaboration between researchers and end users; and support EI/BDM (Brownson and Jones 2009). Knowledge brokers are part of the knowledge to action cycle in healthcare (Granham et al. 2006; Strauss et al. 2009). Prior studies on knowledge brokers and brokering have emphasized either the impact of the social intermediation and networks positions (*the social function*) (Granovetter, 1973; Hansen, 1999; Burt, 1992; Burt, 2005) or the impact of knowledge integration and processing (*the cognitive function*) (Rogers, 1995; Hargadon and Sutton, 1997; Hargadon, 2002) in order to explain the acquisition, dissemination, integration, translation and implementation of knowledge into new or improved products, services and practices. These studies consider the cognitive function and the social function as the two basic functions of knowledge management achieved by knowledge brokers. However, the issues of how resources influence the ways knowledge brokers perform these two critical functions have been largely under-explored. This is the first contribution of this exploratory study. Furthermore, prior studies that emphasize those two core functions are useful for describing network positions and knowledge processing, but not for understanding how individual and organizational resources of knowledge brokers influence the role profiles they adopt, like this study does. Moreover, given the fact that the position of knowledge brokers is not yet a well established formal position in most organizations, a large number of prior studies have focused their effort on documenting the roles of knowledge brokers and brokering (Howells, 2006). Most prior empirical studies have tended to rely on a case study approach and had explored these functions separately (Howells, 2006; Hargadon and Sutton, 1997; Hargadon, 2002). A literature review on intermediaries and intermediation also shows that most studies adopt the organization as their unit of analysis (Howells, 2006). This paper aims to contribute to advance knowledge by taking the individuals as its unit of analysis, to explore how the resources available to individuals operating in different types of healthcare organizations influence the way they perform, with respect to the two core functions: *the cognitive function and the social function,* separately and combined. Taken together, these shortcomings of the existing literature led us to address the following questions: How the two core functions can be integrated to derive a typology of knowledge brokering profiles? What are the determinants of these profiles? What are the practical implications deriving from findings on the determinants of these knowledge brokering profiles?

http://dx.doi.org/10.5772/54802

1.1. Method

1.1.1. Population under study

The population of this study consists of the members of the knowledge brokerage community of practices (CoP) under the initiative of the Canadian Health Services Research Foundation (CHSRF). The purpose of this CoP is to share knowledge and expertise on knowledge brokerage, focus on learning and furthering the practice of knowledge brokerage, develop and share a collective repertoire of communal resources, including activities and means of participation, and operate as an interdependent network defined by the collaborative efforts of the members. This CoP has been operating since 2003. Since its inception, members of the CoP have participated in national or regional workshops, and have shared knowledge brokering resources (through forums and directories of experts) during these face-to-face activities, as well as on the virtual platform of the CoP supported by CHSRF (http://www.chsrf.ca/brokering/). This population was composed of 441 individuals in October 2005. We decided to exclude 12 individuals from the study, who work for CHSRF, in order to avoid response biases. The final population of the study was therefore made up of 429 individuals.

1.1.2. Conceptual framework and measures

1.1.2.1. Dependant variables

The dependent variable is composed of four KB profiles measured using two function indexes: the cognitive function and the social function. The first index included four items assessing how frequently, over the last twelve months, the KB had: 1) read research information, studies and research reports; 2) understood research findings, studies and research reports; 3) cited research information, studies and research reports to his colleagues; and 4) discussed research information, studies and research reports with colleagues. For each statement, a 5-point scale ranging from 1 (never) to 5 (very often) is used. The cognitive function index is the sum of the scores of the items corresponding to the responses of the knowledge brokers to these four statements. Hence, this index can range from 4 to 20. The construction of the social function index was based on the same logic. More specifically, this index was created by adding the scores of four items corresponding to the answers of the respondents to assess, on a 5-point scale ranging from 1 (never) to 5 (very often), how frequently, over the last twelve months, they had: 1) facilitated the involvement of individuals from their organizational unit into research projects; 2) facilitated the creation of research projects' advisory committees; 3) facilitated person-to-person contact between people in their administrative unit and researchers; and 4) organized seminars, meetings, conferences or other events to provide opportunities for exchanges between people in their organizational unit and researchers. Thus, the social function index can range from 4 to 20. Considering that these two indices were based on multiple-item scales, we conducted a principal components factor analysis (PCFA) on the construct scales to assess their unidimensionality. For the index reflecting the cognitive function, the results of the PCFA indicated that one factor explained 65.17% of the original variance of the phenomenon studied, with an initial Eigenvalue of 2.61. Likewise, a PCFA on the construct scales of the index capturing intensity of the social function indicated that one factor explained 66.20% of the original variance of the phenomenon studied with an initial Eigenvalue of 2.65. In addition, Cronbach's alphas for the two indices were, respectively,.82 and.77, indicating that the items in each index are reliable (Ahire and Devaray, 2001; Nunally, 1967, 1978) (Figure 1).

1.1.2.2. The copula approach

The construction of the dependent variable used in this paper was based on these two indexes and was derived in a two-step process. Firstly, we used the copulas approach to profile knowledge brokers' (KBs) critical functions. Copula has been first introduced by Sklar (1959) in surveys on random metric spaces, and is defined as a joint distribution function of standard uniform random variables. That is:
$C(u_1, \ldots, u_p) = Pr\{U_1 \leq u_1, \ldots, U_p \leq u_p\}$,

where

$$U_i \sim U(0,1) \; for \, i = 1, \ldots, p. \qquad (1)$$

Copulas allow the modelling of the dependency relationships among random variables independently of their marginal distributions. This is of great relevance for two reasons. Firstly, copulas can handle dependency between random variables without the limitations of other dependency measures, e.g., the normality assumption in linear correlation coefficient (Nelson, 1999; Basrak and al., 2004, Gagliardini and Gouriéroux 2006). Secondly, the thresholds calculated with copulas allow determining with high precision the limits for the four profiles conceptually defined in Figure 1.

We used copulas to evaluate the correlation between the cognitive function index (COG_FUN) and the social function index (SOC_FUN), and to determine with 95% of precision the cutting-

Figure 1: Conceptual Framework

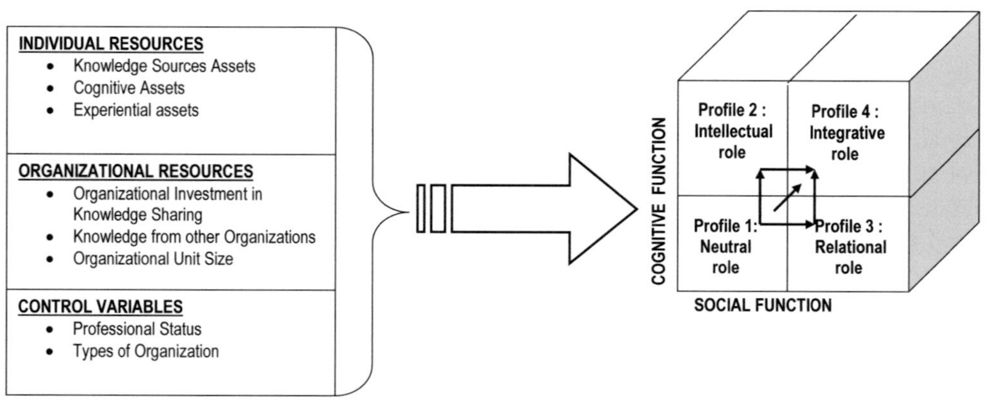

Figure 1. Conceptual Framework

points (thresholds) that limit the different KBs' profiles. The marginal distribution for COG_FUN is bounded and has an exponential form, thus the Beta distribution is used for this fit. SOC_FUN index follows a normal distribution. More specifically, we calculated the joint conditional probability of the variable COG_FUN knowing SOC_FUN, and we found that the effect of the variable SOC_FUN is more significant for the values superior to 15. This threshold corresponds to a probability in the 72% non-overtaking. The threshold obtained for COG_FUN is 17, which corresponds to a probability in the 73% non-overtaking. The crossing of these two thresholds was used to classify the KBs in their appropriate role profile. This is illustrated by Figure 1 where the four KBs' profiles constructed according to the copulas approach are shown by the four quadrants separated by the bold lines. Figure 1 also illustrates the huge difference between the KBs' profiling based on the copulas approach and an alternative profiling based on medians given by the four quadrants separated by the narrow lines. Indeed, medians are good measures of central tendency, but are less precise than thresholds calculated through copulas (Clemen and Reilly, 1999; Amara et al., 2005).

Secondly, the four KBs' role profiles were characterized by combining the cutting points (thresholds) of the two indexes as follow (Figure 2):

- Neutral role (low cognitive and low social): COG_FUN ≤ 17 and SOC_FUN ≤ 15
- Relational role (low cognitive and high social): COG_FUN ≤ 17 and SOC_FUN > 15
- Intellectual role (high cognitive and low social): COG_FUN > 17 and SOC_FUN ≤ 15
- Integrated role (high cognitive and high social): COG_FUN > 17 and SOC_FUN > 15

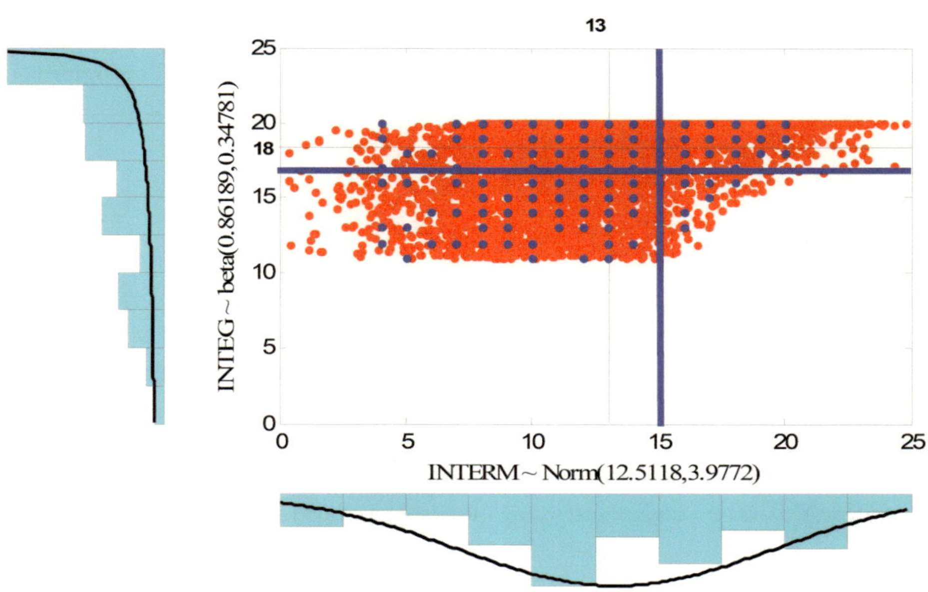

Figure 2. Joint distribution of cognitive (INTEG) and social (INTERM) functions of knowledge brokers

2. Independent variables

In this exploratory study, we build on the resource-based view of the firm (Barney, 1991; Kogut and Zander, 1992; Conner and Prahalad, 1996; Grant, 1996) to argue that KBs' idiosyncratic resources determine how they will achieve their brokering role. The overall exploratory hypothesis of this paper is that the particular role profile that KBs perform will depend on the resources they can mobilize to achieve their brokering activities, in respect to the cognitive function and the social function (see the left hand side of Figure 1).

2.1. Individual resources

2.1.1. Knowledge sources assets

The primary resources inputs of the KB are made up of the ideas and information that they acquire from sources external to their organizations (Hargadon, 2002). One may hypothesize that the larger the variety of the knowledge sources on which the KBs can rely on, the better their opportunities to assess not only the value of external knowledge, but also its validity and reliability. In this paper, broker's knowledge sources assets (SOURCES) were measured in reference to the acquisition by the KBs of studies and research reports from 15 sources of information.

2.1.2. Cognitive assets

The literature on KBs does address the impact of education on how knowledge intermediaries perform their different roles. However, one may hypothesize that individuals engaged in brokering need to have the capabilities required to assess the information collected for its quality, relevance and applicability to a given problem. In this paper, KBs' cognitive assets were measured with a binary variable, to precise the level of education, defined with regard to the most advanced completed degree.

2.1.3. Experiential assets

KBs with more experience has had more opportunities to develop their ability to search, select, integrate and recombine appropriate pertinent knowledge into practical solutions for their organizations (Hargadon, 1998). Similarly, more experience may be instrumental in providing more opportunities to interact with research organizations and therefore to develop more interactions with researchers. Furthermore, experience may generate the production of idiosyncratic knowledge resulting from the history of the relations developed over time between the KBs and the researchers and knowledge users of their organizations. This rationale suggests that more experienced individuals are more likely to play a role of integrative role than the three other roles, or alternatively to adopt an intellectual role or a relational role rather than a neutral role. In this paper, the experience of KBs (EXPER) was measured by the number of years of relevant experience that the KB has in his current job.

2.2. Organizational resources

2.2.1. Organizational investment in knowledge sharing

Individual resources are necessary, but might not be sufficient to explain how KBs perform their roles. Organization's investments in mechanisms for knowledge sharing may leverage the sharing of the knowledge that KBs have accumulated (Ipe, 2003; Huysman and de Wit, 2004; Berends et al., 2006). Based on this rationale, one may hypothesize that the higher the organizational investments in knowledge sharing mechanisms, the higher the capabilities of KBs to score well on the social function. In this paper, organizational investments in knowledge sharing (SHARE) were measured by using a five-item index regarding the importance of the investment of the broker's organizations in knowledge sharing activities.

2.2.2. Knowledge assets from other organizations

The knowledge assets accumulated by KBs are built on two types of knowledge sources: firstly, they are built on the proactive knowledge search activities of the KBs when they attempt to access knowledge from various sources; secondly, they are also built on the knowledge that KBs receive from people who carry out their professional activities in other organizations. One may hypothesize that the larger the variety of the categories of organizations and people from which the KBs receive ideas, information and reports, the larger is their knowledge assets. In this paper, KBs' knowledge assets provided by people from other organizations (KOTHE) were measured by a variety index referring to ten categories of people from other organizations that have provided the KBs with ideas, information and research reports.

2.2.3. Organizational unit size

As organizations increase in size, KB may face increasing difficulty to recognize and recombine appropriate knowledge, as well as increasing difficulty to share what they know with the appropriate individuals in their organizations (Hargadon, 2002:75-76; Spenser, 2003; Cillo, 2005). Furthermore, as organizations increase in size, they become more specialized, and separations that help organizational units to keep focus also hamper communication and information sharing across organizational units (Hargadon and Sutton, 2000). In this paper, organizational unit size (LNSIZE) was measured by the total number of employees in the KB's organizational unit. This variable was matched with the normal distribution using a logarithmic transformation.

2.3. Control variables

Two control variables were added: the professional status of the KBs and the type of organizations where the KBs carry out their professional activities. The professional status was measured with a series of binary variables defined in reference to the current professional status of the KB. The types of organizations where the KBs primarily carry out their professional activities were measured with a series of binary variables.

3. Data collection

All individuals included in the population were contacted for an interview. The questionnaire and the 429 names composing the population were sent to a private survey firm using the CATI (computer-assisted telephone interviewing) technology, which allows embedding data coding and data entry simultaneously within the data collection phase. The survey was administered by telephone between November 24, 2005 and February 08, 2006. Out of the 429 individuals, 17 respondents were found to be ineligible (e.g., individuals not involved in knowledge brokering activities, or had changed jobs and were no longer involved in professional activities related to knowledge brokering), 63 respondents could not be reached after many telephone calls. In order to increase the response rate, 169 individuals were contacted by email to inform them about the study, its objectives and its sponsors. A total of 39 individuals refused to participate in the study (after a recall). Finally, the survey generated 301 usable questionnaires for a net response rate of 74.69%.

The questions used to survey the respondents never mentioned the expressions "knowledge brokers" and "knowledge brokerage" in order to avoid suggesting that there were good or bad answers. Furthermore, the approach used in this study did not attempt to associate knowledge brokerage activities to a particular definition of knowledge brokerage. Instead, the research strategy used in this study relied on an empiricist approach which led us to ask respondents what they do, how they do it and why they do what they do regarding knowledge management in terms of the acquisition, adaptation, and exchange of knowledge. Therefore, individual respondents could not, in advance, be considered as knowledge brokers or non-knowledge brokers. The research strategy developed for this study aimed at capturing the diversity of the respondents' practices regarding their activities associated to knowledge brokering as part of the knowledge management strategy of Canadian healthcare organizations.

4. Results

4.1. Descriptive statistics

As can be seen in the first part of Table 1, the results of the copulas approach classified the respondents in the four different profiles as follows: 111 respondents or 37.4% of the sample in the neutral role, 17 respondents or 5.7% in the relational role, 111 respondents or 37.4% in the Intellectual role, and 58 respondents or 19.5% in integrative role. The integrative role is the gold standard for knowledge brokering.

The descriptive statistics of the explanatory variables used in this study are reported in Table 1. The average number of knowledge sources from which the 297 KBs acquired studies and research reports in their day-to-day professional activities was 5.68 sources, with a standard deviation of 3.40 sources. The average experience of the respondents, as measured by the number of years of relevant experience in their current job, was 8.64 years, with a standard

Dependent variable: Knowledge Broker's role profile		**Number of cases**		**Percentage**		
• Neutral role		111		37.4		
• Relational role		17		5.7		
• Intellectual role		111		37.4		
• Integrative role		58		19.5		
Total		**297†**		**100.0**		
Independent Variables	**Type of variables**	**Min.**	**Max.**	**Mean**	**Standard deviation**	**Cronbach's ∝**
Continuous variables:						
• Knowledge Sources Assets	Continuous: number	0	15	**5.68**	3.40	--
• Experiential Assets	Continuous: number	0	36	**8.64**	7.56	--
• Organizational Investment in Knowledge Sharing	Index: 5 items	5	25	**17.38**	5.06	.86
• Knowledge from other Organizations	Continuous: number	0	10	**2.74**	2.32	--
• Organizational Unit Size	Continuous: number	1	2700	**44.43**	183.84	--
Categorical variables:						
• Cognitive Assets	• Bachelor's and less degree • Master's degree • PhD degree					16.5% 55.9% 27.6%
• Professional Status	• Top (or executive manager): • Middle manager: • First-line manager: • Professional:					25.6% 29.3% 7.1% 38.0%
• Types of organizations	• Health Care Administrations: • Health Care Settings Organizations: • Universities & Other Research Organizations • Foundations & Funding Agencies: • Private Firms:					38.0% 17.8% 28.4% 10.4% 5.4%

† 4 observations in the one or the two indices used to construct the four profiles were missing data. Hence the total number of observations dropped from 301 to 297

Table 1. Descriptive Statistics

deviation of 7.56 years. As for the average number of employees in the respondents' organizational unit, it was 44.43, with a standard deviation of 183.84. On average, the respondents scored 17.38 out of a possible maximum of 25 on the index of organizational investments in knowledge-sharing. The descriptive statistics also show that 16.5% of the respondents have completed a bachelor's or less degree, 55.9% have completed a master's degree, and 27.6% have completed a PhD degree. As for the current professional status of the respondents, the figures of Table 1 show that 25.6% were top managers, 29.3% middle managers, 7.1% were first-line managers, and 38% professionals. Finally, the answers to the question about the type of organizations where the respondents primarily carry out their professional activities indicated that out of the 297 respondents, 38% worked in healthcare administrations, 17.8% in healthcare settings organizations, 28.4% in universities or other research organizations, 10.4% in non-profit foundations or funding agencies, and 5.4% in private firms.

We checked the correlation matrix between the continuous independent variables used in the regression models to test for multi-collinearity (Table 2). Our results indicate absence of multi-collinearity problems.

	SOURCES	EXPER	SHARE	KOTHE	LNSIZE
SOURCES	1	.099	.300	.452	.040
EXPER		1	.094	.040	.147
SHARE			1	.376	.166
KOTHE				1	.066
LNSIZE					1

Table 2. Correlations between continuous explanatory variables

4.2. Analytical plan

Five situations were considered relevant in our investigation aiming to identify the factors which would increase the likelihood that individuals would adopt a higher-value-adding-role profile rather than a lower-value-adding-role profile: 1) a profile of knowledge broker rather than one of neutral role; 2) a profile of integrative role rather than one of relational role; 3) a profile of integrative role rather than one of the Intellectual role; 4) a profile of relational role rather than one of neutral role; and 5) an Intellectual role rather than one of neutral role. A multinomial Logit regression was estimated to ascertain the first three situations, while two bivariate logit regressions were estimated to identify the factors increasing the likelihood that a neutral role adopts a relational role and an intellectual role.

4.3. Specification of the multinomial logit model

For the multinomial logit regression, the qualitative dependent variable used is the KBs' roes determined by the copulas approach presented previously. The four alternative roles are 1, 2, 3 and 4, with 1) being the assessment that the respondent adopted a neutral role (low in cognitive functions and low in social functions); 2) the assessment that the respondent adopted

http://dx.doi.org/10.5772/54802

a relational role (low in cognitive functions and high in social functions); 3) the assessment that the respondent adopted an intellectual roe (high in cognitive functions and low in social functions); and 4) the assessment that the respondent adopted an integrative role (high in cognitive functions and high in social functions), identified as the reference category in our model.

The probability of choosing a profile category k (k=1,2,3,4) is given by:

$$Prob_{ik} = \frac{e^{\beta_k X_i}}{1 + \sum_{k=1}^{4} e^{\beta_k X_i}} \tag{2}$$

where X_i is the matrix of profile attributes and β_k is m x 1 vector of parameters.

As is the case of bivariate logit models, coefficients for reference choice are set equal to zero. Such normalization will be taken into account when interpreting the rest of model coefficients. In our case, the profile corresponding to integrative role is seen as the gold standard and taken as a reference category and, as a consequence, the estimated parameters will be interpreted in the following sense:

$$\begin{aligned}
&\frac{\text{Prob}_{i1}}{\text{Prob}_{i4}} = \frac{e^{\beta_1 X_i}}{e^{\beta_4 X_i}} = e^{(\beta_1 - \beta_4)Xi} = e^{\beta_1 X_i} \\
&\frac{\text{Prob}_{i2}}{\text{Prob}_{i4}} = \frac{e^{\beta_2 X_i}}{e^{\beta_4 X_i}} = e^{(\beta_2 - \beta_4)Xi} = e^{\beta_2 X_i} \\
&\text{and} \\
&\frac{\text{Prob}_{i3}}{\text{Prob}_{i4}} = \frac{e^{\beta_3 X_i}}{e^{\beta_4 X_i}} = e^{(\beta_3 - \beta_4)Xi} = e^{\beta_3 X_i}
\end{aligned} \tag{3}$$

or

$$\begin{aligned}
&Ln(\frac{\text{Prob}_{i1}}{\text{Prob}_{i4}}) = (b_1 - b_4)X_i = b_1 X_i \\
&Ln(\frac{\text{Prob}_{i2}}{\text{Prob}_{i4}}) = (b_2 - b_4)X_i = b_2 X_i \\
&\text{and} \\
&Ln(\frac{\text{Prob}_{i3}}{\text{Prob}_{i4}}) = (b_3 - b_4)X_i = b_3 X_i
\end{aligned} \tag{4}$$

From (3), the estimated coefficients, for instance, β_{1j} (j = 1,....,m), are interpreted as the marginal change in the logarithm of the odds that the respondents were profiled as adopting a neutral role over the category indicating that they were profiled as adopting an integrative role, due to a marginal change in the attribute j. However, while marginal changes in the logarithm of the odds are not always intuitively understandable, we can use the exponential of parameters also referred to as odds ratios. They offer a straightforward model interpretation. Indeed, $\exp(\beta_{1j})$ is the factor by which the odds change when the jth independent variable increases by one unit. If β_{1j} is positive, this factor, i.e., $\exp(\beta_{1j})$, will be higher than 1, which means that the odds are increased. On the contrary, if β_{1j} is negative, $\exp(\beta_{1j})$ is less than 1, implying that the odds are decreased. And if β_{1j} is 0, $\exp(\beta_{1j})$ is equal to 1, which leaves the odds unchanged. For example, for a continuous variable such as the organizational unit size, $\exp(\beta_{1j})$ measures the factor by which the odds of being profiled as neutral role instead of integrative role changes when the organizational unit size is increased by one unit. In an analogous way, if attribute j is a dummy variable, the exponential of parameters, i.e., $\exp(\beta_{1j})$, measures the factor of change in the odds with respect to the reference variable.

4.4. Results of the multinomial logit regression

The regression results of the Multinomial Logit model are summarized in the first part of Table 3 (Panel A). The model has acceptable predictive power, with 59.5% of correct predictions. The value of the Nagelkerke R^2 is.425, which is very good for qualitative dependent variable models. Furthermore, the computed value of the likelihood ratio (i.e., 143.15) is much larger than the critical value of the chi-squared statistic at the 1 percent level, with 39 degrees of freedom. This suggests that the null hypothesis, that all the parameter coefficients (except the intercept) are all zeros, is strongly rejected. Consequently, the model is significant at the 1 percent level. With regard to the variables explaining the likelihood that the respondents adopt a profile of integrative role rather than any of the three other profiles, the three individually controlled resources variables, namely knowledge sources assets, experiential assets, and cognitive assets, have a significant impact in the three situations considered in the Multinomial Logit model. More specifically, increases in the index of respondents' knowledge sources assets (SOURCES) and increases in their experiential assets (EXPER) increase the likelihood that respondents play an integrative role rather than a neutral role, a relational role, or an intellectual role. Likewise, respondents who have completed a PhD degree are more likely to play an integrative role than those who have completed lower degrees. Two out of the three organizationally controlled resources variables do not explain the likelihood that respondents play an integrative role rather than a neutral role, a relational role, or an Intellectual role. However, increasing the index of acquisition of knowledge from other organizations (KOTHE) increases the probability that respondents play the integrative role rather than the Intellectual role.

Finally, regarding the control variables, the results reported in Panel A of Table 3 also show that being a top or middle manager (MANAG), instead of being a professional, decreases the likelihood that respondents play an integrative role rather than a relational role, whereas being a first-line manager (FIRST), instead of being a professional, decreases the likelihood that respondents adopt an integrative role rather than a neutral role or a relational role. As for the

http://dx.doi.org/10.5772/54802

	PANEL A: Multinomial Logit Estimation						PANEL B: Binary Logit Estimation			
Dependant variables	Neutral to Integrative		Relational to Integrative		Intellectual to Integrative		Neutral to Relational		Neutral to Intellectual	
Independent variables	*Coeff. β*	*EXP (β)*	*Coeff. β*	*EXP (β)*	*Coeff. β*	*EXP (β)*	*Coeff. β*	*EXP (β)*	*Coeff. β*	*EXP (β)*
Individual Variables										
Knowledge Sources Assets [SOURCES]	.482***	1.619	.210**	1.234	.262***	1.299	.176***	1.193	.210***	1.234
Cognitive Assets:										
Bachelor's Degree [BACH] [a]		.352	-2.465***	.085	-1.027**	.358	1.196	3.305	-.075***	.928
Master's Degree [MAST] [a]	-1.120***	.326	-2.082***	.125	-1.044***	.352	.810	2.248	-.055***	.947
Experiential Assets [EXPER]	.073***	1.075	.139***	1.149	.071***	1.073	-.053**	.948	.002	.935
Organizational variables										
Organizational Investment in Knowledge Sharing [SHARE]	.035	1.035	-.050	.951	-.015	.985	.109*	.468	.050*	1.051
Knowledge from other Organizations [KOTHE]	.040	1.041	-.091	.913	.141*	1.151	.102	1.108	-.077	.354
Organizational Unit Size [LNSIZE]	-.029	.971	-.107	.898	-.108	.898	.046	1.047	.087	.457
Control Variables										
Professional Status:										
• Manager [MANAG] [b]	-.326	.722	-1.120**	.326	-.151	.860	.650	1.915	-.236	.790
• First-line [FIRST] [b]	-2.142**	.117	-1.887**	.151	-.835	.434	-.544	.580	-1.312**	.269
Types of Organization:										
• Health Care Administrations [ADM] [c]	-.248	.780	.636	1.889	-.238	.788	-.759	.468	-.029	.971
• Universities & Other Research Organizations [RESEAR] [c]	1.060**	2.866	1.725**	5.612	.368	1.445	-.253	.777	.742*	2.100
• Foundations & Funding Agencies [FUND] [c]	1.077*	2.936	.723	2.061	1.360**	3.896	-.012	.988	-.227	.797
• Private Firms [PRIVATE] [c]	-.317	.728	.183	1.201	-.687	.503	-1.924	.146	.272	1.312
Intercept	-4,338		1.583		-2.479		-5.522			
Number of cases: (Total = 291)	110/58		17/58		106/58		110/17		110/106	
Chi-square (d.f.):			143.15 (39)				22.92 (13)		35.70 (13)	
Nagelkerke R^2(Pseudo *R* Square):			.425				.303		.203	
Percentage of correct predictions:			59.5%				88.2%		69.4%	

[a] PhD Degree is the reference category. [b] Professional is the reference category. [c] Health Care Settings Organizations is the reference category. *, ** and *** indicate that variable is significant at 10%, 5% and 1% level respectively.

Note: Exp(β) is the factor of change in the odds of the dependent variable, due to one unit increase in the specific independent variable.

Table 3. Analytical results

types of organizations, the respondents who primarily carry out their professional activities in universities or other research organizations (RESEAR) are more likely than those employed by healthcare settings organizations (hospitals and private clinics) to adopt an integrative role rather than a neutral role or a relational role. Likewise, respondents who primarily carry out their professional activities in non-profit foundations or funding agencies (FUND) are more likely than those employed by healthcare settings organizations to play the integrative role rather than the neutral role or the Intellectual role.

4.5. Specification of the binary logit models

Since the Multinomial Logit regression permits comparison only with regard to one reference category like we did by using the integrative role as reference category, two bivariate logit regressions are also estimated to capture two other relevant situations that refer to the likelihood that the respondents in the neutral role be either in the relational role or in the intellectual role group.

For each of these two situations, the following equation was estimated:

$$Log(P_i / 1 - P_i) =$$

$$b_0 + b_1 SOURCES + + \ b_2 BACH + b_3 MAST + \ + b_4 EXPER + b_5 SHARE + b_6 KOTHE +$$

$$+ \ b_7 LNSIZE + b_8 MANAG + b_9 FIRST + b_{10} ADM + b_{11} RESEAR + b_{12} FUND + b_{13} PRIVATE$$

where, $b_i (i = 0 \ldots \ldots .13)$ are the coefficients.

Log (P_i/1-P_i) is the logarithm of the ratio of the probability that a neutral role be in the profile of a relational role or in that of the Intellectual role, relative to the probability that the same neutral role would be in none of these two profiles.

4.6. Results of the binary logit regressions

The regression results of these binary Logit models are summarized in Panel B of Table 3. The computed value of the Chi-square statistics for each of the two Logit regressions is greater than its critical value (i.e., 27.69) with 13 degrees of freedom at the 1% level. The two equations have good predictive power, with 88.2% and 69.4% of overall correct predictions for the situation corresponding to being in a relational role rather than in one of neutral role, and for the situation corresponding to being in an Intellectual role rather than in one of neutral role. Finally, the value of Nagelkerke pseudo R^2 is.303 for the first binary Logit regression and.203 for the second one, which is quite reasonable for qualitative dependent variable models. The variable individual knowledge sources assets was the only one that significantly explains the likelihood that respondents have of being in a profile of relational role rather than in one of neutral role, and of being in an Intellectual role rather than in one of relational role. Moreover, the positive sign of this variable suggests that increases in the index of the respondents' knowledge sources assets (SOURCES) increase the probability that respondents adopt a relational role or an intellectual role rather than a neutral role. Likewise, the respondents who have completed a PhD degree are more likely than others to adopt the Intellectual role instead of adopting a neutral role. However, the respondents' cognitive assets were not found significant to explain the likelihood that the respondents perform a relational role rather than a neutral role. Finally, increases in the index of the respondents' experiential assets (EXPER) decrease the probability that respondents perform a relational role rather than a neutral role. The variable organizational investments in knowledge-sharing (SHARE) is the only organizationally controlled resources variable that was found to be positively and significantly related to the likelihood of respondents being relational role or the Intellectual Profile rather than neutral role. With regard to the control variables, the results reported in Panel B of Table 3 show that being a first-line manager (FIRST) decreases the likelihood who the respondents adopt an Intellectual role rather than neutral role, whereas the respondents that primarily carry out their professional activities in universities or other research organizations are more likely than those employed by healthcare settings organizations to adopt the Intellectual role rather than neutral role.

5. Discussion and conclusion

The purpose of this paper was exploratory and it aimed to inspire more conceptual and quantitative studies on knowledge brokering core functions, not to validate or invalidate particular conceptual approaches. Instead of adopting a particular definition of knowledge brokers and knowledge brokering, we have conceptually and empirically defined the concept of knowledge broker in reference to two dimensions that literature present as being tightly interdependent but have never explored empirically in a quantitative study: Theses dimensions are the social function and the cognitive function on which KBs can achieve a high or low performance. The combination of these functions generated four KBs role profiles: neutral role, relational role, Intellectual role, and integrative role. The individuals who adopt the integrative role in carrying out their professional activities are the ones who contribute the most significantly to effectively manage knowledge 9internal to their organization and external) and improve the creation of value for their organizations. Such a perspective invites to consider factors that would help individuals to move from one profile to another, up to the profile of the integrative role. Such factors were considered in terms of resources controlled either by individuals or the organizations where they primarily carry out their professional activities.

The results of the regression models suggest that individually controlled resources such as the proactive role of KBs in searching for ideas, information and reports from various sources located in other organizations, their level of education and experience, are the major drivers of knowledge brokering activities. Organizationally controlled resources do not seem to help individuals as much to improve their knowledge brokering performance. Indeed, organizational investments only help to move from a profile of neutral role to a profile of relational role or intellectual role: in other words, these investments help only to move from the lowest performance to a slightly better knowledge brokering performance. Furthermore, increasing the variety of external organizations that provide ideas, information and reports to KBs helps these individuals to evolve from an Intellectual role to one the integrative role. Finally, it is worth pointing out that the number of employees in the respondents' organizational units had no impact on their performance in performing the KBs core functions. The fact that individually controlled resources are the major drivers of knowledge brokering activities suggests that knowledge brokering is still an emerging role that is not yet formally institutionalized, even in large healthcare organizations. In such an informal context, individuals engaged in knowledge brokering activities have to rely primarily on resources that are individually, rather than organizationally, provided. The resource-based approach to knowledge brokering adopted in this study has implications for how organizations might enhance their knowledge brokering capabilities by better exploiting the resources that contribute to improve and value the cognitive and social function of KBs in healthcare organizations. By focusing the attention on resources as explanatory variables of knowledge brokering, the results of this paper allow to derive implications for how healthcare organizations might improve their knowledge brokering capabilities. Hence, the results of this study suggest that managers would improve the knowledge brokerage capability of their personnel by investing resources to:

- Reinforce the cognitive function and its related knowledge absorptive capability by relying on individuals who have completed doctoral degrees, the so-called highly qualified personnel (HQP);
- Increase the knowledge capability of neutral role, relational role and Intellectual role by relying on individuals that have many years of experience;
- Facilitate the graduation of individuals from neutral role, relational role and Intellectual role to the integrative role by supporting the effort of individuals to expand their sources of ideas, information and reports from other organizations.
- Support organizational investments in various knowledge-sharing mechanisms.

In devising their policy interventions, managers of healthcare organizations should also keep in mind that professionals are more likely to improve the cognitive and social function capabilities than top, middle and first-line managers, and that individuals that primarily carry out their professional activities in universities, research organizations, foundations and funding agencies are also more likely to improve the networking and learning functions than the professionals carrying out their professional activities in other types of organizations.

Our results offer some interesting information for those who are involved in human resources management. We have identified critical criteria that may be used as indicators to select a knowledge broker during a job interview. We name here: 1) intellectual assets or qualifications (holding a PhD), 2) number of years in the organization (local experience), 3) past experience in universities, research organizations, foundations and funding agencies (research experience), 4) social assets (extend and variety of personal network) and 5) Research skills (scientific and governmental databases knowledge). However, individual skills and capabilities need an organizational infrastructure to help them perform in their role, especially the integrative role. Organizations have to invest in knowledge management and brokering through the improvement of access to information (databases, internet...) and the implementation of sustainable diversified mechanisms of knowledge sharing (organization of workshops, training courses and continuing professional education credits; and attendance to conferences and colloquiums as well as the scientific one as the professional ones).

http://dx.doi.org/10.5772/54802

This exploratory study suffers form limitations that could inspire future research. First, our survey was based on a self-reported questionnaire that may imply a social desirability. However, we used some strategies to reduce its impact on the validity of the collected data. We did not precise that the questionnaire was targeting the exploration of KBs role neither their performance in this role. In such way they were not feeling as being assessed. Second, the minor role played by the organizational resources that support knowledge brokerage should be considered as an invitation to consider other types of organizational investments in future research. Third, although our quantitative study revealed factors that explain why individuals adopt different brokering profiles, the study does not provide a temporal perspective on the development of brokering. Fourth, the study covered healthcare organizations and may therefore reflect the idiosyncrasies of this particular sector of activity. Fifth, knowledge brokering may fail. The outputs of knowledge brokers can be ignored or rejected. One limit of this study is that it did not take into account the recipient's (in)ability to value, assimilate and apply the knowledge translated by the KBs, in short, this paper did not consider the knowledge absorptive capacity of the recipients (Cohen and Levinthal, 1990; Zahra and George, 2002). Future research could be inspired by these limits and may help to improve knowledge about key attributes and responsibilities of KBs, and give more suggestions for improving this role in healthcare organizations.

The central role of KBs is to provide policy, decision-makers and managers with the best (accurate, relevant and feasible) information available on how to redesign the healthcare structures and processes to efficiently respond to the challenge of decision-making in a dynamic political, economic, epidemiologic and demographic environment. The novelty of the KB role in healthcare organizations provide a unique opportunity to assess the need for and reaction to clarify precisely its associated activities and the requested skills and conditions for the performance of its critical functions, and clearer direction on how to move forward with it to leverage knowledge management in knowledge based organizations. This research has practical implications for public health organizations in Canada and elsewhere in the world. Public health decision makers and managers are facing systemic challenges and constraints. Thus, they need to adequately understand the critical factors (individual and organizational) of knowledge management to foster their organization's performance. Knowledge brokers (KB) are seen as major KT strategic agents for fostering EI/BDM in public health organizations. Our results show that attention should be placed on organizational openness to innovation and innovative approaches, strategic KB recruitment and KB's professional stability in the organization. Knowledge brokering performance is tightly related to supportive mechanisms. Nevertheless, our results are context sensitive (Canadian organizations); they shed light on what is strategically to be undertaken in public health organizations in general. Thus, we clearly show that top-managers have to identify a middle manager with at least a 10 year experience in the organization, holding a PhD and having an extended relational capital (in and out of their organization and as well as in governmental as in private organizations and universities). Moreover, research competencies are highly requested (in terms of timely and relevant evidence acquisition, synthesis, adaptation and communication). This skilled professional has then to be trained as a KB (specific training and continued education for systematic reviews, policy briefings and communication skills).The organization has to provide the KB with 1) an electronic infrastructure (Internet and registration to electronic academic databases) to access and manage information and maintain social links with academia and knowledge users, and 2) adequate and sustained resources to attend relevant conferences and workshops (to be up-to-date with new evidence and extend his social network). Once these prerequisite are made available and operational in the organization, an effective monitoring and process and outcomes evaluations are needed to identify determinants of KB performance in terms of quality and cost-effectiveness of their role in public health organizations.

Acknowledgements

Dr. Jalila Jbilou contribution was supported by the CIHR Team in Familial Risks of Breast Cancer Grant (CRN-8752-1) and the Ministry of Economic Development, Innovation and Export Trade of Quebec – Supporting grant (PSR-SIIRI-701). This work is of the CIHR/CHSRF innovation and knowledge transfer chair directed by Pr Réjean Landry and co-directed by Pr Nabil Amara. We also thank Irving Gold and Julie Villeneuve from the CHSRF for their advice and support at the different stages of this project.

Author details

Réjean Landry[1], Jalila Jbilou[2*], Nabil Amara[1] and Salaheddine El Adlouni[3]

*Address all correspondence to: jalila.jbilou@umoncton.ca

1 Department of Management, Université Laval, Quebec, Canada

2 Centre de formation médicale du Nouveau Brunswick/Family medicine Unit, Vitality Health Network, Moncton, Canada

3 Department of mathematic and statistics, Université de Moncton, New Brunswick, Canada

Authors declare no conflict of interest.

References

[1] Acedo, F. J, Barroso, C, & Galan, J. L. (2006). The Resource-Based Theory: Dissemination and Main Trends. *Strategic Management Journal*. 27(7), 621-636.

[2] Amara, N, Landry, R, & Ouimet, M. (2005). Milieux innovateurs: Determinants and Policy Implication. *European Planning Studies*. 13(6), 939-965.

[3] Andersen, E. W. (2005). Two-stage Estimation in Copula Models Used in Family Studies. *Lifetime Data Anal.* 11(3), 333-350.

[4] Barney, J. (1991). Firm Resources and Sustained Competitive Advantage. *Journal of Management*. 17(1), 99-120.

[5] Barney, J. (2001). Resource-Based Theories of Competitive Advantage: A Ten-Year Retrospective on the Resource-Based View. *Journal of Management.* 27(6), 643-650.

[6] Bartram, S. M, Taylor, S. J, & Wang, Y. H. (2007). The Euro and European Financial Market Dependence. *Journal of Banking & Finance.* 31(5), 1461-1481.

[7] Basrak, B, Klaassen, C. A. J, Beekman, M, Martin, N. G, & Boomsma, D. (2004). Copulas in QTL Mapping. *Behavioural Genetics.* 34(2), 161-171.

[8] Berends, H, Van Der Bij, H, Debackere, K, & Weggeman, M. (2006). Knowledge Sharing Mechanisms in Industrial Research. *R&D Management*. 36(1), 85-95.

[9] Bhargava, H. K, & Choudhary, V. (2004). Economics of an Information Intermediary with Aggregation Benefits. *Information Systems Research.* 15(1), 22-36.

[10] Brownson, R. C, & Jones, E. (2009). Bridging the gap: translating research into policy and practice. *Prev Med,* 49(4), 313-315.

[11] Burt, R. S. (2005). *Brokerage and Closure*, Oxford University Press, New York;

[12] Cillo, P. (2005). Fostering Market Knowledge Use in Innovation: The Role of Internal Brokers. *European Management Journal.* 23(4), 404-412.

[13] Clemen, R. T, & Reilly, T. (1999). Correlations and Copulas for Decision and Risk Analysis. *Management Science.* 45(2), 208-224.

[14] Cohen, W, & Levinthal, D. A. (1990). Absorptive Capacity: A New Perspective on Learning and Innovation. *Administrative Science Quarterly*. 35(1), 128-152.

[15] Conner, K. R, & Prahalad, C. K. Theory of the Firm: Knowledge versus Opportunism. *Organization Science*. 75(5), 477-501.

[16] Dobbins, M, Robeson, P, Ciliska, D, Hanna, S, Cameron, R, Mara, O, Decorby, L, Shawna, K, & Mercer, S. (2009). A description of a knowledge broker role implemented as part of a randomized controlled trial evaluating three knowledge translation strategies. *Implementation Science* 4 (April), , 1-9.

[17] Fernandez, E, Montes, J. M, & Vazquez, C. J. (2000). Typologies and Strategic analysis of Intangible Resources: A Resource-Based Approach. *Technovation*. 20(2), 81-92.

[18] Gagliardini, P, & Gouriéroux, C. (2006). *An Efficient Nonparametric Estimator for Models with Nonlinear Dependence.* Journal of Econometrics. 137(1), 189-229.

[19] Gagnon, M. L. (2011). Moving knowledge to action through dissemination and exchange. *Journal of Clinical Epidemiology*. 64(1), 25-31.

[20] Gould, R. V, & Fernandez, R. M. (1989). *Structures of Mediation: A Formal Approach to Brokerage in Transaction Networks.* Sociological Methodology. 19(1), 89-126.

[21] Graham, I, Logan, J, Harrison, M. B, Straus, S. E, Tetroe, J, Caswell, W, & Robinson, N. (2006). Lost in knowledge translation: Time for a map? *The Journal of Continuing Education in the Health Professions,* 26(1), 13-24.

[22] Granovetter, M. (1973). The Strength of Weak Ties. *American Journal of Sociology.* 78(6), 1360-1380.

[23] Grant, R. M. (1996). Toward a knowledge-based theory of the firm. Strategic. *Management Journal.* 17(Special (109-122), 109-122.

[24] Howells, J. (2006). Intermediation and the role of intermediaries in innovation. *Research Policy.* 35(5), 715-728.

[25] Hull, J. C, & White, A. D. (2006). *Valuing Credit Derivatives Using an Implied Copula Approach.* Journal of Derivatives. 14(2), 8-28.

[26] HuysmanM & de Wit, D. (2004). Practices of Managing Knowledge Sharing: Towards a Second Wave of Knowledge Management. *Knowledge and Process Management.* 11(2), 81-92.

[27] Ipe, M. (2003). Knowledge Sharing in Organizations: A Conceptual Framework. *Human Resource Development Review.* 2(4), 337-359.

[28] Jbilou, J, Amara, N, & Landry, R. (2007). Research-based-decision-making in Canadian health organizations: A behavioural approach. *Journal of Medical Systems.* 31(3), 185-196.

[29] Kimble, C, Hildreth, P, & Wright, P. (2000). Communities of practice: Going Virtual. In *Knowledge Management and Business Innovaion.* Hershey PA USA: Idea Group Publishing.

[30] Kogut, B, & Zander, U. (1992). Knowledge of the firm, combinative capabilities,and the replication of technology. *Organization Science.* 3(3), 383-397.

[31] Landry, R, Amara, N, Pablos-mendes, A, Shademani, R, & Gold, I. (2006). Knowledge Translation- Conceptual Framework and Approaches. *Bulletin of the World Health Organization.* 84(8), 597-602.

[32] Nelsen, R. B. (1999). *An Introduction to Copulas,* Springer, New York.

[33] Newbert, S. C. (2007). Empirical Research on the Resource-Based View of the Firm: An Assessment and Suggestions for Future Research. *Strategic Management Journal.* 28(2), 121-146.

[34] Obstfeld, D. (2005). Social Networks, the Tertius Lungens Orientation, and Involvement in Innovation. *Administrative Science Quarterly.* 50(1), 100-130.

[35] Owzar, K. Jung, Sin-Ho, & Sen, P.K. ((2007). A Copula Approach for Detecting Prognostic Genes Associated With Survival Outcome in Microarray Studies. *Biometrics.* 63(4), 1089-1098.

[36] Peng, L, & Fine, J. P. (2007). Regression Modeling of Semicompeting Risks Data. *Biometrics*. 63(1), 96-108.

[37] Petersen, L, Sorensen, T. I, et al. (2006). Inference Methods for Correlated Left Truncated Lifetimes: Parent and Offspring Relations in an Adoption Study. *Lifetime Data Anal.* 12(1), 5-20.

[38] Shaw, W. T, & Lee, K. T. A. (2007). *Copula Methods vs Canonical Multivariate Distributions: the Multivariate Student T Distribution with General Degrees of Freedom*, Working Papers. Departement of Mathematics King's College, London, UK. http://www.mth.kcl.ac.uk/~shaww/web_page/papers/MultiStudentc.pdf

[39] Sklar, A. (1959). *Fonctions de répartition à n dimensions et leurs marges*, Publications de l'Institut de Statistique de l'Université de Paris 8. , 229-231.

[40] Strauss, S, Tetroe, J, & Graham, I. (2009). Knowledge translation in health care: Moving from evidence to practice. London, UK: Wiley-Blackwell.

[41] Van Kammen, J, De Savigny, D, & Sewankambo, N. (2006). Using Knowledge Brokering to Promote Evidence-based Policy-Making: the Need for Support Structures. *Bulletin of the World Health Organization*. 84(8), 608-612.

[42] Verona, G, Prandelli, E, & Sawhney, M. (2006). Innovation and Virtual Environments: Towards Virtual Knowledge Brokers. *Organization Studies.* , 27(6), 765-788.

[43] Wenger, E. (2000). Communities of practice and social learning systems. *Organisation* 7(2), 225-246.

[44] Zahra, A. S, & George, G. (2002). Absorptive Capacity: A Review, Reconceptualization, and Extension. *Academy of Management Review*. 27(2), 185-203.

Chapter 7

The Need to Measure and Manage the Cumulative Impacts of Resource Development on Public Health: An Australian Perspective

Susan Kinnear, Zobaidul Kabir, Julie Mann and Lisa Bricknell

Additional information is available at the end of the chapter

http://dx.doi.org/10.5772/54297

1. Introduction

Australia is home to several resource-intensive regions that feature vast mineral, ore and/or coal deposits pooled in one physical location (Figure 1). These areas are usually characterised by multiple medium- to large-scale extraction and processing facilities, and typically include extensive road, rail and port infrastructure. The Australian resources sector has been defined by the Commonwealth of Australia [1] as:

'mining, oil and gas operations, including operating mines, quarries, oil and gas wells, as well as constructing those operations…

(and) mining support activities such as fee-for-service activities and exploration'.

Australia's resource regions are already of significant economic value, with the latest estimates for exports in resources and energy being placed at approximately $200 billion for 2011-12 [2]. Ongoing growth is also expected, particularly in the states of Western Australia and Queensland, and this is being driven by the strong relationship between Australian and Chinese markets, together with the rise of the Indian and Chinese middle class; a high demand for natural resources (coal, power, water) and the mobility of the international skilled workforce [3].

The socio-economic and other changes associated with large-scale mineral resource extraction are key issues for regional development in Australia, and well as for other nations whose regions are undergoing a similar transition from rural-based to resource-based (for example Canada and Mongolia). In Australia, public interest and discussion on these issues has been accelerated by a Parliamentary Inquiry underway since 2011 into the use of fly-in, fly-out (FIFO) and drive-in, drive-out (DIDO) workforce practices in the regional resource sector. For example, the terms of reference for this Inquiry includes exploring the 'impacts, costs and benefits' related to the use of non-resident labour; acquiring information about services and infrastructure provision; and developing of strategies to maximise the benefits of FIFO/DIDO arrangements for employees, their families, their communities and the resources industry.

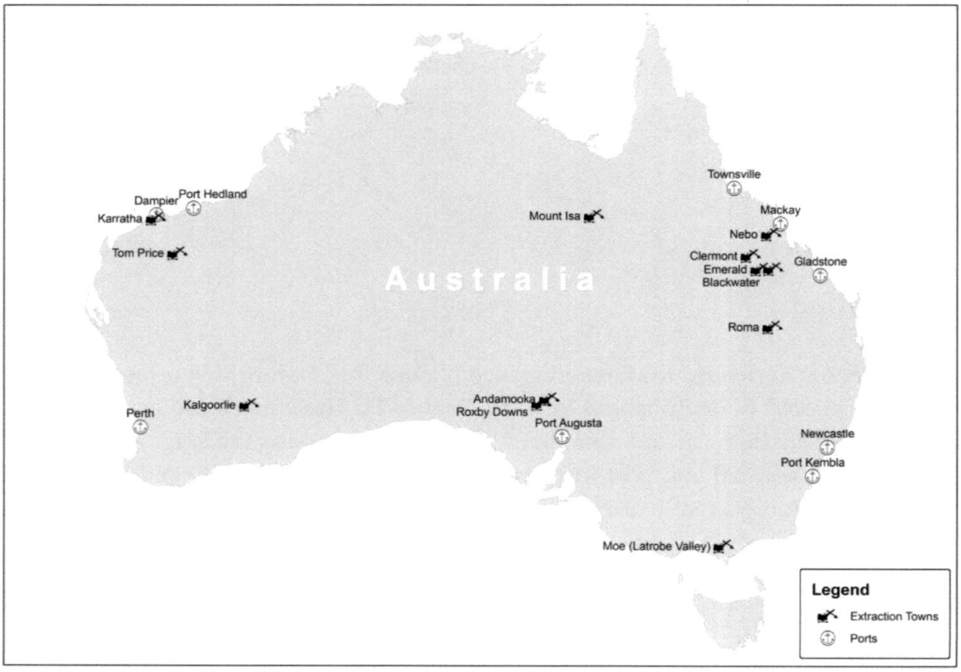

Figure 1. Examples of mining communities and ports underpinning key resource regions in Australia

Clearly, ensuring the best possible public health outcomes in resource regions is of critical importance for employers, employees and mining families as well as the broader community. However, most data relating to public health impacts - including the majority of evidence lodged in submissions to the Inquiry - are anecdotal. This likely reflects the lack of an agreed and comprehensive methodology for identifying, monitoring or managing health impacts in the context of Australian (and other) resource regions. To address this gap, this chapter explores the current evidence for public health impacts related to cumulative resource activity in regional Australia, and highlights the possible mechanisms by which this emerging health issue can be better studied and addressed.

2. Cumulative public health impacts associated with the resource sector

Large scale natural resource extraction activities (for example, mining, oil and gas) can have significant impacts on the health and well-being of both resource sector employees, as well as the communities living in surrounding areas. For the purposes of this chapter, the definition of '*cumulative impacts*' shall be adopted from that provided in [4]:

'cumulative impacts are the successive, incremental and combined impacts of one, or more, activities on society, the economy and the environment... (these) may be the product of past, present or future activities... can be both positive and negative and can vary in intensity as well as spatial and temporal extent'.

Cumulative impacts can therefore occur at the project-level (for example where repeated activities are undertaken at the same site); regional-level (for example multiple projects in close proximity); or even be of wider manifestation (for example global climate change). Cumulative impacts arise from both natural events as well as human activities [5], but the most critical part of the definition is that the impacts are associated with more than one activity over time. As noted by [5]: 'one impact by itself may not be a cause for concern; it might even seem insignificant. However, the addition of many small impacts over time adds to the end result – cumulative effects and an increase for concern. Cumulative impacts can also arise from interactions between issues, which may trigger a new 'tipping point' and the transition to a substantially different situation [4].

With respect to public health issues, a range of cumulative impacts can (and are) emerging due to rapid growth in the Australian resource sector. The range of public health concerns associated with the resources sector in Australia can be considered under the categories of direct and indirect impacts for resource sector employees; and direct and indirect impacts to communities that host mining operations; as well as positive impacts and other linkages. Whilst the extent of public health impacts of the resource sector could also be extended to include the potentially negative and flow-on consequences associated with global climate change [6]; this is outside the scope of this chapter.

2.1. Health impacts for resource sector employees

The health impacts for resource sector employees can be roughly divided into two categories: one, the direct risks or hazards related to performing activities on site, or in travelling to a worksite; and two, the indirect impacts that may be related to sleep, nutrition and other lifestyle patterns related to rostering arrangements.

2.1.1. Direct impacts

According to [7], the mining industry reported 14.9 compensation claims for serious injuries per 1,000 employees in 2009-10, which is well above the average rate for all industries combined (at 12.6 claims/1,000 employees). Furthermore, these data may under-represent the actual rate for resource-extraction activities, as many people within the mining industry are employed by construction firms, and thus their claims are logged to the construction sector. Fatalities for the mining industry occurred at a rate of 3.5/10,000 employees, which is also substantially higher than the average for all workers (at 1.9/10,000 employees) [7].

Accidents and injuries associated with the movement of large vehicles and/or the transport of materials remain as the key issue for mining workforces. Data from [8] indicates body stressing represented almost half of the workplace health and safety claims lodged in Australia in 2010-11. Within this, occupations such as machinery operations/drivers, technician/trade workers and labourers recorded amongst the highest number of insurance claims. Conservative predictions indicate that labour force requirements for mining operations in Australia will increase by 44 per cent between 2010 and 2016, and that growth is likely to be in the at-risk occupations including machinery operators and drivers, followed by technicians and trade workers [9]. As the mining workforce grows to meet production targets and expanded industry activity, it could reasonably be expected that so too, the number of workplace incidents in this category will increase in Australia. On the other hand, the mining sector is also increasing the use of simulation and automation, which may reduce employee exposure to hazards.

There are also a range of other direct health impacts likely to be associated with employment in the resource sector, including exposures to hazardous substances such as silica, dust, caustic products and other substances used in resource extraction, raw materials transport, and minerals processing. A detailed exposition of these is not possible within the limits of this chapter; furthermore, it would appear that statistics on worker exposures are relatively limited, especially in terms of being regionally specific.

2.1.2. Indirect health impacts

Occupational fatigue is of particular concern for resource industry workers. The indirect effects of shift-rostering and commuting have received much attention, particularly in Queensland and Western Australia, where there is now a growing a trend for greater proportions of the workforce to be non-resident employees. This requires a commute to the worksite via drive-in, drive-out (DIDO) or fly-in, fly-out (FIFO) arrangements; whereupon (typically) twelve-hour block shifts are undertaken, before returning to mining camps where meals and accommodation are provided. Employees return to their homes located in other centres during the intervening off-shift periods. A recent review [10] synthesized a wide range of available literature and concluded that shift work was associated with higher risk of both coronary and cerebrovascular events, with shift employees having a 23 per cent increased chance of suffering a heart attack and 5 per cent increased chance of experiencing a stroke. These risk factors were maintained after adjustment for socio-economic status, however, the study was conducted across all shift work types (including mining, transport, healthcare and others). An earlier analysis [11] specific to Australian fly-in fly-out mining shift workers, reported that interruptions to sleep and circadian rhythms represented very real safety risks, with the performance effects exceeding that of a 0.05% blood alcohol concentration, particularly near the end of night shifts.

There have been reports of problems with workers binging on alcohol and drugs either at work camps, or within the general community, from Australia as well as internationally (for example [12]). The true extent of vulnerability to drug and alcohol abuse remains difficult to judge given that some reports are anecdotal rather than empirical. States such as Queensland have already identified that high levels of unhealthy behaviours are a key challenge to improving public health [13]; but the contribution of the burgeoning resource-sector to this has never been measured.

There have been some reports to suggest that mining employees are placed at higher risk of contracting infectious disease, as a result of living in close quarters with others in mining camps, as well as the high mobility of the non-resident workers, who may carry diseases into the community from far afield [14].

Mental health concerns appear to be poorly understood in the mining sector [15]. There have been few statistically rigorous empirical studies, but the weight of anecdotal evidence is large and growing. One group has reported a range of mostly negative impacts of FIFO and DIDO arrangements on employee wellbeing, albeit from a small sample size [16]. Here, impacts included implications for primary relationships, inability to participate in organised sport, loneliness, mood swings and disturbed sleep. Indeed, the lack of support that non-resident employees have, sometimes combined with a culture of non-disclosure amongst 'macho' males, is likely to be compounding mental health issues at worksites [15]. By contrast, problems in psychosocial health and wellbeing have been less commonly cited for the resident mining employees. It appears that, compared with non-residents, resident employees enjoy better shift arrangements and report greater job satisfaction and wellbeing levels [17], presumably linked with the ability to receive better support from family and friends, as well as avoiding the strain of travelling.

Finally, the issue of negative reproductive health outcomes for mining workers remains contentious. There have been assertions that mining lifestyles featuring high disposable incomes and extended periods of time away from family can prompt the use of paid sex, triggering rising rates of gonorrhoea, syphilis and chlamydia. However, this has also been argued against, with several authors pointing to a lack of any real evidence, as well as misconceptions about the real nature of sex work and its linkages to sexually transmitted diseases [18-19].

2.2. Direct impacts on resource regions

A range of direct health impacts are already known from in communities that host minerals extraction and processing activities. Each phase in the lifecycle of coal production is associated with pollutants that affect human health [6]. In America, residents of coal-mining areas face increased risk of cardiopulmonary disease, chronic obstructive pulmonary disease, hypertension and lung and kidney diseases, compared with populations of non-mining regions [20, 21]. The burning of coal for electricity generation is also hazardous to human health, including workers and community residents. For example, the Australian Academy of Technological Sciences and Engineering [22] estimated that coal burning in Australia was associated with some $AU2.6 billion in impacts to the national health burden. This included the problems associated with particulate matter as well as NOx and SOx emissions. The modelling used in this report showed the damage cost for both primary and secondary pollutants, and illustrated that the damage costs are roughly proportional to the regional population density [22]. Consequently, as regional populations are swelled by growth in resource-sector jobs, it follows that the regional health burden is also likely to grow.

2.3. Indirect impacts on resource regions

2.3.1. Flow-on impacts to partners and families

The partners and families of resource sector employees can experience a wide range of adverse health impacts which may be related to having a member of the household working in the resource sector, and/or to living in the resource regions themselves. For example, there are anecdotal reports that child mental health in resource communities is of concern; often, this is linked with the perception that increased rates of marital separation and conflict are associated with shiftwork arrangements in the mining sector. However, [23] reported that the psychosocial wellbeing of children from FIFO families was not adversely impacted by work-related parental absence; rather it more often the remaining parent (typically the mother) who reported difficulties, especially the need to manage family cohesion during long periods of separation. This was echoed by [16] who recorded difficulties for FIFO/DIDO partners, including depression and other emotional challenges that emerge from having to cope whilst the employee was absent during shifts. Noted elsewhere was anecdotal evidence that suggests '...depression, anxiety, post-traumatic stress disorder, social phobias and substance abuse disorders are almost as likely to be found in the stay-at-home partner as they are in the FIFO worker' [15]. Thus, problems of isolation, cultural change and difficult social environments emerge within family units, as well as in the wider community [24]. It is important to note also that FIFO/DIDO arrangements introduce the potential for negative public health outcomes to be experienced beyond resource-region townships, extending instead into the source communities from which the FIFO/DIDO labour is supplied.

Health issues relating to mining 'boom' periods in Canada run in the themes of family health, women's health, mental health, worker's health and health and social services [25]. Specific impacts included concerns about divorce, violence, stress, increased rates of pregnancies (presumably unwanted) and sexually transmitted diseases; sexual harassment and addictions. For women's health, the availability and accessibility of transition housing and maternity care were key issues. The gender imbalance and progressive masculinisation of the workforce is also linked with increasing levels of violence and overconsumption of alcohol [26]. In a recent submission to the Australian Parliamentary Inquiry on DIDO/FIFO work practices, a regional Alcohol, Tobacco and Other Drugs

Service (ATODS) reported an increase in alcohol-related injuries in Queensland townships [27]. They also recorded a higher incidence of workplace referrals for employees returning positive drug or alcohol tests.

2.3.2. Flow-on impacts to the wider regional community

2.3.2.1. Increased demand for health infrastructure and services

Almost all resource-rich areas are located in regional and rural parts of Australia [28]. This is a critical factor when considering the public health implications of resource extraction, because regional areas are already challenged by a broad spectrum of issues related to health services and infrastructure. For example, regional Australia is often challenged by under-resourced health systems, with low service provision, issues of accessibility and quality of care, difficulties in staff attraction/retention, skills shortages, high workloads, a much higher cost of service delivery, and unique case mixes [27, 29]. People living in rural and remote areas also tend to have higher levels of disease risk factors and illness than those in major cities [30]. In particular, rural and remote residents have higher rates of injury mortality, especially road accidents; higher rates of communicable diseases, disability and homicide; and higher rates of smoking and alcohol consumption; with Aboriginal and Torres Strait Islander wellbeing being a particularly challenging issue. Consequently, the cumulative impacts of resource sector development often manifest as additional stress being placed on the aspects of regional health systems that are already under strain.

The increased demand represented by the non-resident workforce is probably the most critical of the impacts that resource sector development has on health services and infrastructure in regional Australia. The key problem here is that the FIFO/DIDO workforce are typically not included in regional statistics, and thus are not accounted for as part of the baseline population loads used to forecast need and allocate government expenditure in resource townships [31]. Unpublished research at Central Queensland University shows regional demographics calculations can substantially underestimated expected growth if the multiplier effects of the mining workforce are not considered. Consequently, health services and infrastructure in resource communities is often inadequate to cater for the rapidly growing populations associated with increased mining activity [32]. This is true for Australia as well as other countries: in Canada, development of the oil sands of northern Alberta has been linked with poor community health outcomes associated with infrastructure deficits, where the municipalities that host mining score worse than the provincial average for health indicators [33].

There are many examples available that illustrate the problems of providing health services and infrastructure in burgeoning resource communities. Recent modelling work done by [34] indicated that health and emergency services provision within Queensland's Bowen Basin is significantly undersupplied because of the combined resident and non-resident demand linked with growth in the resources sector. General practitioners [14] have noted that Central Queensland had the highest doctor-to-patient ratio in the state in July 2009 (1: 1,824), and that this was being exacerbated by the influx of population related to the resources boom. Records from their private practice at Moranbah (a key centre servicing the Bowen Basin) demonstrate clear increases in the number of non-resident patients seeking care: almost one-quarter of the patients serviced in 2011 were non-resident (that is, had home postcodes outside of the immediate local area), compared with only 18 per cent in 2007. This overburdening means the practice can no longer offer same-day service to the resident population [14]. The authors also highlighted that non-resident patients offer a more challenging case mix, for example, presenting with emergencies due to workplace accidents, fatigue-related road incidents, and/or reckless behaviour (for example drug/alcohol abuse). Furthermore, treating these patients is challenged by the lack of existing relationship with the medical staff, which can result in low cooperation, the danger of drug interaction and/or unidentified allergy risks; and dissatisfaction with perceived 'small town' medical services [14]. The increased burden on health in resource regions is particularly challenging considering that workloads for general practitioners in rural and remote settings are already higher than metropolitan areas [35].

The resource sector is also notable in the ways in which it influences the patterns of demand for health and community services. For example, in Central Queensland, the difficulties in recruiting for the mining labour force from rural and regional Australia has led to an increase in the employment of staff on 457 (skilled migrant) visas. This multicultural influx brings with it new demands in the areas of community wellbeing, such as having access to appropriate places of worship, bilingual counselling, and increased (anecdotal) incidence of mental illness due to isolation from family, and abandonment of the home country (Centacare, personal communication, August 2012). Reference [25] also noted that mining booms can pressure regional health services by changing community demographics.

2.3.2.2. Attraction and retention challenges for health-related roles

A number of challenges are faced in attracting staff to regional health and community services, particularly in resource communities. There are already recognised skills shortages in disability, physicians, nurses and allied health professionals in states such as Queensland, which house a large proportion of Australia's mining activities [36, 37]. The ratio of allied health professionals to the general population of regional centres is approximately half that of metropolitan areas, where staff retention is already a key issue [38]. This arises predominantly because of concerns about the high costs of accommodation, because regional centres that host mining activity often experiencing inflated housing prices [31, 39]. It also reflect a combination of other (often pre-existing) concerns about rural and remote health practice, including high workloads due to pre-existing low staffing levels, mandatory on-call duties, frequent overtime, limited opportunities for professional development, and poor supervision and management support [40]. Each of these can contribute to high stress levels and staff exhaustion ('burnout'), thus prompting staff to leave, and the development of a self-perpetuating cycle. The difficulties in staff attraction/retention due to high costs of living, perceived poor liveability and other issues also has negative flow-on effects in terms of the (lack of) continuity of patient care, brought about by the high staff turnover. This may manifest at both administrative (tracking of medical records) and personal levels (personalised follow-up) [41].

2.3.2.3. Economic and social costs of service delivery in resource regions

Rural and regional health services in Australia, especially primary health, already suffer from difficulties in the proper costing of service delivery. In particular, service providers are faced with tricky decisions about local service provision compared with 'outreach' services; this includes not only the economic costs but also other considerations such as employee safety, the likelihood of good patient outcomes, and the challenge of filling positions with appropriate workforce experience and skills. In servicing the burgeoning resource regions of Australia, health sector employees themselves can operate on FIFO/DIDO arrangements. However, there are already concerns about the health and safety of outreach services employees, who may experience similar issues to resource sector shift workers (as mentioned above). Staff may have the need to travel long distances to service resource-based communities, and this places them at safety risks, including extended hours of travel by road in rural areas where mobile coverage is poor; visits to the homes of (unfamiliar) clients in isolated areas; fatigue due to long days and long periods away from home; and challenges finding suitable accommodation, particularly in mining areas where much of the accommodation is booked out months in advance [37, 42].

2.3.2.4. Other impacts in resource regions

The indirect impacts of resource development may also manifest through effects on the natural environment, leading to lost ecosystem services, and the potential for flow-on impacts to human health. For example, in 2011, an outbreak of diseased fish occurred in the Gladstone harbour in Central Queensland, which is currently undergoing extensive dredging and development as part of the growth of the coal seam gas industry. A temporary ban on fishing was enacted, and there was much local concern about whether the fish were fit for human consumption, and the reason(s) for the outbreak. The Queensland government commenced a fish sampling and water quality program, including an investigation into human health concerns and the establishment of a Scientific Advisory Panel [43]; but debate continues as to whether the dredging program is responsible, with other stressors including natural parasites and the entry of floodwaters into the nearshore environment also being cited as possible contributors.

A new term was coined [44] - *solastalgia* - to represent the "distress that is produced by environmental change impacting upon people while they are directly connected to their home environment". The authors studied the community supporting the Hunter Valley, a region of New South Wales that was experiencing rapid growth in mining and power station developments, and found that resource sector developments can have a substantial impact upon emotional health of regional residents. Here, the residents were reported to experience emotional stress and mental health problems linked with a sense of powerlessness and injustice over the region's development. This problem appears to be particularly acute for those with strong connections to the land (such as generational farming families, or Indigenous Australians) [44].

2.4. Positive impacts and other linkages

The potential for positive health outcomes from resource development has hardly been studied. It was identified that increased awareness of health and safety was one possible positive outcome of cumulative development [4]. Furthermore, some workers have described the lifestyle and wellbeing benefits that a generous mining salary can provide, and point to strong camaraderie within the workplace as a positive impact of their employment [17]. The higher wages paid to mining employees could also be linked with an increased ability to purchase foods with better nutrition, access higher-quality health care, and spend discretionary income on participation in organised sport and recreational activities. Such linkages have rarely been reported in the literature, but it would seem a reasonable conclusion given that, in some instances, over half the population of resource towns can receive double the national average weekly wage [31]. The apparent lack of any published material in this area may represent a research bias towards reporting of health problems of resource regions, rather than health and wellbeing benefits.

Developed nations such as Australia also have a comparatively tight regulatory environment regarding mining sector operations, and these should reduce the potential for the direct impacts of development on local populations, such as through water or air pollution. This avoids the situation being experienced by some countries, such as Africa, rapid and poorly managed industrialisation is presenting new risks termed modern environmental health hazards (MEHHs). These MEHHs are 'products of rapid development in the absence of health and environment safeguards, as well as the unsustainable consumption of natural resources', and contribute significantly to the environmental disease burden [45].

Another encouraging sign is that there continues to be a strong focus on workplace safety in the resource sector, with particular areas of focus including being fatality-free, recording a minimum of lost time injury, and experiencing low incidence of disease [46]. In demonstrating this commitment, in recent years, the Australian Coal Association Research Program (ACARP) has funded wide-ranging health projects including exploring the dust risks for open cut mining, exhaust emissions from alternative diesel fuels, human health impacts related to the growth of toxic blue-green algae in mining-related water bodies, injury risks with underground coal mining equipment (including ergonomics and high pressure injection injuries), and mine safety regulations [47].

There are already reports of surging growth in businesses in health care and social assistance, for those regions that host resource activity. In Queensland, the health and community services sector is already the state's largest industry employer, representing 11.7 per cent of the state's total labour market [48]. In Central Queensland's Bowen Basin, Australia's premier coal-producing region, data from the Australian Bureau of Statistics shows that the number of health and social services businesses operating in this industry division has grown by almost 20% over 2008/09 to 2010/11 – the second-fastest growth sector overall, and far greater than the baseline population growth for the same period.

Finally, the last possible health benefit linked with the resource sector is the potential for improvements to health infrastructure and services, funded from mining royalties. However, it is peculiar to note that proposed trials for the National Disability Insurance (NDI) Scheme were declined by both the Western Australia and Queensland governments – despite those two states hosting the greatest proportions of resource activity in Australia; and the NDI scheme being funded from the newly introduced Minerals and Resources Rent Tax.

3. Monitoring and measuring cumulative health impacts

Health Impact Assessments (HIAs) are important tools in policy development and can be used in a wide range of planning and development applications. In their early iterations, health impacts were included as part of broader environmental impact assessment (EIA) processes, and assessments were often limited to quantitative, as opposed to qualitative, risk assessments. This process overlooked broader considerations such as cumulative impacts, intergenerational effects and broader determents of health [49]. Gradually, however, public health assessment has become more inclusive and far-reaching. This occurred first through the change in interpretation of 'environment' to include not only the biophysical elements, but also wider considerations around social, cultural and human health perspectives. Secondly, at the urging of the World Health Organisation, there was a transition for 'health' to imply not only physical health, but also the general state of wellbeing. This allowed for the health components of EIA to include not only disease-related effects, but also all impacts on human wellbeing. In this more 'mature' state, impact assessment approaches have changed with the recognition that physical and social environments are critical determinants of health overall, compared with the earlier focus for risks assessments to quantify the carcinogenic potential of single toxins. However, it can be concluded [50] that environmental health issues were not being sufficiently treated in EIA processes; in particular, while physical health impacts directly caused by environmental change were afforded some consideration, other health determinants in the social sphere were rarely, and often poorly, considered. Additionally, they noted that there is "little evidence to suggest that health concerns, particularly issues associated with social health and quality of life, carry over to the post-decision monitoring stages of the EIA" [50].

3.1. Health impact assessment in Australia

Australia has conducted HIA work for over fifteen years [51]. In 1994, a National Health and Medical Research Council (NHMRC) report emphasised that health impacts deserved special attention within EIA processes; this was followed by the publication of enHeath HIA guidelines [52] and later, the development of an equity-focused HIA framework [53, 54]. In the latter, the 'equity' approach acknowledges that vulnerable groups have special health needs, and may experience particular health impacts; it also recognises that health and wellbeing are linked with where people live, work and play [55]. Australia is now considered a leading nation in considering equity within HIAs [56].

Specific tools to identify and manage health impacts in their own right have been developed only relatively recently (since the 1990s onwards); and decision-making tools for HIA emerged in the early 2000s [49]. Most recently, in 2007, the Australian Government published a practical guide of HIA, which encourage a scope beyond environmental health, and into the broader perspectives of health determinants [56, 57]. Unfortunately, the good progress that Australia appears to have been made with HIAs overall does not appear to have been translated into managing health impacts specifically related to resource development activities.

3.2. Impact assessment for resource development activities

The disruptive nature of extractive resource activity means that particular care must be taken to understand the likely impacts of project development, and to manage them throughout the various phases of activity (construction, operations, and decommissioning). In Australia, EIA tools have been used as part of mining development applications since the pre-1980s. Whilst health impacts can be assessed and monitored within the EIA process, this is typically limited to physical risks and hazards, and rarely do the terms of reference for EIAs actually prescribe a section on health impacts. For example, current EIA statements typically include an assessment of impacts across areas such as land, water or air contamination; noise and vibration; traffic and transport and largely ignore the health and social issues [58, 59]. Project proponents are also required to prepare environmental management plans (EMPs), which partly cover health impact issues, albeit with an environment focus.

Social Impact Assessments (SIAs) have also been introduced into Australian planning and development processes. Here, the SIA process sets out to analyse the potential social consequences of projects on demographics, behaviours, social services and aspects of community wellbeing and lifestyle. Therefore, similarly to EIAs, the use of SIA tools could include some consideration of broader health impacts, particularly the indirect effects to community infrastructure and services (as described above). In Queensland, a key state for resource activity, this now includes the preparation of a companion Social Impact Management Plan (SIMP). However, undertaking HIA appears to be still at the experimental stage, being undertaken on an ad hoc basis if at all [60]. Confusingly, there is no clear guidance as to whether health impacts should be monitored within EMPs or SIMPs, or instead, whether a purpose-built Health Impact Management Plan (HIMP) is required. The issue of assessing cumulative impacts also remains unresolved, with no standard methodology for the assessment of cumulative impacts as part of either EIS or SIA reports; and nor are there specific legislative requirements as to how cumulative impacts should be addressed. In part, this may reflect the complex nature of cumulative impacts, which vary in severity and duration, depending on the timing, duration and number of concomitant construction and operational activities. Nevertheless, the weight of evidence relating to cumulative impacts clearly demonstrates the need for innovative methodological approaches to be developed, such that the range of impacts, including health impacts, can be properly accounted for during planning, approvals and operational phases.

http://dx.doi.org/10.5772/54297

4. Developing better systems to monitor, predict and manage cumulative health impacts from resource activity

The rapid pace of resource development in many Australian regions means that suitable frameworks and monitoring tools for public health impacts need to be developed urgently. Already, current data suggest that regional health infrastructure and services are overburdened and unable to cope with the rapid population growth that accompanies growth in the resource sector; let alone able to cater for new case mixes related to cumulative impacts. Despite this, adoption of cumulative health impacts has yet to be fully supported, particularly in legislation, across the varying levels of government in Australia [51] (Table 1).

Legislation and/or Terms of Reference	Relevant areas
Commonwealth Environment Protection and Biodiversity Conservation Act 1999 (March 2010)	No specific mention of cumulative impacts; though the Act requires consideration of 'reasonably foreseeable indirect impacts' by third parties. Impact is defined to include direct, indirect and reasonably foreseeable consequences of actions. Federal court rulings have interpreted the act to include cumulative impacts. The Hawke review of the EPBC act has signalled that cumulative impacts will be a focus of reform.
Queensland Environmental Protection Act 1994	The Act makes no distinction between cumulative or other impacts, but expects an EIS to assess all such impacts. The draft ToR must be 'in the approved form.' In practice this means that project ToR must be based on the generic ToR developed by the Department of Environment and Natural Resource Management.
Qld Department of Environment and Resource Management, Generic Terms of Reference for impact assessment statements (2010)	The generic ToR does not require a separate section for cumulative impacts, but rather requires them to be assessed in issue-related sections, such as those for ecology, social impacts, or noise. For example, indicative extracts from the generic ToR include: "Describe any cumulative impacts on environmental values caused by the project, either in isolation or by combination with other known existing or planned development or sources of contamination." "The cumulative impacts of the project must be considered over time or in combination with other (all) impacts in the dimensions of scale, intensity, duration or frequency of the impacts". "Where impacts from the project will not be felt in isolation to other sources of impact, it is recommended that the proponent develop consultative arrangements with other industries in the proposal's area to undertake cooperative monitoring and/or management of environmental parameters.
State Development and Public Work Organisation Act 1971	This Act addresses impacts associated with State Significant projects (as defined under the Act. However, there is no specific mention of cumulative aspects (except in environmental assessment of fishing activities).

Table 1. Examples of legislative considerations related to the assessment and monitoring of cumulative impacts in Australia and Queensland (ToR = Terms of Reference).

Monitoring programs for cumulative health effects are already in effect in regions of Canada (for example in Saskatchewan), where the focus is on detecting air, water and food web contamination. However, in Australia, monitoring programs could be designed to provide data that underpins decision-making across a broad range of health objectives. For example, these might include developing healthy lifestyles and social cohesion, and ensuring good housing quality, accessibility to health services, safety, equity, and appropriate air and water quality [61]. It could also cater for wider community development issues linked with good health outcomes, such as impacts on regional health workforce planning. It's been recommended [62] that HIAs associated with extractive industries should include a wide description of the environmental health areas impacted upon by the development, the extent of impact, as a spatial delineation of the potentially affected communities. For example, this would include traditional indicators such as communicable diseases; vector-borne illnesses; soil, water and waste-related diseases; sexual and reproductive health; food and nutrition related issues; as well as accidents and injury, hazardous exposures. Most importantly, the authors also noted the importance of considering social determinants of health, cultural health practices and health system issues as being important, and developed an innovative HIA methodology for how these could be considered in a developing-nations context [62].

Once key classes of impacts have been identified, it also would be particularly useful to determine how many people are likely to be affected. Considering the rapid and ongoing growth of the resources sector, and the regional population growth that often accompanies economic booms, it is likely that an increasing number of regional Australians will be affected by the health impacts of resource development. For example, unpublished research by CQUniversity suggests that future projections might be prepared based on expected industry growth (nature and volume of project expansion), as well as the multiplier effect that this creates for regional population growth.

Understanding and predicting cumulative effects is a challenging science, requiring both spatial and temporal considerations [5]. For cumulative public health, this also means understanding the dynamics of exposed (or potentially exposed) population groups and subgroups. It is particularly important to recognise that some population cohorts are likely to be at greater risk and disadvantage with respect to cumulative health impacts of resource development. For example, 'social apartheid' can develop in resource regions, where people with a disability, Indigenous and culturally and linguistically diverse (CALD) communities experience greater difficulty in accessing services (such as health services), compared with the general population [63]. Also, migrants have already been identified as being of greater risk of mental health disorders in resource regions [15]. This is of note given that some 18.5% of Australians have a disability [64], and 20.4% identify as CALD (speaking more than one language at home [65]. Other key groups that may be impacted include women, sole parents and the aged; and people who fit into more than one of the above categories would be considered to be at greater and more complex disadvantage. Unfortunately, there is a paucity of empirical data regarding the impacts on such groups, with work on the effects of mining on First Nations people in Canada being a notable exception [66]. Here, the concerns included issues around pollution of traditional food and water sources (by arsenic and mercury for example), and departure from the traditional diet to favour processed foods because of fears about hunting and/or gathering nearby to mining shafts, processing equipment and tailings ponds [66]. Others [12], have explored the effects of resource-extraction specifically on young people's health in the oil and gas communities of British Colombia, reporting that low education levels, addictions (alcohol, drugs) and high costs of housing were key impact areas. In Australia, new evidence is also emerging from the Parliamentary Inquiry mentioned above: for example, the following comments were made by [67]:

"...medical and dental services across Whitsunday, Isaac and Mackay have become increasingly difficult to access, particularly for low to middle income earners. The deficits include only one dentist in Moranbah, which is currently at risk of closure due to tenancy/rental issues; no pre-natal services in Bowen; (and) no full bulk billing GP surgeries in Mackay and Whitsunday or Moranbah. This significantly disadvantages youth, people with a disability, older people and low income earners."

In Australia, the options for introducing health impact assessments specifically for resource sector development in regional areas appear to be either (a) include better articulation of health impacts in the existing terms of reference for EIA or SIA processes; or (b) introduce a third impact assessment approach that specifically addresses health concerns. In both cases, overlap amongst the approaches may be a problem; and it must also be noted that both would represent an increased reporting and administrative burden on proponents and the government planning and development departments. Incorporating cumulative health impacts into existing management plans may help to streamline the process, but it must also be noted that this could result in the work being done by non-health specialists.

In considering new approaches for cumulative health impact assessments, the potential contribution of strategic-level assessments is also important for good health outcomes, given that strategic assessments are often promoted as a tool that more effectively accounts for cumulative impacts. For example, the advantages of undertaking health assessments at the wider (policy and planning) level, include:

- early consideration of health matters in planning processes
- greater certainty to the local communities and developers over future development
- reduced administrative burden for proponents and government
- capacity to achieve better health outcomes and
- the ability address cumulative impacts at the regional level.

Evaluation of impacts and communication with stakeholders about the impacts outcomes is an important aspect of managing cumulative health impacts. The number of parameters to be monitored will depend upon the potential likelihood and magnitude of the health impacts. At the same time, coordination with stakeholders particularly between the proponents, government agencies (for example health and environment agencies) and the affected community is important [68] to effectively manage the cumulative impacts. While monitoring is the responsibility of proponents, routine surveillance from environment and health sectors is also warranted. Furthermore, if health, allied health and social community/services sectors are to be properly integrated into this processes, it would be useful to identify (or in some cases, establish) peak representative groups for the key subsectors, so that consultation during development approvals can be done effectively, rather than proponents trying to engage with individual service providers.

With respect to engaging the mining sector itself, there is already strong motivation for their interest and participation in health impact assessments, even if these remain outside of current regulatory requirements. Improving employee health and wellbeing is of direct benefit to mining proponents, who may experience improved morale, reduced absenteeism, reduced staff turnover and improved productivity [15]. Engagement in the health area is also likely to pay dividends in terms of the 'social licence to operate'. Recommendations from north-west Queensland [69] encourage the use of the Framework for Health Promotion to help engage with resource sector employees and begin identifying and addressing workplace health and safety issues. Direct partnerships between mining companies and health service providers has also been suggested as one way to address the public health concerns linked with 'mining booms', particularly in the areas of health promotion and health education [12]. For example, some authors [25] have noted 'mine(s) and health authorities could engage in joint training (for) healthy living, workplace safety, nutrition ... a focus on a preventative approach'. A close examination of shift schedules and the impacts of these on worker's health, as well as flow-on impacts to partners and families, has also been called for [25].

Finally, the use of zoning may be useful in facilitating the monitoring and measurement of health impacts of a particular regional area, in a cost-effective fashion. For example, a Cumulative Management Area has been established within the Surat Basin for the purposes of managing groundwater impacts arising from the multiple coal seam gas leases now in operation [70].

5. Areas for further study

There is a severe lack of peer-reviewed material regarding environmental health from Australian resource regions [6]. There are a paucity of studies on the health impacts of existing industry, let alone the possible health benefits of new technologies used in the mining sector, or even or alternative industry sectors altogether. Furthermore, the research that has been done to date often appears constrained by relatively low sample sizes or a focus on physical safety and physical health. The lack of empirical evidence presented to the Australian Parliamentary Inquiry is of particular note, with most submissions reliant on anecdotal reports of impacts. This lack of data has implications for record-keeping, data collection and/or data availability for EIA and/or SIA practitioners; as in many cases, understanding of impacts could be significantly improved through the collection of relatively simple data. An extraordinarily good example of this is recording the postcode of residence for patients being treated in resource-regions, as done by Moranbah Medical [14], as this is a good indicator of the pressures that resource-sector employees add to regional health services. Comparing incidence rates of key issues, such as mental and reproductive health problems, in the pre-boom and post-boom phases of construction and operation may also help to identify particular health issues that are heavily linked with resource sector activity.

Specific research challenges in the area of cumulative health effects from resource development activity therefore include:

- a need for systematic and comprehensive data collection on environmental health concerns, both for employees as well as residents;
- a need to understand the role of cumulative impacts on not only physical health, but also mental health, community wellbeing;
- the development of appropriate techniques for assessing cumulative human health impacts, which has been severely lacking to date [58, 71].

The latter includes the need to model and forecast the likely influence of resource sector development on regional development dynamics, especially with respect to population growth, and the expected trends for disadvantaged groups who may require specialised services and infrastructure.

Each of these are complex issues: whilst it is already well known that the mining boom has been generating social and economic impacts, the patterns of impacts appear to vary across communities depending on the size of the impact, community structure and history, and the extent to which a non-resident workforce is involved [72]. Furthermore, as noted by [29]: 'rural and remote health is complex … (a) web of individual actions, community control, local culture, government regulation from several levels, risk management in various ways and a combination of autonomy and surveillance at all levels'.

Two further areas of study should also revolve around what constitutes good practice for the assessment of cumulative health impacts, as well as how the division of responsibility for health should be tackled between project proponents, government and community. For the former, A Good Practice Guidance on Health Impact Assessment is already available [73], but it not clear that this adequately considers cumulative impacts, especially in the context of resource sector development.

Finally, in addition to the establishment of a framework (legislation, administrative guidelines, and infrastructure) for applying HIA, the development of appropriate training, workforce development programs and broader capacity within organisations to undertake HIA is of growing concern. There is a case to ensure that cumulative impacts are identified in the training curriculum so that practitioners are aware of this emerging issue. The general visibility of environmental health requires consideration in Australia; these skill sets are needed across a range of career domains including occupational health and safety, psychology, environmental science, nursing and regional planning, so there is the potential for wider teaching of environmental health across a range of undergraduate and postgraduate programs.

The incorporation of environmental health experts into committees and panels responsible for preparing, and/or approving the impact assessments drafted for resource sector activities, has been a missing element in the past [74]. Introducing this in Australia (and elsewhere) would help to ensure that the plethora of direct and indirect health impacts linked with resource development are better identified, and generate a focus on mitigating negative outcomes as well as maximising any opportunities for public health benefits.

6. Conclusions

The cumulative health impacts of large-scale resource development are emerging as a key challenge for regional Australia. Mining employees, their partners and families, and the residents of resource regions each face a multitude of public health challenges linked with the resource sector. However, there is a lack of research data regarding employee and public health impacts in resource communities. This is a critical information gap in preparing social and environmental impact assessments, and is likely to be a key constraint in developing the accompanying management and mitigation plans. The severity of this problem is particularly highlighted when the lack of empirical data is contrasted with the large quantity of available anecdotal data, as shown by the recent submission to an Australian Parliamentary Inquiry.

The health impacts experienced by resource regions are further exacerbated by the fact that resource development activity in Australia is almost entirely located in rural and remote settings where there are already health service and infrastructure constraints, as well as fewer opportunities to access preventative health care and public health education. The expected ongoing and rapid growth in the mining sector, and the potential for multiple developments to occur in close physical and temporal proximity, introduces a further level of complexity to this challenge.

Introducing stronger and clearer requirements for the identification of cumulative health impacts within planning and development processes would be useful way to begin tacking the range of effects experienced by resource-regions. This should include a consideration of whether health impacts can be properly accommodated in existing processes (EIAs or SIAs) or whether a de novo health assessment process for resource sector activity is required. Regardless of which option is selected, there a number of mechanical issues that must be worked through, including how best to simultaneously streamline the process, ensure rigour, engage effectively with stakeholders and ensure that assessments are effective for capturing cumulative, regional-level impacts. In the short term, one practical recommendation is to ensure that EIA/SIA teams included environmental health experts.

Highlighting the cumulative health impacts of resource sector activity is an important step in working to improve the health of the population in regional Australia. It represents a good channel to increase the policy focus on regional health impacts; which may include better consideration within the 'health' portfolio, but also a number of others including those for workforce development, community services and regional development more generally. It represents a good opportunity to develop a sound business case for investment of the wealth created by the resources industry, in order to avoid adverse public health outcomes that accompany resource development.

Author details

Susan Kinnear[1*], Zobaidul Kabir[1], Julie Mann[1] and Lisa Bricknell[2]

*Address all correspondence to: s.kinnear@cqu.edu.au

1 CQUniversity Australia, Centre for Environmental Management, North Rockhampton, Australia

2 CQUniversity Australia, School of Health and Human Services, North Rockhampton, Australia

References

[1] DEEWR. Resourcing the future National Resources Sector Employment Taskforce Discussion Paper, March 2010. Department of Education, Employment and Workplace Relations: Commonwealth of Australia; 2010.

[2] BREE. Resources and Energy Quarterly, March Quarter 2012. Bureau of Resources and Energy Economics: Australian Government: Canberra; 2012.

[3] Shan D. Maximising growth in a mining boom. Minerals Council of Australia; 2012.

[4] Franks DM, Brereton D, Moran CJ, Sarker T, Cohen T. Cumulative impacts - a good practice guide for the Australian Coal Mining Industry. Centre for Social Responsibility in Mining & Centre for Water in the Minerals Industry: Sustainable Minerals Institute: The University of Queensland: Australian Coal Association Research Program: Brisbane; 2010.

[5] INAC. A Citizen's Guide to Cumulative Effects. Department of Renewable Resources and Environment: Indian and Northern Affairs Canada; 2007.

[6] Castleden W, Shearman D, Crisp G, Finch P. The mining and burning of coal: effects on health and the environment. Medical Journal of Australia 2011;195(6) 333-335.

[7] Safe Work Australia. Key Work Health and Safety Statistics Booklet 2012. Safe Work Australia; 2012.

[8] SRCC. Compendium of OHS and Worker's Compensation Studies December 2011. Safety, Rehabilitation and Compensation Commission: Commonwealth of Australia: Canberra: ACT; 2011.

[9] Skills Australia. Employment Growth Projections in Mining Operations (less oil and gas), 2010-2016. Australian Workforce Productivity Agency; 2011. http://www.awpa.gov.au/sector-specific-skill-needs/resource-sector-skills/employment-estimates/employment-estimates.html (accessed August 2012)

[10] Vyas MV, Garg AX, Iansavhicus AV, Costella J, Donner Al, Laugsand LE, Janskzy I, Mrkobrada M, Parraga G, Hackam DG. Shift work and vascular events: systematic review and meta-analysis. British Medical Journal 2012; 345.

[11] Muller R, Carter A, Williamson A. Epidemiological diagnosis of occupational fatigue in a fly-in fly-out operation of the mineral industry. Annals of Occupational Hygiene 2008;52(1) 1-10.

[12] Goldenberg SM, Shoveller JA, Koehoorn M, Ostry AS. And they call this progress? Consequences for young people of living and working in resource-extraction communities. Critical Public Health 2010;20(2) 157-168.

[13] Queensland Health. The Health of Queenslanders 2010, Third Report of the Chief Health Officer. Queensland Government: Brisbane; 2010.

[14] Scholtz J, Nieuwoudt R. Medical Services in Moranbah and the impact of non-resident workers, submission to the House of Representatives Standard Committee on Regional Australia, Inquiry into the use of 'fly-in, fly-out' (FIFO) workforce practices in regional Australia by Moranbah Medical. September 2011. http://aphref.aph.gov.au/house/committee/ra/fifodido/subs.htm (accessed August 2012)

[15] Bowers J. Mental health is critical to safety and productivity in Australian mining operations. In: Brereton D, Pesce D, Abogabir X. (eds.) Proceedings of the First International Seminar on Social Responsibility in Mining, 19-21 October 2011, Santiago, Chile; 2011.

[16] Torkington AM, Larkins S, Gupta TS. The psychosocial impacts of fly-in fly-out and drive-in drive-out mining on mining employees: A qualitative study. Australian Journal of Rural Health, 2011;19 135-141.

[17] Mclean KN. Mental health and well-being in resident mine workers: Out of the fly-in fly-out box. Australian Journal of Rural Health 2012;20 126-130.

[18] Scott J, Minichiello V. Mining, sex work and STIs: why force a connection? The Conversation; 8 August 2012. http://theconversation.edu.au (accessed August 2012)

[19] Scarlet Alliance. Submission to the House of Representatives Standard Committee on Regional Australia, Inquiry into the use of 'fly-in, fly-out' (FIFO) workforce practices in regional Australia. Scarlet Alliance; October 2011. http://aphref.aph.gov.au/house/committee/ra/fifodido/subs.htm (accessed August 2012)

[20] Hendryx M. Mortality from heart, respiratory, and kidney disease in coal mining areas of Appalachia. International Archives of Occupational and Environmental Health 2009;82 243-249.

[21] Hendryx M, Ahern MM. Relations between Health Indicators and Residential Proximity to Coal Mining in West Virginia. American Journal of Public Health 2008;98 669-671.

[22] ATSE. The Hidden Costs of Electricity: Externalities of Power Generation in Australia. The Australian Academy of Technological Sciences and Engineering; 2009.

[23] Kaczmarek EA, Sibbel AM. The psychosocial well-being of children from Australian military and fly-in/fly-out (FIFO) mining families. Community, Work and Family 2008;11(3) 297-312.

[24] Lovell J, Critchley J. Women living in a remote Australian mining community: exploring their psychological well-being. Australian Journal of Rural Health 2010;18(3) 125-30.

[25] Janis AS, Marcello MV, Jean S, Malcolm S, Mieke K. Perspectives on community health issues and the mining boom–bust cycle. Resources Policy 2011;36 178-186.

[26] RSDC. Social issues relating to permanent and non-permanent residents in the Moranbah mining community, report on behalf of Isaac Regional Council. Regional Social Development Centre; 2011.

[27] QNU. Queensland Nurses' Union Submission to the House of Representatives Standard Committee on Regional Australia, Inquiry into the use of 'fly-in, fly-out' (FIFO) workforce practices in regional Australia. Queensland Nurses' Union; October 2011. http://aphref.aph.gov.au/house/committee/ra/fifodido/subs.htm (accessed August 2012)

[28] Carrington K, Pereira M. Assessing the social impacts of the resources boom on rural communities. Rural Society 2011;21(1) 2-20.

[29] Bourke L, Coffin J, Fuller J, Taylor J, Editorial for the Rural Health Special Issue of Rural Society. Rural Society 2010;20(1) 1-9.

[30] AIHW. Health status of population groups, Australia's health 2010, Australian Institute of Health and Welfare, June 2010. Canberra: Australian Government; 2010.

[31] ABS. Catalogue 4102.0 - Australian Social Trends, 2008 - Towns of the Minerals Boom. Australian Bureau of Statistics; 2008. www.abs.gov.au (accessed August 2012)

[32] Schandl H, Darbas T. Surat Basin Scoping Study: Enhancing regional and community capacity for mining and energy driven regional economic development, Report to the Southern Inland Queensland Area Consultative Committee and Australian Government Department of Infrastructure, Transport, Regional Development and Local Government. CSIRO Sustainable Ecosystems: Canberra; 2008.

[33] Gosselin P, Hrudey SE, Naeth MA, Plourde A, Therrien R, Van Der Kraak G, Xu Z. Environmental and health impacts of Canada's oil sands industry. The Royal Society of Canada Expert Panel: December 2010.

[34] KPMG. Redefining regional planning: managing change, measuring growth (Abridged report for Isaac Regional Council). KPMG; 2011.

[35] McGrail MR, Humphreys JS, Joyce CM, Scott A, Kalb G. How do rural GPs' workloads and work activities differ with community size compared with metropolitan practice? Australian Journal of Primary Health 2011;18(3) 228-233.

[36] HACSWC. Health and community services industry skills report: August 2011. Health and Community Services Workforce Council: Brisbane; 2011.

[37] NRHA. Submission to the House of Representatives Standard Committee on Regional Australia, Inquiry into the use of 'fly-in, fly-out' (FIFO) workforce practices in regional Australia. National Rural Health Alliance; October 2011. http://aphref.aph.gov.au/house/committee/ra/fifodido/subs.htm (accessed August 2012)

[38] Chisholm M, Russell D, Humphreys J. Measuring rural allied health workforce turnover and retention: What are the patterns, determinants and costs? Australian Journal of Rural Health 2011;19 81-88.

[39] Rolfe J, Miles B, Lockie S, Ivanova G. Lessons from the Social and Economic Impacts of the mining boom in the Bowen Basin 2004-2006. Australasian Journal of Regional Studies 2007;13(2) 134-153.

[40] Opie T, Dollard M, Lenthall S, Wakerman J, Dunn S, Knight S, MacLeod M. Levels of occupational stress in the remote area nursing workforce. Australian Journal of Rural Health 2010;18 235-241.

[41] NSW Rural Doctor's Network. Submission to the House of Representatives Standard Committee on Regional Australia, Inquiry into the use of 'fly-in, fly-out' (FIFO) workforce practices in regional Australia. New South Wales Rural Doctor's Network; September 2011. http://aphref.aph.gov.au/house/committee/ra/fifodido/subs.htm (accessed August 2012)

[42] Autism Queensland. Submission to the House of Representatives Standard Committee on Regional Australia, Inquiry into the use of 'fly-in, fly-out' (FIFO) workforce practices in regional Australia, April 2012. 2012. http://aphref.aph.gov.au/house/committee/ra/fifodido/subs.htm (accessed August 2012)

[43] DAFF. Expanded fish health survey interim report June/July 2012. Department of Agriculture, Fisheries and Forestry: Queensland Government: Brisbane; 2012.

[44] Albrecht G, Sartore G, Connor L, Higginbotham N, Freeman S, Kelly B, Stain H, Tonna A, Pollard G. Solastalgia: the distress caused by environmental change. Australasian Psychiatry 2007;15 S95-8.

[45] Nweke OC, Sanders WH. Modern Environmental Health Hazards: A Public Health Issue of Increasing Significance in Africa. Environmental Health Perspectives 2009;117(6) 863-870.

[46] Mineral Council of Australia. MCA Annual Report 2011. Mineral Council of Australia: Australia; 2011.

[47] ACARP. Australian Coal Association Research Program Reports. Australian Coal Association Research Program; 2012. www.acarp.com.au (accessed August 2012)

[48] Queensland Government. The health and community services industry – building a stronger economy and a fairer Queensland, The Queensland Compact towards a fairer Queensland. Heath and Community Services Workforce Council; February 2012.

[49] Harris P, Spickett J. Health impact assessment in Australia: A review and directions for progress. Environmental Impact Assessment Review 2011;31 425-432.

[50] Noble B, Bronson J. Integrating Human Health into Environmental Impact Assessment: Case Studies of Canada's Northern Mining Resource Sector. Arctic 2005;58(4) 395-405.

[51] Harris P. Health Impact Assessment: the State of the Art. Impact Assessment and Project Appraisal 2012;30(1) 43-52.

[52] National Public Health Partnership. Health Impact Assessment Guidelines. Commonwealth of Australia; 2001.

[53] Mahoney M, Simpson S, Harris E, Aldrich R, Stewart-Williams J. Equity Focused Health Impact Assessment Framework. Australasian Collaboration for Health Equity Impact Assessment: Newcastle; 2004.

[54] Harris-Roxas B, Simpson S, Harris E. Equity Focused Health Impact Assessment: A literature review. CHETRE: Sydney; 2004.

[55] Vohra S. International perspective on health impact assessment in urban settings. NSW Public Health Bulletin year;18(9-10) 152-154.

[56] Harris B, Viliani F, Bond A, Cave B, Divall M, Furu P, Harris P. Overview of Health Impact Assessment Practice in Australia, World Congress on Risk 2012: Risk and Development in a Changing World, 18-20 July, Sydney, Australia, 2012.

[57] Mahoney M. Health Impact Assessment in Australia. NSW Public Health Bulletin 2007;16(7-8) 113-114.

[58] Steinemann A. Rethinking human health impact assessment, Environmental Impact Assessment Review, 2000;20(6) 627-45.

[59] Kabir SMZ, Momtaz S. The quality of Environmental Impact Statements and the environmental impact assessment practice in Bangladesh. Impact Assessment and Project Appraisal 2012;30(2) 94-99.

[60] Morgan RK. Health and impact assessment: Are we seeing closer integration? Environmental Impact Assessment Review 2011;31(4) 404-411.

[61] Barton H, Tsourou C. Healthy urban planning: a WHO guide to planning for people. Spon Press on behalf of the World Health Organisation: Regional Office for Europe: London; 2000.

[62] Winkler MS, Divall MJ, Krieger GR, Balge MZ, Singer BH, Utzinger J. Assessing health impacts in complex eco-epidemiological settings in the humid tropics: Advancing tools and methods. Environmental Impact Assessment Review 2010;30 52-61.

[63] Goggin G, Newell C., editors. Disability in Australia: Exposing a Social Apartheid. UNSW Press: Sydney; 2004.

[64] ABS. Catalogue 4430.0 - Disability, Ageing and Carers, Australia: Summary of Findings, 2009. Australian Bureau of Statistics; 2009. www.abs.gov.au (accessed August 2012.

[65] ABS. Census QuickStats Australia profile. Australian Bureau of Statistics; 2001 and 2012. www.censusdata.abs.gov.au (accessed August 2012).

[66] IHRC. Bearing the burden: the effects of mining on First Nations in British Columbia. International Human Rights Clinic: Harvard Law School: 2010.

[67] Regional Social Development Centre, Submission to the House of Representatives Standard Committee on Regional Australia, Inquiry into the use of 'fly-in, fly-out' (FIFO) workforce practices in regional Australia. New South Wales Rural Doctor's Network; September 2011. http://aphref.aph.gov.au/house/committee/ra/fifodido/subs.htm (accessed August 2012)

[68] Kabir SMZ. A critical review of environmental impact assessment system in Bangladesh using a holistic approach. University of Newcastle; 2012.

[69] Devine SG, Muller R, Carter A. Using the Framework for Health Promotion Action to address staff perceptions of occupational health and safety at a fly-in/fly-out mine in north-west Queensland. Health Promotion Journal of Australia 2008;19(3) 196-202.

[70] Department of Environment and Heritage Protection, Cumulative Management Area, 2012, http://www.ehp.qld.gov.au/management/coal-seam-gas/cumulative-management.html (accessed September 2012).

[71] Mcintyre L, Petticrew M. Methods of Health Impact Assessment: a literature review. Occasional Paper: MRC Social & Public Health Sciences Unit: University of Glasgow: UK; 1999.

[72] Petkova V, Lockie S, Rolfe J, Ivanova G. Mining developments and social impacts on communities: Bowen Basin case studies. Rural Society 2009;19(3) 211-228.

[73] ICMM. Good Practice Guidance on Health Impact Assessment. International Council on Mining and Metals; 2010. http://www.icmm.com/library/hia (accessed August 2012)

[74] Goldstein BD, Kriesky J, Pavliakova B. Missing from the Table: Role of the Environmental Public Health Community in Governmental Advisory Commissions Related to Marcellus Shale Drilling. Environmental Health Perspectives 2012; 120(4) 483-486.

Chapter 8

Health Care Waste Management – Public Health Benefits, and the Need for Effective Environmental Regulatory Surveillance in Federal Republic of Nigeria

Nkechi Chuks Nwachukwu, Frank Anayo Orji and Ositadinma Chinyere Ugbogu

Additional information is available at the end of the chapter

http://dx.doi.org/10.5772/53196

1. Introduction

Waste generated by health care activities includes a broad range of materials, from used needles and syringes to soiled dressings, body parts, diagnostic samples, blood, chemicals, pharmaceuticals, medical devices and radioactive materials (WHO, 2011).

Poor management of health care waste potentially exposes health care workers, waste handlers, patients and the community at large to infection, toxic effects and injuries, and risks polluting the environment. It is essential that all medical waste materials are segregated at the point of generation, appropriately treated and disposed of safely(WHO, 2011). Health-care waste (HCW) is a by-product of healthcare that includes sharps, non-sharps, blood, body parts, chemicals, pharmaceuticals, medical devices and radioactive materials.

WHO Programme activities include developing technical guidance materials for assessing the quantities and types of waste produced in different facilities, creating national action plans, developing national healthcare waste management (HCWM) guidelines and building capacity at national level to enhance the way HCW is dealt with in low-income countries (LICs).

Classification of Health Care wastes shows that

1. Of the total amount of waste generated by health-care activities, about 80% is general waste.

2. The remaining 20% is considered hazardous material that may be infectious, toxic or radioactive.
3. Every year an estimated 16 000 million injections are administered worldwide, but not all of the needles and syringes are properly disposed of afterwards.
4. Health-care waste contains potentially harmful micro organisms which can infect hospital patients, health-care workers and the general public.

Health-care activities protect and restore health and save lives. But what about the wastes and by-products they generate

Types of waste

Waste and by-products cover a diverse range of materials, as the following list illustrates (percentages are approximate values):

Infectious waste: waste contaminated with blood and its by-products, cultures and stocks of infectious agents, waste from patients in isolation wards, discarded diagnostic samples containing blood and body fluids, infected animals from laboratories, and contaminated materials (swabs, bandages) and equipment (such as disposable medical devices); are considered as infectious waste, all wastes that are susceptible to contain pathogens (or their toxins) in sufficient concentration to cause diseases to a potential host. Examples of infectious waste include discarded materials or equipment, used for the diagnosis, treatment and prevention of disease that has been in contact with body fluids (dressings, swabs, nappies, blood bags…). This category also includes liquid waste such as faeces, urine, blood or other body secretions (such as sputum or lung secretions).

Pathological waste: recognizable body parts and contaminated animal carcasses; Pathological waste consists of organs, tissues, body parts or fluids such as blood. Even if pathological waste may contain healthy body parts, it has to be considered as infectious waste for precautionary reasons.

Anatomical waste is a sub-group of pathological waste and consists in recognisable human body parts, whether they may be infected or not. Following the precautionary principles, anatomical waste is always considered as potential infectious waste.

Pharmaceutical wastes: expired, unused, and contaminated drugs; vaccines and sera; Pharmaceutical waste includes expired, unused, spilt and contaminated pharmaceutical products, drugs and vaccines. In this category are also included discarded items used in the handling of pharmaceuticals like bottles, vials, connecting tubing. Since various ministries of health or their equivalents usually put in place specific measures that will reduce the the wastage of drugs, Health care facilities should deal only with small quantities of pharmaceutical wastes. This category also includes all the drugs and equipment used for the mixing and administration of cytotoxic drugs. Cytotoxic drugs or genotoxic drugs are drugs that have the ability to reduce/stop the growth of certain living cells and are used in chemotherapy for cancer. Cytotoxic waste is dealt with under a separate heading.

Genotoxic waste: highly hazardous, mutagenic, teratogenic or carcinogenic, such as cytotoxic drugs used in cancer treatment and their metabolites; Genotoxic waste derives from drugs generally used in oncology or radiotherapy units that have a high hazardous mutagenic or cytotoxic effect. Faeces, vomit or urine from patients treated with cytotoxic drugs or chemicals should be considered as genotoxic. In specialised cancer hospitals, their proper treatment or disposal raises serious safety problems.

Radioactive waste: such as glassware contaminated with radioactive diagnostic material or radiotherapeutic materials; Radioactive waste includes liquids, gas and solids contaminated with radionuclides whose ionizing radiations have genotoxic effects. The ionizing radiations of interest in medicine include X- and g-rays as well as a- and b- particles. An important difference between these types of radiations is that X-rays are emitted from X-ray tubes only when generating equipment is switched on whereas g-rays, α- and β- particles emit radiations continuously.

The type of radioactive material used in HCF results in low level radioactive waste. It concerns mainly therapeutic and imaging investigation activities where Cobalt 60Co, Technetium 99mTc, Iodine 131I and Iridium 192Ir are most commonly used.

With the noticeable exception of Cobalt 60Co, their half-life is reasonably short (6 hours for 99mTc, 8 days for 131I and 74 days for 192Ir) and the concentrations used remain low. A proper storage with an appropriate retention time is sufficient to prevent radioactivity spillage in the environment.

Infectious and anatomic wastes together represent the majority of the hazardous waste, up to 15% of the total waste from health-care activities. Sharps represent about 1% of the total waste but they are a major source of disease transmission if not properly managed. Chemicals and pharmaceuticals account for about 3% of waste from health-care activities while genotoxic waste, radioactive matter and heavy metal content account for around 1% of the total health-care waste.

The major sources of health-care waste are:

1. hospitals and other health-care establishments
2. laboratories and research centres
3. mortuary and autopsy centres
4. animal research and testing laboratories
5. blood banks and collection services
6. Nursing homes for the elderly.

High-income countries generate on average up to 0.5 kg of hazardous waste per bed per day; while low-income countries generate on average 0.2 kg of hazardous waste per hospital bed per day. However, health-care waste is often not separated into hazardous or non-hazardous wastes in low-income countries making the real quantity of hazardous waste much higher.

Laboratory waste: This is also high risk category waste. This includes chemicals used in the pathological laboratory, microbial cultures and clinical specimens, slide, culture dish, needle, syringes, as well as radioactive waste such as Iodine-125, iodine -131.

Health impact

Health-care waste contains potentially harmful micro-organisms which can infect hospital patients, health-care workers and the general public. Other potential infectious risks may include the spread of drug-resistant micro-organisms from health-care establishments into the environment.

Waste and by-products can also cause injuries, for example:

1. radiation burns;
2. sharps-inflicted injuries;
3. poisoning and pollution through the release of pharmaceutical products, in particular, antibiotics and cytotoxic drugs;
4. poisoning and pollution through waste water; and
5. Poisoning and pollution by toxic elements or compounds, such as mercury or dioxins that are released during incineration.

Sharps

WHO estimates that, in 2000, injections with contaminated syringes caused 21 million hepatitis B virus (HBV) infections, two million hepatitis C virus infections and 260 000 HIV infections worldwide. Many of these infections were avoidable if the syringes had been disposed of safely. The re-use of disposable syringes and needles for injections is particularly common in certain African, Asian and Central and Eastern European countries.

In developing countries, additional hazards occur from scavenging at waste disposal sites and the manual sorting of hazardous waste from health-care establishments. These practices are common in many regions of the world. The waste handlers are at immediate risk of needle-stick injuries and exposure to toxic or infectious materials.

Vaccine waste

In June 2000 six children were diagnosed with a mild form of smallpox (vaccinia virus) after having played with glass ampoules containing expired smallpox vaccine at a garbage dump in Vladivostok (Russia). Although the infections were not life-threatening, the vaccine ampoules should have been treated before being discarded.

Radioactive waste

The use of radiation sources in medical and other applications is widespread throughout the world. Occasionally, the public is exposed to radioactive waste, which originates from radiotherapy treatment, which has not been disposed of properly. Serious accidents have been documented in Brazil in 1988 (where four people died and 28 had serious radiation burns), Mexico and Morocco in 1983, Algeria in 1978 and Mexico in 1962.

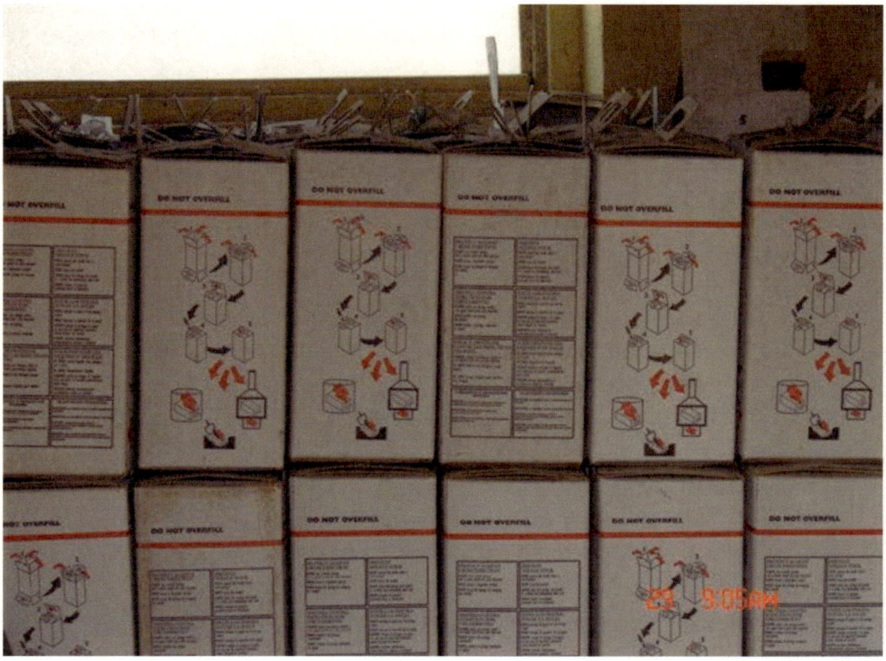

Figure 1. Boxes for sharps disposal (AIHPPRP, 2007)

Risks associated with other types of health-care waste, in particular blood waste and chemicals, may be significant but have not been fully assessed. In the meantime, precautionary measures should be taken.

Risks associated with waste disposal

Although treatment and disposal of health-care waste reduces risks, indirect health risks may occur through the release of toxic pollutants into the environment through treatment or disposal.

1. Landfills can contaminate drinking-water if they are not properly constructed. Occupational risks exist at disposal facilities that are not well designed, run, or maintained.

2. Incineration of waste has been widely practised but inadequate incineration or the incineration of unsuitable materials results in the release of pollutants into the air and of ash residue. Incinerated materials containing chlorine can generate dioxins and furans, which are human carcinogens and have been associated with a range of adverse health effects. Incineration of heavy metals or materials with high metal content (in particular lead, mercury and cadmium) can lead to the spread of toxic metals in the environment. Dioxins, furans and metals are persistent and bio-accumulate in the environment. Materials containing chlorine or metal should therefore not be incinerated.

3. Only modern incinerators operating at 850-1100 °C and fitted with special gas-cleaning equipment are able to comply with the international emission standards for dioxins and furans.

Alternatives to incineration are now available, such as autoclaving, microwaving, steam treatment integrated with internal mixing, and chemical treatment.

Waste management: reasons for failure

Lack of awareness about the health hazards related to health-care waste, inadequate training in proper waste management, absence of waste management and disposal systems, insufficient financial and human resources and the low priority given to the topic are the most common problems connected with health-care waste. Many countries either do not have appropriate regulations, or do not enforce them. An essential issue is the clear attribution of responsibility for the handling and disposal of waste. According to the 'polluter pays' principle, the responsibility lies with the waste producer, usually the health-care provider, or the establishment involved in related activities. To achieve the safe and sustainable management of health-care waste, financial analyses should include all the costs of disposal.

Steps towards improvement

Improvements in health-care waste management rely on the following key elements:

1. building a comprehensive system, addressing responsibilities, resource allocation, handling and disposal. This is a long-term process, sustained by gradual improvements;
2. raising awareness of the risks related to health-care waste, and of safe and sound practices;
3. selecting safe and environmentally-friendly management options, to protect people from hazards when collecting, handling, storing, transporting, treating or disposing of waste.

Government commitment and support is needed for universal, long-term improvement, although immediate action can be taken locally.

World Health Organisation response

The first global and comprehensive guidance document, *Safe management of wastes from health-care activities*, originally released by WHO in 1999, addresses aspects such as regulatory framework, planning issues, waste minimization and recycling, handling, storage and transportation, treatment and disposal options, and training.

It is aimed at managers of hospitals and other health-care establishments, policy makers, public health professionals and managers involved in waste management. It is accompanied by a *Teacher's guide*, which contains material for a three-day workshop aimed at the same audience.

Additionally, WHO guidance documents on health-care waste are now available including:

1. a monitoring tool

2. a cost assessment tool
3. a rapid assessment tool
4. a policy paper
5. guidance to develop national plans
6. management of waste from injection activities
7. management of waste at primary health care centres
8. management of waste from mass immunization activities
9. Management of waste in emergencies.

Poor management of health care waste potentially exposes health care workers, waste handlers, patients and the community at large to infection, toxic effects and injuries, and risks polluting the environment. It is essential that all medical waste materials are segregated at the point of generation, appropriately treated and disposed of safely.

However in most countries including Nigeria, such wastes are not given appropriate treatment, thus it is impacting negatively on the environment.

2. Medical and pharmaceutical waste in Europe and America

In Europe, wastes are defined by their European Waste Catalogue (EWC) Codes. EWC Codes are 6 digits long, with the first two digits defining the overarching category of waste, the next two defining the sub-category, and the last two defining the precise waste stream. Clinical waste comes under the "18" codes, for example: "18 01 01" corresponds to healthcare waste (18), from humans (01), that is sharp and not infectious [01].

United Kingdom

In the UK, clinical waste and the way it is to be handled is closely regulated Applicable legislation includes the Environmental Protection Act 1990 (Part II), Waste Management Licencing Regulations 1994, and the Hazardous Waste Regulations (England & Wales) 2005, as well as the Special Waste Regulations in Scotland.

United States

In 1988 the Federal government passed The Medical Waste Tracking Act which set the standards for governmental regulation of medical waste. After the Act was repealed in 1991, States were given the responsibility to regulate and pass laws concerning the disposal of medical waste. All fifty states vary in their regulations from no regulations to very strict. Disposal of this waste is an environmental concern, as many medical wastes are classified as *infectious* or *biohazardous* and could potentially lead to the spread of infectious disease. Examples of infectious waste include blood, potentially contaminated "sharps" such as needles and scalpels, and identifiable body parts. Sharps include used needles, lancets, and other devices capable of penetrating skin. Infectious waste is often incinerated. The most common method of sterilization is an autoclave. The autoclave uses steam and pressure to sterilize the waste. Additionally, medical facilities produce a variety of hazardous chemicals, including radioactive materials. While such wastes are normally not infectious, they may be classified as hazardous wastes, and require proper disposal.

In the United States, there are three main methods for medical waste generators to dispose of their waste: On-site, truck service, and mail-back disposal. On-site treatment involves the use of very expensive equipment, and is generally only used by very large hospitals and major universities who have the means to afford such equipment. Truck service involves hiring of a medical waste disposal service whose employees are trained to collect and haul away medical waste in special containers (usually cardboard boxes, or reusable plastic bins) for treatment at a facility designed to handle large amounts of medical waste. Mail-back medical waste disposal is similar, except that the waste is shipped through the U.S. postal service instead of by private hauler. Although currently available in all 50 U.S. states, mail-back medical waste disposal is limited to very strict postal regulations (collection and shipping containers must be approved by the postal service for use) and only available by a handful of companies.

3. Health care waste in Nigeria

In developing countries like Nigeria, where many health concerns are competing for limited resources, it is not surprising that the management of healthcare wastes has received less attention and the priority it deserves (Abah and Ohimain, 2010). Unfortunately, practical information on this important aspect of healthcare management is inadequate and research on the public health implications of inadequate management of healthcare wastes are few and limited in scope (Abah and Ohimain, 2010). Although reliable records of the quantity and nature of healthcare wastes and the management techniques to adequately dispose of these wastes has remained a challenge in many developing countries of the world, it is believed that several hundreds of tones of healthcare waste are deposited openly in waste dumps and surrounding environments, often alongside with non hazardous solid waste (Alagoz and Kocasay, 2007; Abah and Ohimain, 2010).

A near total absence of institutional arrangements for HCW in Nigeria has been reported by others (Coker et al., 1998). Various methodologies have been used all over the world to assess and quantify HCW. They include the use of physical observation, questionnaire administration and quantification (Adegbita et al., 2010; Olubukola, 2009; Phengxay et al., 2005), as well as checklists (Townend and Cheeseman, 2005) and private and public records (Coker et al., 2009). Recent studies in Nigeria has estimated waste generation of between 0.562 to 0.670 kg/bed/day (Abah and Ohimain, 2011) and as high as 1.68 kg/bed/day (Abah and Ohimain, 2011). As reported in the literature, there may not be much of a difference in the way and manner wastes generated in various health care institutions are managed in Nigeria. A good example is given by the findings of the study in Lagos by Olubukola which reported the similarity in waste data and HCW management practices in two General hospitals, characterized by a lack of waste minimization or waste reduction strategies, poor waste segregation practices, lack of instructive posters on waste segregation and disposal of HCW with general waste (Olubukola, 2009). The mismanagement of healthcare waste poses health risks to people and the environment by contaminating the air, soil and water resources. Hospitals and healthcare units are supposed to safeguard the health of the community. However, healthcare wastes if not properly managed can pose an even greater threat than the original diseases themselves (PATH, 2009).

A study of Health Care Waste management in Jos Metropolis, Nigeria has demonstrated that the waste management options in the hospitals did not meet the standard practices (Ngwuluka *et al.,* 2009). Waste management with safe and environmentally sound methods cannot be over-emphasized. The hospital management board and the hospitals should make a conscious and deliberate effort to ensure they do not contribute to the present and future threats to human health and the environment by poor waste management practices. In order to execute standard waste management, an understudy of a healthcare establishment with standard waste management practices in or outside the country may be the first practical step to undertake (Ngwuluka *et al.,* 2009). A waste management team should be constituted which will prepare waste management plan, policy documents and technical guidelines and in addition supervise waste management activities (Ngwuluka *et al.,* 2009).

In another study in Port-Harcourt metropolis, Nigeria carried out to assess hospitals waste management practice (Ogbonna, 2011). The study enquired into waste generation rates and various waste disposal options by different categories of hospital. It was further evident in this study that hospital waste management issues and problems are not peculiar to Port Harcourt metropolis alone. Solid waste disposal methods indicated that open dump sites is most preferred while incineration was non existent in the hospitals, clinics. Most other hospitals do not segregate wastes into marked or colour coded containers for the different waste streams neither do they keep records of waste generation and disposal (Ogbonna, 2011). In addition, the survey revealed that both hospital waste generators and handlers treat hospital wastes as a usual domestic waste (Ogbonna, 2011).

Therefore disposal of ashes containing toxic metals from Hospital waste incineration can be done through solidification-stabilization of fly and bottom ash with cement because it appears to be the best method to render ash less toxic. Similarly, the concentration of toxic heavy metals in the ash of hospital waste incinerator can be avoided to some extent through segregation of the waste prior to incineration. Lack of relevant training and protective equipment for waste handlers was a common feature in the survey. Generally, Port Harcourt, as a fast growing city in Nigeria, like most developing countries, lacked the infrastructure, as well as institutional capacity necessary to effectively manage medical wastes as part of the effort to enhance protection of human life and the environment from health hazards arising from improper management of hazardous waste (Ogbonna, 2011).

It was further observed that open dump sites are not even engineered or treated, thus expose the entire public to risks of infection. Ogbonna (2011) reported that except for the oil company clinics such as the SPDC, all the other hospitals sampled do not have any unit or department responsible for waste management. Knowledge, attitude and practices towards environmental issues are relatively low among the various actors in the tasks of hospital waste management.

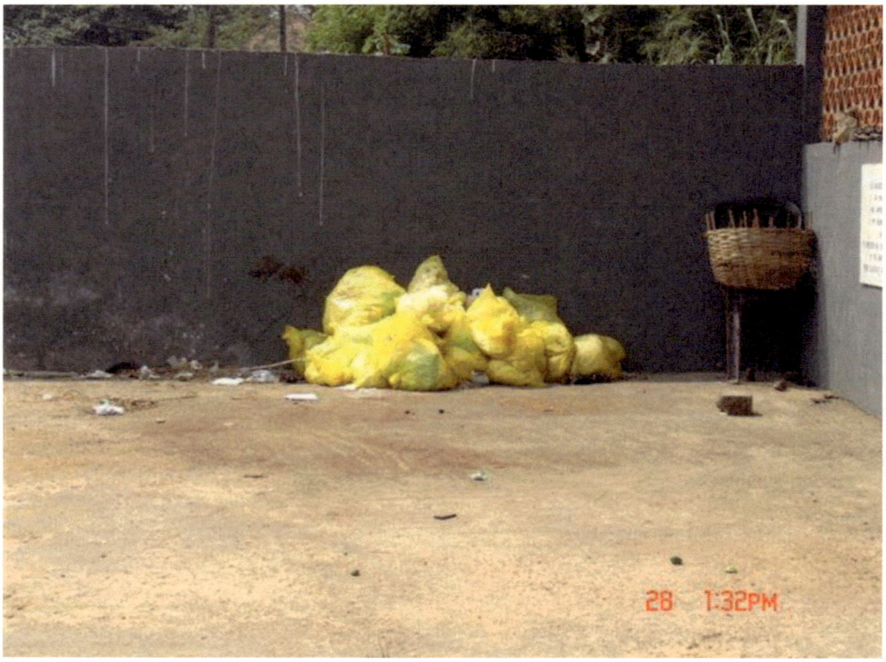

Figure 3. Temporary storage area at NOH, Igbobi (AIHPPRP, 2007)

4. Microorganisms associated with health care waste

The following groups of persons are at the risk of health care waste Medical staff: doctors, nurses, sanitary staff and hospital maintenance personnel; In and out-patients receiving treatment in healthcare facilities as well as their visitors. Workers in support services linked to healthcare facilities such as laundries, waste handling and transportation services; Workers in waste disposal facilities and the general public. Presence of various microorganisms such as pathogenic viruses and bacteria have been investigated by both cultivation and by (RT)-PCR assays. A number of (opportunistic) pathogenic bacteria, including *Pseudomonas* spp., *Lactobacillus* spp., *Staphylococcus* spp., *Micrococcus* spp., Kocuria spp., *Brevibacillus* spp., *Microbacterium oxydans*, and *Propionibacterium acnes*, were identified and reported from the various medical wastes. In addition, pathogenic viruses such as noroviruses and hepatitis B virus have been also detected in human tissue wastes. Commonly identified bacterial and viral pathogens such as *Pseudomonas* spp., *Corynebacterium diphtheriae, Escherichia coli, Staphylococcus* spp., and respiratory synctial virus (RSV) have been reported to be part of the medical wastes. Medical waste should be carefully controlled and monitored to prevent nosocomial infection associated with the exposure to these wastes (Nascimento *et al.*, 2009)

Health service waste gives rise to controversy regarding its importance for human, animal and environmental health (Nascimento *et al.*, 2009). Occurrences of clinically relevant bacteria in piles of health service waste in a sanitary landfill and their antimicrobial susceptibility profile have been previously studied by Nascimento *et al.*, 2009. Nascimento *et al.*, 2009 reported that aliquots of leachate from health care waste in Brazil contained pathogenic strains of *Staphylococcus* sp, Gram-negative rods of the *Enterobacteriaceae* family and non-fermenters. Bacterial resistance to all the antimicrobials tested was observed in all microbial groups, including resistance to more than one drug. This makes it possible to suggest that viable bacteria in health service waste represent risks to human and animal health. Furthermore, occurrences of multi-resistant strains support the hypothesis that health service waste acts as a reservoir for resistance markers, with an environmental impact. The lack of regional legislation concerning segregation, treatment and final disposal of waste may expose different populations to risks of transmission of infectious diseases associated with multi-resistant microorganisms.

S/N	Microbial Group	Type of Disease caused
1	Bacterial	Tetanus, gas gangrene and other wound infection, anthrax, cholera, other diarrhoeal diseases, enteric fever, shigellosis, plague etc
2	Viral	Various hepatitis, poliomyelitis, HIV-infections, HBV, TB, STD rabies etc.
3	Parasitic	Amoebiasis, Giardiasis, Ascariasis, Ancylomastomiasis, Taeniasis, Echinococcosis, Malaria, Leishmaniasis, Filariasis etc.
4	Fungal infections	Various fungal infections like Candidiasis, cryptococcoses, coccidiodomycosis etc.

Table 1. Microbial diseases associated with health care waste (Akter, 2010)

5. Dangers of improper disposal of health care waste

Transmission of disease through infectious waste is the greatest and most immediate threat from healthcare waste.

If waste is not treated in a way that destroys the pathogenic organisms, dangerous quantities of microscopic disease-causing agents—viruses, bacteria, parasites or fungi—will be present in the waste. These agents can enter the body through punctures and other breaks in the skin, mucous membranes in the mouth, by being inhaled into the lungs, being swallowed, or being transmitted by a vector organism (World Health Organization,

1992).People who come in direct contact with the waste are at greatest risk. Examples include healthcare workers, cleaning staff, patients, visitors, waste collectors, disposal site staff, waste pickers, drug addicts and those who knowingly or unknowingly use "recycled" contaminated syringes and needles. Although sharps pose an inherent physical hazard of cuts and punctures, the much greater threat comes from sharps that are also infectious waste. Again, healthcare workers, waste handlers, waste pickers, drug addicts and others who handle sharps can, and have, become infected with HIV/AIDS and hepatitis B and C viruses through pricks or reuse of syringes/needles. These infections may be fatal (Johannessen, 2000). Contamination of water supply from untreated healthcare waste can also have devastating effects. If infectious stools or bodily fluids are not treated before being disposed of, they can create and extend epidemics, since sewage treatment in Africa is almost nonexistent.

For example, the absence of proper sterilization procedures is believed to have increased the severity and size of cholera epidemics in most parts of Africa during the last decade.

Chemical and toxic threats

Chemical and pharmaceutical wastes, especially large quantities, can be health and environmental threats. Since hazardous chemical wastes may be toxic, corrosive, flammable, reactive, and/or explosive, they can poison, burn or damage the skin and flesh of people who touch, inhale or are in close proximity to them. If burned, they may explode or produce toxic fumes. Some pharmaceuticals are toxic as well (Johannessen, 2000).

When chemical and pharmaceutical waste is disposed of in unlined landfills, especially unlined pits, these wastes may contaminate ground and surface water—particularly when large quantities are disposed of. This can threaten people who use the water for drinking, bathing and cooking, and damaging plants and animals in the local ecosystem. Burning or incinerating healthcare waste, while often a better option than disposal in an unlined pit, may create additional problems. Burning or incineration of healthcare waste may produce toxic air pollutants such as Nitrogen Oxides (NOx), particulates, dioxins and heavy metals and distribute them over a wide area. Dioxins and heavy metals are of particular concern (Prüss and Townend, 1998). Dioxins believed to be potent cancer-causing agents, do not biodegrade, and accumulate in progressively higher concentrations as they move up the food chain (WHO, 1999).

Heavy metals such as mercury and cadmium are toxic and/or cause birth defects in small quantities and can also concentrate in the food chain.

Disposable pressurized containers pose another hazard for incineration, as they can explode if burned.

In fact, disposal of large quantities of hazardous chemicals and pharmaceuticals is a serious problem. In most of Africa, no methods are available to small-scale facilities that are safe and affordable (Prüss and Townend, 1998).

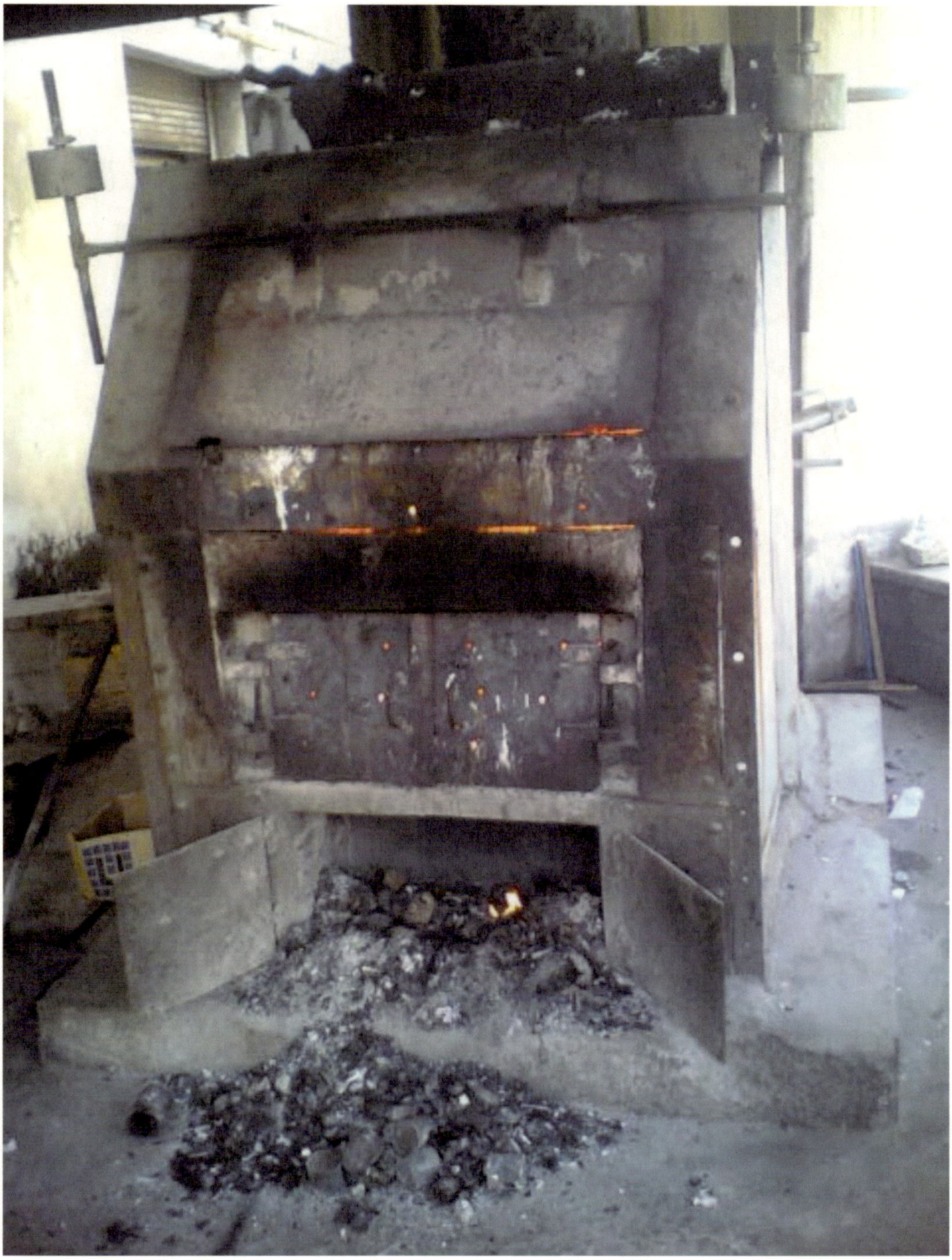

Figure 4. Improvised incinerator at UCH, Ibadan

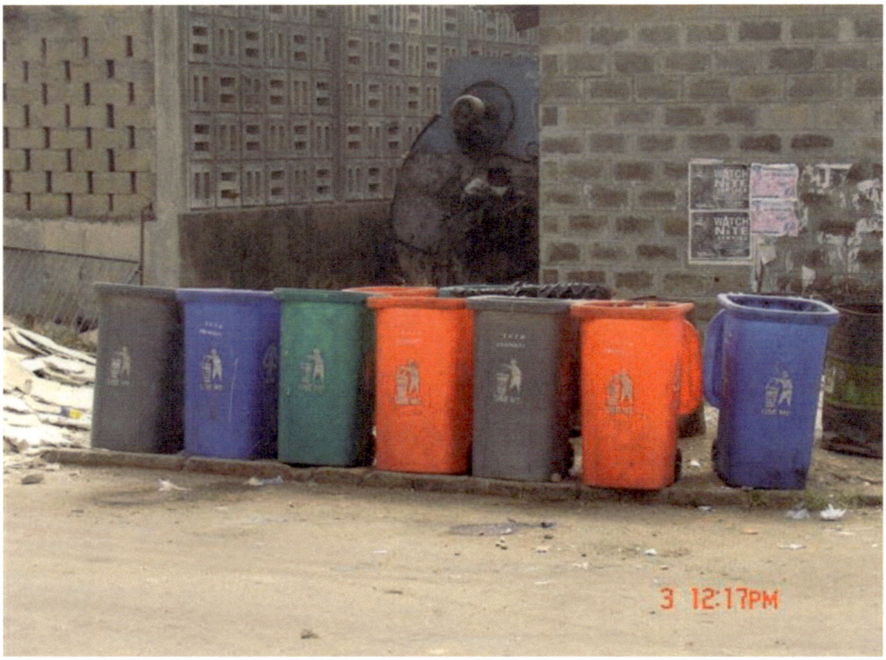

Figure 5. Medical waste storage area at LUTH, Lagos, Nigeria without proper symbols to differentiate wstes into categories (AIHPPRP, 2007)

Antibiotic resistance spread in the Environment through improperly disposed Health Care Wastes

Antimicrobial resistance (AMR) is resistance of a microorganism to an antimicrobial medicine to which it was previously sensitive. Resistant organisms (they include bacteria, viruses and some parasites) are able to withstand attack by antimicrobial medicines, such as antibiotics, antivirals, and anti-malarials, so that standard treatments become ineffective and infections persist and may spread to others. AMR is a consequence of the use, particularly the misuse, of antimicrobial medicines and develops when a microorganism mutates or acquires a resistance gene (WHO, 2012). In places like Nigeria most families become financially distressed after hospitalization of members of their families. Many infectious diseases risk becoming uncontrollable and could derail the progress made towards reaching the targets of the health-related United Nations Millennium Development Goals set for 2015. When infections become resistant to first-line medicines, more expensive therapies must be used. The longer duration of illness and treatment, often in hospitals, increases health-care costs and the financial burden to families and societies (WHO, 2012). Multidrug resistance is described as a phenomenon where a microbial pathogen resists at least three groups of antibiotics (CDC, 2005). Healthcare liquid wastes are the reservoirs of harmful infectious agents such as the pathogens and multiple drug resistant microorganisms (Sharma *et al.*, 2010). Potential infectious risks include the spread of infectious diseases and microbial resistance from healthcare establishments into the environment and thereby posing risks of getting infections and antibiotic resistance in the communities (Sharma *et al.*, 2010).

Therefore, even if the hospitals are discharging their healthcare liquid waste into Sewage system, it is mixed with the sewage and gets in surface water without proper treatment. If the hospital effluents are not treated, concentrated forms of infectious agents and antibiotic resistant microbes are shed into communities resulting in water borne diseases such as cholera, typhoid fever, dysentery and gastroenteritis. Antibiotics, disinfectants and bacteria resistant to them have been detected in the environmental compartments such as waste water, surface water, ground water, sediments and soils (Kummerer, 2004). Studies have discovered trace level concentrations of antibiotics in waste water treatment plant effluents and surface waters (Kolpin et al, 2002). Long term exposure of microorganisms to low concentrations of antibiotics in wastewater and surface water has the potential for the development of antibiotic resistance in these organisms (Smith *et al.*, 1999).

The concerns about antimicrobial resistance are increasing. In a report by the United Kingdom, House of Lords, it is stated that the resistance to antibiotics and other anti-infective agents constitutes a major threat to public health and ought to be recognized (HLSCST, 1998). Input of resistant bacteria as well as of antibiotics can disturb the established well balanced and important interdependencies (Hiraishi, 1998). The input of resistant bacteria into the environment seems to be an important source of resistance in the environment.

Therefore, the development of antibiotic resistance in bacteria and their dissemination in the environment is of serious public health concern because an individual patient can develop an antibiotic resistant infection by contacting a resistant organism and spread in the communities. Hospitals and public health care units must safeguard the health of the community. However, the waste produced by the health care centres if disposed of improperly, can pose an even greater threat than the original diseases themselves due to the presence of concentrated forms of numerous risks including pathogenic and antibiotic resistant microorganisms (Sharma *et al.*, 2010).

In Nepal, where several thousand die due to infectious diseases and several more, losing quality of lives, untreated hospital liquid waste discharge into surface water directly or indirectly must have been adding more problems. It is our common observation that majority of the healthcare facilities do not practice safe healthcare liquid waste treatment and disposal.

6. International agreements and principles on health care management

Basel convention

This convention is a global agreement, ratified by some 178 member countries to address the problems and challenges posed by hazardous waste. Nigeria is a signatory to this convention.

The Secretariat, based in Geneva (Switzerland) is administered by UNEP. It facilitates the implementation of the Convention and related agreements. It also provides assistance and guidelines on legal and technical issues and conducts training on the proper management of hazardous waste.

The key objectives of the Basel Convention are:

1. to minimize the generation of hazardous wastes in terms of quantity and hazardousness;
2. to dispose of them as close to the source of generation as possible;
3. to reduce the movement of hazardous wastes.

A central goal of the Basel Convention is "environmentally sound management" (ESM), the aim of which is to protect human health and the environment by minimizing hazardous waste production whenever possible. ESM means addressing the issue through an "integrated life-cycle approach", which involves strong controls from the generation of a hazardous waste to its storage, transport, treatment, reuse, recycling, recovery and final disposal. Health Care Related Wastes (HCRW) is one of the **categories of hazardous wastes covered by the Convention**. It was adopted in 1989. During its first decade, the Convention's principal focus was the elaboration of controls on the "transboundary" movement of hazardous wastes that is the movement of such wastes across international frontiers and the development of criteria for environmentally sound management of the wastes. More recently the work of the Convention has emphasized full implementation of treaty commitments, promotion of the environmentally sound management of hazardous wastes, a lifecycle approach, and minimization of hazardous waste, generation. The Convention entered into force 5 May 1992. (HCWC, 2007).

The **Basel Convention** (Article 4) requires each Party to minimize waste generation and to ensure, to the extent possible, the availability of disposal facilities within its own territory. The Conference of the

Parties at its sixth meeting in December 2002 adopted a Strategic Plan for the implementation of the Basel Declaration to 2010 building on and using the framework of the 1999 Ministerial Basel Declaration on Environmentally Sound Management. The **Basel Convention** covers wastes that are listed in Annex I, if they display the hazardous characteristics listed in Annex III. Hazardous wastes are those wastes that are: explosive, flammable, poisonous, infectious, corrosive, toxic, or ecotoxic.

The Stockholm convention on persistent organic pollutants

This Convention is a global treaty to protect human health and the environment from persistent organic pollutants (POPs). POPs are chemicals that remain intact in the environment for long periods, become widely distributed geographically, accumulate in the fatty tissue of living organisms and are toxic to humans and wildlife. Persistent Organic Pollutants (POPs) circulate globally and can cause damage wherever they travel. In implementing the Convention, Governments will take measures to eliminate or reduce the release of POPs into the environment. The countries that have signed these conventions are Afghanistan, Albania, Algeria, Andorra, Angola, Antigua and Barbuda Argentina, Armenia, Australia, Austria, Azerbaijan, Bahamas, Bahrain, Bangladesh, Barbados, Belarus, Belgium, Belize, Benin, Bhutan, Bolivia, Bosnia, and Herzegovina, Botswana, Brazil, Brunei, Darussalam, Bulgaria, Burkina Faso, Burundi, Cambodia, Cameroon, Canada, Cape Verde, Central African Rep, Chad,

Chile, China, Colombia, Comoros, Congo, Costa Rica, Cote d'Ivoire, Croatia, Cuba Cyprus, Czech Republic, Dem. Rep. of Korea, Dem. Rep. of the Congo, Denmark, Niger, Nigeria and many more other countries.

The Stockholm Convention was adopted in 2001. POPs are chemicals that are highly toxic, persistent, bio-accumulate and move long distance in the environment. The Convention seeks the elimination or restriction of production and use of all intentionally produced POPs (i.e. industrial chemicals and pesticides). It also seeks the continuing minimization and, where feasible, ultimate elimination of the release of unintentionally produced POPs such as dioxins and furans. The Convention entered into force17 May 2004 (HCWC, 2007).

The Rotterdam convention

The Rotterdam Convention was adopted in 1998. In the 1980s, UNEP and FAO developed voluntary codes of conduct and information exchange systems, culminating in the Prior Informed Consent (PIC) procedure introduced in 1989. The Convention replaces this arrangement with a mandatory PIC procedure and information exchange mechanism on hazardous chemicals and pesticides. The Convention entered into force 24 February 2004.

The **Rotterdam Convention** (Article 5), obliges Parties to notify the secretariat of final regulatory actions taken in respect of banned or severely restricted chemicals, for the information of other Parties and possible listing under the Convention. Developing countries and countries with economies in transition may also propose the listing of severely hazardous pesticide formulations (Article 6).

TheRotterdam Convention apply to any chemical that is banned or severely restricted by a Party. The Prior Informed Consent procedure applies to the following 28 hazardous pesticides: 2,4,5-T, aldrin, binapacryl, captafol, chlordane, chlordimeform, chlorobenzilate, DDT, 1,2- dibromoethane (EDB), dieldrin, dinoseb, DNOC and its salts, ethylene dichloride, ethylene oxide, fluoroacetamide, HCH, heptachlor, hexachlorobenzene, lindane, mercury compounds, monocrotophos, parathion, pentachlorophenol and toxaphene, plus certain formulations of methamidophos, methyl-parathion, monocrotophos, parathion, phosphamidon and a combination of benomyl, carbofuran and thiram. It also covers 11 industrial chemicals: asbestos (actinolite, anthophyllite, amosite, crocidolite, tremolite), polybrominated biphenyls (PBBs), polychlorinatedbiphenyls (PCBs), polychlorinated terphenyls (PCTs), tris (2,3 dibromopropyl) phosphate and tetraethyl lead (TEL) and tetramethyl lead (TML).

World conventions and Principles of Health Care Waste management

1. Duty of care principle

This principle stipulates that any organisation that generates waste has a **duty to dispose of the waste safely**. Therefore it is the HCF that has ultimate responsibility for how waste is containerized, handled on-site and off-site and finally disposed of.

2. Polluter pays principle

According to this principle all **waste producers are legally and financially responsible for the safe handling and environmentally sound disposal of the waste they produce**. In case of an accidental pollution, the organisation is liable for the costs of cleaning it up. Therefore if pollution results from poor management of health-care waste then the HCF is responsible. However, if the pollution results because of poor standards at the treatment facility then the HCF is likely to be held jointly accountable for the pollution with the treatment facility. Likewise this could happen with the service provider. The fact that the polluters should pay for the costs they impose on the environment is seen as an efficient incentive to produce less and segregate well.

3. Precautionary principle

Following this principle **one must always assume that waste is hazardous until shown to be safe**. This means that where it is unknown what the hazard may be, it is important to take all the necessary precautions.

4. Proximity principle

This principle recommends that **treatment and disposal of hazardous waste take place at the closest possible location to its source** in order to minimize the risks involved in its transport. According to a similar principle, any community should recycle or dispose of the waste it produces, inside its own territorial limits.

Five fundamental principles for handling health care wastes

These principles include Minimization and Recycling, Sorting receptacles and handling, Collection and Storage, Transportation, and Treatment and Disposal (ICRC, 2011).

Minimization and recycling

The reduction of waste generation must be encouraged by the following practices: Reducing the amount of waste at source, Choosing products that generate less waste: less wrapping material, for example, Choosing suppliers who take back empty containers for refilling (cleaning products); returning gas cylinders to the supplier for refilling, Preventing wastage: in the course of care, for example, or of cleaning activities, Choosing equipment that can be reused such as tableware that can be washed rather than disposable tableware (Bassey *et al.*, 2006; ICRC, 2011).

Sorting receptacles and handling

Sorting consists of clearly identifying the various types of waste and how they can be collected separately. There are two important principles that must be followed. The simplest way to identify the different types of waste and to encourage people to sort them is to collect the various types of waste in separate containers or plastic bags that are colour-coded and/or marked with a symbol (ICRC, 2011).

Waste sorting must always be the responsibility of the entity that produces them. It must be done as close as possible to the site where the wastes are produced. There is no point in sorting wastes that undergo the same treatment process, with the exception of sharps, which must at all times be separated at source from other wastes (Longe and Williams, 2006).

Collection and storage

Waste must be collected regularly - at least once a day. It must never be allowed to accumulate where it is produced. A daily collection programme and collection round must be planned. Each type of waste must be collected and stored separately with different known signs on the containers (Longe and Williams, 2006).

Infectious wastes must never be stored in places that are open to the public.

The personnel in charge of collecting and transporting wastes must be informed to collect only those yellow bags and sharps containers which the care staff have closed. They must wear gloves. The bags that have been collected must be replaced immediately with new bags (Longe and Williams, 2006).

Transportation

This means of conveyance must meet the following requirements: they must be easy to load and unload; they must not have any sharp corners or edges that might tear the bags or damage the containers; they must be easy to clean; (with a 5% active chlorine solution); they must be clearly marked.

Furthermore, off-site means of transport must meet the following requirements: they must be closed in order to avoid any spilling on the road; they must be equipped with a safe loading system (to prevent any spilling inside or outside the vehicle); they must be marked according to the legislation in force if the load exceeds 333 kg (for some countries). The entity producing the waste is responsible for packaging and labelling the waste to be transported outside the hospital. Packaging and labelling must be in conformity with national legislation on the transport of dangerous substances and with the Basel Convention in the case of cross-border transport. If there is no national legislation on the subject, the [United Nations] Recommendations on the Transport of Dangerous Goods1312or the European Agreement on the International Carriage of Dangerous Goods by Road (ADR) 1413 should be referred to. If a vehicle is carrying less than 333 kg of medical waste entailing the risk of contamination (UN 3291), it is not required to be marked. Otherwise it must bear sign plates

Treatment and disposal

Choices of treatment and disposal technique depend on a number of parameters (Bassey *et al.,* 2006). These include the quantity and type of waste produced, availability of waste treatment site near the waste generating facility, availability of reliable means of transport, availability of National legislation on health care waste management, climate conditions, groundwater level, regular supply of electricity in the area etc. The handling and treatment of waste entails health risks for staff throughout the chain. The purpose of protective measures is seriously recommended. The purpose of protective measures is to reduce the risks of accident/exposure or the consequences (Sharma *et al.,* 2006; Longe and Williams, 2006).

7. Environmental regulatory agencies in Nigeria with health care wastes related mandates

Federal Ministry of Environment (FMENV)

The need to protect the environment in Nigeria started with the pronouncement prohibiting water pollution through the colonial hygiene of public health inspectors. In 1975, a Division was created in the Federal Ministry of Economic Development to deal with pollution and other industrial matters. Lack of effective implementation of its mandate led to the relocation of the Division from one Ministry to another (Rain Forest, 2012; FMenv, 2012)

The discovery of six ship loads of toxic waste of Italian origin in Koko, Delta State in 1988, exposed the need for stringent environmental laws and its effective enforcement with monitoring mechanism put in place. The Federal Government promulgated the Harmful Wastes Criminal Provision Decree 42 of 1988, which made it a criminal offence to import or trade in toxic waste. The Federal Environmental Protection Agency (FEPA) was created by Decree 58 of 1988 as a parastatal of the Ministry of Works and Housing. The agency authority was strengthened through Decree 59 of 1992 and October 12th, 1999 saw the creation of the Federal Ministry of Environment (FMEnv) (FMenv, 2012). The Federal Ministry of Environment is charged with the overall responsibility of protecting the Nigerian environment including biodiversity, conservation and sustainable development of natural resources (Rain Forest, 2012).

The National Environmental Protection (Pollution Abatement in Industries & Facilities Generating Waste) Regulation S. I 9 of 1991,

- Prohibits the release of hazardous or toxic substances into the environment beyond the limits approved by the Agency,
- Solid, liquid and gaseous discharge should be analyzed and reported to their nearest office,
- The factory is required to submit yearly environmental audit report within 90 days of demand by the Agency(FMenv, 2012).

Waste Management and hazardous Waste Regulations of 1991,

- Regulates the collection, treatment and disposal of solid and hazardous wastes from municipal and industrial sources (FMenv, 2012).

Guidelines and Standards for Environmental Pollution Control in Nigeria 1991,

- Directs industries to improve the quality of the environment.
- Serves more or less as recommended standards of environmentally good behaviour for industries.

The Federal Government of Nigeria also passed into law the Environmental Impact Assessment (EIA) Act No 86 of 1992, which is summarized below,

http://dx.doi.org/10.5772/53196

- Requires the government, its agency and private enterprises to carry out EIA study of a proposed project,
- The study also covers for proposed expansion of existing project or facility/ industry(FMenv, 2012).

In November 1989, the present Nigeria Environmental Policy was launched to guide environmental activities in Nigeria. The main objective of the policy is to achieve sustainable development which can be achieved by;

1. Securing for all Nigerians a quality of Environment adequate for their health and well being;
2. Conserving and using the natural resources for the benefit of the present and future generations;
3. Restoring, maintaining and enhancing the ecosystem and ecological process essential for the preservation of biological diversity;
4. Raising public awareness and promoting understanding of the essential linkages between environment and development;
5. Co-operation with other countries and international organizations and agencies to achieve the above specific goals, and prevent transboundary environmental pollution(FMenv, 2012)..

National Environmental Standards and Regulation Enforcement Agency (NESREA)

The basis of environmental policy in Nigeria is contained in the 1999 Constitution of the Federal Republic of Nigeria. Section 20 of the Constitution empowers the state to protect and improve the environment; and safeguard the water, air and land, forest and wildlife of Nigeria. Hitherto, various laws and regulations have been enacted to safeguard the Nigerian environment. These include:

- National Environmental Protection (Effluent Limitation) Regulations;
- National Environmental Protection (Pollution Abatement in Industries and Facilities Generating Wastes) Regulations; and
- National Environmental Protection (Management of Solid and Hazardous Wastes) Regulations.

- National Environmental Health Practice Regulations 2007; and

- Nigerian Radioactive Waste Management Regulations 2006.

- Environmental Impact Assessment Act of 1992 (EIA Act).
- The Petroleum (Drilling and Production) Regulations 1969, made pursuant to The Petroleum Act.
- Harmful Wastes (Special Criminal Provisions etc.) Act of 1988 (Harmful Wastes Act).

- The National Oil Spill Detection and Response Agency (Establishment) Act 2006 (the NOSDRA Act).
- Nigerian Radioactive Waste Management Regulations 2006 issued pursuant to the Nuclear Safety and Radiation Protection Act 1995
- The National Environmental Standards and Regulations Agency 2007 (NESREA Act).

The NESREA Act was enacted on the 31st July, 2007 to provide for the establishment of the National Environmental Standards and Regulations Agency (NESREA). This Act repealed the Federal Environmental Protection Agency Act (the FEPA Act) pursuant to which the FEPA which was formerly charged with the protection and development of the environment in Nigeria was established. However all regulations, authorizations and directions made pursuant to the FEPA act and which were in force at the commencement of the NESREA Act shall continue to be in force and have effect as if made by the NESREA Act. The NESREA Act applies to the regulation and the protection and development of the environment in Nigeria with the exception of the oil and gas sector. The NESREA is responsible for the protection and development of environmental standards, regulations, rules, laws, policies and guidelines within Nigeria. The NESREA's functions do not however include enforcement of environmental standards, regulations, policies and guidelines in the oil and gas sector of Nigeria. The NESREA Act give authorized officers of the NESREA powers to:

1. enter and search any land, building, vehicle, tent, vessel, floating craft or any inland water; for the purpose of conducting inspection, searching and taking samples for analysis which are reasonably believed to be carrying out activities or storing goods which contravene environmental standards or legislation
2. seize or detain for such a period as may be necessary articles which are reasonably believed to contravene provisions of the legislation or any of its regulations; and
3. Obtain an order of a court to suspend activities, seal and close down premises including land, vehicle, tent, vessel, floating craft or any inland water and other structure.

Functions of NESREA Act

1. Under the NESREA Act, the Minister charged with the responsibility of the environment is empowered by regulations to prescribe any specific removal methods and reporting obligations on the owners or operators of vessels discharging harmful substances and waste into the environment.
2. Public authorities are statutorily required to inform the public of Environment-related issues. The NESREA Act requires NESREA to enforce compliance with environmental regulations, to create public awareness, provide environmental education on sustainable environmental management and to publish data resulting from the performance of its functions.
3. The NESREA Act provides that a person who breaches the provisions of the Act commits an offence and shall on conviction be liable to a fine, or imprisonment, or both.

4. The NESREA Act also provides that where there has been a discharge of any hazardous substance in violation of environmental laws/permits, the person responsible for the discharge will bear the liability of the costs of removal and clean up.

5. In executing its functions, the NESREA is required to conduct environmental audits and establish a data bank on regulatory and enforcement standards.

The following are environmental impacts associated with the improper disposal of medical wastes:

Pollutants from medical waste (e.g. heavy metals and PCBs) are persistent in the environment

Accumulation of toxic chemicals within soil (proximity to agricultural fields, humans, soil organisms, wildlife, cattle) ground water contamination, decrease in water quality bio-accumulation in organism's fat tissues, and biomagnify through the food chain

Repeated and indiscriminate application of chemicals over a long period of time has serious adverse effects on soil microbial population - reducing the rate of decomposition, and generally lowering the soil fertility.

Pathogens leads to long term accumulation of toxic substances in the soil specimens collected for analysis have the potential to cause disease and illness in man, either through direct contact or indirectly by contamination of soil, groundwater, surface water, and air wind blown dusts from indiscriminately dumping also have the potential to carry hazardous particulates with domestic animals being allowed to graze in open dumps, there is the added risk of reintroducing pathogenic micro-organisms into the food chain.

Public nuisance (e.g. odours, scenic view, block the walkway, aesthetics, etc.)

Improper sterilization of instruments used in labour room may cause infection to mother and child

Combination of both degradable and non-degradable waste increase the rate of habitat destruction due to the increasing number of sites necessary for disposal of wastes (degradation of habitat)

Plastic-bags, plastic containers, if not properly destroyed may contaminate the soil and also reduces the chance for water percolation into the soil during precipitation.

Open air burning does not guarantee proper incineration, and releases toxic fumes (dioxin) into the atmosphere from the burning of plastics i.e., PCB's (Atkin, 2010).

Medical waste management has received very little attention in waste management process in Nigeria. Neither the government nor hospital authorities pay proper attention to its management. Unwholesome waste disposal by many hospitals, clinics and health centers in Abuja pose serious health hazard to the city dwellers in general and people living within the vicinity of the health care institutions in particular (Bassey *et al.*, 2006).

Almost all the health care institutions surveyed dispose every kind of waste generated into municipal dumpsites without pre-treatment, leading to an unhealthy and hazardous environment around the health institutions, affecting patients and staff (Bassey *et al.*, 2006).

Scavengers who collect waste from dustbins are at risk of injury from sharp instruments and direct contact with infectious materials. Liquid medical wastes are disposed directly into the municipal sewer system by all the institutions surveyed (Bassey *et al.*, 2006). Direct disposal of faces and urine of infectious patients in municipal sewer system may cause outbreak of epidemic diseases. The scavengers that engage in recycling operations are unaware of the harmful consequences of exposure to contaminate and hazardous waste (Bassey *et al.*, 2006).

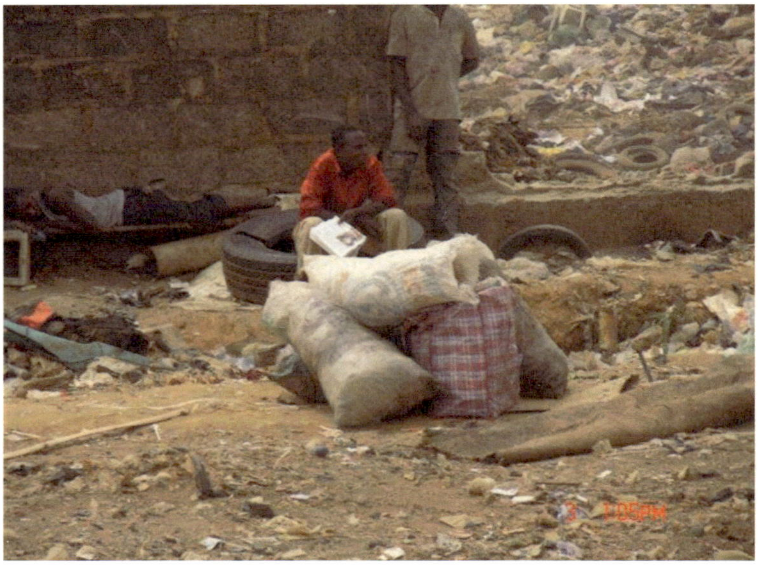

Figure 6. Scavenging at Ojota dumpsite in Lagos, Nigeria

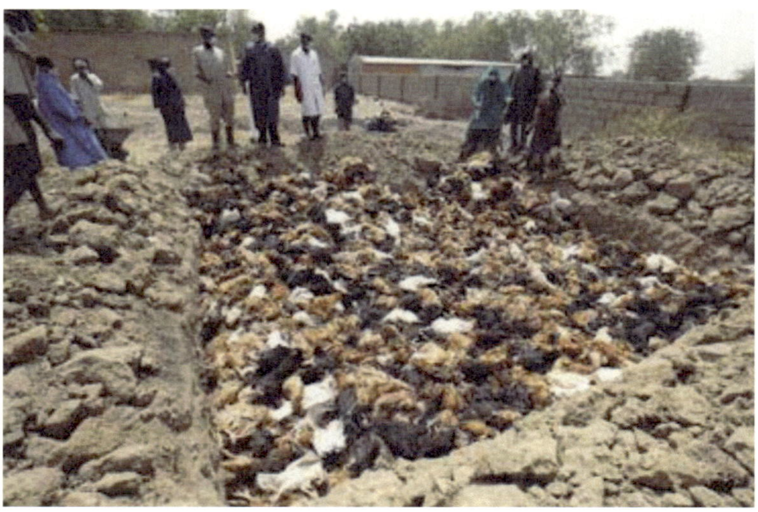

Figure 7. Infected carcasses gathered in a dump for burning (AIHPPRP, 2007)

Most at times, the absence of Environmental impact assessments before commencement of public health and pharmaceutical industry projects is responsible for the archive of challenges associated waste management in the developing worlds including Nigeria. Nigeria lacks both effective and adequate waste management facilities and an inadequate Government policy to guide health providers and punish offenders. There is great need to incorporate standard EIA processes into the Nigerian regulatory documents for Public health institutions and pharmaceutical industries. These regulatory bodies need to establish mitigatory measures especially on waste management during the EIA process of Health care facility in Nigeria.

Incidentally, lapses on these bodies have resulted in no or poor implementation of hazard/ risk/ waste management processes in health care institutions.

NESREA and FMEnv are required to follow-up medical laboratories, hospitals, Pharmaceutical companies springing up all over Nigeria on laboratory waste, and Industrial effluent treatment and disposal.

Without this strict implementation of impact mitigation and management of health care waste, Sustainable development is far from being attained.

Health care waste should be treated with utmost attention, since the wastes could be virulent, pathogenic, carcinogenic, mutagenic, and teratogenic. This shows that its impact on environment and human and plant's health is greater than that of petroleum hydrocarbon spill.

8. Emerging issues of health care waste management

There is no proper waste management system in place in most developing countries. On-site incineration, autoclaving, and steam disinfection are a few processes currently in use for treating very small amounts of hazardous wastes.

Countries found to practice incineration are Brazil, Argentina, Peru, India, Pakistan and Bangladesh etc. Clinical waste incinerators, particularly in developing and poorer countries, often operate under sub-optimal conditions. Most of the cases the percentage of incinerators that were functioning poorly or not operational (HCWH, 1999). Most medical administrations usually focus on installing disposal technologies such as incinerators and do not implement a "practice" of waste management within the hospital. Over 6500 incinerators were installed in the US alone in the 1980s (Agarwal, 1998). Chronic problems both relating to very high toxic levels as well as difficulties in operating a sophisticated engineering technology in a medical setting have given rise to a debate which attempts to define a clean technology for medical waste disposal. There are some techniques practiced by different countries all over the world such as: Incineration, Autoclave Disinfection, Microwave Disinfection, and Mechanical/Chemical Disinfection. Each of this technique has limitations in terms of technological aspect, environmental condition and waste composition. Burning and incineration of medical and municipal waste have been linked to severe public health threat and pollution resulting in the release of toxic dioxin as well as mercury and other toxic substances. These substances produce a remarkable variety of adverse affects in humans at extremely low doses (Basset *et al.,* 2006). Putrefaction occurs in portions of refuse, which have not been fully burnt and add to air pollution through foul smells. Sanitary landfill can lead to pollution of ground water if not properly managed.

However, most of the developed countries have defined policy and regulations to handle and manage medical waste such as Germany, France, Canada, and USA. Unfortunately, health care waste management is not yet carried out with a satisfactory degree of safety in many parts of the globe especially in the underdeveloped world (Stanley *et al.,* 2011).

In Nigeria, the lack of will by policy makers and implementation groups to adopt current technology in Health Care Waste management is an emerging challenge towards HCW management. The Health Care system is not developed in Nigeria, and by extension Health Care Waste Management.

9. Environmental impact assessment for public health and pharmaceutical institutions

In Nigeria Health Care facilities are constructed and flagged off in terms of operations without due considerations to Environmental Impact Assessment (EIA). Its hazards are numerous to be counted. The regulatory agencies in Nigeria on the Environment such as NESREA, FMEnv etc must rise to the challenges of environmental pollution coming from health care facilities. Community engagement during the process of establishing Public health institutions and pharmaceutical companies is also advisable. This will ensure the development of robust Terms of Reference, EIA document, Environmental Management Plan (EMP). The EMP should address the issues or negative impacts of the health care facility on the bio-physical, social environment and health.

It is worthy to note that some health care facilities such as medical and Environmental Laboratories are small projects and may not require full blown EIA. However, the regulatory agencies should develop a module of monitoring their waste disposal to avoid pollution. The situation is bit different in developed countries, where there is integrated Health management system; medical laboratories are usually part of large health care facilities. It is good to state categorical that laboratory wastes are among the most infectious group of health care waste. They contain live virulent pathogens and mutagenic, teratogenic chemicals including dyes. Laboratories must be forced to have a standard waste tracking protocol, in line with the international convention called Polluters Pay Principles (PPP).

10. Conclusion

Federal Republic of Nigeria will gain a lot from the battery of Public health benefits of Health Care waste Management. It is still not well understood why Nigeria at its level of development, Health Care Waste management is not well legislated and thus proper attention has not been given to it by Environmental regulators and Health Care operators. The issues are to be treated as urgent and very critical by Government. Immediate interventions are also required. All hands including the National Orientation Agencies and communities must be on deck to get over this challenge.

11. Recommendation

There is great need for effective Environmental regulatory Surveillance in Nigeria. National laws on Health Care waste management should be established and be moved to an act.

This is the best time for Nigerian Government to establish a regulatory agency to effectively monitor medical wastes and its treatment in Nigeria. Otherwise, the FMEnv and NESREA are to be strengthened to establish a well funded unit (Finance and good Human Resources) for monitoring of Health Care Institutions over Health Care Wastes.

Author details

Nkechi Chuks Nwachukwu[1*], Frank Anayo Orji[2*] and Ositadinma Chinyere Ugbogu[1*]

*Address all correspondence to:

1 Department of Microbiology, Faculty of Biological and Physical Sciences, Abia State University, Uturu, Abia State, Nigeria

2 Enzymes and Genetics Division, Department of Biotechnology, Federal Institute of Industrial Research, Oshodi, Lagos State, Nigeria

References

[1] Abah, S. O., & Ohimain, E. I. (2010). Assessment of Dumpsite Rehabilitation Potential using the Integrated Risk Based Approach: A case study of Eneka, Nigeria. *World Appl. Sci. J.,*, 8(4), 436-442.

[2] Avian Influenza Control and Human Pandemic Preparedness and Response Project. (2007). Final report on Medical Waste Management Plan, Environquest, Nigeria.

[3] Adegbita, M. A., Nwafor, S. O., Afon, A., Abegunde, A. A., & Bamise, C. T. (2010). Assessment of dental waste management in a Nigerian tertiary hospital. *Waste. manag. Res.,*, 28, 769-777.

[4] Alagoz, B. A. Z., & Kocasoy, G. (2007). Treatment and disposal alternatives for health-care wastes in developing countries- A case study in Istanbul, Turkey. *Waste Manag. Res.,*, 25, 83-89.

[5] Coker et al. (2009). Medical waste management in Ibadan, Nigeria: Obstacles and Prospects. *Waste Manag.,*, 29(2), 804-811.

[6] Olubukola, B. O. (2009). Comparative Analysis of Health Care Waste Management Practice in Two General Hospitals in Nigeria. Available at, http://www.eco-web.com/edi/index.htm., Accessed August 10, 2012.

[7] PATH. (2009). Achieving effective sharps waste management in GAVI host countries. A proposed approach with estimates of cost 2006. Available at, http://.www.Path.org/files/TS_ach_eff_swm.pdf., Accessed 6th April, 2012.

[8] Phengxay, S., Okumura, J., Miyoshi, M., Sakisaka, K., Kuroiwa, C., & Phengxay, M. (2005). Healthcare Waste Management in Lao PDR: A case study,. *Waste. Manage. Res.,*, 23, 571-581.

[9] The Hazardous Chemicals and Wastes Conventions (HCWC). (2007). http://www.healthcarewaste.org/fileadmin/user_upload/resources/UNEP-3Conventions-2007-EN.pdf, Accessed August 15, 2011).

[10] Park, H., Lee, K., Kim, M., Lee, J., Seong, S. Y., & Ko, G. . (2009). Detection and hazard assessment of pathogenic microorganisms in medical wastes. *Environ Sci Health A Tox Hazard Subst Environ Eng.,*, 44(10), 995-1003.

[11] Nascimento, T. C., Januzzi, W. A., Leonel, M., Silva, V. L., & Diniz, C. G. (2009). Occurrence of clinically relevant bacteria in health service waste in a Brazilian sanitary landfill and antimicrobial susceptibility profile,. *Rev. Soc. Bras. Med.Trop.*, 42(4).

[12] Rain Forest. (2012). Nigerian Regulatory bodies. Available at, http://www.rainforestlimited.com/contactus.html., Accessed on 20 August, 2012).

[13] Federal Ministry of Environment (FMEnv). (2012). Vision Statement of the Ministry. available on, http://directory-nigeria.org/federal-ministry-of-environment-housing-and-urban-dev.html, Accessed on 20th August, 2012.

[14] Akter, N. (2010). Medical Waste Management: A Review,. Asian Institute of Technology, Thailand,, 25.

[15] Agarwal, R. (1998). Medical waste Disposal. *Issues, Practices and Policy.*, An Indian and International Perspective. Seminar on Health and the Environment. Centre for Science and Environment. New Delhi. India.

[16] BAN & HCWH. (1999). Medical Waste in Developing Countries. *An analysis with a case study of India, and A critique of the Basel-TWG guidelines.*, Basel Action Network (BAN) secretariat, Asia_Pacific Environmental Exchange, 1827 39th Ave. E., Seattle, WA. 98112, USA.

[17] WHO. (1999). Health Care wastes. Available at:, http://www.who.int/water_sanitation_health/Environmental_sanit/MHCWHanbook.htm.

[18] Prüss, A., & Townend, W. K. (1998). Teacher's Guide- Management of wastes from health-care activities,. World Health Organization, Geneva, 227 pages. Available at:, http://www.who.int/environmental_information/Information_resources/worddocs/HCteachguid/health_care_wastes_teacher.htm.

[19] Johannessen, L. M. (2000). Healthcare Waste Management Guidance Note. Anchor Team, The World Bank,, 68, Available at:, http://wbln0018.worldbank.org/hdnet/hddocs.nsf/c0d65c5ea6fcb4688525670c004d14c2/0d87e869807f2f69852568d20054e66b.

[20] World Health Organization, Geneva. (1992). Managing medical wastes in developing countries: report of a Consultation on Medical Wastes Management in Developing Countries, Geneva,. Available at:, http://whqlibdoc.who.int/hq/1994/WHO_PEP_RUD_94.1.pdf.

[21] Ngwuluka, N., Ochekpe, N., Odumosu, P., & John, S. A. (2009). Waste management in healthcare establishments within Jos Metropolis, Nigeria,. *African Journal of Environmental Science and Technology,*, 3(12), 459-465.

[22] Ogbonna, D. N. (2011). Characteristics and waste management practices of Medical wastes in healthcare institutions in Port Harcourt, Nigeria,. *Journal of Soil Science and Environmental Management,*, 2(5), 132-141.

[23] Abah, S. O., Ohimain, E. I., & (2011, . (2011). Healthcare waste management in Nigeria: A case study,. *Journal of Public Health and Epidemiology,*, 3(3), 99-110.

[24] Stanley, H. O., Okpara, K. E., Chukwujekwu, D. C., Agbozu, I. E., & Nyenke, C. U. (2011). Health care waste management in Port Harcourt Metropolis. *American Journal of Scientific and Industrial Research*, 2(5), 769-773.

[25] Bassey, B. E., Benka-Coker, M. O., & Aluyi, H. S. A. (2006). Characterization and management of solid medical wastes in the Federal Capital Territory, Abuja Nigeria. *African Health Sciences,*, 6(1), 58-63.

[26] WHO. (2012). Antimicrobial resistance. Available on, http://www.who.int/mediacentre/factsheets/fs194/en/, Accessed 24tth August, 2012.

[27] Sharma, D. R., Pradhan, B., & Mishra, S. K. (2010). Multiple drug resistance in bacterial isolates from liquid wastes generated in central hospitals of Nepal. *Kathmandu University Medical Journal*, 8(29), 40-44.

[28] Kümmerer, K. (2004). Resistance in the environment. *Journal of Antimicrobial Chemotherapy*, 54, 311-20.

[29] Kolpin, D. W., Furlong, E. T., Meyer, M. T., Turman, E. M., Zaugg, S. D., & Barber, L. B. (2002). Pharmaceuticals, Hormones, and Other Organic Waste water Contaminants in U.S. Streams, 1999-2000: A National Reconnaissance. *Environmental Science and Technology,*, 36(6), 1202-11.

[30] Smith K E, Besser J M, Hedberg C W, Leano F T, Bender J B, & Wicklund J H. (1999). Quinolone resistant Campylobacter jejuni infections in Minnesota, 1992-1998,. *The New England Journal of Medicine,*, 340, 1525-32.

[31] House of Lords Select Committee on Science and Technology (HLSCST). (1998). 7th Report of House of Lords (UK). London: The Stationery Office.

[32] Hiraishi, A. (1998). Respiratory quinone profiles as tools for identifying different bacterial populations in activated sludge. *Journal of General and Applied Microbiology,*, 34, 39-56.

[33] International Committee of the Red Cross (ICRC). (2011). Medical Waste Management,. 19, avenue de la Paix 1202 Geneva, Switzerland., 164, Available at, http// www.icrc.org., (Accessed 26th August, 2012).

[34] Longe, E. O., & Williams, A. (2006). A preliminary study on medical waste management in Lagos Metropolis, Nigeria. *Iranian Journal of Environmental Health Sciences and Engineering,*, 3(3), 1333-139.

Chapter 9

Characterisation of Dental Waste in Tertiary Dental Hospitals: A Third World Example

Michael Adewole Adedigba,
Isaiah Adesola Oke and Regina Arobieke

Additional information is available at the end of the chapter

http://dx.doi.org/10.5772/53194

1. Introduction

Dental (Medical) waste has been defined as all wastes generated from health care or health related facilities. The waste generated from the dental hospital are of various materials, sizes, shades and shapes and are therefore regarded as heterogeneous [1]. There are dental liquid wastes such as X-ray (developer and fixer) wastes and other chemicals and drugs generated within the dental or medical facilities in general. The waste can also be in form of solid generated from the diagnosis, investigations and treatment of human beings and or in animal trials [2,3]. The solid waste generated from the dental hospital can be broadly categorised into two, namely; infectious and non-infectious wastes. The mode of treatment of these waste differ sharply for the safety of man and his environment. Generators of medical/dental wastes are defined as those producing more than 23 kg of regulated medical/dental waste per month [4]. For generators who manage their waste by shipping to offsite disposal facilities, they are supposed to separate, package, label, mark, and track the waste according to regulations [2, 5]. In Nigeria, generators have, for long time, assumed treatment methods based on techniques suitable for treatment of municipal solid waste.

Infectious wastes include blood on swabs or dressings and used sharps (needles, probes, endodontic reamers and files etc.) are considered non-hazardous waste. This can be mixed with routine rubbish if such are properly treated to become non-infectious. Any untreated waste should be properly labelled and handled by a waste hauler [6]. Contaminated sharps must be placed in a puncture-resistant rigid container and treated prior to disposal. It is also must be submitted that untreated containers of sharps cannot be compacted.

Dental waste can lead to infection and or transmission of infectious diseases. This is done because of the micro-organisms content namely bacteria, fungi and viruses. These micro-organisms can cause disease or mirage of health related conditions [7]. The level of infectiousness of any agent will grossly depend on the dose of micro-organism introduced in to the body, portal of entry (intravenous, aerosol, oral-faecal etc.), virulence factor of the micro-organism (production of enzymes, waste products and other toxins capable of damaging host tissues) and the state of host immune resistance. The quantity of infectious waste generated in health care facility is in the range of 10 to 25% of the total generation [8, 9, 10, 11].

Dental waste has been demonstrated to contribute significantly to pollution of the environment if poorly treated [12] and that it can lead to cross-infection risks [13] such as deadly HIV and Hepatitis among others [14]. Heavy metals such as Chromium, Cadmium and Amalgam are frequently generated from the dental hospitals and are known to be hazardous. These metals have been known to cause diseases in humans such as liver, kidney and respiratory damage by Chromium while cadmium may cause kidney disorders and lung cancer [15].

Dental treatment involves the use of consumables such as gloves, face masks, rubber dams, protective cellophane and other chlorine containing items which are disposed off by incineration. The process of incineration leads to release of dioxin, Hydrogen Chloride (HCl) and Chlorofluorocarbon (CFC) which has been implicated in reproductive defects, neurological problems, cancer formation, hormonal and immune disorders [16]. Also, food remains and glass wares should be sort out of dental waste because they adversely affect the performance of incinerator. Although, dental waste do not generally contain food remains to any large extent as this is not a common practice within the clinics, but more of plastics (Polyvinyl Chloride PVC, Polyethylene, (PE), polypropylene (PPE). This can be mixed with routine rubbish if such are properly treated to become non-infectious. Any untreated waste should be properly labelled and handled by a waste hauler [6]. Contaminated sharps must be placed in a puncture-resistant rigid container and treated prior to disposal.

The proper and standardized management of dental waste will assist in controlling health risks among humans and safe environment. These are the main reasons for proper managing of dental waste.i.e. to render such non-infectious /hazardous. It is the sole responsibility of generators of (dental) waste to dispose them adequately and so it is for the handlers as well. The standard practice for dental waste are: designation and identification, segregation, packaging, storage, transport and handling, treatment techniques, disposal of treated waste, contingency planning and continued staff training [2,17]. The cost of mishandling of dental waste is another question that must be answered by dental waste generator. Their goal would be to minimize such cost to the lowest possible.

There is a sharp difference in the way dental waste should be handled compared with that of Municipal waste. The traditional way of handling Municipal waste are such as landfilling, composting, recycle and waste-to-energy technologies (WTE); but these cannot be applied directly to dental waste except recycling and WTE system. Dental waste will require special treatment due to infectious nature and common incineration (as is the case with municipal wastes). This cannot be performed except staff of such device are properly trained. During the process of incineration, dioxins and furans can be controlled or reduced by the incineration

http://dx.doi.org/10.5772/53194

temperature. However, under start-up conditions, dioxins and furans can be stopped from entering the atmosphere by use of wet scrubbers [4]. Dental wastes consist of extracted teeth and other human parts which are usually loaded with micro-organisms and hence Dental waste must be rendered non-infectious before disposal which is regarded as the process of waste treatment. If this is not achieved the dispersal of dangerous infectious materials will ensue. Waste treatment is determined by waste type and the type of treatment appropriate for it. Incineration is just appropriate for dental waste. The volume and weight of incinerated dental waste is reduced to above 90% making the eventual disposal of a less problem when compared with other methods. Incineration is the best technology to date yet it has its own short comings such as high capital and running cost, operating charges, sterilisation efficacy, maintenance and operator skills, control of air and water emissions. Lastly, it cannot take care of radioactive materials from X-ray rooms. Management of dental waste can be done by treatment first, recovery of useful materials such as Mercury, Silver and other metals, modification of characteristics of the waste, making exposure free of harm and environmental friendly. Basically there are two types of incineration namely large and small scale systems. The large scale systems utilises any of the followings: fluidized bed combustors [18], starved and excess air incineration and rotary kilns; while the small scale systems uses chambers which can be single or double chambers. Incineration can be used to heat water for the use of both the patients and hospital. Dental local anaesthetic cartridges, ampoules, glass wares that are not combustible can be treated with steam autoclaving, microwave irradiation, chemical treatment and radiofrequency irradiation [2].

Van Veen [5] was of the opinion that medical waste must be monitored so that the where about of such is known at all times, this can be achieved by proper controls put in place. The control can be done through policy and adequate empowerment for the policy to work. Only by this, will our environment be free and fear of harm from medical wastes. At this point, little is known about policy and implementation of medical waste in Nigeria as compared to that of advanced countries. Even if the policy is there little is known about the implementation and it's monitoring. "Regulation myopia" which means failure to look beyond the immediate issue to see the full effects of the regulatory actions [4] must be avoided when policy on waste management are put in operation. There are various current ways to manage dental waste, this include reduction of waste generated, this is done by eliminating or substituting substances that increase or expose individuals to health risks e.g. use of digital X-rays compared to the conventional film, developer/fixer combination [12]. Another way is to segregate and recycle useful materials from the dental waste such as mercury from amalgam, Silver from fixer/ developer. Noncombustible items in dental waste should not be fed into incinerators and waste-to-energy system (WTE). This is because they give rise to continuous smoke which will hinder complete combustion of the waste components. To recycle dental hospital waste poses some challenges of harm to handlers of such unlike the municipal waste. This is why dental (like the medical) recyclables are highly discriminated at [4]. Hence there is a need to prove to the general recycling market that dental waste has great prospect.

Previous studies in Africa have reported non-conformity to standard ways of disposing of dental (medical) waste [19,3,13,12]. The majority of studies carried out on dental waste centred on knowledge, attitude and practice of Dental Health Care Workers [19], infection control [20, 21], composition of dental waste [22] and management of mercury and dental amalgam [23]. This study therefore aims at sorting, characterizing and quantifying wastes generated in selected eight clinics of a Dental Hospital in third world nation. This is with a view to providing information on waste classification in dental hospitals in developing nations. It is expected that such information will aid sustainable dental waste disposal in the study area and beyond.

2. Materials and methods

Waste generation and management were monitored daily for a month at the eight dental clinics of Obafemi Awolowo University (OAU), Ile-Ife, Nigeria. The choice of dental Hospital OAU Ile-Ife for this study is influenced by some factors. First, it serves as the referral centre for dental patients from Osun, Ekiti, Ondo and part of Kwara states, in southern part of Nigeria. Other dental tertiary hospitals in the region lack such regional coverage. In addition, it's the only one located in the sub-urban area peculiar to the third world environment.

Wastes at the source were characterised, classified by the authors into the two main categories by weight and by volume infectious and non-infectious. Waste collection polythene bags were placed in each of the two waste baskets (one for infectious and the other for non-infectious) in all the eight clinics and the X-ray room of Obafemi Awolowo University Dental Hospital for collection of waste from each unit. On many occasions there was a necessity for sorting of the wastes into the two categories. The sorting was done with the use of disposable gloves and facemasks and duck lip forceps by the authors, this sorting method was similar to that used by [13]. Measurement of solid wastes was carried out using a weighing scale of sensitivity of 0.01g weight. The breath, height and length of the tied solid waste inside waste disposal bags were measured in metres. The measurement was done by the principal investigator and two other assistants at the close of each clinic day and before the waste were carried away by haulers. Statistical information on the waste generations and classifications were determined through number of patients and measurement of necessary parameters.

2.1. Results and discussion

Results from study are discussed in the following categories: characterisation, generation and application of the results.

Characterisation: It is well known that the wastes generated from the treatment of patients suffering from infectious diseases may spread infection either through direct contact or indirectly through the environment. In Nigeria the management of these infectious waste materials is regulated under Decree 42 of November 1998 [2]. It was reported that injections undertaken with contaminated syringes caused about 23 million infections of Hepatitis B, Hepatitis B and HIV worldwide [2]. Report from Tanzania, was that during immunization campaigns the medical waste management staff needs to take an extra care and the wastes generated during such campaigns have different classes depending on the mode of classification [1]. The classification of sharps and softs on weight and volume bases shows that sharps

http://dx.doi.org/10.5772/53194

are still a small portion of the waste, which requires special care compared to the softs [2]. Tables 1 and 2 show the typical waste composition from the clinics and the characterisation of the waste studied based on the weight and volume, respectively.

Clinic	Mass of the waste per patient (g)				Volume of the waste per patient (cm^3)				Density of the waste per patient (g/cm^3)			
	Maximum	Minimum	Standard Deviation	Mean	Maximum	Minimum	Standard Deviation	Mean	Maximum	Minimum	Standard Deviation	Mean
Oral Diagnosis	119.50	1.00	30.33	22.39	20254.00	6.00	4468.57	1568.72	0.1667	0.0005	0.0506	0.0213
Conservative	113.00	0.00	34.21	29.53	3300.00	0.00	947.21	728.26	2.0000	0.0000	0.4444	0.1149
Periodontology	104.00	0.20	28.44	43.33	4620.00	1.20	1081.25	1266.42	0.0355	0.0012	0.0109	0.0131
Paedodontics	173.33	0.00	48.07	51.35	9240.00	0.00	2389.19	1774.59	0.0833	0.0000	0.0233	0.0183
Orthodontics	64.86	0.00	20.44	33.63	3736.86	0.00	890.76	956.82	0.0833	0.0000	0.0252	0.0190
X-RAY	129.00	0.00	29.94	18.69	2372.53	0.00	553.05	423.47	0.1128	0.0000	0.0338	0.0163
Prosthetics	150.00	0.00	45.91	52.28	6562.50	0.00	1499.00	1000.76	3.0588	0.0000	0.6782	0.1804
Oral Surgery	112.00	0.00	24.13	32.55	3480.00	0.00	996.21	1043.18	6.2381	0.0000	1.3919	0.3255

Table 1. Statistical information on infectious waste generation

Clinic	Mass of the waste per patient (g)				Volume of the waste per patient (cm^3)				Density of the waste per patient (g/cm^3)			
	Maximum	Minimum	Standard Deviation	Mean	Maximum	Minimum	Standard Deviation	Mean	Maximum	Minimum	Standard Deviation	Mean
Oral Diagnosis	72.50	0.00	15.72	7.15	7245.00	0.00	1589.82	593.73	0.166667	0.000000	0.050847	0.018091
Conservative	40.00	0.00	12.27	16.11	3045.00	0.00	870.46	832.61	2.750000	0.000000	0.612814	0.148557
Periodontology	47.50	0.01	13.77	21.37	6375.00	1.20	1548.16	1915.26	0.033333	0.000654	0.009942	0.007505
Paedodontics	50.00	0.01	15.34	25.39	7245.00	3.00	2016.11	2529.82	0.083333	0.000700	0.024514	0.013248
Orthodontics	68.00	0.01	18.26	25.49	10657.50	3.00	2541.14	2627.27	0.083333	0.001308	0.024607	0.011846
X-RAY	120.00	0.00	27.20	13.59	3990.00	0.00	1030.05	616.96	0.083333	0.000000	0.025575	0.011189
Prosthetics	110.00	0.00	25.19	13.39	2800.00	0.00	830.34	546.47	2.291667	0.000000	0.509659	0.129943
Oral Surgery	62.00	0.00	17.05	17.34	4914.00	0.00	1087.43	1105.23	0.083333	0.000000	0.025008	0.010657

Table 2. Statistical information on non- infectious waste generation

The Oral surgery clinic was the highest generator of infectious waste (density= 1.392) while Prosthetic clinic was in the same category for non-infectious waste (density=0.130). The amount of waste generated from the Oral Surgery clinic was not unexpected in view of the procedures involved in tooth extraction, biopsies and other surgery routines. From the tables it can be seen that waste generation and characterisation are functions of clinics and number of patients. Table 3 presents statistical data on the patients per clinic.

Clinic	Oral Diagnosis	Conservative	Periodontology	Paedodontics	Orthodontics	X-RAY	Prosthetics	Oral Surgery
Maximum (Number of patients)	30	24	25	10	10	31	25	18
Minimum (Number of patients)	1	0	1	1	2	0	0	0
Standard Deviation	8.48	7.10	5.33	2.45	2.58	10.73	5.93	5.55
Mean	12.4	7.4	6.1	3.9	4.35	11.7	5.55	8.9

Table 3. Statistical data on the patients

From the tables maximum waste per patient for infectious waste was 173.33g/ day and maximum volume per patient was 20254.00 cm^3 / day. For non-infectious waste maximum mass per patient is 120.00 g/day and volume per patient is 10657.50 cm^3 with maximum patient per clinic of 31 per day. The dental wastes are managed as the municipal wastes in the present study similar to the findings of [1,12] which was contrary to international standard practice.

Application of the results: The current waste management techniques consist of generation, storage, transporting and final disposal, which indicates that there is a need of having treatment facilities for infectious and non- infectious wastes individually. For infectious waste proposed waste treatment period is weekly (5 working days in a week) using locally developed facilities as Figure 1, 2 or Figure 3.

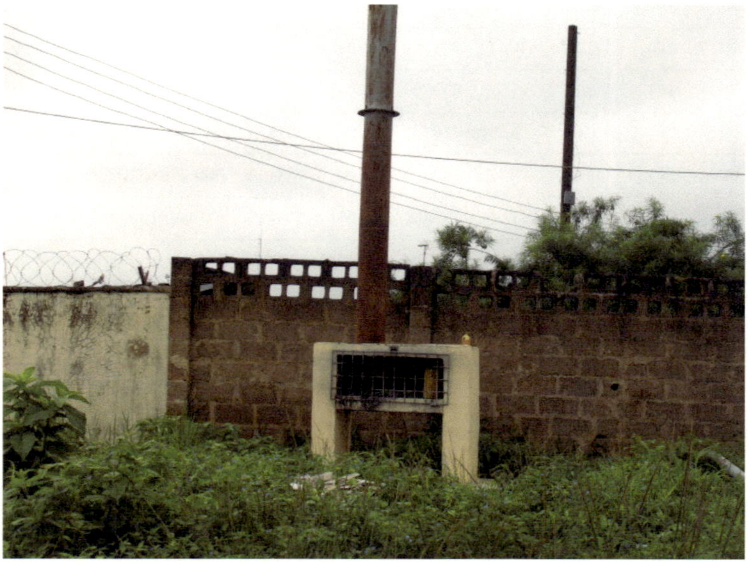

Figure 1. Locally developed incinerator using concrete

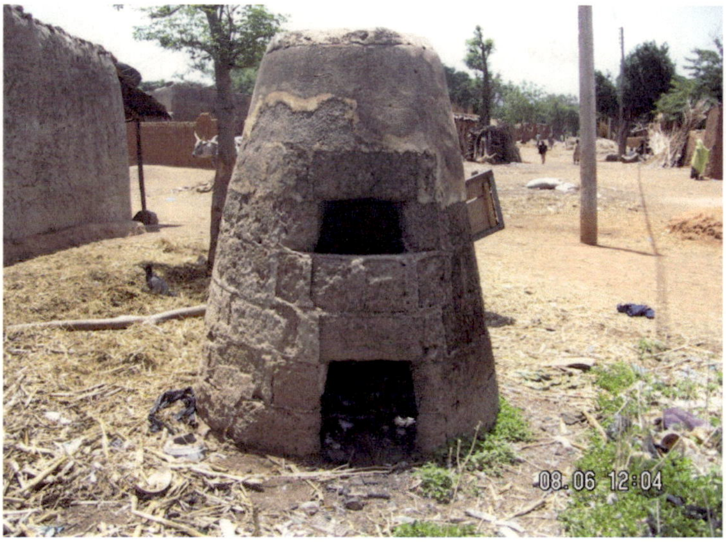

Figure 2. Locally developed incinerator using sandcrete

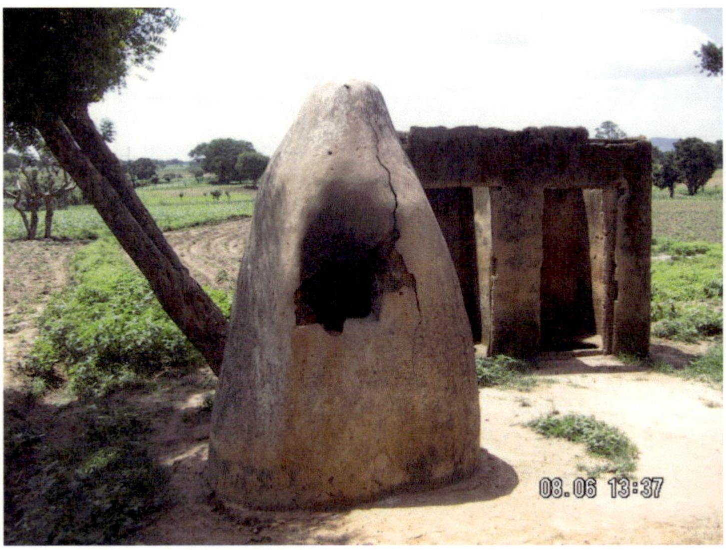

Figure 3. Locally developed incinerator using mud blocks

The expected volume is 3.14 m^3 (20254 x 5 x 31 cm^3). The expected volume for non-infectious waste is 3.3 m^3 (10657.50 x 10 x 31 cm^3). The non-infectious waste should be disposed twice in a month (10 working days). From these calculations, the provision of 3.5 m^3 or above of locally developed incinerators will help in dental waste treatment technique.

2.2. Medical waste elsewhere in nigeria

Waste generation and characterization in Ibadan: Coker et al [13] reported that the nature and amount of healthcare waste (HCW) generated in the various Health Care Facilities (HCFs) is presented in Table 4.

MW Component	Generated waste in each HCFs category (kg/d)					
	Tertiary (n= 1)	Secondary (n= 19)	Primary (n= 1)	Diagnostic (n= 9)	Total wastes for all surveyed HCFs	Percentage of total waste (%)
Human anatomical part	766.5	6279.3	1693.6	-	8739.4	4.0
Plastic, PVC, syringes	1412.6	40233.4	1109.5	1461.2	44216.7	20.1
Swabs, absorbents	36.5	8509.4	9820.7	613.6	18980.2	8.6
Alcohol, disinfectant	-	2094.0	57.9	-	2151.9	0.9
Animal infected anatomical	-	1232.9	-	-	1232.9	0.6
Glass	203.7	54202.5	3082.6	10.5	57599.3	26.1
Bedding, shavings, paper, faecal matter	10.9	9224.5	973.6	0.32	10209.3	4.6
Gauze pads, garments, cellulose	98.6	39109.3	2892.3	-	42100.2	19.1
Sharps, needles	30.3	24551.0	269.9	0.41	14851.6	11.3
Fluids, residues	-	1002.5	1232.1	0.41	2235.0	1.0
Infectious wastes	20.1	8085.6	52	2.0	8112.9	3.7
Daily total generation (kg/d)	2579	194524	21137	2088	220329	100
Generation / facility (kg/d)	2579	10238	919	232		

Source: Coker et al., 2009

Table 4. Nature and mean generation rate of medical waste (MW) in various HCFs surveyed in Ibadan, Nigeria (on a weight/ facility basis.

The bulk (39%) of total solid medical waste materials comprise of plastics, PVC, syringes, gauze pads, garments, and cellulose. Other main solid medical wastes were sharps and needles (11.3%), swabs and absorbents (8.6%), and beddings, shavings, paper and faecal matter (4.6%). Overall, infectious wastes constituted only 3.7% of total waste. A similar study by [24] in Bangladesh reported 10.5% infectious waste. With the exception of the tertiary HCFs, there was no proper segregation in most HCFs. In fact, the study team had to implement waste sorting and segregation at source by providing coded separate receptacles for each identified components of waste. Previously, waste which otherwise could have been handled and disposed as household waste, would end up being mixed together with HCW, thus increasing the amount of waste regarded as medical waste. This supports the argument that waste segregation does reduce waste volumes. It was opined that only waste capable of initiating infectious diseases should be considered infectious, such that the presence and virulence of

http://dx.doi.org/10.5772/53194

pathogens, entry portal and host susceptibility should be overriding considerations when estimating risk [25]. Their study (at the University Hospital Freiburg, Germany) revealed that up to 70% of the content of infectious waste consisted of household waste (such as journals, newspapers; packaging, paper, and glass) without risk for infection.

In Ibadan, the non-sorting approach at many HCFs causes contamination of materials with blood, which promotes unnecessary waste items in the waste stream. In this case, many benefits would accrue (both environmental and financial) if some materials were reprocessed and reused without risking patient health. The peak average rate of waste generation/facility was from the secondary HCFs whose value of 10,238 kg/d was almost quadruple of the tertiary HCF, ≈11 times the primary HCFs and≈ 25 times the 232 kg/d rate of diagnostic centres (Table 4). Similarly, in Karachi, Pakistan, another developing nation, secondary HCFs generate more solid medical waste than other HCFs [26]. Indeed, secondary HCFs have greater patronage of patients than any other kind in Ibadan. In such HCFs, the management allows home-cooked food and other essentials to be brought-in for patients. Thus, general household waste all too easily becomes mixed with medical waste destined for the waste stream. Waste sorting and segregation, practiced at the tertiary HCF, has aided substantial reductions in what would otherwise eventually end up in the waste stream. This is because pro-active recycling of some materials is employed. Unlike elsewhere in Ibadan, the hospital (UCH) is known to uniquely follow standard international practices of patient care and hygiene. However, treatment costs at UCH, which are beyond the reach of many patients, have forced many people to patronize secondary HCFs. The declining patronage of UCH seems intrinsically linked with government expenditure reductions on health-related programmes. For instance, percentage of government expenditure spent on healthcare dropped from 33.5% in 2000 to 25.6% in 2002, with private sector expenditure accounting for the other 66.5% and 74.4%, respectively [27]. However, as with other nations, the private sector is profit-driven. Meanwhile, the primary HCFs chiefly attend to outpatients and, as such, have a much-reduced generation/facility rate. However, that said, diagnostic laboratories have the least amount of waste generation because patients mostly come to drop-off specimens.

In Lagos metropolis (Nigeria) medical waste generation in selected hospital are as presented in Tables 5 and 6. From the tables, medical waste generation in surveyed hospitals (kg/ bed. day) and the total waste generation (kg/day) can be obtained.

Designation	Hospital Type	Number of beds	Total waste generated (kg/day)	Waste generated rate (kg/bed/day)
A	Private	40	22.5	0.563
B	Private	50	28.1	0.562
C	Public	600	399.6	0.666
D	Public	378	161.3	0.427
Total		1068	611.5	0.573
Average rate = 0.573 kg/bed/day (Source: Longe and Williams, 2006)				

Table 5. Medical waste generation in selected hospital in Lagos, Nigeria

Waste category	Hospital A (Private 1)	Hospital B (Private 2)	Hospital C (Public 1)	Hospital D (Public 2)	Average
Regulated waste	51	66	50	50	54
Infectious	34	19	37	37	32
Sharps/Pathological	11	10	10	10	10
Chemical	2	4	3	3	3
Others	2	1	-	-	1
Total	100	100	100	100	100

Source: Longe and Williams, 2006

Table 6. Composition of medical waste generation in selected hospital in Lagos, Nigeria

It was discovered that most hospitals had no record of the volume of waste being generated by them. The amount of wastes generated is easily expressed in volume as most storage facilities are in litres aside those at depot centres [28]. Medical waste generation rates ranged between 0.427 and 0.666 kg / bed. day was obtained. The total volume of medical waste generated in all the hospital was 611.5 kg/day. This translates to 17.19 kg/bed month and calculated total waste volume of 18345.00 kg/ month by all hospitals. Out of this infectious waste was 5, 870.4kg/month, sharps, 1845 kg/month and chemical waste 550.35 kg/ month. Regulated domestic waste constitutes 54% of the total medical waste stream. Another noticeable inference is that the proportion of medical waste from the two public hospitals was more than 91% of the total volume of waste stream. The percentages by weight of infectious waste generated by these hospitals are also of higher magnitudes compared with others. The only explanation for this has to do with the number of available medical services and facilities in the two public hospitals [28]. Based on the data from [29] presented in Table 7(a) and 7(b), it was discovered that 65% of hospitals/clinics do not segregate waste generated in their clinics.

Serial Number	Name of hospital and clinics in Akure	Number of beds	General	Infectious	Hazardous
1	State Specialist Hospital	110	13.055	3.48	0.87
2	Optimum clinic	8	4.2	1.12	0.28
3	City Hospital	8	3.6	0.96	0.24
4	Royal Medical Centre	6	2.55	0.68	0.17
5	Don Bosco Health Centre	4	2.775	0.74	0.185
6	St John and Mary Hospital	10	7.65	2.04	0.51
7	Sijuwade Specialist Hospital	12	3.975	1.06	0.265
8	St Michael Hospital Pol. HQ	10	3.975	1.06	0.265
9	Banjo Memorial Hospital	30	2.45	0.66	0.165
10	Adetade Hospital Ondo Rd	10	1.875	0.5	0.125
11	First Mercy Hospital Gbogi	42	14.071	3.92	0.98

12	FUTA Gate Clinic	4	4.05	1.08	0.27
13	Oludare Hospital Fanibi	12	11.755	3.14	0.785
14	Abitoye Hospital Ijapo	22	2.926	0.78	0.195
15	University Health Centre	6	4.5	1.2	0.30
16	Faith Clinic Oke Aro	6	1.95	0.52	0.13
17	Abitoye Hospital, Ijoka	15	0.75	2.6	0.65
18	Crown Hospital	17	10.725	2.86	0.715
19	Hope Hospital Ijoka	6	3.225	0.86	0.25
20	Momaak Specialist Hospital	10	4.65	1.24	0.31

(a)

Serial Number	Name of hospital and clinics in Akure	Total waste/day (kg)	Daily waste generation (kg/day)		
			General (75%)	Infectious (20%)	Hazardous (5%)
1	State Specialist Hospital	17.4	13.05	3.44	0.87
2	Optimum clinic	5.6	4.2	1.12	0.28
3	City Hosiptal	4.8	3.6	0.96	0.24
4	Royal Medical Centre	3.7	2.78	0.74	0.18
5	Don Bosco Health Centre	3.4	2.55	0.68	0.17
6	St John and Mary Hospital	10.2	7.65	2.04	0.51
7	Sijuwade Specialist Hospital	6.6	4.95	1.32	0.33
8	St Michael Hospital Pol. HQ	5.3	3.975	1.05	0.265
9	Banjo Memorial Hospital	3.3	2.475	0.66	0.165
10	Adetade Hospital Ondo Rd	2.5	1.875	0.5	0.125
11	First Mercy Hospital Gbogi	19.61	14.708	3.922	0.981
12	FUTA Gate Clinic	5.4	4.05	1.08	0.27
13	Oludare Hospital Fanibi	15.7	11.775	3.14	0.785
14	Abitoye Hospital Ijapo	3.9	2.925	0.78	0.198
15	University Health Centre	6.0	4.5	1.2	0.3
16	Faith Clinic Oke Aro	2.6	1.95	0.52	0.13
17	Abitoye Hospital, Ijoka	13.0	9.75	2.6	0.65
18	Crown Hospital	14.3	10.725	2.86	0.715
19	Hope Hospital Ijoka	4.3	3.225	0.86	0.215
20	Momaak Specialist Hospital	6.2	4.65	1.24	0.31

(b)

Source: Babatola (2008)

Table 7. (a): Daily Waste Generation (kg/day) and the Numbers of Beds in Each Hospitals/Clinics (b): Waste Generation by Waste type

However, 30% do segregate infectious waste as recorded. Waste segregation is the only key step to hospital waste management. Unlike in other developing countries, waste segregation is virtually not being carried out in Nigeria. The present study also confirms this. The composition study is based on field sorting events around hospitals/clinics in Akure main town. The waste samples were analysed and survey.

It is apparent that average waste generation rate per bed per day was 2.782 kg/bed/day. Generation rate (Total weight) per health institution is as follows: National Hospital, 3.59kg; Garki General Hospital, 2.86kg; Wuse General Hospital, 2.50kg; International Diagnostic Centre, 1.98kg and National Institute for Pharmaceutical Research and Development, 2.18kg. Non– hazardous waste ranged from 1.48kg/bed/day at International Diagnostic Centre (IDC) to 3.14kg/bed/day at National Hospital, while hazardous waste ranged from 0.15kg at National institute for pharmaceutical research and development to 0.50kg/bed/day at IDC. The average of hazardous and non-hazardous waste generated from the five health care institutions amounted to 0.346kg and 2.276kg respectively. There was a significant variation in the volume of hazardous and non-hazardous wastes generated at P=0.05. General waste had a mean percentage of 73.5%; infectious waste (spent cultures/swabs/cotton wool), 19.5% and paper/cellulose 2.5%, Sharps (needles, blades, syringes, scalpel, broken glass, and nails), 4.5%. Figures showing variation in the volume of waste generated from each health care institution and solid wastes generation rate per kg/bed/day from the five selected institutions in the Federal Capital Territory, Abuja are presented on Table 8 [30]. Results obtained from investigation on generation rate per/bed/day are presented on Table 9 [30].

Institutions	**Generation rate kg/ bed/ day (%)**		
	Non-Hazardous	**Hazardous**	**Total**
National Hospital (NHA)	3.14 (87)	0.45 (13)	3.59
Garki Gen. Hospital (GGH)	2.45 (85)	0.41 (15)	2.86
Wuse Gen. Hospital (WGH)	2.28 (91)	0.22 (09)	2.50
International Diagnostic Centre (IDC)	1.48 (75)	0.50 (25)	1.98
Nat. Inst. Pharm. Res. & Dev. (NIPRD)	2.03 (93)	0.15 (07)	2.18
Total	11.28	1.73	13.91
Average	2.276	0.346	2.782
Source: Bassey et al., (2006)			

Table 8. Solid waste generated from selected health care institutions in the Federal Capital Territory, Abuja

Ward/ Unit	Garki Gen. Hospital (GGH)	National Hospital (NHA)	Wuse Gen. Hospital (WGH)	Nat. Inst. Pharm. Res. & Dev. (NIPRD)	International Diagnostic Centre (IDC)
Out patient	0.68	0.88	0.23	-	0.13
Female medical	1.84	1.37	1.24	-	0.80
Male medical	1.00	0.88	0.90	-	0.14
Dressing Room	0.83	0.64	0.34	-	0.33
Male Surgical	0.97	0.82	2.90	-	0.42
Female Surgical	1.02	0.79	1.33	-	0.81
Theater	1.89	0.94	2.07	-	1.32
Post natal	3.11	3.35	2.81	-	2.03
Neo natal	2.33	2.71	2.00	-	1.88
Eye clinic	0.21	0.11	-	-	-
ENT	0.08	0.18	-	-	-
Physiotherapy	-	0.22	-	-	-
Psychiatric	-	-	-	-	-
Orthopaedic	-	1.28	-	-	-
Laboratory	2.51	1.89	3.01	-	1.93
Pharmacy	0.69	0.43	0.85	-	0.83
Casualty / Emergency	0.33	0.41	0.66	-	0.14
Labour Room	2.59	4.08	5.67	-	3.03
Ante-natal	0.18	0.10	-	-	0.14
Pharmacology	-	-	-	5.03	-
Microbiology	-	-	-	1.14	-
Diagnostic	-	-	-	1.32	-
Biochemistry	-	-	-	1.67	-
Average	1.261	1.151	1.862	2.290	1.053

[1]A plot is equal to 25m x 50 m

Source: Bassey et al., (2006)

Table 9. Ward/Unit wise distribution of wastes generated in kg/bed/day

In Garki General Hospital generation rate ranges from 0.08kg/bed/day in Ear Nose and throat (ENT) unit to 3.11kg/bed/day in post natal unit. In the National Institute for Pharmaceutical Research and Development, Idu, waste generation rate ranges from 1.14kg in microbiology unit to 5.03kg in the Pharmacology unit. Generation rate in National Hospital ranges from 0.10kg/ bed/day in antenatal unit to 4.08kg/bed/day in the labour ward. In Wuse General Hospital generation rate ranges from 0.23kg/bed/day in the outpatient unit to 5.67kg/ bed/day in the labour unit. At the International diagnostic centre generation rate ranges from 0.13kg/bed/day in outpatient unit to 3.03kg/bed/day in the labour ward.

Tables 10 to 13 present composition of the waste into: generated per department (Table 11), infectious and non-infectious (Table 12) and combustible and non- combustible (Table 13). Table 11 shows generation of waste from the selected hospitals. From the table the waste generated by these hospitals ranged from 1.16 to 1.95 kg/bed.day with overall mean of 1.49 kg/bed. day with standard deviation of 0.235.

Hospitals	Locations as per Residential area	Size (plot'of land)	Outpatient section	Wards, inpatient, Nursing section	Medical records	Laboratory/ pathology section	Waste Transport section	Pharmacy/ administration section	Radiography (X-ray, ultra sound etc)	Environmental section	Consulting rooms	Emergency ward	Nature of the premises
A	Low dense	8	Present	Present	Present	Absent	Absent	Present	Present	Absent	Present	Present	Fenced
B	Residential area	>10	Present	Present	Present	Present	Present	Present	Present	Present	Present	Present	Fenced
C	Medium dense	2	Present	Present	Present	Present	Absent	Present	Absent	Absent	Present	Absent	Fenced
D	Residential area	2	Present	Present	Present	Absent	Absent	Present	Absent	Absent	Present	Absent	Fenced
E	Residential area	8	Present	Present	Present	Absent	Absent	Present	Absent	Absent	Present	Absent	Fenced
F	Residential area	2	Present	Present	Present	Absent	Absent	Present	Present	Absent	Present	Absent	Fenced
G	Residential area	3	Present	Present	Present	Absent	Absent	Present	Absent	Absent	Present	Absent	Fenced
H	Low dense	2	Present	Present	Present	Absent	Absent	Present	Absent	Absent	Present	Absent	Fenced
I	Residential area	2	Present	Present	Present	Present	Absent	Present	Absent	Absent	Present	Absent	Fenced
J	Dense	3	Present	Present	Present	Present	Present	Present	Present	Present	Present	Present	Not Fenced

[2]Some of the patients transport their waste directly to the final disposal unit

[3]Specialist hospitals with clinics on Mondays and Thursdays

(source: Oke et al., 2011)

Table 10. Classification and characteristics of the selected hospitals

http://dx.doi.org/10.5772/53194

These results were similar to results obtained in literature but have different magnitude. Tables 14 showed on average basis, infectious waste was 79.4 kg and 0.053 m^3 by weight and volume, respectively, while non-infectious waste was 34.1 kg and 0.073 m^3 by weight and volume, respectively. This indicates that 0.077 x 44 (3.388) m^3 and 0.053 x 44 (2.332) m^3 of non-infectious and infectious, respectively, were generated during each of the EPI campaigns in Kano state [3].

Hospitals	Outpatient Department (kg/day)	Wards, inpatient, Nursing Department (kg/day)	Medical records (kg/day)	Laboratory/ pathology Department (kg/day)	Waste Transport Department (kg/day)	Pharmacy/ administration Department (kg/day)	Radiography (X-ray, ultra sound etc) Department (kg/day)	Environmental Department (kg/day)	Consulting rooms (kg/day)	Emergency Department (kg/day)	Total weight (kg/day)	Total waste generated (kg/bed. day)
A	2.2	8.5	2.5	-	-	4.7	3.0	-	2.7	2.5	26.0	1.73
B[1]	4.4	16.9	4.9	4.4	4.4	9.4	5.9	4.4	5.4	5.1	65.1	1.45
C	1.7	6.8	2.0	1.7	-	3.7	-	-	2.2	-	18.2	1.30
D[2]	2.2	8.5	2.5	-	-	4.7	-	-	2.7	-	20.5	1.33
E[3]	2.6	10.2	3.0	-	-	5.6	-	-	3.3	-	24.6	1.76
F[3]	1.6	6.1	1.8	-	-	3.4	2.1	-	2.0	-	16.9	1.41
G	2.1	8.1	2.4	-	-	4.5	-	-	2.6	-	19.7	1.52
H	1.8	7.1	2.1	-	-	3.9	-	-	2.3	-	17.2	1.32
I	1.7	6.8	2.0	1.7	-	1.9	-	-	2.2	-	16.3	1.16
J	3.9	15.2	4.4	3.9	3.9	8.4	5.3	3.9	4.9	4.6	58.6	1.95

(source: Oke et al., 2011)

Table 11. Generation of solid waste from selected hospitals

Hospitals	Characteristics of the wastes	Outpatient Department (kg/day)	Wards, inpatient, Nursing Department (kg/day)	Medical records (kg/day)	Laboratory/pathology Department (kg/day)	Waste Transport Department (kg/day)	Pharmacy/administration Department (kg/day)	Radiography (X-ray, ultra sound etc) Department (kg/day)	Environmental Department (kg/day)	Consulting rooms (kg/day)	Emergency Department (kg/day)	Total weight (kg/day) (%)
A	IFW	0.1	0.4	-	-	-	3.0	2.5	-	-	2.5	8.5 (32.7)
	NIFW	2.1	8.1	2.5	-	-	1.7	0.4	-	2.7	0.1	17.5 (67.7)
B	IFW	0.2	0.8	-	3.8	0.2	6.0	5.0	0.2	-	4.9	21.2 (32.7)
	NIFW	4.2	16.1	4.9	0.6	4.2	3.3	0.9	4.2	5.4	0.2	43.9 (67.3)
C	IFW	0.1	0.3	-	1.5	-	2.6	-	-	-	-	4.5 (24.9)
	NIFW	1.7	6.5	2.0	0.2	-	1.2	-	-	2.2	-	13.6 (76.1)
D	IFW	0.1	0.4	-	-	-	3.2	-	-	-	-	3.7 (19.1)
	NIFW	2.1	8.1	2.5	-	-	1.5	-	-	2.7	-	16.8 (80.9)
E	IFW	0.1	0.6	-	-	-	4.3	-	-	0.1	-	5.1 (20.7)
	NIFW	2.5	9.6	3.0	-	-	1.3	-	-	3.1	-	19.5 (79.3)
F	IFW	0.1	0.3	-	-	-	2.6	1.8	-	-	-	4.9 (29.0)
	NIFW	1.5	5.8	1.8	-	-	0.7	0.3	-	1.9	-	12.0 (71.0)
G	IFW	0.1	0.3	-	-	-	3.5	-	-	-	-	4.0 (20.3)
	NIFW	2.0	7.9	2.4	-	-	1.0	-	-	2.6	-	15.7 (79.7)
J	IFW	0.1	0.2	-	-	-	3.4	-	-	0.2	-	3.9 (21.3)
	NIFW	1.7	6.9	2.1	-	-	0.5	-	-	2.1	-	13.3 (78.7)
H	IFW	0.1	0.3	-	1.5	-	1.7	-	-	0.2	-	3.8 (20.9)
	NIFW	1.6	6.5	2.0	0.2	-	0.2	-	-	2.0	-	12.5 (79.1)
I	IFW	0.3	0.8	-	3.4	0.2	7.7	4.7	0.2	0.3	4.4	22.2 (37.9)
	NIFW	3.6	14.4	4.4	0.5	3.7	0.7	0.6	3.7	4.5	0.2	36.4 (62.1)

(source: Oke et al., 2011)

Table 12. Classification of the waste into infectious and non- infectious wastes

Hospitals	Characteristics of the wastes	Outpatient Department	Wards, inpatient, Nursing Department	Medical records	Laboratory/pathology Department	Waste Transport Department	Pharmacy/administration Department	Radiography (X-ray, ultra sound etc) Department	Environmental Department	Consulting rooms	Emergency Department	Overall
A	NCBW (%)	5.5	5.8	1.0	-	-	65.5	86.0	-	1.5	97.5	33.7
	CBW (%)	94.5	94.3	99.0	-	-	34.5	14.0	-	98.6	2.6	66.3
B	NCBW (%)	5.7	6.1	1.6	88.0	5.8	66.0	86.9	5.6	2.6	97.8	34.0
	CBW (%)	94.3	93.9	98.4	12.0	94.2	34.1	13.1	94.4	97.5	2.2	66.0
C	NCBW (%)	3.5	6.1	1.6	88.0	-	70.2	86.9	-	2.6	97.9	26.1
	CBW (%)	96.5	93.9	98.4	12.0	-	29.8	13.1	-	97.5	2.1	73.9
D	NCBW (%)	4.5	6.2	1.5	-	-	69.1	-	-	2.6	-	19.3
	CBW (%)	95.6	93.8	98.5	-	-	30.9	-	-	97.5	-	80.7
E	NCBW (%)	3.6	6.8	1.6	-	-	78.3	-	-	6.6	-	22.1
	CBW (%)	96.5	93.2	98.4	-	-	21.7	-	-	93.4	-	77.9
F	NCBW (%)	5.0	7.0	1.8	-	-	80.1	86.4	-	3.6	-	30.5
	CBW (%)	95.0	93.0	98.2	-	-	19.9	13.6	-	96.5	-	69.5
G	NCBW (%)	7.5	4.7	1.7	-	-	80.1	-	-	3.6	-	21.7
	CBW (%)	92.5	95.3	98.3	-	-	19.9	-	-	96.5	-	78.3
J	NCBW (%)	7.4	4.7	1.6	-	-	88.3	-	-	9.2	-	24.3
	CBW (%)	92.6	95.3	98.4		-	11.7	-	-	90.8	-	75.7
H	NCBW (%)	7.7	5.7	1.4	88.0	-	91.1	-	-	9.2	-	24.8
	CBW (%)	92.3	94.3	98.6	12.0	-	8.9	-	-	90.8	-	75.2
I	NCBW (%)	9.6	6.8	1.2	88.7	6.4	93.4	90.4	6.1	9.2	97.8	39.3
	CBW (%)	90.4	93.2	98.8	11.3	93.6	6.6	9.6	93.9	90.8	2.2	60.7

(source: Oke et al., 2011)

Table 13. Classification of the waste into combustible and non- combustible wastes

Stations	Outpatient Department	Wards, inpatient, Nursing Department	Medical records	Laboratory/ pathology Department	Waste Transport Department	Pharmacy/administration Department	Radiography (X-ray, ultra sound etc) Department	Environmental Department	Consulting rooms	Emergency Department
Non-infectious waste (kg)	31.2	22.4	36.5	20.4	13.9	55.1	60.2	32.9	272.6	34.1
Infectious waste (kg)	70.4	52.3	82.5	44.6	34.8	116.7	125.3	108.5	635.1	79.4
Total (kg)	101.6	74.7	119	65	48.7	171.8	185.5	141.4	907.7	113.5

Source: Oke et al., (2011)

Table 14. Waste generation in the surveyed sites and overall average (wt%)

Tables 12 and 13 show the characterization of the wastes (infectious and non-infectious) into combustible and non-combustible, and type (glass, cloth, etc.) by weight. From the results compositions of the waste ranged from 23.3% to 32.5% (average 29.9%) for non-infectious waste and from 67.6% to 76.7% (average 70.1%) for infectious waste by weight. Compositions ranged from 53.9% to 64.0% (average 59.9%) for non-infectious waste and from 36.0% to 46.1% (average 40.1%) for infectious waste by volume [31].

3. Conclusion

The study has shown that there was no mechanism put in place towards sorting of dental wastes in the study area. This has made its characterisation cumbersome and sorting hazardous. The research also revealed that 3.3m^2 of waste were generated in a month by the eight dental clinics. Along this line, the study concludes that the dental waste generation in the third world dental hospitals especially in the study area are poorly sorted. Based on the report of the present study, the followings are recommended: Provision of a standard waste management must be put in place (segregation, storage, transportation and final disposal); locally designed Incinerators should be constructed to manage the wastes after the wastes were treated to render them non-infectious and hazardous. This pre-incinerator treatment should be in form of recycling of heavy metals such as Ag, Pb, Sn, Hg etc from the waste and the use of digital X-rays will reduce wastes generated from the X-ray rooms.

http://dx.doi.org/10.5772/53194

Author details

Michael Adewole Adedigba[1*], Isaiah Adesola Oke[2] and Regina Arobieke[1]

*Address all correspondence to: adedigba@oauife.edu.ng

1 Faculty of Dentistry, Department of Preventive & Community Dentistry, Nigeria

2 Department of Civil Engineering, Obafemi Awolowo University, Ile-Ife, Nigeria

References

[1] Manyele, S.V., H. Anicetus, and M.H. Bilia, "Globalization and its Effects on Medical Waste Management in Tanzania", IET Annual Conference and General Meeting, 4th-5th December, 2003, AICC Arusha, Tanzania, (2003), 76-92.

[2] Blackman, W.C., Jr., "Basic Hazardous Waste Management", 2nd Ed., Chapter 12, Lewis Publishers, CRC Press, NY, 1996.

[3] Oke, I. A. Management of Immunization Solid Wastes In Kano State, Nigeria. Journal of Waste Management 2008; 28, 2512-2521

[4] Manyele S.V. Medical Waste Management In Tanzania: Current Situation And The Way Forward. AJEAM-RAGEE 2004; 8 (1) 74-99

[5] Van Veen, F., Definition of Hazardous Waste: The Issues of Western Europe", in "Hazardous Waste: Detection, Control and Treatment", R. Abbou, (Ed.), Elsevier, Oxford 1998, pp. 75-100.

[6] Colorado Department of Public Health and Environment. Compliance Bulletin for Hazardous Waste, Photographic, X-ray and Dental Wastes. 7/97 CHW-012. http://www.cdphe.state.co.us/hmi/ Accessed 20/04/2007.

[7] U.S. Environmental Protection Agency. EPA Guide for Infectious Waste Management. Office of Solid Waste and Emergency Response, Washington, D.C. EPA 1986; 530-SW-86-014.

[8] WHO (Pruss, A., Giroult, E. & Rushbrook, P. (eds)). Safe Management of Wastes from Health-care Activities. World Health Organisation, Geneva, Switzerland, 1999.

[9] Adsavakulchai, S. Study on waste from hospital and clinics in Phitsanulok. Online Journal of Health Allied Sciences, 2002; 3, 3–11.

[10] Muhlich, M., Scherer, M. & Daschner, F.D. Comparison of infectious waste management in European hospitals. Journal of Hospital Infection, 2003; 55, 260–268.

[11] Chaerul M., Tanaka, M. & Shekdar, A.V. Resolving complexities in healthcare waste management: a goal programming approach. Waste Management & Research, 2008; 26, 217–232.

[12] Adedigba, M.A., Afon, A.O., Abegunde, A.A., Nwhator, S.O., Bamise, C.T.. Assessment of dental waste management in a Nigerian tertiary hospital. Waste Management & Research 2010; 28: 769–777

[13] Coker, A, Sangodoyin, A. Sridhar, M., Booth, C., Olomolaiye, P. & Hammond, F. Medical waste management in Ibadan, Nigeria: obstacles and prospects. Waste Management, 2009; 29, 804–811.

[14] Rao, P.H., Report: Hospital Waste management – awareness and practices: a study of three states in India. Waste Management and Research, 2008; 26, 297–303.

[15] Punchanuwat K., Drummond, B.K. & Treasure, E.T.. An investigation of the disposal of dental clinical waste in Bangkok. International Dentistry Journal, 1998; 48, 369–373.

[16] Floret, N., Mauny, F., Challier, B., Arveux, P., Cahn, J.-Y. & Viel, J.F. Dioxin emissions from a solid waste incinerator and risk of non-Hodgkin lymphoma. Epidemiology, 2003; 14, 392–398.

[17] Griffin, R.D., "Principles of Hazardous Materials Management", Lewis Publishers Inc., Michigan, USA, 1989.

[18] Lee, C.C. and G.L. Huffman, "Medical Waste Management/ Incineration", Journal of Hazardous Materials, 1996; 48, 1996, 1-30.

[19] Osamong, L.A., Gathece, L.W., Kisumbi, B.K. & Mutave, R.J. Management of dental waste by practitioners in Nairobi, Kenya. African Journal of Oral Health, 2005; 2, 24–29.

[20] Taiwo, J.O. & Aderinokun, G.A. Assessing cross infection prevention measures at the Dental Clinic, University College Hospital, Ibadan. African Journal of Medicine & Medical Science, 2002; 31, 213–217.

[21] Adedigba, M.A., Ogunbodede, E.O., Fajewonyomi., B.A., Ojo O.O. & Naidoo, S. Gender differences among oral health care workers in caring for HIV/ AIDS patients in Osun state, Nigeria. African Health Sciences, 2005; 3, 182–187.

[22] Ozbek, M. & Sanin, F.D. A study of the dental solid waste produced in a school of dentistry in Turkey. Waste Management, 2004; 24, 339–345.

[23] Mohapatra, S.P., Nikolova, I. & Mitchell, A. Managing mercury in the great lakes: An analytical review of abatement policies. Journal of Environmental Management, 2007; 83, 80–92.

[24] Akter, N., Trankler, J. An analysis of possible scenarios of medical waste management in Bangladesh. Management of Environmental Quality: An International Journal 2003; 14 (2), 242–255.

[25] Daschner, F.D., Dettenkofer, M. Protecting the patient and the environment – new aspects and challenges in hospital infection control. Journal of Hospital Infection 1997; 36 (1), 15–17.

[26] Waseem, A., Igbal, A., Hasan, Z. Field investigation on characterization and management of Karachi hospital wastes. Environmental News 1995; 3 (1), 2–6.

[27] Falola, T., Heaton, M.M. (Eds.). Traditional and Modern Health Systems in Nigeria. Africa World Press, Inc., Trenton, NJ, 2006; pp. 1–9.

[28] Longe, E.O., Williams, A. A preliminary study of medical waste management in Lagos Metropolis, Nigeria, Iran. Journals Environmental Health Sciences Engineering 2006; 3 (2), 133–139.

[29] Babatola, J.O.. A Study of Hospital Waste Generation and Management Practices in Akure, An International Multi-Disciplinary Journal, 2 (3) 2008, 292-305.

[30] Bassey, B.E; Benka-Coker, M.O and Aluyi, H.S. Characterization and management of solid medical wastes in the Federal Capital Territory, Abuja, Nigeria. African Health Sciences 2006; 6(1), 59-63

[31] Oke, I. A.: J.A Otun; D.B. Adie; M. A. Asani; S. Lukman and A. Ismail : Chapter 7: Characterisations and Management of Medical Solid Wastes from Selected Private Hospitals in Ile-Ife, Nigeria, In a) Solid Waste Management and Environmental Remediation. ISBN: 978-1-60741-761-3. Editor: Timo Faerber and Johann Herzog. © 2011 Nova Science Publishers, Inc. New York.

Chapter 10

Nursing and Public Health in Developing Countries

Carmen Luisa Betancur P.

Additional information is available at the end of the chapter

http://dx.doi.org/10.5772/53452

1. Introduction

The nursing profesional has an important role in public health, highly relevant in developing countries, as their interventions as caregivers are addressed, not only to sick individuals, but above all to the communities of the families of the patients. When they engage in the recuperation process, they are of high value for the implementation of distinct management alternatives.

The transformation of the people toward a better quality of life and long-lasting health, according to the available conditions for each community, are viable only when, through education, the promotion of health and the prevention of sickness impact their behaviors and change their habits.

The nurse has the possibility to walk with the communities, taking a permanent step, independent of creeds, idiosyncrasies, morals, and development. The permanent closeness of vulnerable people in need of care and support is a central axis in the actual role of the nursing professional, who has abandoned hospital caregiving to move their interest to housing sites, and to work for different people. Continuing to work in the areas of labor, teaching, administration, and politics, they make this change, not only for the image of this profession, but also for the evident impact of their social projection in the transformation of the health of the communities.

The capacity for empathy toward people, even in the worst circumstances, leads the nursing professional to position themself safely and committed to actions that allow interventions and projections in rated health, most significantly for the leaders of the communities, and for the members thereof, since they represent the possibilities of bettering the quality of life of people in different life cycles. The interdisciplinary and trans disciplinary skills, and the permanent incursion in the development of the themes on community health, project the nursing professional as a permanent leader of activities and interventions toward the health of the population.

Public health is not only a tool of work for our profession; it's also a context of development in professional and personal influence, and an opportunity to interact with other disciplines that, like this, project toward the accomplishment of representative changes in the countries that, for their contexts, are forced into difficult conditions in relation to coping with risk factors that somehow directly or indirectly affect the health of different groups of people.

Public health for the nursing professional, like that for other health professionals, is an enterprise occupied by the health of the people, their environment, quality of life, and the possibilities of development in terms of bettering living conditions.

2. Historic role of public health and nursing in developing countries

Historically, public health has evolved from a relationship between environmental conditions, socio-economics, and healthy living. Because of this, the situation of health and the development of a community are conditional to the characteristics of the economy, social structure, and the environmental conditions in a determined moment in its history. An intimate relationship exists between these factors, each one becomes the reflection of the other and therefore a society, its environment, and its economy reflect in its state of health and vice versa. Undoubtedly, the state of the health of a given community reflects the state of development of the country in to which it belongs, and in these aspects, the contributions of the Nursing professional are important to address specific actions for social transformation.

Like that which complements and advances social structures, in this globalized world, also makes the health systems, and in a relevant manner in developing countries in which presently exist parallel systems of private health, oriented toward distinct social groups, in accordance with the predominant population in each country and depending on their level of development. Equally, this approach to health care determines the approximation of nursing care as to the population of each one of the countries, and even the region within them. In the majority of the countries, the ministry of health is the organization in charge of ensuring the health of the population, based on socio-economic, demographic, and environmental indicators. With these, ensuring the project plans, health programs and policies, which in all cases include the Nursing Professional.

The purpose of both the ministries and health institutions, like health professionals, especially of the nurse, is to try to accomplish the equity of Access to the health services of the people, as with the extension of coverage, especially to vulnerable populations. Many developing countries are finding an epidemiological transition process in which coexist communicable diseases with diseases caused by violence and other chronic no communicable diseases; situations that the majority of the time is based on inequities that should stir the communities to face the accessibility of the health systems.

Currently the countries of Latin America and the Caribbean face distressing problems social, including poverty and marginalization and translation issues basic rights of education, health and housing. Seeking to diminish the gaps and establish the development of public health to offer equality of opportunities, overall to the communities of developing nations, the(Banco Interamericano de Desarrollo) BID, [1,2,3] performed in a categorization of Latin American and Caribbean countries, which were classified in the following categories:

Groups	Countries	Developed in public health
Group A	Ecuador, Bolivia, Guatemala, El Salvador, Honduras, Haití.	• Several factors against the health • Necessity of priority care • Attention to the elimination of eradicable and reducible diseases • Conscience of the importance of a community organization for the development of health • Interventions in environmental health (zoonotic diseases) • Expansion of public health programs • Maintaining of existing plans
Group B	Paraguay, República Dominicana, Colombia, Nicaragua, Brasil.	• Expansion of environmental health plans • Expansion of basic health services to the national level for the most vulnerable • Development of basic health plans executed by interdisciplinary teams • Health care from care units • Increased competence in public health services for healthcare staff • Implement plans of nutritional health, diminution of psycho-social and laboral risk for vulnerable groups of the population.
Group C	Argentina, Uruguay, Venezuela, Chile, Panamá, México, Costa Rica.	• Maintainment and bettering planning and management of public health services. • Solving specific problems related to industrialization. • Development of centers of investigation of public health. • International alliances the allow providing support for the development of public health to the countries in categories A and B.

Table 1. Classification of Latin American and Caribbean countries in their health development by the (Banco Interamericano de Desarrollo), BID.

In accordance with this classification, it is evident that there are various Latin American and Caribbean countries that conform the large group of developing countries and that require economic and logistic support, along with human talent, in order to better the public health conditions for their populations. In this context, the Nursing Professionals, like other professionals in the area of health, contribute permanently and continue the strength of the work that facilitate the accomplishment of this objective.

3. Current challenges in the face of public health for the Nursing Professional

World-wide life expectancy increases, even for the communities of developing countries. In the last five decades, it has increased the number of years that each person lives. Between 1950 and 1990 the life expectancy at birth was 46.5 years on average, and by 2002 it was 65.2 years. In 2011 the life expectancy for countries like Monaco was 90 years, and for developing countries, like South Africa, it varies according to the public between 39 and 48 years. For the region of Latin America and the Caribbean it varies between 68 and 75 years. The average life expectancy has important differences between developing countries with high morality and those with low morality. The life expectancy has increased in recent decades for almost all the countries of the world. The socio-economic support of each one of the nations has a direct relationship with the conditions of public health and the quality of life that their residents can access. Congruently with this, the actions of the Nurse also have links to the technological and scientific developments in each country, which in turn interacts with the distribution that is intended for public health care. [4]

The increase in life expectancy registered in the first half of the 20th century in developing countries was a result of a rapid descent in the rates of mortality, particularly of mother and child, and attributable to infectious diseases in infancy and the first steps of adulthood. The access to a dwelling, some sanitation services, and an education of the best quality, the tendency to form more reduced families, increased income and the adoption of public health measures, like the immunization against various infectious diseases, contribute in an important way to what Public Health has called an epidemiological transition. In many developing countries this change began approximately 100-150 years ago. In some places, for example in Japan, the transition began later, although more recently their rhythm has advanced rapidly. And in many developing countries, it began even later and still has not concluded, as is the case in the majority of developing countries. [5]

This population dynamic has implied, for the public health professional, a better and greater scientific foundation to everything related to public health practices, tending to preserve the conditions of health, controlling the conditional factors, and tending to actions that favor the development of actions in public health for the prevention of diseases and the promotion of health. The increase of the quality of life has a profound relationship with the academic plans of the universities to fortify the Nursing Professional from their undergraduate formation. Especially in developing countries, practice has been backed and supported by the

World Organization of Health. This panorama leads to the attention of the nurse currently projected to the elderly population, since its mandatory increase brings care to the chronic and degenerative diseases which undoubtedly constitutes one of the major challenges to the nursing professional.

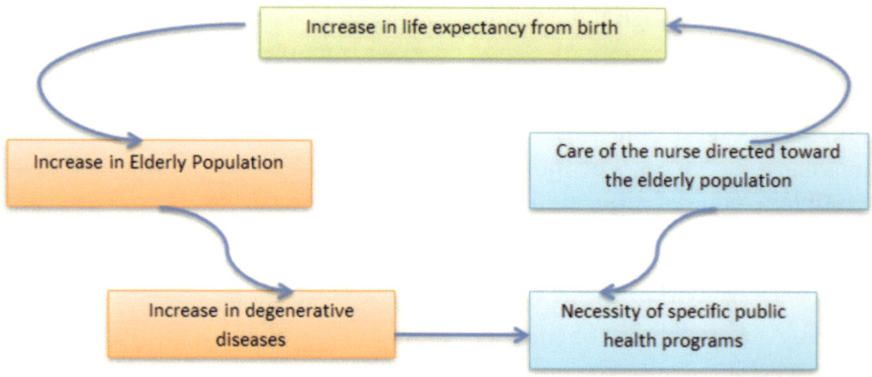

Figure 1. Repercussions of the increase in life expectancy from birth over the activities of the public health professional.

Other current challenges to public health and in the development of nursing care to the populations should face statistics about mortality that many developing countries considerably underestimate the attributable weight of no transmissible diseases in adults, excluding the health problems of nonfatal consequences like depression or vision disorders. In the case of depression, more than that of vision, they can cause an increase in mortality. One method of utility to synthetically express the burden consists of calculating the number of years adjusted to the disability (AVAD), indicator that combines years of life lost due to premature death (APP) and the years lost to the disability (APD) [6]. It could be said that one AVAD is equivalent to one year of "Healthy Life" lost, and the burden and that the burden of disease as well as indicates the difference between the state of health of a given population and a global population normative reference with high life expectancy in perfect health. In terms of AVAD, 35% of the total years of healthy living lost in 2011 in the world should have been to diseases, injuries, and from external causes suffered by children less than 15 years, many of them preventable, nearly 50% of the pathologies and external injuries suffered by adults between 15 and 59 years. [6]. All of these components permit review and make new propositions to better the indicators through direct interventions to these specific populations, without losing sight of the rest of the population.

It has also constituted an important challenge for public health in developing countries, infantile supervision that currently continues to play an important role in the international health agenda. [7]. Since about 91% of deaths of children under 15 that occur in the world occur in children who have not completed five years, and in developing countries. Equally, international forces have aimed to comprehend the magnitude of the sanitary challenges that that face adults in developing countries, even those that do not accomplish changes in the epidemiological profiles that are expected and projected, while the health of the adult population has had a broad advance in rich countries, which have also reduced, remarkably, premature mortality in children. Undoubtedly so many in developing countries as in the nations in development of health professionals have participated, with the rest of the disciplines of health sciences, in the marathon task of combatting preventable diseases, many of those no preventable, through the programs, plans, and policies of public health that imply the direct work with the communities and addresses from planning and projection of the institutions and health authorities.

The formulations of these policies, plans, and programs for health workers and for involved populations can only are sized by indicators of public health. The construction and management of training required from undergraduate education, however in many developing countries, the nursing professional is found as limiting the inadequate record management which is based on the construction of the indicators. This situation in many developing countries as another of the challenges for the nursing professional, that works in public health, not only as a proposal of betterment to the quality of information, but rather, as the projection of reliable data in which they can base the making of governmental decisions to solve the difficulties of the health of the community.

4. Actions of the nursing professional in the monitoring of public health

The monitoring of public health for the majority of developing countries involves oriented actions for the changes in the management of intervention strategies for the pathologies of major prevalence in each one of them. The nursing professional, as a leader of many of the work teams that develop this monitoring, know and size the pertinent ways and effective activities that favor the factors of protection for the subject population of the monitoring.

The nursing professional, in conjunction with other health professionals, performs an analysis of the situation of health of the population, figure 2. To start the process with this public health surveillance of a particular event, it takes a first step to review the available scientific literature on the event, given the evidence shown so far to manage the disease in question. Then, analyses data collected product information on the population being monitored with this information produces a statistical analysis in order to formulate a diagnosis of the situation and proposals for intervention, which must be accepted from the political, by administrators public health, from the technical to facilitate the planning and execution finally implemented by the operating personnel monitoring, implemented the proposed intervention program or intervention is made of its effectiveness that triggers a new decision-making on the event subject to public health surveillance.

Each of the countries annually conducts a review of its health indicators, in order to establish the conditions that during the next year will be the subject of public health surveillance. According to WHO guidelines, World Health Organization, every nation does tracking

http://dx.doi.org/10.5772/53452

events most prevalent during the previous year, indicating that for many of these, such surveillance may differ from year to year and between different developing countries. While analyzing the different surveillance systems in public health, is often found that among them, there are periods in which the monitoring pathologies are very similar, or at least of the same group.

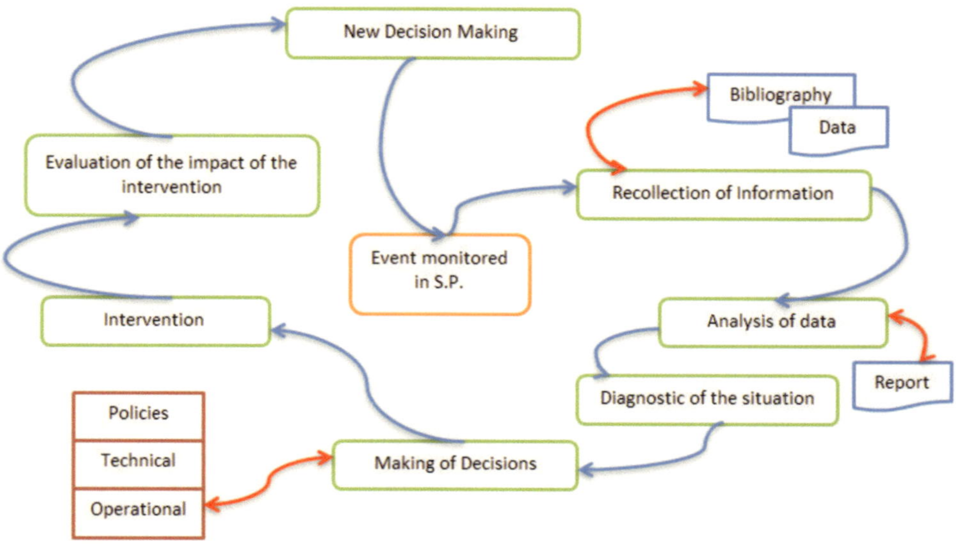

Figure 2. Sequence of the monitoring in public health.

These types of interventions contribute significantly in changing handling the morbidity and mortality, and also promote relevant changes in the behavior of populations which ultimately leads to better quality of life, greater number of years of healthy life and productive impact on the social and economic transformation. [8]

5. The determinants of public health in developing countries

The determinants are a set of conditions of health and disease in individuals and communities. In 1974 when the Minister of Health Canada, (developed country), Lalonde analyzed the determinants of health, created a public health model, to improve the health of its inhabitants, which was later extended to the other countries. [9]. According to this model is considered that the level of health of a community is determined by four variables:

Determinants of Health	Components of the determinant
Human Biology	Genetic and aging
Environmental:	• Biological contamination • Virus • Micro-organisms • Bacteria
	Atmospheric Contamination • Noise • Vibrations • Radiations
	Chemical Contamination • Sulfur Oxide • Fertilizers • Pesticides • Heavy Metals
	Psycho-Social & Socio-Cultural Contaminations • Stress
Lifestyles (Unhealthy Habits or Behaviors)	Sedentariness Consumption of drugs, including tobacco Excessive consumption of foods rich in fats and carbohydrates Dangerous or reckless driving Misuse of health care services Aggressiveness
Health care assistance system	Quality Gratuity Coverage

Table 2. Determinants of the health and its components, according to Lalonde.

Among these determinants of health, which currently provides more weight to determine the presence of health or disease in the context of public health especially in developing countries, is the behavioral or lifestyle, and is in this in which nursing professionals have greater opportunity to achieve major changes. Habits such as sedentary lifestyle can be changed when the professional who leads the activities of prevention and promotion does impact the transformation of personal and community behaviors towards developing guidance and exercise routines and physical activity, for weight loss, improving physical functions and therefore reduction of chronic diseases such as hypertension, diabetes, musculoskeletal problems. Also against the use of drugs and the nurse is of high importance in developing countries, where often vulnerable community has no easy access to medical specialist or general practitioner, is when the professional nursing can deploy activities established in the public health policies of each country, in order to minimize the use of these drugs, in no way easy, but certainly in which we must continue working to make an impact. Undoubtedly many times with little or community receptiveness of the individuals involved in the process. As for the excessive consumption of foods high in fats and carbohydrates, every day the situation becomes more complex, since developed countries have high experience in this matter and its impact on developing countries make greater proportion through mass media. There are a growing number of people involved in processes of malnutrition, mostly by overweight, which ends in a high proportion suffering from preventable diseases such as hypertension and diabetes, whose morbidity is increasing every day with dire consequences on individuals and communities. Reckless attitudes, both when driving as aggressive, increasingly number within the young population, are one of the causes of high morbidity and mortality, as many of these actions are outcome externally caused injury to lethality, or in many cases with severe and irreversible damage to those who are involved in such actions, which is not always a direct relationship between the injured and recklessness, as the injuries often have nothing to do with the process and suffer damage, being close to the subject reckless. In addition to the above, the nursing professional is a low adherence to the programs established in each of the countries and few support tools to increase it or motivate. However, given the professional scientific technical preparation in nursing, is always ready to ride new strategies, develop innovative new plans or promote public health policies aimed at decreasing the risks and harms associated with these.

Undoubtedly the best actions against determinants of public health should be geared toward the prevention of disease and promotion of health and the professional in this field has been developing permanent nursing actions, primary health care has a high impact on developing countries, actions addressed by properly targeted and highly competent professionals in the field, make an impact in a relevant and timely information on the magnitude of the problem.

The greatest weight in determining public health, such as behavioral, environmental and the system or health services are largely modifiable factors, at least theoretically, and therefore the actions of public health should be routed to this change. Another important feature of these determinants is that they are influenced by social, within which the economy, culture and social development are highly relevant. [10].

6. Relevance current of the environmental determinant

Environmental risks and their impact on health are becoming increasingly important. In the twentieth century, the UN in 1984 structured the commission for the Environment Management and Development was held in 1987 and the Tokyo Declaration, which was attended by most of the countries interested in environmental preservation and implementation of preventive measures this level, the publication of the Brundtland, Gro Harlem, in the Rio summit, 1992, gave guidelines in Agenda 21, sustainable development project that enabled decisive actions for developing countries such as sustainable cities and towns, 1994. By 2002 at the Johannesburg summit, it became clear the negative impact of many of the measures proposed and implemented by the various nations.

Given the importance of ozone for the protection of the health of the population in 1985 was conducted Vienna Convention for the Protection of the Ozone Layer. In 1987 and looking to delve on the issue and improve control strategies on the environment was held the Montreal Protocol. In 1992 took place the framework convention on climate change. In 2000 was held the Millennium Summit goals within this one was directed to the proper environmental management. In 2005, achieving the Paris Declaration and the Kyoto Protocol, making each of these conventions and protocols important advances in the analysis of the risks that the environment can offer to the health of the population and in the population decisively vulnerable. Within the management of environmental issues and their relationship to community health, waste sub has taken a leading role, the Basel in 1989, with amendments in 2011, Rotterdam in 1998, Stockholm in 2001. [11] Parallel to this international action each country has developed its own rules, as support and adjustment to international component. From this collaboration have also developed a series of international cooperation agendas that directly or indirectly benefit the health of communities.

The 61st World Health Organization, in 2008, noting with concern the findings of the Intergovernmental Panel on Climate Change regarding the effects of rising temperatures on the planet and their involvement in some aspects of human health; besides providing estimated that climate change begins to have negative net global effect on human health, especially in developing countries, small island developing States and least vulnerable local communities capacity to prepare for such a change and adapt to it; and that the estimated exposure to climate change affects the health status of millions of people as a result of increased malnutrition, mortality, morbidity and injury due to extreme weather events, the burden of diarrheal disease and the frequency of cardiopulmonary diseases, as altering the distribution of some infectious disease vectors; also found that climate change hinders the achievement of the Millennium Development Goals, including the goals for health, undermining the efforts of the Secretariat of the 60th World Conference and Member States to improve public health and reduce all health inequalities globally. It recognized the importance of addressing timely health consequences of climate change due to the cumulative effects of emissions of greenhouse gases, and recognized that solutions to the health impacts of climate change should be seen as a joint responsibility of all States, and that developed countries should assist developing countries in this regard. The conference found the importance of strengthening health systems in order to provide them with the ability to address both gradual changes and sudden shocks is a key priority for the correction of direct and indirect effects of climate change on health. [12]

Certainly the environment is a very important factor in the development of strategies and public health, both understood in the traditional sense (physical and biotic environment), as in the socio-cultural sense. One of the outstanding features of the new public health is the attention given to environmental factors and their relationship to human health.

Environmental management has been a rediscovery of community needs, which has allowed public health to explore and understand the importance of prompt and effective intervention to facilitate the development of a balanced and healthy relationship. In these respects, the story has changed since a few decades ago the environmental component was completely ignored and roomy ignorance of its effects on the development of certain diseases. [13]

Models	Description
Biocentrism	Currently the environment is understood as part of the conditions around the man, who is an element of the context, in interaction with all the biotic (living) and physical surrounding
Systemic view	Conception of the environment as a system with different levels of complexity: • Biosphere: relates to the nature and everything which has life • Technossphere: system of man-made structures that assist the biosphere • Sociosphere: set of institutions to regulate human creation developed internal relations, social (public, religious, etc.).
Development of an environmental ethic	In recent years environmental ethics has emerged as the everyday moral philosophy. It is a line of thought and action experienced as commitment for action in contravention of the system balance. This ethic is based on solidarity in which the man found with the privilege level of nature, should be responsible for it.
Sustainable development model	Facing the expansionist model of unlimited growth of the industrial product and technology development, new knowledge of the natural resource exhaustibility and irreversible dynamics of any system, requires rethinking and growth patterns of behavior, not substantiated exclusively economic parameters, but more consistent with respect to all forms of life and the development of greater quality of education.

Table 3. Environmental Models.

For the XXI century one of the biggest environmental challenges the decision of what constitutes equitable North-South, or what in other contexts is called operator-exploited.

The social, cultural and health of the various treaties, conventions and international agendas have shown the importance of resolving the Needy present without compromising the ability of future generations' development, thus giving the opportunity for each company to resolve their own conflicts towards the environment. [14] According to this approach should be a basic balance between the environment and community health, to achieve this is essential, consider some elements:

- Population Stabilization: population control
- Efficient use of natural resources
- Reduction of residual contamination

- Reduction of greenhouse effects and climate changes
- Implementation of situational benefit to everyone
- Define environmental limits
- Debugging the concept of market economy
- Formation and social/cultural changes

It is perhaps this last element in which greater prominence has taken the role of public health and with it the number of commitments and activities to be performed by the nursing professional in each of the developing countries. One of the most important things is education consisting of habitat management in children and young populations, which in most cases constitute multipliers at family and community.

Caring for the environment as part of public health responsibility involves some approaches of social, environmental activities and programs must address ecological variability, sustainability in the social, economic viability as a sustainable solution in the short, medium and long term.

Global environmental problems should be assessed against public health. The environmental issue is not limited to pollution, however covers a range of circumstances in which most of the time, people generate damage on the environment, which may be irreversible and against which you have to face the consequences and suffer damage from these.

Some of the most relevant issues regarding health of people are, the population explosion, the human being on the planet has grown in an uncontrolled dimension and most people on earth live in developing countries. About 1.4 million people lack food, which leads to major health problems as malnutrition triggers a series of important diseases in the human population. Deforestation, in which between 60 and 70% of the world's forests have been destroyed, with the unfortunate consequences that it brings to the environment and health of people. The increasing desertification, with consequences such as reduced water, the extinction of animal and plant species, increased mineral consumption, increased air pollution, destruction of natural heritage, cultural and technical-artistic, increased armed conflicts and the use of weapons that also affect the environment.

From the perspective of public health must take into account that people like all living things depend on a complex set of environmental factors. Humans occupy various environmental systems with characteristics and specific environmental characteristics:

- The environment is not only physical and biological, but also sociocultural.
- The human being is capable of modifying the physical and biological environment to suit your needs.

These changes may be accompanied by alterations of the natural balance with environmental damage and extent of individual and community health as well as quality of life.

Against this background the institutions public health regulators propose lines of action to minimize the damage and initiate protection activities, for which studies are required to strengthen the evidence and to protecting the environment, such research should be oriented physical health and the environment, integrating aspects as abiotic air Pollution, contamination of water, soil and food, contamination by radiation, noise pollution, health studies and biological environment as subtopics biotic pollution, communicable diseases and the study of health and socio-cultural environment. This interaction supported policies that will raise the level of quality of life. In relation to this issue include the great interest of the professional training institutions in Nursing, for educational interventions to strengthen knowledge and stewardship of the environment. [14]

7. International cooperation for public health

It is clear that at present the only way forward in health policies and programs of adequate and timely scope is establishing cooperation networks. In the case of public health, cooperation must answer a global need, where the greatest needs are located in developing countries. Their viability depends on the strengthening and integration of countries and organizations assigned by them to support processes that manage work schedules and coordinated sets. The internationalization of needs and finding a solution encourages technological development, common economic interests and interaction processes, if international cooperation is conceived as a strategy to strengthen each of the countries, the possibility of financial support, technical and scientific and logistics by developed states, to developing countries, improve public health perspective in the current context. [15]

Shared knowledge between countries, given that between them there are different degrees of development over public health is an aspect that motivates the approach for the development of projects in which the consideration of collective agreements, is seen as a point of starting to close the gap between actors, international cooperation in order to strengthen public health milestones evaluates and transforms impact on communities, especially the vulnerable, for obvious reasons that belong to the neediest countries.

It should be noted how the experience of international cooperation in public health has allowed this to be inserted into other activities on international scientific cooperation, networking of knowledge about health issues, as their understanding of the ethical issues and the appropriation of knowledge have led to the accompaniment of cooperative work in several developing countries, and on whose initiative has worked to expand such cooperation.

The importance of expanding international cooperation areas to strengthen relations development and integration of public health with the scientific community in several countries is a matter of the internationalization policy not only health but also of science and that be taken as strategic perspective and long range. This internationalization strategy favors public health community institutions like health administrators and forming human resources, which is important to include all disciplines in the health sciences. Internationalization in public health is a context that relates unfailing capacity of each country, its institutions and networks that are formed between them for a more effective dialogue, however refers therefore to a scenario international cooperation highly competitive and complex. [16]

In the process of international cooperation in public health include the generation of new ways of working around the synergy of processes that encourage interaction and communication of each of the countries involved. This implies that for health care organizations as well as for generating knowledge in public health aspects, integration into the opportunities and international scientific cooperation mechanisms represent a strategic position within the multilateral schemes and initiatives within each country to work together around the national public health agendas.

Many national research networks in Health Policy and Systems, at the level of individual developing countries are interested in advancing their maturation and consolidation processes for each of their countries. Within the process of international cooperation for public health has been proposed to increase the efficiency of capacity to respond effectively to those in need of intervention and research and participatory development in achieving national and international studies of the impact of health policies with social relevance.

Although the network approach achieves through its leadership role in the determination of public policy in the sector, it is proposed to endogenously maintain permanent meetings, forums and meetings with experts, using various scenarios academics to discuss health issues public in the country.

Each of developing countries has been developing an agenda for international cooperation that facilitates individually and jointly meets the challenges facing the public health and promoting management processes supported by most developed countries, thus opening opportunities innovation associated with research, innovation, technology and therefore the scientific development related to public health. Vitalize the national agendas from scenarios decision making process and stakeholders with high social commitment, since this interaction of the endogenous progresses toward the exogenous, when strengthens systematization of processes of each country, as evidence for informed consolidated action and social management, to develop public health research at the national level, can move easily in the interaction with other states. Many of these developing countries, through international cooperation involving public health in their agendas, issues like: The Millennium Development Goals, the fight against the world drug problem, environmental protection, reproductive health, nutrition, occupational health, social reconciliation and governance. The search for the consolidation of domestic and international alliances to achieve reduces social inequalities and promotes the development of public health, has become a joint effort. As evidenced by the needs of these populations the work of professional nursing responsibly supports the development of themes through actions relevant to each community. Reducing poverty, achieving full coverage in health and education, and the decline of the unemployment rate in developing countries achieve progress in development of production and competitiveness, not only in meeting the eradication of extreme poverty and hunger, but generally towards achieving higher levels of economic and social development with equity and without exclusion, which ultimately benefits significantly to rural communities, the poverty belt, displaced by violence, natural events or social injustice. [17]

8. Trajectory of public health

Only in the mid-eighteenth century the concept of health acquired a public dimension, although there are indications of community care since antiquity. The concept of public health, as it says Gómez Arias, integrates two basic concepts, the health and "public", historically evolved and it was necessary to gather at one time in his career.

Stage	Evolutionary conception	Moments
Primitive	Survival requires collective experiences. [18] Commits primitive communities and ancient civilizations. Emerging notions of individual and the public. The disease comes to the community despite its supernatural origin. Collective healing rituals. Hammurabi's Code of Laws.	The historical relationship of primitive health. The Jews in the twelfth century BC had religious rituals of disease management and its determinants. The Egyptians, Assyrians, Babylonians and Mesopotamians, at the same time made similar processes versus disease management. Other primitive societies connected the disease with cosmic events and thus addressed his management from conception religious magic.
Old	It develops the notion of the public, but the disease and health issues remain purely individual. Religious magical character. Illness as a result of the forces of nature or the spiritual powers. Health practices preventive, had a religious magic lasso. Using amulets, restrooms, food or sex vetoes. [18]	Paleolithic: Individual disease management consistent with the nomadic life. Diseases caused by excessive physical activity or atmospheric exposure. Neolithic: appearance of inactivity, change in the epidemiological profile, pest outbreaks, malnutrition. The Mayas: health resulting from the coexistence with the laws of nature and society. Diseases are the product of the transgression of these. Prevention is done through religious rituals and medicinal plants. The Jews: connection with the performance of religious codes, standards of prevention. Greece: management terms as epidemic, endemic, community health. Use of curative and preventive medicine. Hippocrates forerunner of medical

Stage	Evolutionary conception	Moments
		practice and medical code first recognized to date. Rome: Followers of the Greek medical doctrines, innovative environmental and community health. China: Important development in environmental health, individual and collective hygiene, preventive health.
Middle Age	Setback in terms of public health, through the influence of the dominant church. Major pandemics, leprosy, smallpox, cholera, bubonic plague in Europe, China, India, the Middle East, during the XI-XIII centuries.	Phase of average age: largest urban concentration, development of land and sea routes, church influence on the care component, war situations, poor socioeconomic conditions, malnutrition Renaissance Stage: XVII-XVIII centuries, awakening of humanity against the dogmas. Expansion of geographic knowledge. Invention of printing. New philosophical systems. Flowering of art. Trade expansion. Industry appearance: appearance of anatomy, physiology, experimental medicine, first scientific investigations, including the field of preventive medicine and disease control.
Modern Age	Develops between the XIV and XV, in the Renaissance period. Appears recognition of some conditions of risk and protection against diseases of the time. Despite the scientific, public health does not receive any direct benefit during this period.	Inequality of health from other scientific technical developments, boom of sexuality and thus sexually transmitted diseases. Discovery of the natural process of some diseases such as scarlet fever, increased assertive diagnoses by clinical observation and epidemiological. Checking the relationship between cause effects such as scurvy. Work began addressed social interventions.
Contemporary	It extends from the Industrial Revolution to the present day. Important advances in public health, research, treatment, and prevention. Commodification of health services.	In Germany, Rudolf Virchow, deepened the study of typhus. We conducted the first international conference on health, which culminated a century later with the establishment of the World Health Organization. They originated professions

Stage	Evolutionary conception	Moments
	Ownership rights of citizens against the concept of health care from the state, through public assistance. The epidemiological transition and health transition. Rise of multiple-causality. Regulatory changes and development of social movements against the requirement of public health. Alma Ata: Health for All by the Year 2000 Development and renewal of primary health care and family medicine. Development of community nursing. Investment of the population pyramid. Three demographic transitions.	such as medicine and nursing. Koch gave rise to the creation of bacteriology microscope. Fleming discovered penicillin and all its possibilities starting the... Medical era: understanding of the disease as a preventable condition, to reduce morbidity and mortality and improve the living conditions. Psycho-Social Era: advances in psychological components, social and ecological function of disease control. Epidemiological Era: development of research on health determinants. Epidemiology as a method of knowledge to approach the study of diseases, their prevention and control. Statement by WHO on the health of communities, most especially on developing countries. Revaluation of the impact of environmental health in the development of public health.

Table 4. Stages of evolutionary development of public health

Within the evolutionary development of public health this has gone through many different stages, from the ignorance of their importance in the health-disease process, with a magical religious development, to implementation policivas connotations for control of communicable diseases, or the commodification of health services. It is now when public health has attracted interest from all kinds of thinkers and administrators, some with the encouragement to expand services to all communities at low cost and with high quality, in terms of expanding other economic power, some social.

But for decades to developing countries to enable them to plant objectives, reduce the health burden from communicable diseases such as HIV-AIDS, tuberculosis, vaccine-preventable diseases, acute respiratory infections and reduce the social and economic impact of theseReduce disease, disability and premature mortality, noncommunicable diseases such as hypertension, diabetes, kidney failure, cancer, dental gold diseases, mental illness and injuries from external causes such as domestic violence, accidents transfixed, the trauma. Reduce the risk factors associated with the disease burden, through habits and healthy lifestyles, healthy nutrition, reduction or elimination of smoking habits, alcohol, psychoactive substance use, increased physical activity, weight control, sexual behavior safe and responsible. Reduce morbidity and mortality through all life cycles. [19, 20, 21] Reduce inequalities in health for the entire population. Protect the health of the population through the improvement of the environmental conditions and the assurance of food safety. Strengthen psycho-social protection for the entire population. Strengthen the institutional health. Improve the quality of health care for all communities, with priority for the vulnerable. Strengthen the health sector response to disasters, emergencies and epidemics. Strengthen public health components for the entire population. Governments are committing to free health, public and affordable and accessible to all. [22, 23, 24]

9. The nursing professional in public health

Nursing care is the science of human health. The nurse dedicated his professional life to providing care to people in order to maintain health and reduce the risks or potential, compared to this. The singular focus of nursing as profession and art, focusing on the study of the response of the individual or community to a health problem as it can be presented or looming on the situational analysis of the community, from another perspective, in addition to the need of every human being to take care of yourself from the biological, emotional, social and spiritual, i.e., from a holistic projection. Critical thinking is formed in which the nurse is based on the foundation of the search for answers to questions and challenges facing a complex situation and how to deal with this situation. Nursing practice provides mechanisms by which the nurse uses their views, knowledge and skills to diagnose and treat diseases wings needs or problems facing individuals or groups of the population.

Nursing care encompasses autonomous and collaborative, which lend to people of all life cycles, families, groups and communities, sick or well, in all contexts, broadly include advocacy health, disease prevention, diagnosis and interventions to community care for the sick, disabled and dying people, as well as for populations at risk or pathology community. Essential functions are nursing or patient advocacy community from the bioethics field, promoting a safe environment, research, participation in health policy and management of the resources needed to promote recovery and rehabilitation strategies of patients and healthcare systems. [25, 26]

The first theory is born with Florence Nightingale nursing, and this theory is precisely what is closer to public health, the theorist of nursing care of the environment to provide a safe environment for patients, explores the importance of habits hygiene to prevent disease and preserve health, structure management plans of patients according to the support of their families and communities. From there arose new models each with new philosophical and epistemological contributions to understanding the nursing and care as science. Nursing in its historical development has gone through several stages, as yet been able to focus on the acquisition of technical and scientific knowledge in other historical moments were delegates in other professions, has been moving in the categorization of the profession. With the publication of the book "Notes on Nursing" by Florence Nightingale in 1852, laid the basis of nursing as a profession, in her book Florence attempt to define the specific contributions of nursing to health care both individual and community. Her spirit of inquiry is based on pragmatism. The objective of the model is to preserve the patient's vital energy and based on the action exerted by nature on individuals place it in the best possible conditions to act on it. Her theory focuses on the environment; she believed that a healthy environment was necessary to apply a suitable nursing care. She says "there are five key points to ensure health: clean air, pure water, efficient drainage, cleanliness and light." Another of her contributions refers to the need for home care nurses provide services in home care, should teach patients and their families to help themselves to maintain their independence. Nightingale's theory has significantly influenced other theories: Adaptation Theory, Theory of Needs Theory and Stress.

The basis of the theory of Nightingale is the environment: all conditions and external forces affecting the life and development of an organism. Nightingale describes five major components of a positive or healthy environment: adequate ventilation, adequate lighting, sufficient heat, the fumes control and noise control. To Nightingale physical environment consists of the physical elements in which the patient is treated, such as ventilation, temperature, hygiene, light, noise and elimination. For Nightingale psychological environment can be adversely affected by stress and Nightingale as the social environment that includes clean air, water and proper disposal involves collecting data about the disease and prevention of it, which is one of the most important contributions to the development of epidemiological studies in public health. [27, 28]

Another important theorist for public health nursing is Nola Pender with her "model of health promotion". This theory identifies the individual cognitive-perceptual factors that are modified by situational characteristics, personal and interpersonal, which results in participation in health-promoting behaviors, when there is a pattern for action. The model of health promotion concepts used to identify behaviors relevant to health promotion and to integrate research findings so as to facilitate the generation of hypotheses affordable.

This theory continues to be refined and expanded in its ability to explain the relationships among the factors thought to influence health behavior change at the community level. In the context of this theory health is a highly positive. The definition of health is more important than any general statement. The person is the individual and theorizes center. Each person is defined in a unique way by its own pattern and cognitive-perceptual variables factors. The environment described accurately with the representation of the interactions between the factors and perceptual, cognitive-modifying factors that influence the occurrence of health-promoting behaviors at the individual and collective.

The nurse on this theory has the responsibility to provide basic health care as care for the communities, from the aspects of disease prevention and health promotion.

A theoretical level most nursing programs develop public health issue as a central axis with practical theoretical approach, by raising awareness of models of public health work, the historical evolution of this, including the primary health care, effective participation in the development of policies, programs and health plans for communities. Paradigm shifts in coping with the risk factors and protective factors and the determinants of health, come together for a secure training of nurses with expertise in being, knowing and doing, which facilitate development of strengths that allow populations to manage their health components from its own needs. [29, 30, 31]

Nursing as a profession, in a holistic way is inclusive of the strengths, opportunities, needs and threats to the community is exposed, evaluates to base diagnoses and plans to raise from the educational interventions, the practical and political order improve the quality of life of the population to their work. It strengthens trans interdisciplinary work, as in the inter integration.

10. Conclusion

Nursing professionals within our academic role, research, and administrative assistance, we focus on the daily work to the attention of the people to provide public health care consistent with the needs of communities, the environment and the conditions existing at the time participate in the work. One of the opportunities that are currently nursing professionals is fresh out of training and development of skills in all matters relating to primary health care, including education as a tool to strengthen social development, is a permanently open door.

Public health has been established for professional nursing in a working strategy with wide projection. Population dynamics, environmental, socio-economic conditions, among many others offer the possibility of deepening concretely and specifically against the background of each of the populations, their needs and finding efficient solutions to achieve the desired changes and eventually support the prolonging life years in good condition and excellent quality of life.

However for all this possibilities into the profession and the public health, we cannot ignore the social weight that represents the life conditions of communities into development countries specially all the topics related with health, education, work and housing. These components also are affected by environmental conditions, inequality and inequity facing health services and the precarious conditions to resolve the situations of risk that they face daily.

It is important to look at the context of the work of professional nurse into public health in a prospective of development, integrity and support in which development the self-sufficient countries can support through economic and scientific-technical alliances to those most vulnerable. The economy, which finally can be the more important factor for health development support, investigation, technology, social responsibility between others, should have redistribution which benefits needy population to achieve the benefits of a better quality of life.

Acknowledgements

- A very special thanks to Dr. Alfonso Javier Rodriguez, for inviting me to be part of this project.

http://dx.doi.org/10.5772/53452

- To all my colleagues, because they have been a source for obtaining information and the achievement of the document structure.
- To the patients, their families and communities, throughout my working life I have been led to skills for work like this.
- To my undergraduate and graduate students, because they are the engine of my current activity
- To my family, which is a permanent inspiration in all things personal

Author details

Carmen Luisa Betancur P.

Teachers associated Pereira Technological University (Pereira, Colombia), Teachers associated Andean University Foundation, Sectional Pereira (Pereira, Colombia), Coordinating expertise in epidemiology, FUAA, sectional Pereira, Colombia

References

[1] Banco Interamericano de desarrollo. Paises agrupados según el índice de desarrollo humano 2008, revisado julio 30 2012 en: http://hdr.undp.org/en/media/HDR_20072008_SP_paises.pdf

[2] Betancur P. Carmen Luisa, Castrillón B. Dora María, Cardona G. Dora. Apoyo social percibido por personas en situación de desplazamiento en los municipios de Risaralda, excepto área metropolitana. EN: Aspectos psicosociales del desplazamiento forzado en Risaralda: factores de riesgo, Resiliencia y apoyo social [compiladora Granada Patricia], 2012. ISBN 978-958-722-135-0 Universidad Tecnológica de Pereira – Colciencias.

[3] Albornoz Mario. Situación de la Ciencia y la Tecnología en las Américas. 2002. Centro de Estudios sobre Ciencia, Desarrollo y Educación Superior Buenos Aires, revisado julio 26 del 2012 en: http://www.science.oas.org/Doc/Policy/Situacion_CT_Americas.pdf

[4] Index Mundial. Expectativa de vida al nacer, en todos los países, Revisado julio 31 del 2012 En: [http://www.indexmundi.com/map/?v=30&l=es

[5] Betancur P. Carmen Luisa. Gerencia del cuidado hospitalario. 2011. Editorial Ecoe. Bogota, Colombia. ISBN 9789586487405.

[6] Organización mundial de la Salud. Estadisticas Sanitarias mundiales. 2011. Revisado agosto 3 del 2012 En: http://www.who.int/whosis/whostat/ES_WHS2011_Full.pdf

[7] Organización mundial de la Salud. Indicadores sanitarios mundiales. 2011. Revisado agosto 4 del 2012En: http://www.who.int/whosis/whostat/ES_WHS2011_Full.pdf

[8] Organización mundial de la salud. Declaración de Adelaida sobre la Salud en Todas las Políticas Hacia una gobernanza compartida en pro de la salud y el bienestar. 2010. En: http://www.who.int/social_determinants/publications/isa/spanish_adelaide_statement_for_web.pdf (revisado julio 20 2012)

[9] Organización mundial de la salud. commission on social determinants of health. estrategia de participacion de las organizaciones de la sociedad civil de america latina 2006 – 2008 En: http://www.who.int/social_determinants/resources/america_civil_society_strategy.pdf (revisado junio 30 de 2012)

[10] Edgar C. Jarillo Soto y Oliva López Arellano. Salud Pública: Objeto de Conocimiento, Prácticas y Formación. Revista de salud pública. N° 9 (1):140-154, 2007.

[11] Torres Cristina, Mujica Oscar. Salud y equidad en Los Objetivos de desarrollo del milenio. En: Rev Panam Salud Publica/Pan Am J Public Health 15(6), 2004. (revisado septiembre 14 del 2012) http://www.scielosp.org/pdf/rpsp/v15n6/22178.pdf.

[12] Organización Panamericana de la Salud. Determinantes de la salud pública. Revista Salud Publica.

[13] Colombia. Ministerio de medio ambiente. Revisado el 26 de julio del 2012 en: http://www.minambiente.gov.co/contenido/contenido.aspx?conID=1292&catID=556.

[14] Organización Mundial de la Salud, 61ª Conferencia mundial. Ginebra, mayo 2008. Revisado junio 26 del 2012 EN: http://apps.who.int/gb/ebwha/pdf_files/WHA61-REC1/A61_REC1-sp.pdf

[15] Organización mundial de la salud. Conferencia de las Naciones Unidas sobre el Desarrollo Sostenible (Río+20). Río de Janeiro, Brasil, 20 al 22 de junio de 2012. Revisado agosto 3 del 2012 en: http://www.who.int/mediacentre/events/meetings/2012/sustainable_development/es/index.html

[16] Organización panamericana de la salud. Salud pública y desarrollo sostenible. 2012, revisado junio 30 del 2012 En: http://www.un.org/esa/sustdev/documents/WSSD_POI_PD/Spanish/POIspChapter6.htm

[17] Martínez H Eliana, Franco M Diego F, Villa V Liliana. Las redes de conocimiento en salud pública y el fortalecimiento de capacidades a través de estrategias de cooperación. Rev. Fac. Nac. Salud Pública [serial on the Internet]. 2009 Sep [cited 2012 Aug 20] ; 27(3): 349-355. Available from: http://www.scielo.org.co/scielo.php?script=sci_arttext&pid=S0120-386X2009000300013&lng=en.

[18] Organización Panamericana de la Salud/Organización Mundial de la Salud. Red Colombiana de Investigación en Políticas y Sistemas de Salud. Logros y limitaciones a Julio de 2007: sistematización de las experiencias en desarrollo de políticas de investigación en salud pública de la Red Colombiana de Investigación en Políticas y Siste-

mas de Salud. [Sitio en Internet]. Bogotá: 2007 [acceso el 11 de agosto de 2012]. Disponible en:http://redalyc.uaemex.mx/redalyc/src/inicio/ArtPdfRed. jsp? iCve=92430815.

[19] Frenk Julio, Chen Lincoln, Bhutta Zulfiqar A, Cohen Jordan, Crisp Nigel, Evans Timothy et al . Profesionales de la salud para el nuevo siglo: transformando la educación para fortalecer los sistemas de salud en un mundo interdependiente. Rev Peru Med Exp Salud Publica [serial on the Internet]. 2011 June [cited 2012 Sep 12] ; 28(2): 337-341. Available from: http://www.scielosp.org/scielo.php?script=sci_arttext&pid=S1726-46342011000200023&lng=en. http://dx.doi.org/10.1590/S1726-46342011000200023.

[20] Sachs Jeffrey D.. Rev Panam Salud Publica [serial on the Internet]. 2002 Aug [cited 2012 Sep 12] ; 12(2): 143-144. Available from: http://www.scielosp.org/scielo.php?script=sci_arttext&pid=S1020-49892002000800017&lng=en. http://dx.doi.org/10.1590/S1020-49892002000800017.

[21] Republica de Colombia. Ministerio de Salud. Objetivos para el decenio 2010 – 2020

[22] Republica de Chile. Objetivos sanitarios década 2011-2020 revisado agosto 22 del 2012. Disponible en: http://www.slideshare.net/CesfamMTC/objetivos-sanitarios-decada-2011-2020

[23] Cruz Rojo Concepción. Apuntes sobre Evolución historica de la salud publica. Universidad de Sevilla. 2011, revisado julio 11 del 1012 disponible en: http://personal.us.es/cruzrojo/EVOLUCION-SALUD-PUBLICA.pdf

[24] Cruz Rojo C. "Modelos biologicista y social en el campo de la salud". 2007. Revisado julio 11 del 2012. Disponible en: http://www.personal.us.es/cruzrojo/

[25] Krieger Krieger N. Emerging theories for social epidemiology in the 21st century: an ecosocial perspective. Int J Epidemiol 2001;30:668-677.

[26] R. L. Wesley (1997): Teorías y modelos de enfermería. McGraw-Hill Interamericana, México.

[27] Juana Hernández Conesa (1995): Historia de la Enfermería. Un análisis histórico de los cuidados de Enfermería, McGraw-Hill Interamericana, Madrid.

[28] Florence Nightingale (1990): Notas sobre Enfermería. ¿Qué es y qué no es?, Masson – Salvat Enfermería, Barcelona.

[29] Betancur, op cit pag. 75

[30] Leddy, Susan. Pepper J. Mae. Bases Conceptuales de la Enfermería Profesional. Organización Panamericana de la salud. New York 1989

[31] Universidad Nacional de Colombia. Facultad de enfermería. Dimensiones del Cuidado. Unibiblos. Bogotá. 1998. Liliana González Juárez. Profesor de Carrera ENEO/UNAM

Chapter 11

The Financing of Public Health

Jason S. Turner, Simone Singh,
Connie Evashwick and Steve Eastaugh

Additional information is available at the end of the chapter

http://dx.doi.org/10.5772/54572

1. Introduction

The provision of public health depends on the availability of adequate resources. In most nations, financing is composed of a combination of public and private funding that provides direct support to the public health system and indirect support through the healthcare delivery system. How much and in what ways funding is provided affects the types and effectiveness of public health activities.

This chapter considers private and public financing of public health and the various mechanisms used to foster both from an economics perspective. This then leads to a brief description of the way in which public policies can be used to affect change in financing public health and subsequently in the services provided.

Public health is "the science and art of preventing disease, prolonging life, and promoting health through the organized efforts of society." [1] The health system should be thought of as a broad construct that includes the political and institutional framework of each country. More formally, the healthcare system is "the ensemble of all public and private organizations, institutions and resources mandated to improve or restore health. Health systems encompass both personal and population services, as well as activities to influence the policies and actions of other sectors to address the social, environmental and economic determinants of health." [2] Although in some developing nations the public health and healthcare delivery systems are difficult to differentiate, in most countries the public health and healthcare delivery systems are distinct. Yet, what happens is one affects the other. For the purposes of this chapter, public health encompasses the activities described by the World Health Organization (WHO) in its essential Public Health Services Framework (Table 1).

1. Surveillance of diseases and assessment of the population's health and well-being
2. Identification of priority health problems and health hazards in the community
3. Preparedness for and planning for public health emergencies
4. Health protection operations (environment, occupational, food safety and others)
5. Disease prevention
6. Health promotion
7. Assuring a competent public health and personal health care workforce
8. Core governance, financing and quality assurance for public health
9. Core communication for public health
10. Health-related research.
Source: World Health Organization, www.who.org

Table 1. Ten essential public health operations (EPHOs)

This chapter conceptualizes public health financing using two economic theories: supply and demand and resource/health optimization. The supply/demand theory maintains that as the price of health services declines the consumption of that service will increase. The converse is also true. If the price of a good increases the consumption of services will decrease. Resource/ health optimization refers to the idea that there is a point where the private and public benefits (both monetary and non-monetary) from the consumption of services are exactly offset by private and public costs (both monetary and non-monetary). Movement away from this point means that the public health services are not worth the cost or countries would benefit from spending more on health.

The financing of both public health and healthcare activities is essential, complex, and subject to substantial variation. In 2010, spending data on public health expenditures alone are not available for multi-national comparisons. By using the broad WHO definition of public health, the data on total health expenditures can be employed as an indication of public health expenditures, as it encompasses both public health activities and direct health services. Spending ranged from lows of $16 (US$) per person per year in the African nations of Ethiopia and the Congo to over $8,000 (US$) per person per year in Luxemburg and the United States of America. [3, 4] Figure 1 shows the substantial variations in per capita health expenditures by region in 2010. The role that the public sector adopts in financing health-related activities is also highly uneven. For example, in 2010, government expenditures as a percentage of the overall spending ranged from just over 11% in Afghanistan to more than 90% in Cuba, Micronesia, and Tuvalu. [3, 4]

Not surprisingly, the substantial variations in health financing reflect the history, culture, income, and political will of the respective countries. [5] Some opt for active participation of the government in the organization, planning, and financing of health activities, while others look to maximize market forces. [6] Most countries lie somewhere between the two ends of the spectrum, where some activities like physician education or disease surveillance are managed by the government, while others, like drug development or insurance, are left to individual market players.

http://dx.doi.org/10.5772/54572

Regardless of position on the market maximization/minimization spectrum, both overall and government support of public health are related to the wealth of the respective countries, as shown in Figure 2. Wealthier countries spend more on health than poorer countries. Early estimates indicate that for every 10 percent increase in per capita gross domestic product (GDP) health related spending increases by approximately 13 percent. [7] Similar results are demonstrated in Figure 2, although not to the same magnitude.

2. Mechanisms for financing

In general, health expenditures can be financed through five mechanisms- general tax revenues, social insurance, voluntary insurance, charitable donations (also referred to as financial aid), and individual out-of-pocket expenses. Figure 3 shows the 2007 world health financing mechanisms by category.

Financing public health with **general tax revenues** is most common in more affluent, Western countries with substantial stability. [5] In more developed countries, productivity and income allow financing with tax revenues to occur that may exclude important educational or infrastructure financing in less developed countries. The tax revenues generated in poor countries are smaller and must be spread over other, important public goods. As a result, public health efforts might be lower priority than activities pertaining to education, infrastructure, and economic development. Moreover, the tax base and consistency required for developing, administrating, and sustaining public health efforts often excludes very poor or transitional economies from financing public health activities with general tax revenues.

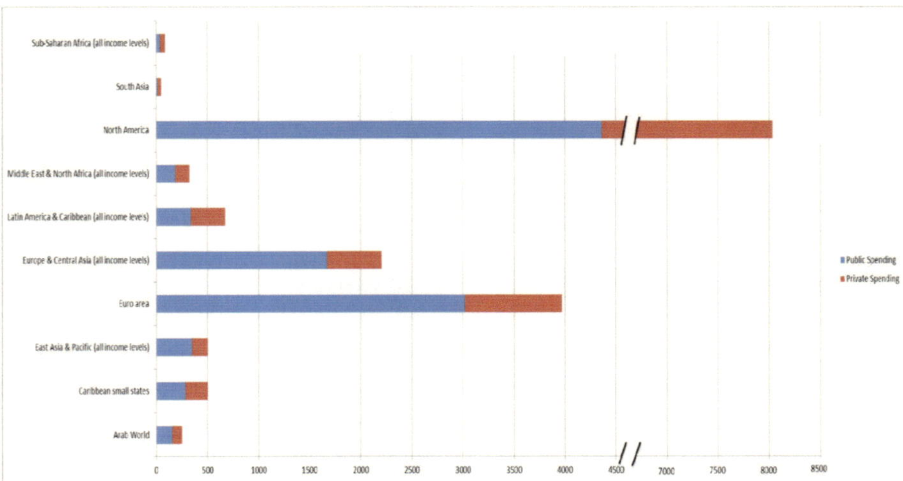

Data source: WHO Global Health Data Repository, 2011)

Figure 1. Total Health Expenditures per Capita in 2010 (Public & Private Expenditures)

When used to pay for public health activities, the taxes themselves are considered *direct, indirect, or excise taxes*. **Direct taxes** are paid by individuals to governments and cannot be avoided by behavioral or consumption decisions. By virtue of citizenship or ownership of property, individuals must pay direct taxes. **Indirect taxes** are taxes on transactions that occur within a government's purview. Indirect taxes can be considered a tax on consumption. At the point of sale or service the seller collects the tax from the consumer and later delivers the tax revenue to the government. Sales taxes, value added taxes (VAT), and goods and services taxes (GST) are examples of common indirect taxes. While indirect taxes apply to all goods or services, excise taxes are much more specific. **Excise taxes** are taxes that are placed on the production or sale of certain goods or services. They can be used by governments to change the population's consumption behavior by increasing the cost of a particular good or service. For example, an excise tax on cigarettes increases the price to consumers and can be used to generate additional tax revenue.

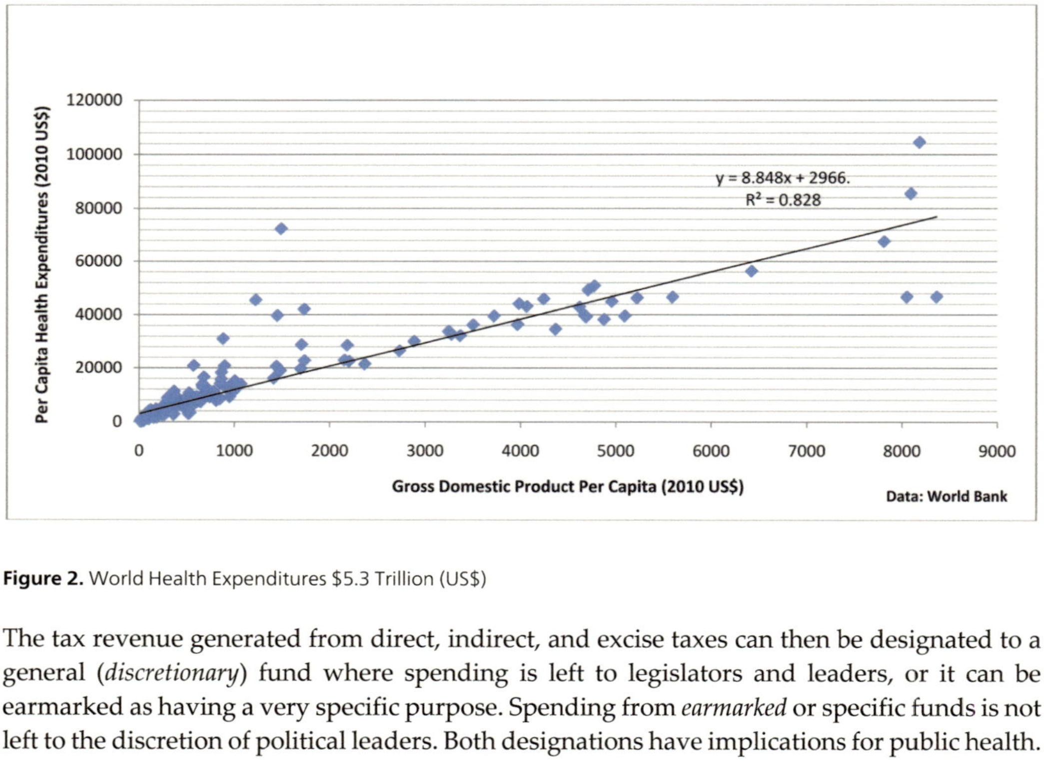

Figure 2. World Health Expenditures $5.3 Trillion (US$)

The tax revenue generated from direct, indirect, and excise taxes can then be designated to a general (*discretionary*) fund where spending is left to legislators and leaders, or it can be earmarked as having a very specific purpose. Spending from *earmarked* or specific funds is not left to the discretion of political leaders. Both designations have implications for public health. In instances where legislators are periodically replaced, the priorities for government spending also change. When incumbents who favored funding public health from discretionary funds are replaced by challengers who do not favor those initiatives, the resulting instability in public health financing may create substantial barriers to long-term success. Financing with earmarked funds avoids the disruption caused by periodic changes to government leadership but can be subject to substantial variations in the revenue generated by taxes. For example, anti-

http://dx.doi.org/10.5772/54572

smoking initiatives that are financed by an excise tax on high-sugar drinks may experience decreased funding if public consumption of sugary drinks declines. Finally, when economies are healthy, government programs, including public health programs, have a tendency to expand in both scope and scale. However, given the cyclical nature of economies, tax revenues often decline in periods of less robust growth or recession. Unless governments clearly place public health high in the importance queue, then in periods of slower growth and reduced tax revenues, public health initiatives may be crowded-out in favor of other activities.

Social insurance programs are mandatory insurance systems that are contributed to by employers and employees. Rather than using primarily general tax revenues to finance health, many developed countries have established social insurance systems for this purpose

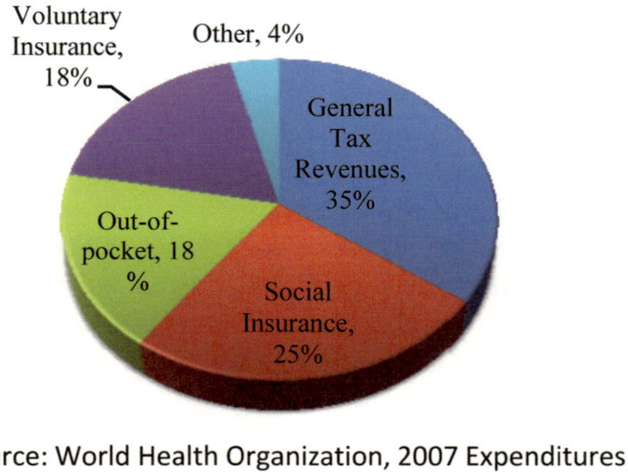

Figure 3. Relationship Between National Health Expenditures and National Gross Domestic Product

Often cited as a classical example of a social insurance system, Germany has developed a minimum level of economic protection for its citizens in the form of a comprehensive system of health, retirement, long-term care, and unemployment insurance. Financed jointly by employers and employees, Germany's social health insurance plays an important role in the public health system through the advancement of disease prevention, health promotion, resource and capital planning, and the participation in and management of disease registries, all of which are components of the essential health operations as determined by the World Health Organization (see Table 1). [8]

Voluntary insurance occurs when employers and/or individuals opt to purchase insurance from private firms to mitigate a potential loss of income associated with illness or the costs of healthcare consumption. In some countries, voluntary insurance systems are used instead of social insurance systems to finance the health needs of large shares of the population. In the United States, for example, voluntary insurance covers about two-thirds of the non-elderly working population, but the exact percentage varies at any given time and tends to decrease during periods of slow economic growth.

Both social and voluntary insurance financing mechanisms are more associated with the delivery of acute healthcare services than the essential operations of public health. However, in addition to the disease management and health promotion functions mentioned in association with social insurance, insurance (social or voluntary) provides other contributions such as health education and the potential for public/private partnerships. For example, AIDS/HIV prevention and treatment require close collaboration of health care providers and public health. Without the support from private insurers that pay private practitioners to treat those who are ill, the tax revenue designated to AIDS/HIV alone would be insufficient to manage this condition at the individual patient level.

Charitable donations, financial aid, and the work of **non-profit organizations** in the development and financing of public health cannot be understated. All countries, regardless of wealth, history, or where they reside on the market maximization vs. market minimization spectrum, rely at least to some extent on charity and non-profit organizations. Some non-profit organizations provide the same or similar services as for-profit organizations or the government, while others are the sole provider of services targeting needs inadequately addressed by for-profit organizations and government. For example, the American Diabetes Association promotes health, educates the population and serves as a catalyst for additional research. Similar roles are filled by the European CanCer Organization or the Heart and Stroke Foundation of Canada. These organizations meet a need in generating awareness of diseases and providing education and resources beyond that which local and national government entities are able to provide. Without the financial and expertise assistance provided by these non-profit organizations, the burden placed on governments to meet domestic needs would increase substantially on the very countries that can least afford to designate substantial government funds to public health.

Also important, in particular for developing countries, are international financial assistance and charity work. The funding of the international charitable work comes in three forms: *non-governmental organizations* (NGOs), *bilateral assistance*, and *multilateral assistance*. NGOs are specifically organized to be independent of government agencies and can provide everything from acute care to financial aid and technical assistance for a particular health need or community outreach project. Project Hope, for instance, an international NGO founded in 1958, spent $205M (US$) in 2011 to provide health education and humanitarian assistance throughout the world. [9] The largest of the health-related NGOs, Oxfam, is an international organization that spent €991M in 2010-2011 to remedy injustice and address the concerns of the poor, including many public health projects. Over €660M was spent directly on program implementation, development, and maintenance throughout the world with the highest percentage of expenditures (12.8%) focused on Central America, Mexico, and the Caribbean followed by South Asia (11.9%) and East Asia (9.2%). [10]

Bilateral assistance comes directly from a government agency within a single country. The largest source of bilateral aid comes from the United States Aid for International Development (USAID), which spent over $8.6B in 2011. [11] However, the United States is not alone in providing aid. Most developed countries have agencies that provide technical assistance or financial support. Today, many of those bilateral aid relationships are prod-

http://dx.doi.org/10.5772/54572

ucts of historical associations that resulted from the colonialism of the 19th and 20th century. Japan continues to support its former East Asian colonies, while England and France provide aid to countries in Africa. Although it has not been borne out in recent years, [12] it is thought that continued pressure on global economic markets may force government agencies to revisit expenditure levels moving forward. Austerity measures coupled with slower economic growth may compel developed countries to balance global public health needs with immediate and local demands.

When health financing is contributed to by multiple countries, the financial support transitions from being a bilateral relationship to a *multilateral relationship.* Examples of institutions implementing multilateral aid include the World, Asian and African Banks; UNICEF; and the foremost international public health body, the World Health Organization (WHO). In 2012-13, the WHO is projected to spend US$3.9B on public health initiatives ranging from reducing HIV/AIDS and malaria in Africa, to education for leaders and technicians needed to achieve the Millennium Development Goals and improved public health throughout Asia and South America. [13] Initiatives in Africa, the Eastern Mediterranean, and Southeast Asia account for the majority of WHO expenditures, with Europe, the Americas and the Western Pacific receiving substantially less aid.

Despite the considerable amount of money contributed bilaterally, multilaterally, or via NGOs, it is estimated that the contributions from developed countries account for less than 5% of the total funding sources for health in developing countries. [11] Nonetheless, their importance and impact cannot be overstated. In low-income countries (Gross National Income < $1,025 per capita), general tax revenue covers less than 40% of healthcare costs. [3] The balance of costs in these low-income countries is made up by charitable donations, NGOs, and financial assistance. Considering that there are no voluntary or mandatory social insurance programs in many developing countries, external funding contributes over 50% of the total health financing in some countries. In Sub-Saharan Africa, for example, 54% of healthcare is provided by NGOs, multinational health efforts, or individual government development agencies. [3]

Finally, even in developed countries with universal or near universal health coverage, **individual or out-of-pocket payments** represent an important mechanism of health financing. These payments can take the form of payment-in-full for a particular service, or they can be related to cost sharing instituted by insurance or government plans (in the form of deductibles, copayments, and coinsurance). The economic theory of supply and demand mentioned earlier applies here. By instituting or increasing out-of-pocket payments for health, individuals will consume fewer services. Moreover, and more problematic for consumers, out-of-pocket payments require consumers to weigh the potential benefits of a good or service with the costs in an uncertain environment where there are multiple, competing priorities. Consumption may make the individual healthy or it may not. Figure 4 shows how the price paid by individuals shifts from P* to P** as individuals face a higher price. The higher price intersects the demand curve at a point closer to the vertical axis. This point is associated with fewer services being consumed and a decrease in the total healthcare expenditures. The desire to hold down health costs must be balanced with providing access if the health service being offered is a normal, **private good**. When the good is considered private, the consumption of the good reduces the availability to others and can even exclude individuals who do not have the ability to pay. For example, in a country where markets are used to disperse healthcare, an individual who injures his or her knee and requires an x-ray is consuming a private good. By using the x-ray machine and spending time with the doctor, the availability of the doctor and x-ray to screen other patients becomes more limited. Direct out-of-pocket payments further limit (or exclude) those who are unable to pay for services or those who place greater weight on other priorities. As a result, direct, out-of-pocket payments for healthcare services can be a substantial barrier to obtaining services and improving health. Research indicates that out-of-pocket payment can become a substantial barrier when they exceed 20% of total health expenditures.

	Excludable	**Non-excludable**
Rivalrous	Private Goods (Example: Acute care where individuals are responsible for a portion of the cost of care)	Common Goods (Example: Clean water campaign where the demand for clean water is greater than the supply)
	Desirable Financing: Tax, Social Insurance, Voluntary Insurance, Financial Aid (Charity), and Out-of-Pocket (limited)	Desirable Financing: Tax, Social Insurance, Financial Aid (Charity)
Non-Rivalrous	Club Goods (Example: Healthy eating campaign that specifically targets breast feeding mothers)	Public Goods (Example: Radio campaign increasing the awareness of the dangers associated with smoking)
	Desirable Financing: Tax, Social Insurance, Voluntary Insurance, Financial Aid (Charity), and Out-of-Pocket (limited)	Desirable Financing: Tax, Social Insurance, Financial Aid (Charity)

Table 2. Classification of healthcare goods

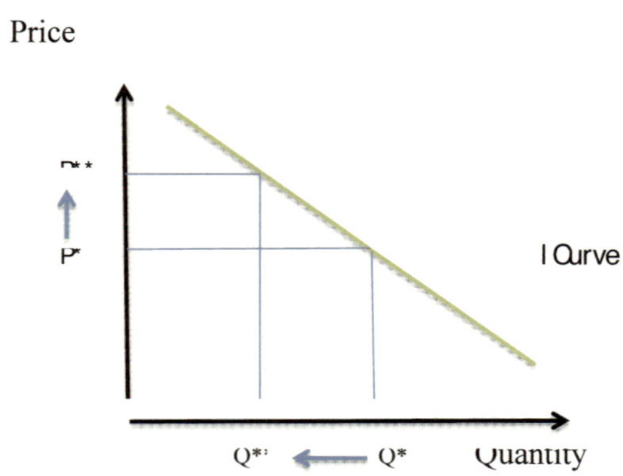

Figure 4. Impact of Rising Prices on Consumption of Public Health Goods

Financing public health initiatives with out-of-pocket payments may not lead to the most desirable outcomes. First, many public health enterprises look to maximize consumption (disease management programs, health promotion efforts, or other such activities) by removing the very barriers to participation that out-of-pocket payments present. Second, financing health with out-of-pocket payments indicates what individuals are willing to pay for a service and the consumption at that given price. It does not, however, necessarily optimize the health of the total population served. In fact, there may be no relationship between the level of services consumed and the health outcomes of either an individual or a population. Third, there are public health efforts to improve air quality, disseminate knowledge, protect parks and open spaces that are not normal, private goods but **public goods**. These goods are *non-exclusive* and *non-rivalrous*, which means that all individuals have access to the good and the use of a good by an individual does not reduce the availability for others to consume the same good. Charging individuals for consumption of these public health goods is logistically difficult and doing so would transition the good into having all the respective disincentives to consumption that private goods carry.

The traditional spheres of public health include *common goods* and *club goods* in addition to public and private goods. Table 2 shows how these concepts apply to public health. **Common goods** or services are those to which everyone has access but of which there is a limited supply. The challenge when allocating and financing common goods is to find a mechanism that is equitable or maximizes the utility of the program, or, ideally, both.

Allocating common goods based on what individuals are willing to pay for out-of-pocket carries with it all of the same disincentives discussed earlier. As a result, common and public goods should be financed with tax revenue or some charitable/financial aid.

Public health goods that are considered **club goods** are inversely related to common goods. There is sufficient supply to meet the need but access may be limited. While the limitation may be a result of willingness to pay, the more common scenarios are those where a targeted or vulnerable population would disproportionately benefit from the public health intervention. Rather than canvas an entire population, attempts are made to maximize the effectiveness of efforts by limiting the population to those who derive the greatest benefit. Club goods can and have been financed with out-of-pocket payments (if the perceived benefit clearly outweighs the cost), but participation and program penetration are improved with tax financing, social insurance, and financial aid that does not carry disincentives to participation.

3. Policy implications

If the promises of WHO's *Millennium Development Goals*[1] and improved public health are to be realized, then substantial changes must be made in how countries finance both public health

1 Millennium Development Goals include eradicating extreme poverty and hunger, achieving universal primary education, promoting gender equality and empowering women, reducing child mortality rates, improving maternal health, combating HIV/AIDS, malaria, and other diseases, ensuring environmental sustainability, and developing a global partnership for development (http://www.un.org/milleniumgoals/bkgd.shtml).

and the larger health system. Complicating the change are the sometimes conflicting ideas of "protect [ing] people from the financial consequences of ill-health and paying for health services" while simultaneously "encourage [ing] the optimum use of available resources." [14] This is particularly challenging when one considers that to achieve these goals, developing and developed countries alike must extend healthcare and public health services to populations that are currently not covered. They must also expand the services that are being offered, and cost sharing and fees must be reduced to increase both access and affordability, at least for services where this is desirable (see discussion above). Expansion of covered populations and services in tandem with a reduction in out-of-pocket expenses creates additional pressures on governments, insurance systems, and charitable organizations to increase the resources devoted to public health and healthcare systems. To alleviate the pressure, the WHO has proposed a number of initiatives that target increasing revenue, removing barriers, and increasing efficiencies: [14]

1. *Increase the efficiency of revenue collection*. Tax avoidance and tax minimization plague both developed and developing countries. Similar problems have emerged with the collection of insurance premiums. Moreover, substantial informal, black or grey markets make taxation difficult. Strengthening tax infrastructure and movement away from black and grey markets to a more stable environment where tax avoidance is minimized will increase the financial resources available to governments and thus to financing public health.

2. *Reprioritize government budgets.* When faced with multiple priorities, governments often opt to pursue non-health concerns. An additional $15B (US$) could be raised if 41 of the low-income countries increased health expenditures up to 15% of their government budget. [15] Making public health a top priority would be substantially aided by additional research that explicitly ties improved population health and health infrastructure to improved economic growth and social wellbeing.

3. *Innovative Financing*. Innovative financing for public health could come in the form of new taxes such as an international excise tax on everything from air travel to fees placed on international monetary exchanges. At the national level, additional financing could be derived from an increase of sumptuary taxes (a specific type of excise tax that is also known as a "sin tax"). These taxes target goods or services that may have detrimental effects on individuals or the general population. The increase in sumptuary taxes would have the dual effect of increasing revenues for health while also decreasing the consumption of a good or service that society deems undesirable. This could be an additional tax on tobacco, alcohol, excessively sugary drinks or foods high in saturated fat.

4. *Development assistance*. Even with reprioritized government budgets and an increase in tax revenues, the WHO estimates that 41 of the 49 poorest countries would not be able to meet the health needs of their populations. The result is continued dependence upon charitable organizations to fill the funding gap between the public health that the country is able to provide and the public health need of a country. Charitable organizations and international aid must maintain their current levels of funding and consider increasing future aid.

5. *Promoting efficiency and eliminating waste.* An estimated 20-40% of health expenditures are wasted. [14] Less expensive treatments are bypassed in favor of more expensive therapies, drugs and antibiotics are overused, multiple and different administrative structures create a lack of standardization and decrease interoperability. Moreover, insufficient investment in public health exacerbates the prevalence and severity of disease burdens that could be avoided. Reducing waste and inappropriate use as well as, focusing on prevention rather than acute episodic care have the potential to dramatically improve the effectiveness of healthcare expenditures and thus reduce the need for additional financing.

6. *Improving access equality.* Public health has the responsibility to focus on population-based disease prevention and health promotion. Unfortunately, large scale population initiatives that reduce barriers for all in a given country may not be the most efficient use of resources. Meeting the needs of remote or rural locations can require substantial resources that are being used by relatively few individuals. Those funds may generate more benefit by being concentrated in dense population pockets where more individuals can take advantage of the resources. Clarity of priorities will allow resources to be distributed according to predetermined goals.

7. *Reduction in direct payments.* Direct, out-of-pocket payment for services continues to be a substantial barrier to improving health. Individuals do not seek needed care, and in countries that have little to no existing public health infrastructure, the option to purchase may be prohibitive or not even available. Increased tax revenues and improved efficiencies will enable governments to reduce direct payments for services and should likely be pursued before or concurrently with the reduction of direct payments.

In addition to the WHO proposals there are substantial opportunities to partner with private businesses to increase the funding available for public health activities. These opportunities must balance private sector interests with the goals of improving public health. In general, this will include balancing the costs of public health services provided by the private sector with the benefits derived from these activities. Examples of private-sector actors that may contribute to public health include healthcare systems, health insurance companies, larger employers, foundations, associations, and non-profit community-oriented organizations, as well as individual volunteers. An exhaustive discussion is beyond the scope of this chapter; however, examples of private contributions to the public health system are exemplified by large employers and healthcare systems.

Large employers, for instance, can be important partners for governments when it comes to improving public health. Large employers can easily reach their employees and their employees' families and are thus in an ideal position to implement public health initiatives. Many large employers, for instance, have begun to develop corporate wellness programs. These programs may include health screenings, vaccinations, exercise classes and subsidized fitness clubs, healthy eating options, and smoking cessation support groups, to name but a few. While corporate wellness programs started in the United States and Europe, many multinational companies are now expanding them globally. Employers often have a financial incentive to engage in employee wellness programs as these programs can reduce absenteeism and promote job satisfaction, thus improving efficiency and reducing costly employee turnover. Employers who are self-insured can also experience a decrease in direct healthcare costs.

Another important partner in improving public health are traditional providers of health care services, such as hospitals and health systems. Hospitals and health systems may be well positioned to take over certain public health activities, such as health education, health screenings, immunizations, and community support groups. Since many of these services are not adequately reimbursed and thus money-losing activities, for-profit organizations generally do not have sufficient financial incentives to provide them. Not-for-profit organizations, on the other hand, may consider public health services part of their mission and be able to dedicate financial resources to such activities. [16]

4. Conclusion

The resources needed for an effective public health system depend on private, as well as public, financing. As has been summarized in this chapter, a variety of mechanisms can be used to achieve a combination of public and private contributions. Which mechanisms are used and what the expected effects are drawn from economic theory. It is thus essential that those making policies have a solid understanding of the principles of economics and how local factors influence the behavior of individuals and organizations, including government and private entities. Variations in policies across nations are to be expected, but this then poses a challenge to global efforts to promote population health and support individual countries, as well as world-wide, public health initiatives. Finally, moving forward, an evidence-based approach to resourcing public health would benefit greatly from more refined data on health systems outcomes, which would contribute to choosing between options, as well as data on expenditures that differentiate public health services for populations from healthcare delivery to individuals, which would then permit more sophisticated analysis of supply, demand, and the impact of potential economic policies.

Author details

Jason S. Turner[1], Simone Singh[2], Connie Evashwick and Steve Eastaugh[3]

1 Department of Health Management and Policy, Saint Louis University, St. Louis, MO, USA

2 Department of Health Services Organization and Policy, University of Michigan, Ann Arbor, MI,

3 Department of Health Services Management and Leadership, George Washington University, Washington, D.C., USA

http://dx.doi.org/10.5772/54572

References

[1] Acheson, D., Public Health in England: The Report of the Committee of Inquiry into the Future Development of the Public Health Function, London: HMSO. 103; 1988.

[2] *The Tallinn Charter: Health Systems for Health and Wealth,* W.R.O.F. Europe, Editor. World Health Organization: Copenhagen. p. 1; 2008.

[3] The World Bank. *Data Indicators*. 2012; Available from: http://data.worldbank.org/indicator/all.

[4] World Health Organization. *Global Health Observatory Data Repository*. 2011; Available from: http://apps.who.int/ghodata/?vic=1901.

[5] Fried, B. and L.M. Gaydos, *World Health Systems: Challenges and Perspectives*. 2002: Health Administration Press.

[6] G.F. Anderson, J.P.P., *Health Spending, Access, and Outcomes: Trends in Industrialized Countries.* Health Affairs, 1999: p. 178-92.

[7] Schieber, G., *Health Care Financing and Delivery in Developing Countries.* Health Affairs, 1999: p. 193-205.

[8] WHO, *Self Assessment Tool for the Evaluation of Public Health Services*. 2012.

[9] *Hope is Here: 2011 Annual Report*. 30; 2011.

[10] *Oxfam Annual Report 2010-2011*. 64; 2011.

[11] IMVA. *The Major International Health Organisations*; 2012.

[12] IHME. *Financing Global Health 2011: Continued Growth as MDG Deadline Approaches*; 2011.

[13] WHO. *WHO Programme Budget 2012- 2013*; 2011.

[14] WHO. *Health Systems Financing: The Path to Universal Coverage*. The World Health Report.; 2010.

[15] *More money for health, and more health for the money: final report,* T.o.I.I.F.f.H. Systems, Editor. 2009, International Health Partnership.

[16] IRS, *Tax-Exempt Status For Your Organization (Rev. June 2008)*. 2008. p. 65-66.

Section 3

Evidence-Based Public Health

Chapter 12

Clinical Epidemiology and Its Relevance for Public Health in Developing Countries

Cristian Díaz-Vélez, Víctor Soto-Cáceres,
Ricardo E. Peña-Sánchez,
Moisés A. Apolaya Segura and Edén Galán-Rodas

Additional information is available at the end of the chapter

http://dx.doi.org/10.5772/54901

1. Introduction

The current medical approach must contemplate the application of clinical epidemiology in the health establishments, patients; in general, epidemiologic research with its analytical designs and clinical trials allow the progress in treatments and managements, as well as defining the quality of auxiliary exams ever more sophisticated by means of the test of tests design and its cost-benefit approach [1,2] On the other hand, the field epidemiology is applied through descriptive studies of the population's health situation with their analytical approaches to the Situational Health Analysis (SHA), the study of epidemic outbreaks and evaluation of the respective answer of the community interventions [3,4]. This way, it allows carrying out an integral management of the epidemiology, both communal and individual, which will finally result in preventive medicine and public health

Clinical epidemiology has its application peak in the solution of treatment and management of diseases, contributing the identification of risk factors to certain illnesses and being to date the fundamental part of Evidence Based Medicine, and for that it becomes important the teaching of clinical epidemiology, for it will aid in the education of professionals with judicious capacity and rational use of the best alternatives in diagnostic and treatment, by means of a critical evaluation of the literature [5], as well as helping to stimulate the training of researchers, because it's implied that the execution of the clinical epidemiology will lead to the development of research [6].

Research development makes it necessary to use tools that will make research more efficient, such as GoogleDocs, ZOGO, OneNote, which allow to write and edit online texts, or scientific literature search engines that will let us find evidence for the sustain of our activities in the healthcare systems, and in some cases without even looking for them, like with the applications from Google Reader and the RSS/XML, or obtaining portals dedicated to Evidence Based Medicine, or programs such as the statistical calculator Epidat which can simplify our statistical analysis, without even mentioning the multiple statistical softwares available [7].

Other concepts to consider are social epidemiology, which have been gaining ground these last decades and backing up the analysis of the social determinants of health status. This approach has generated big expectation for its integration and multidisciplinary character, but it's not free of skepticism that relates it with the idealism of a politics' strategic instrument [8].

However, social epidemiology, like field of clinical epidemiology, is based on the positivist paradigm and uses the statistical methods as analysis foundation. Besides, it is important to mention that currently, it has been generated a whole new research line based on the approach of the social determinants, where it is critical the usage of multilevel statistical models and new technologies that pose a new challenge to young researchers [9].

According to what it is stated, the current medical science tendency is focused in the generation of evidence that contributed in its development and has an impact in the patients' health. This approach, of EBM, is expressed mainly in the care, in relation to drugs and medical devices, though it is admitted that community interventions through Public Health deserve to be recognized as significant events that have had an impact in the population's health [10]. In this way, it is necessary to recognize the existence of research that s directed to make evidence of the impact of Public Health's diverse activities.

Evidence Based Public Health keeps the cause-effect logic, and allows adding the determinants of health, such as lifestyles, culture and environment, to the scientific context that often is what characterizes the good or bad execution of an intervention. Evidence Based Public Health is a new tendency that is joining efforts to offer the best information for an efficient politics decision making [11]. When it is oriented to the research of a population's health issues whether in the community or the hospital sphere, it contributes remarkably to the solution of very different local and regional realities, thus making a progress in Public Health, especially in out developing countries.

2. Differences between clinical epidemiology and field epidemiology

2.1. Classic or field epidemiology

Epidemiology is an old discipline with roots on scientific and rational structures, based on experience, on what is real. It is of great importance for Public Health and its impact for clinical medicine has risen in the last decades [12].

The comparison between clinical epidemiology and field epidemiology may demonstrate similarities and differences that can result in a contribution to their final application, which is their common desire: the people's health.

http://dx.doi.org/10.5772/54901

Field epidemiology's primary function is to identify the cause or source of infectious diseases' outbreaks, containing its dissemination and organizing the infected patients' treatment as soon as possible [3].

Information obtaining and action are done «in the field», on the ground, namely, in the epidemic territory, there being a dominance of practice over theory. During an outbreak, the field epidemiologist works long hours until he has control over the outbreak. Another specific feature is that it is not only executed by doctors, but also by other specialties professionals, such as nurses, veterinarians, biologists, technicians, etc. [3].

The Training Programs in Epidemiology and Public Health Interventions Network (TEPHINET), founded in 1997 and currently located in 53 countries around the world, aims to strengthen, at an international level, the field epidemiologists' capacity for Public Health [13]. In Peru, is has been developed the Field Epidemiology Residency Program (PREC), in order to train professionals in different specialties to act in their respect jurisdictions, challenging the lack of epidemiology specialists.

This national Program had 4 stages: I Introduction to Epidemiology (2 months), II Basic Epidemiology (4 months), III Intermediate Epidemiology (6 months) and IV Specialized Epidemiology (12 months). The designated participants for each Regional Health Direction started to take the classes in their own offices, taught by specialists from the General Epidemiology Office and professors from a macro regional level University's headquarters with on line tutoring, as well as field practices. Stages II and III were carried out in the University's headquarters and the selection of the participants to continue on to the next stages were done with a pyramidal system, according to weighted averages and additional exams. The last stage was carried out only Lima-Peru, though it was still open to other provinces [14].

It is discussed that field epidemiology would tend to action without a theoretical framework. This tendency would be based on its most direct reference: the Epidemic Intelligence Service (EIS) of the Center for Disease Control and Prevention (CDC) from the USA government, administrative body of military origin related to the intelligence service, which gives them a more attractive image than a function, closer to a secret agent directed towards the action, the protection of a community against a germ invasion, the avoidance of social alarm and insecurity on the population [4]. Field epidemiology executes its intervention on a daily basis in micro spaces, generally institutional: schools, restaurants, elderly residencies, hospitals whose services can present outbreaks, and uses conventional methods [15].

Thacker SB and Buffington J., who belong to the CDC, call field epidemiology as the 21st century applied epidemiology, based on the philosophy of 'learn by doing', supervised by experienced epidemiologists on field research, database analysis, vigilance system evaluation, presenting and publishing scientific research and answering to public questions. On the other hand, it has to be directed toward action regarding the main Public Health problems, the reduction of social inequality, having a greater consideration for psychosocial elements of the illness process, the incorporation of contents and methods from social sciences and working in multidisciplinary teams [16].

In the case of field or applied epidemiology, which is also denominated general epidemiology, it has as a feature the use of epidemiologic methods for the prevention of diseases and promotion of health in the populations, to achieve in an effective way the Public Health objectives, trying to apply a primary prevention.

3. Clinical Epidemiology

In 1938, Jean Paul coined the term clinical epidemiology, and defined it as: 'a new basic science for preventive medicine'. Therefore, the practical application of clinical epidemiology is a key part of Evidence Based Medicine and clinical decision making [17]. Clinical epidemiology is a discipline that puts into practice the epidemiologic principles into the clinical environment, focusing on patients [18]. What characterizes it is the combination of epidemiologic methods with the objectives of social clinical activity, which are, a good diagnostic and treatment of the ill. The knowledge is integrated with what is obtained from a good bibliographic research and critical reading of scientific reading [1]. It is currently considered the cornerstone of Evidence Based Medicine.

Clinical epidemiology is based mainly on its clinical trials, examining the diagnostic methods, discussing the prognosis, taking part in the evolution of treatments, trying to organize a controlled and randomized study opposite to sick people getting placebos or another indicated drug [1].

Truthfully, it was difficult to distinguish this activity from what would later be called as Evidence Based Medicine (EBM), term introduced in 1992 by the same group that, years before, had founded the discipline called Clinical Epidemiology (CE) [2].

However, both disciplines: field epidemiology and clinical epidemiology share the same methodology and tool, the difference relies on the place where these are applied (Table 1).

The current medical approach must contemplate the application of clinical epidemiology in health establishments, for the benefit of patients, given that epidemiologic research, with its analytical designs and clinical trials, allow the progress in treatments and managements, as well as defining the quality of auxiliary exams ever more sophisticated by means of the test of tests design and its economic approach (cost-benefit, cost-utility, cost-effectiveness), without forgetting the general population. It is in the community where field epidemiology is applied, the descriptive studies of the population's health situation with its analytical approaches to the Situational Health Analysis, the study of epidemic outbreaks and their respective intervention, as well as the posing of hygiene measurements and global prevention for a better quality of life and disease prevention. This way, an integral management is being carried out, both communal and individual, which will finally result in preventive medicine and public health.

David Sackett drew attention over the need to integrate the evidence with the clinical experience and the value of patients in the clinical decision making, referring to it as Clinical

http://dx.doi.org/10.5772/54901

Aspect	Field Epidemiology	Field Epidemiology
Fundamental objectives	To identify the causes or sources of outbreaks. To carry out the prevention of diseases and promotion of health in the population.	To evaluate methods and the quality of diagnostics and patient treatment.
Place of action	Community, population	Health establishments (hospitals, clinics, etc.)
Intervention or study population	General population of the community	Patients in health establishments.
Professionals in charge	Multidisciplinary: doctors, nurses, technicians, veterinarians, biologist, etc.	Multidisciplinary: with a greater emphasis in doctors for carrying out diagnostic and treatment activities.
Methods	Action without an extended theoretical background, it is practice, applied.	Bibliographic research and critical reading, applying Evidence Based Medicine.
Basic prevention	Primary	Secondary and Tertiary
Study type	Observational	Experimental : clinical trial (mostly)
Situation at work	It is dealt with unexpected problems and has to travel and work in the field, giving immediate answers in a limited time.	Hospitalized patients are evaluated; applying the validity and reliability of diagnostic tests and choosing the best alternative for the patient's treatment.

Table 1. Differences between field epidemiology and clinical epidemiology.

Epidemiology and defining it as: *'the application of epidemiologic principles and methods to the problems challenging clinical medicine. The basic aim of clinical epidemiology is to promote the clinical observation and interpretation methods, which result in valid conclusions'* [19].

Clinical epidemiology aims for the production and identification of valid tests, and to its logical extension. It is EBM, which aims for the rational use of evidence in the individual diagnosis and treatment of patients [17]. Clinical Epidemiology represents the way in which classic epidemiology, traditionally directed to general strategies in the public health of communal groups, *has been extended to include* clinical decisions in the care of individual patients (Figure 1) [20].

3.1. Evolution of clinical epidemiology

Clinical epidemiology has perform a center role in 5 recent evolutions (some say revolutions) on the healthcare area: evidence generation, critical evaluation, efficient storage and recovery, evidence based medicine and evidence synthesis (Table 2).

The effect of using epidemiologic principles has not been simply to improve the usage of clinical judgment and to eliminate the implicit element of epistemology from clinical reasoning. Arthur Elstein declared that decades of psychological research in decision making has demonstrated that: clinical judgment from experts was not as expert as we thought it was, that knowledge transference was more limited than we expected, and that judgment errors are not

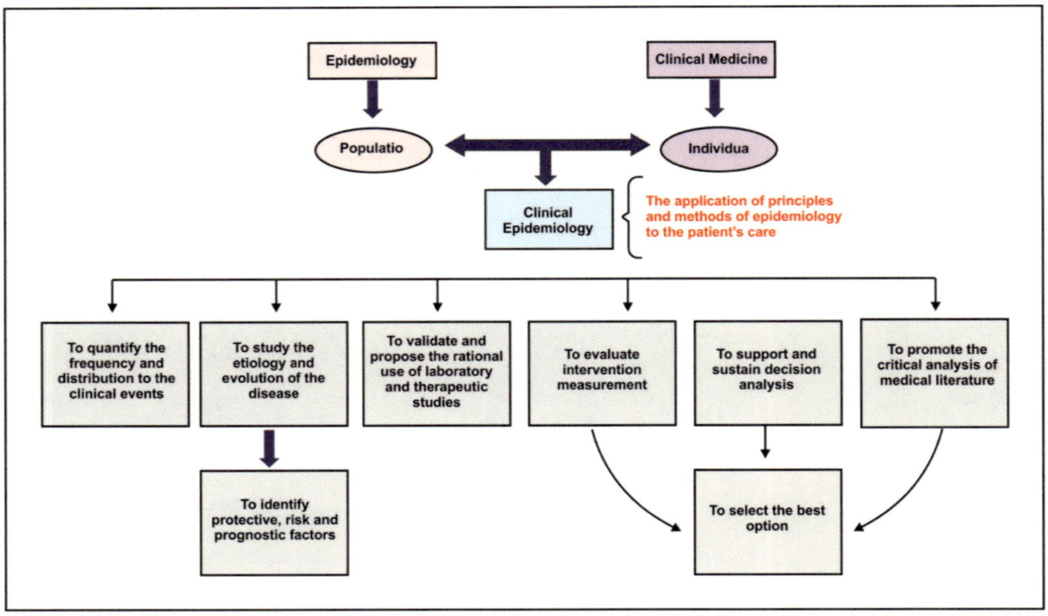

Figure 1. Uses of Clinical Epidemiology.

Evolution	Change	Description
1° Evolution	Evidence generation	Increase of reports, especially clinical trials, followed by prognostic and diagnostic studies.
2° Evolution	Critical evaluation	Critical evaluation of the validity of medical literature.
3° Evolution	Efficient storage and recovery	Implementation of databases and scientific literature search engines.
4° Evolution	Evidence Based Medicine	Number Needed to Harm (NNH)
5° Evolution	Evidence synthesis	Start of the Cochrane Collaboration (http://www.cochrane.org)

Table 2. Evolution of the Clinical Epidemiology (Sackett DL. 2000).

limited to medicine students nor are eradicated by experience, so that, them being the cognitive errors inherent to clinical reasoning, they can be aggravated through the dependency called 'experts opinion' [21].

In 1992, Sackett DL. and Col. decided to substitute the term 'Clinical Epidemiology' for 'Evidence Based Medicine', meaning that every medical action of diagnosis, prognosis and therapy must be sustained in quantitative, solid proofs, based on the best epidemiologic and clinical research [21]. Thereby, Sacket DL., in one of the first definitions of EBM, he mentioned:

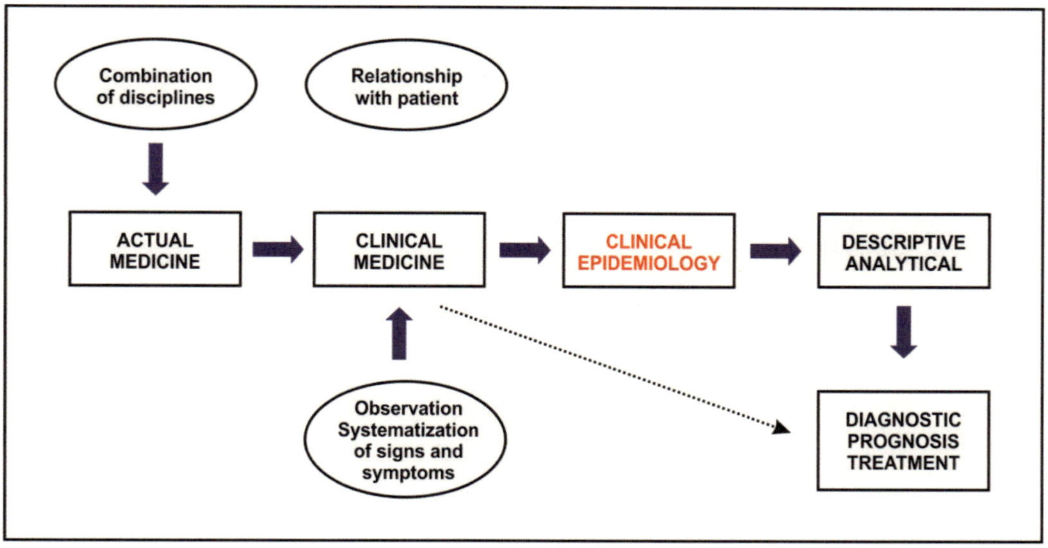

Figure 2. Actual medicine, clinical medicine and clinical epidemiology

'conscious, explicit and reasonable use of the best current evidence to make decisions regarding the care of individual patients' [5].

Sackett DL. mentions the dichotomous existence between the science of epidemiologic reasoning and the art of intuitive judgments of clinical epidemiology. He realized that the application of these epidemiologic principles (plus a bit more of biostatistics) to the beliefs, judgments and intuitions that make up for the art of medicine can considerably improve the accuracy and effectiveness of diagnosis and prognosis [21]. The practice of EBM means to integrate the individual clinical experience with the best external clinical evidence available from systematic research, and recently, in a paper published on 2000, it is described as: 'the integration of the best research evidence, of clinical experience and the patients' values' [5]. Meanwhile, Cuestas E. defines it as 'the discipline that takes care of the study of the happening of medical decisions regarding its determinants' [22].

Broadly, clinical epidemiology takes care of the event of patients', which range from the appearance of the disease to its result in the form of healing, sequels or death. Therefore, the study subjects are ill people who are normally found in health establishments, and their contribution is relevant, especially for diagnosis and secondary and third prevention of the disease.

Clinical epidemiology can be divided into descriptive and analytical. The descriptive part is focused on the variation of clinical prognosis, whereas the analytical is focused on the reasons for this variation, that is to say, the main predictors for the prognosis, diagnosis and treatment, which are key concepts in the clinical epidemiology and the practice of clinical medicine (Figure 2). Also, demographic epidemiology is largely directed to the general population, whereas clinical epidemiology is more focused on the individual [23] (Figure 1).

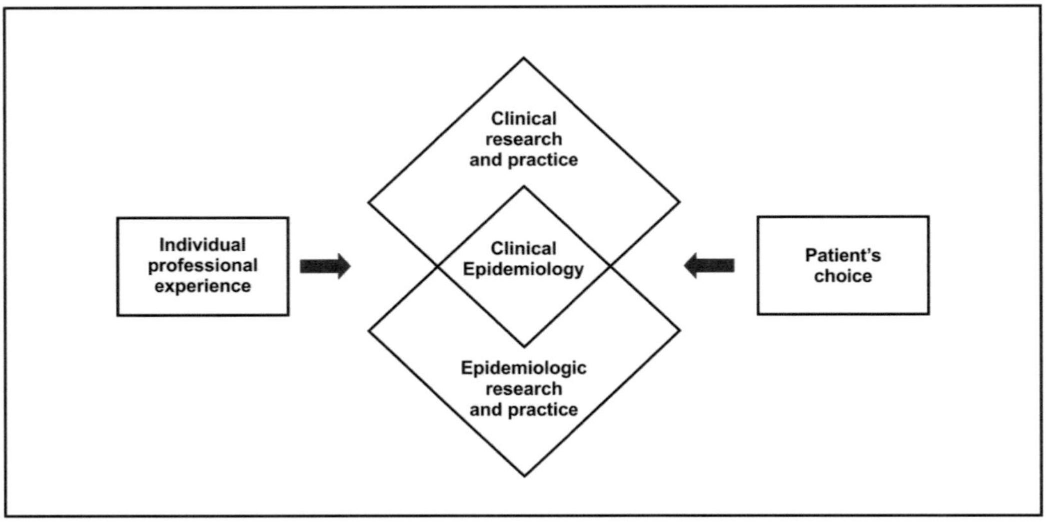

Figure 3. Interactions of the Clinical Epidemiology.

The EBM is driven by the need of confront the surplus of information and the medical practice, the patient's demand for the best diagnosis and treatment, y by the cost control, being known that the world tendency is the rise of costs in healthcare, leading to a stimulus of the critical evaluation of laboratory tests as an attempt for the best use of the limited resources. That means to realize a cost-benefit analysis [5]. In the last years, clinical epidemiology has become 'very important' for the health system, due to the need to perform evaluations in the quality of care, patient's security, health economy and resource usage areas. All these aspects are based on clinical epidemiology's thinking [23].

Nowadays, there have been many misunderstandings about EBM, which arise because it has been adopted by functionaries and academicians in Public Health, and by health managers, who for better or for worse, are 'too far from patients', giving interpretations like 'they remain sitting comfortably in their desks', 'they manage abusively and without a criteria, telling clinical doctors how to treat the patients in cost-effective ways'...; points of view far from what was originally planned for the integral approach of clinical practice and clinical epidemiology [24].

But we also need to bear in mind that the EBM is not a 'cookbook', like some think, for it requires the integration of the best external evidence with the individual professional experience and the patient's choice; the clinical evidence may inform but cannot substitute the individual clinical experience. This knowledge is necessary to evaluate if the external evidence can be applied to the individual subject to decide how to improve the patient's clinical results (Figure 3). In the same manner, the use of EBM as a 'cost reducing' medicine is a misunderstanding, because doctors who practice the EBM, identify and apply the more efficient interventions to achieve the best in terms of patient's quality of life, might increase the cost of healthcare instead of reducing it [5].

3.2. From epidemiology teaching and practice to research

Clinical Medicine, Clinical Epidemiology and EBM have been widely promoted as an improvement in patient's healthcare [25]. For that, doctors must be capable of showing the patient the therapeutic options for a shared decision making [26], using the results obtained in clinical studies [27]. Then it becomes important to correctly interpret the results of a study, to transmit appropriately this information to the patients, and to take the best diagnostic and therapeutic decisions.

Through systematic reviews and meta-analysis, as well as clinical practice guidelines, important progress has been made in the search of scientific literature, evaluation and synthesis. Terms such as 'likelihood ratio' or 'number needed to harm' are used commonly in medical journals [28]. In medical literature it is also used many epidemiologic risk indicators to present the results on the effectiveness of a therapeutic intervention. Between the most used are: relative risk (RR), relative risk reduction (RRR), absolute risk reduction (ARR), hazard ratio (HR) and number needed to harm (NNH). These entire indicators represent different ways to express the same result [29].

Studies done at the beginning of the decade showed that practicing doctors had a limited comprehension of numerical data given by the research results [5,30]. In Estellat C's study, the highest proportions of correct answers were the questions about relative risk reduction (87.7%), sensibility (84.6%) and specificity (80%), whereas the lowest proportions were for the calculus and use of likelihood ratio (16.9% and 9.2% respectively), and the interpretation of the kappa coefficient (19.2%). Though more than 80% of the respondents were able to calculate the sensibility or the specificity of a diagnostic test, only 32% was capable of using it in a clinical context. In the same way, the 30% correctly defined the likelihood ratio, but a percentage lower than 10% was able to use it to approximate the post-test probability of a disease [31].

In the same study, the subjects that had had previous training in statistics, epidemiology or critical evaluation of medical literature scored significantly higher than those who did not have this training. The average score (highest score being 7) was of 5.9 (IC95% 5.3-6.5) and 4.5 (IC95% 4.0-5.0), respectively ($p<0.01$). Therefore, their capacity to interpret quantitative data from medical scientific literature may be limited, which can deplete the information given to the patient for the decision making [31]

The practice of EBM requires the comprehension of five tasks: (1) building of a clinical question, structured on the patient's problem, (2) the acquisition of skills o search in medical literature and obtain the best evidence available, (3) critical evaluation of the evidence, (4) the application and integration of evidence to the patient's healthcare and (5) the evaluation (how to evaluate the process of helping the patient?) [32,33], which have taken EBM to be now part of the undergraduate teaching and the graduate activities of continuous medical education in various countries all over the world [34].

For example, in France, the critical evaluation of a medical article is part of the national residence exam, and for that, most the schools of medicine have incorporated it in their curricula as a formal training in clinical epidemiology. However, in the teaching hospitals most doctors tend to ignore clinical epidemiology and EBM, mainly because it requires the knowledge and comprehension of epidemiology and statistics technical terms, which makes its understanding complex to some, whether for self-sufficiency or lack of interest [34].

This way, when the risk indicators used to inform the results of clinical trials were evaluated in students and residents, it was found that 19.4% didn't recognize any of the indicators and 81.4% wasn't able to calculate them. The relative risk reduction was the most recognized indicator (55.2%), followed by 'number need to harm' (51.6%), absolute risk reduction (26.6%) and hazard ratio (9.5%), concluding that medicine students and residents do not recognize and are incapable of correctly calculating the risk indicators used in clinical trials [35].

In a similar study carried out in faculties of a northern city of Peru (unpublished data), with 139 medicine students, among them a group that had finished a the Clinical Epidemiology course and another group that was finishing Classic Epidemiology; it was found that the most recognized indicator was NNH (number needed to harm) with 58.9%, followed by RRR (relative risk reduction) with 56.8%. Besides, 30.9% of the students recognized at least one indicator and 13.7% didn't recognize anyone. However, this changed when they were asked to calculate the indicators, finding that ARR (35.9%) and RR (30.9%) were the ones with the most correct calculation. Likewise, 11.5% did adequately the calculation of at least one of them, and 56.1% didn't do one of them correctly. A little more than 10% was able to recognize and calculate the risk indicators. Comparing both groups, there was a significant difference ($p<0.05$) at recognizing and calculating the indicators (Table 3)

Indicators	Clinical Epidemiology	Classic Epidemiology	p
Recognizes*	3.12 ± 0.89	0.79 ± 1.19	p<0,05
Calculates&	2.94 ± 0.96	1.45 ± 0.79	p<0,05
Total§	6.06 ± 1.43	2.21 ± 1.53	p<0,05

*Maximum score: 4. &Maximum score: 4. §maximum score: 8.

Table 3. Comparison of mean scores obtained

The medicine students usually start their courses enthusiastically, curious and willing to improve the human condition, but soon find themselves surrounded by a long and passive curriculum, where they have a small direct role in patient healthcare. There are courses that are hard for students to learn and the results tend to have an immediate effect on patient healthcare. Evidently, this goes beyond the fact that students apply the theory to artificial circumstances, situation that would improve if students used the EBM for the choosing of patient's clinical problems, so that then they can locate and evaluate the appropriate articles that will help in the healthcare patients get. These activities might improve their critical skills and experiential approach as a real teamwork [36].

Dunn K. and Col. in the last decade they were already channeling the teaching of EBM, looking to create competences in students such as (1) elaboration of researchable clinical questions, (2) access to the best and most recent literature, (3) evaluation and scoring of the literature for its validity and pertinence, and (4) cost-performance-benefit analysis and the interpretation of meta-analysis [37]. Rucker L also mentions the 'EBM recipe' [38] as a useful tool to bring EBM closer to healthcare, which consisted in posing clinical questions relevant during rounds at hospitals, which would later be solved by the students with the help of teachers. A similar progress occurs at the Canadian Institute of Health Research (http://www.cihr-irsc.gc.ca/), implementing a 'teaching recipe', which allows the resident to take note of the doubts from a concrete clinical case, and answer them following a methodology based on the PICO model (problem/pacient, intervention, comparison and result) and finally designate a date and a person in charge to deliver the answer.

As it has been mentioned, evolution of clinical epidemiology started with the creation of scientific research, which has led to critical reading, database creation and its search engines, EBM and finally, information synthesis (Table 2). That means, in the beginning and in all of its evolution it is surrounded by research. But, what stands out is that, in 2005, in a study we realized in 1484 medicine students from 13 Peruvian faculties, we found that 53.7% had a good knowledge and 71.9% an adequate attitude towards research, as well as a relation between belonging to a research group and having a good knowledge (Díaz-Velez C et al) [39]. This suffered a reduction of 7% and 34.2% respectively in a later study by Cabrera-Enríquez JA et al, where also 68% did not do any extracurricular courses, and those who did, only 3.28% and 6.24% could do critical reading and statistics respectively, finding an association between the level of knowledge and attitude towards research ($p<0.05$) and only 51% had taken part, or was taking part, of a research. [6]

While the Latinamerican context is not the most adequate to train researchers, there are students societies that can help promote research even if one is undergraduate. The research lines in universities institutions are not always adequately developed. Moreover, they are not even clearly stipulated and the primary healthcare research is poorly developed, while hospital research gains more support, especially from pharmaceutical industries. If we add to this that publications at a local level are scarce (as a consequence of what's stated before) and that 75% are done regarding topics which are not a regional or national priority, and knowing the social, ethnic and cultural differences that exist between communities, then what evidence do we have to answer our clinical doubts? [40]

In this context, a good researcher's attitude, with an integral approach of research, represents, in undergraduates and graduates as well, an alternative to build a solid researcher's intelligence and attitude, in terms of capability for scientific work [41]. Besides, we must promote some activities, as the graduation by publication in undergraduate students as an alternative to increase the universities' scientific production, an aspect we have been promoting as university teachers.

Examples of teaching EBM and research exist all around the world. We have the Accreditation Council for Graduate Medical Education, from the University of California, San Francisco, which includes EBM and practice based learning, among other basic competences. For that, the development of the 'PRIME curriculum' program (EBM/clinical research program) which uses didactic lectures, journal club, progress evaluation sessions and active tutoring that allows the residents to carry out a clinical research project during their residence [42].

The first component of the 'PRIME curriculum' program (didactic lectures) motivates the development of topics such as: statistic power calculation, qualitative research methods, survey research, decision analysis and treatment threshold, cost-effectiveness analysis, ethical use of patients in research, community research and research process evaluation with international support, use of administrative data and spreadsheet management. The second component has weekly evening meetings of small journal clubs (diagnostic test evaluation, case-control studies, cohort studies, controlled randomized clinical trials, meta-analysis, decision analysis, cost-effectiveness analysis, clinical practice guidelines, etc.), which are made by students with a 15 minute duration, with a later debate moderated by the tutor. The third component consists on the trimestral presentation of interactive seminars (used to improve the ideas of the project's author) of the projects done by the residents. So far, these experiences have been successful, perhaps due to the fact that residents that take part of the program have the explicit expectative that the results of their research will be published, and with that, teachers are more willing to spend their time as mentors. However, we believe that the exit relays greatly on the structured curricula, the willingness of the mentors and, above all, the enthusiasm of the residents [42].

There are also other experiences in which the student is assigned to a team with a mentor (research team leader), a methodology tutor, expert clinicians and even biostatistics experts; in a research that coincides with the formation interest of the student, in which he learns about the research process. The mentor and the student meet weekly to develop and review the participant's curricula, apart from analyzing the research thesis and clarifying doubts that are generated in the sessions, so that, at the end, the student can have the thesis manuscript ready in the form of an article journal and can be presented [43].

The satisfactory fulfillment of the program gives the student the knowledge of the basic types of research design, including randomized clinical trials, cohort and case-control studies, quasi-experimental studies, concepts of health measurement and evaluation in the epidemiologic studies, capacity to critically evaluate medical literature and to use and interpret the various statistical programs for the data analysis [43].

However, there are limits to the EBM that, according to Cuestas E., might be: a) the frequently conflictive results of randomized and controlled trials (RCT); b) the inexistence of evidence in an enormity of topics; c) the questionable quality of many RCT and meta-analysis; and d) many time the RCT are not easy to conduct due to practical reasons, or impossible to do because of ethical reasons. Besides, it is necessary to integrate the best scientific evidence available with the preferences of the patient, with limits such as economic, social, ethnic, moral, cultural and health organization of the system [24].

In the USA, the Internal Medicine Residence and Postgraduate Curriculum Working Group suggests that the EBM concepts should be an integral part of the undergraduate and residency curriculum, given that medicine students do not necessarily acquire these skills in classrooms or during medical or teaching rounds [44].

http://dx.doi.org/10.5772/54901

3.3. Clinical epidemiology competences [44]

- Understanding of how bias and chance can affect the accuracy of observations in individual patients.
- Evaluation of the validity of original articles over diagnosis, prognosis, treatment and prevention.
- Knowing the strengths and weaknesses of randomized clinical trials, case-control studies, cohort studies (prospective and retrospective) and meta-analysis.
- Using practical strategies to judge the validity of clinical evidence synthesis (i.e. reviews).
- Comprehension of the meaning, uses and limits of the statistic power, the values of 'p' and the confidence interval, relative risk, attributable risk and NNH (number needed to harm).
- Knowing how to measure the patients' preferences.
- Comprehension and usage of the sensibility analysis and the cost-effectiveness analysis.

3.4. Competences for quantitative clinical reasoning [44]

- Comprehension of the way to calculate the pre-test disease probability and how to use the Bayes theorem to calculate the post-test probability.
- Defining and using sensibility, specificity and likelihood ratio of the diagnostic information.
- Knowing and being capable of detecting possible bias in calculations of sensibility and specificity.
- Comprehension of the value of decision trees and decision making.

Opportunities for health professionals to obtain the education and training in clinical epidemiology have extended gradually. In South America, there is a group that promotes its development, LatinCLEN (Latinamerican Clinical Epidemiology Network), regional member of the International Clinical Epidemiology Network (INCLEN Trust http://www.inclen.org/), that is formed by research and Clinical Epidemiology training centers, as well as Clinical Epidemiology units around the world. (Table 4) [45].

With all these things mentioned we can see that both disciplines (field epidemiology and clinical epidemiology) share the same methodology and tools, just that the application of them is done in different locations and the current medical approach must contemplate the application of clinical epidemiology in health establishments, patients, in those who research epidemiology, with its analytical designs and clinical trials allow the progress in treatment and management, as well as defining the quality of the auxiliary exams ever more sophisticated by means of the test of tests and its economic approach (cost-benefit, cost-utility, cost-effectiveness)

One cannot forget the general population, for it is in the community where field epidemiology is applied, the descriptive study of the health situation with the analytical approach of the

Network	Country members	Website
LatinCLEN	South American countries	www.latinclen.org
INCLEN-África	African countries	www.inclenafrica.org
CanUSACLEN	Canada and the USA	www.canusaclen.org
ChinaCLEN	China	www.chinaclen.org.cn
INCLEN – Euro-Med	Europe countries	www.recif.univ-lyon1.fr
IndiaCLEN	India	www.indiaclen.org
INCLEN – Southeast Asia	Asian countries	www.cim.edu.ph

Table 4. Clinical Epidemiology World Network.

Situational Health Analysis, the study of epidemic outbreaks and the respective intervention, as well as the planning of hygiene and global prevention measurements for a better life quality and disease prevention.

Finally, we can say that the importance of clinical epidemiology in clinical research is recognized in ways that the classic epidemiology hasn't been able to achieve, but is prone to the knowledge of health professionals and its constant evolution makes it stay valid, this way an integral manage of the epidemiology will be carried out, both communal and individual, thus resulting in preventive medicine and public health.

4. Informatics tools for health research

During health professionals' daily practice, the need to keep informed about the new scientific evidence comes up as a responsibility towards patients and, of course, to oneself. It is not strange to see yourself in front of a patient with a specific pathology to which certain treatments haven't had effect, and asking yourself: what is new to treat this condition? Or, on the other hand, in front of a research, lecture or speech about any topic, trying to have the most updated information about the topic. Considering its etymologic origin, the word 'investigation' comes from the Latin word *invenio, invenire,* which means 'to find'. By association and as a logical consequence, to find you must first search. And for that, we must know how to and where to search. This searching implies knowing the principal sources of information to which, as professionals, we must access. However, the task does not end there, for, once we find the information, we must do a critical reading of it and select the most relevant, which in the context of a research must be adequately cited [7].

To do research there are informatics tools, mainly through internet, that ease up the daily work of a researcher, from sources of information to friendly interfaces, of easy access and naviga-

http://dx.doi.org/10.5772/54901

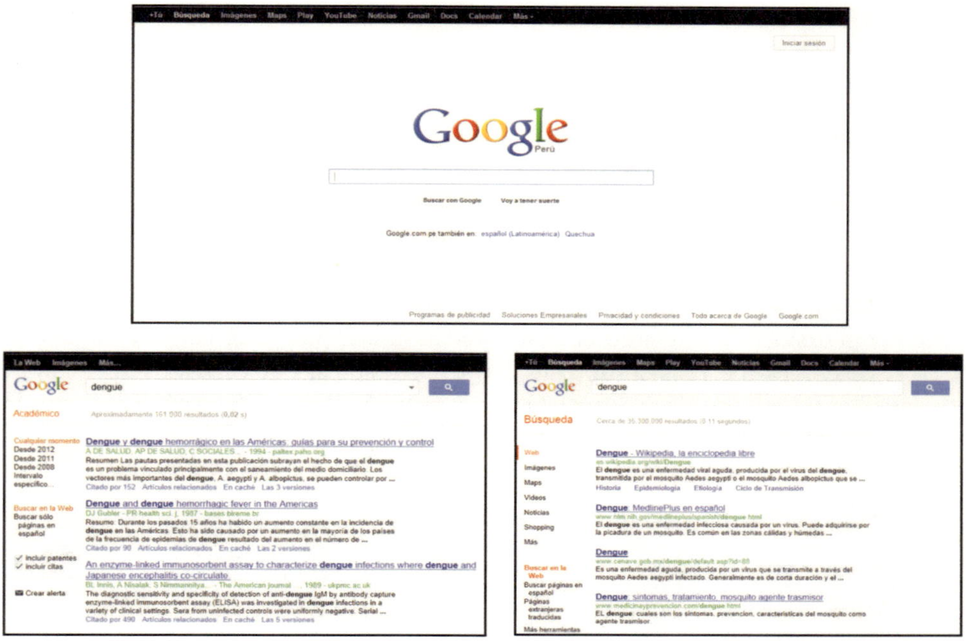

Figure 4. Google y Google Scholar.

tion, bibliographic references managers and statistic applications that allow us to do calculations that would turn very complex if we did it the conventional way.

4.1. Information sources

Search resources to which we normally turn to are general search engines (Google, Yahoo, Altavista, Metacrawler, etc.) Google (http://www.google.com) has the biggest demand, but the health information available in this engines may come from a non-reliable source, so it is important to distinguish which are the most adequate websites to find the health related information, which implies to evaluate the quality of these websites, an activity that sometimes is quite tedious for the researcher [46–49].

Given the wealth of information it retrieves the conventional search engine Google, and considering the existence of dubious sources, Google implemented Google Scholar (Google Scholar) oriented search scientific references (http://scholar.google.es), which are listed in order of relevance, and provide information about the source, year of publication, authors, times the number that have been cited and other versions of the publication, and also, you can access related articles (mentioning or are cited by the text), the content in HTML, PDF, DOC or other format, it is recommended to do the advanced search preference (Figure 4).

Among the great online Medicine bibliographic databases we have MEDLINE, produced since 1966 by the National Library of Medicine (NLM) [50] in the USA. MEDLINE is the largest article bibliographic source in biomedical sciences we have at hand. The database is made up by cited articles by three indexes: Index Medicus, Index to Dental Literature and International Nursing Index. Currently it is the most consulted database by global researchers. A study applied to Spanish speaking biomedical professional researchers referred us to a 34.1% [51].

MEDLINE includes general topics, such as microbiology, health prevention, nutrition, pharmacology and environmental health. However, the covered categories by the database include anatomy, organisms, diseases, drugs, techniques, equipment, psychiatry, biologic sciences, physical sciences, social sciences and education, technology, food, industry, humanities, and communication sciences. All of these related to health. The search is done via PUBMED: http://www.pubmed.gov (Figure 5). Here, the searches are in English base on Boolean operators: AND, intersection, automatic term mapping; OR, conjunction and isolation; NOT, excludes the final term; uses a MeSH (Medical Subject Headings) controlled vocabulary and the subheadings described by the Index Medicus, where most of the abstracts have the link to the editorial where the full text article can be found [52].

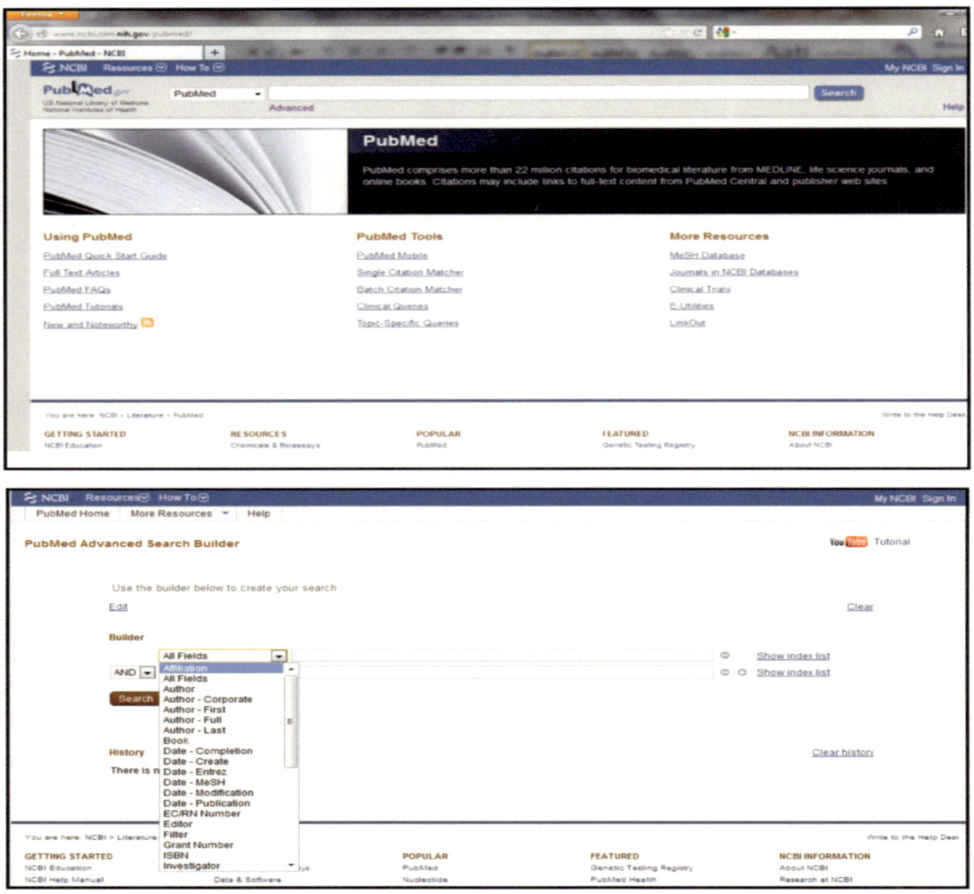

Figure 5. Pubmed specialized search engine of the National Library of Medicine (MEDLINE).

Another large database, not as extensive as MEDLINE, is 'Literatura Latinoamericana y del Caribe en Ciencias de la Salud' (Latinamerican and the Caribbean Literature on Health Sciences - LILACS)[53]. It can be accessed through the Virtual Health Library (Regional Medicine Library – BIREME)[54]: http://www.bireme.br, the same that includes other sources of information in biomedical sciences. One of them is the catalogue of the Library hosting the Panamerican Health Organization (PAHO) and the World Health Organization (WHO). Here you can access full text articles that are included in the Scientific Electronic Library Online (SciELO)[55]: http://www.scielo.org, which includes Argentina, Brazil, Chile, Colombia, Costa Rica, Cuba, Spain, Mexico, Portugal, Venezuela, Public Health, Social Sciences and developing initiatives like Bolivia, Paraguay, Peru, South Africa and Uruguay (Figure 6).

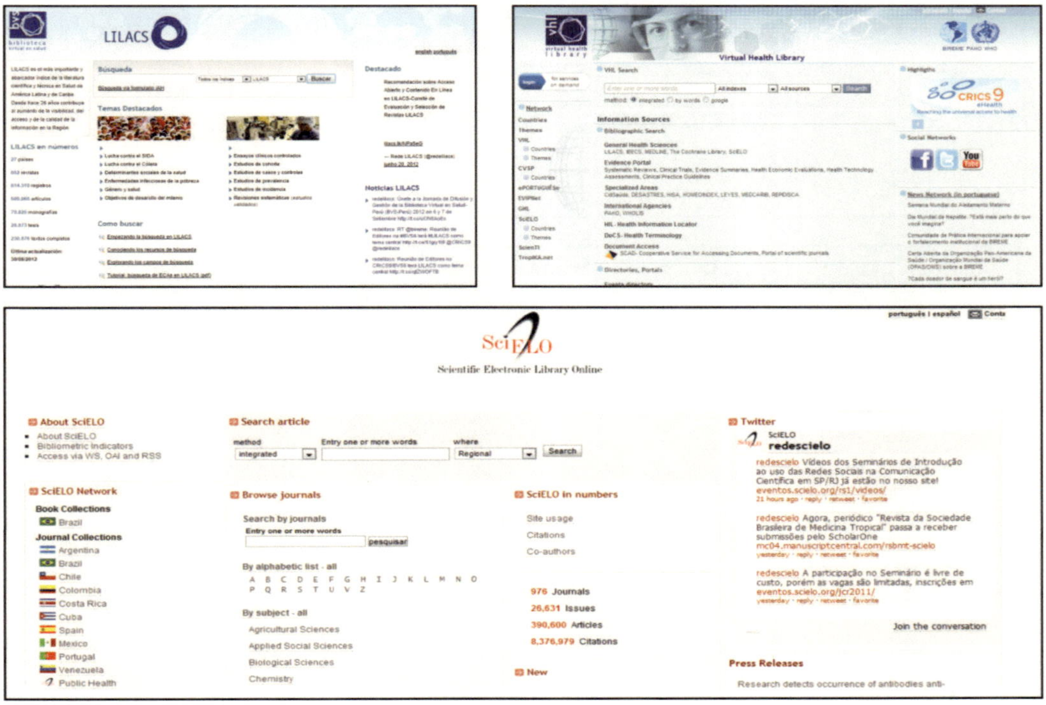

Figure 6. Latinamerican and the Caribbean Literature on Health Sciences (LILACS), Virtual Health Library and Scientific Electronic Library Online (SCIELO).

An important resource is the Cochrane Library: (http://www.bibliotecacochrane.org/) (Figure 7), whose aim is to prepare, keep and spread systematic reviews regarding the effects of healthcare, mostly base on controlled clinical trials, and are highly structured and systematized, for they include the evidence according specific quality criteria.

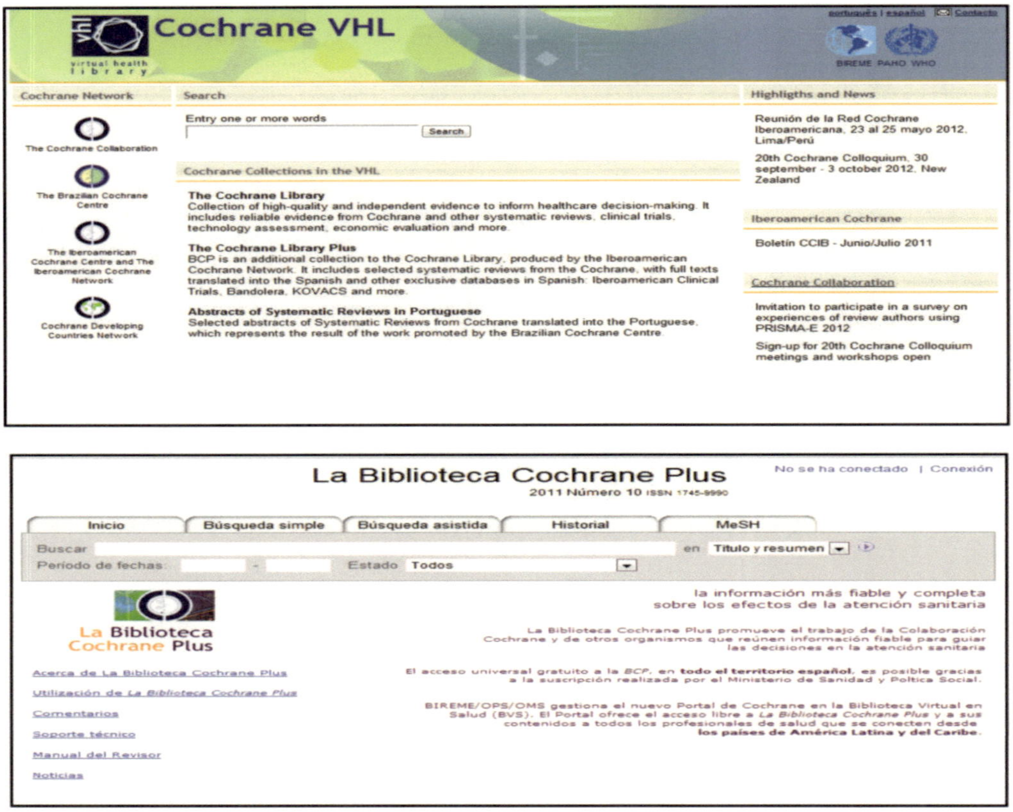
Cochrane VHL
virtual health library
Cochrane Network
Search
Highligths and News
The Cochrane Collaboration
The Brazilian Cochrane Centre
The Iberoamerican Cochrane Centre and The Iberoamerican Cochrane Network
Cochrane Developing Countries Network
Entry one or more words
Search
Cochrane Collections in the VHL
The Cochrane Library
Collection of high-quality and independent evidence to inform healthcare decision-making. It includes reliable evidence from Cochrane and other systematic reviews, clinical trials, technology assessment, economic evaluation and more.
The Cochrane Library Plus
BCP is an additional collection to the Cochrane Library, produced by the Iberoamerican Cochrane Network. It includes selected systematic reviews from the Cochrane, with full texts translated into the Spanish and other exclusive databases in Spanish: Iberoamerican Clinical Trials, Bandolera, KOVACS and more.
Abstracts of Systematic Reviews in Portuguese
Selected abstracts of Systematic Reviews from Cochrane translated into the Portuguese, which represents the result of the work promoted by the Brazilian Cochrane Centre.
Reunión de la Red Cochrane Iberoamericana, 23 al 25 mayo 2012, Lima/Perú
20th Cochrane Colloquium, 30 september - 3 october 2012, New Zealand
Iberoamerican Cochrane
Boletín CCIB - Junio/Julio 2011
Cochrane Collaboration
Invitation to participate in a survey on experiences of review authors using PRISMA-E 2012
Sign-up for 20th Cochrane Colloquium meetings and workshops open
La Biblioteca Cochrane Plus
2011 Número 10
No se ha conectado | Conexión
Inicio
Búsqueda simple
Búsqueda asistida
Historial
MeSH
Buscar
en
Título y resumen
Período de fechas:
Estado
Todos
la información más fiable y completa sobre los efectos de la atención sanitaria
La Biblioteca Cochrane Plus
Acerca de La Biblioteca Cochrane Plus
Utilización de La Biblioteca Cochrane Plus
Comentarios
Soporte técnico
Manual del Revisor
Noticias

Figure 7. Cochrane Library

Health Inter Network Access to Research Initiative (HINARI) in: http://extranet.who.int/hinari/en/journals.php (Figure 8) is a program established by the WHO, in partnership with publisher, and gives an easier access to one of the most extensive biomedical and health literature collections. It contains more than 8 500 information resources, in 30 different languages, which are available for health institutions in more than 100 countries [56].

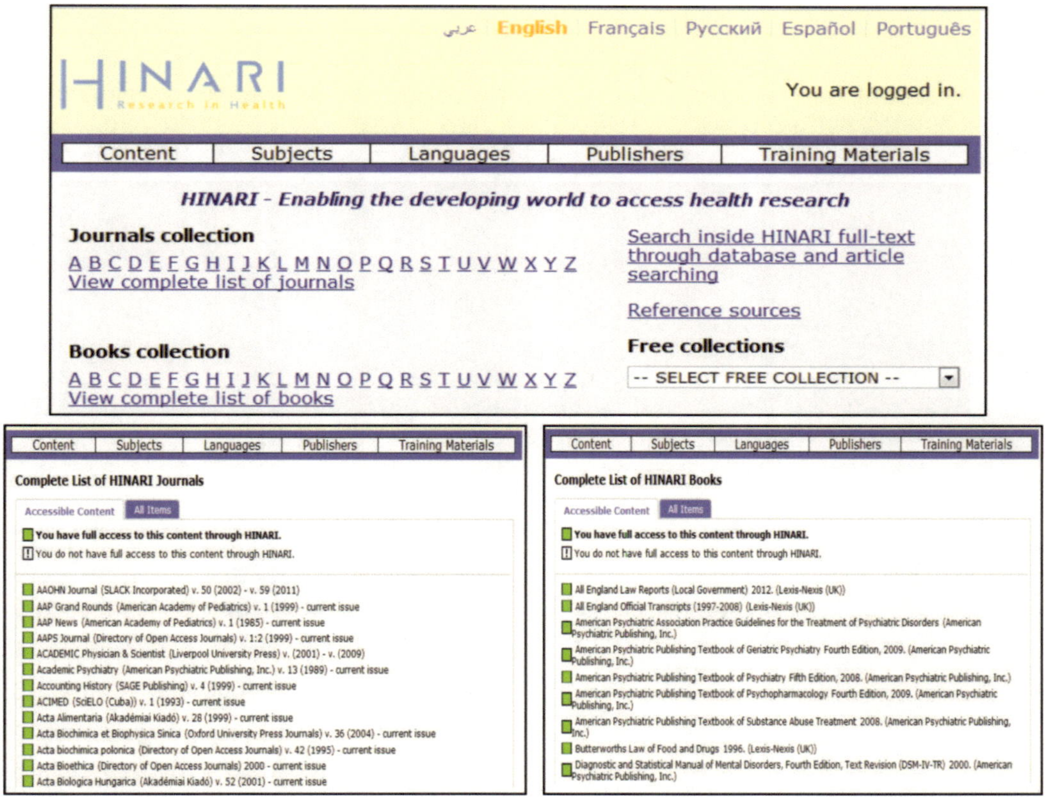

Figure 8. Health Internetwork Access to Research Initiative (HINARI).

Global representative health organizations, such as the PAHO, offer in their website important links, as well as free access to their publications (http://new.paho.org/) [57] (Figure 9). The WHO allows us to access important articles on disease control, vigilance systems and public health. The information is in three languages, including Spanish (http://www.who.int/en/) (Figure 9) [58].

The Center for Disease Control and Prevention (CDC), whose objective is to promote health and wuality of life, gives updated information on the control of disease, lesions and disabilities (http://www.cdc.gov/) (Figure 9)[59].

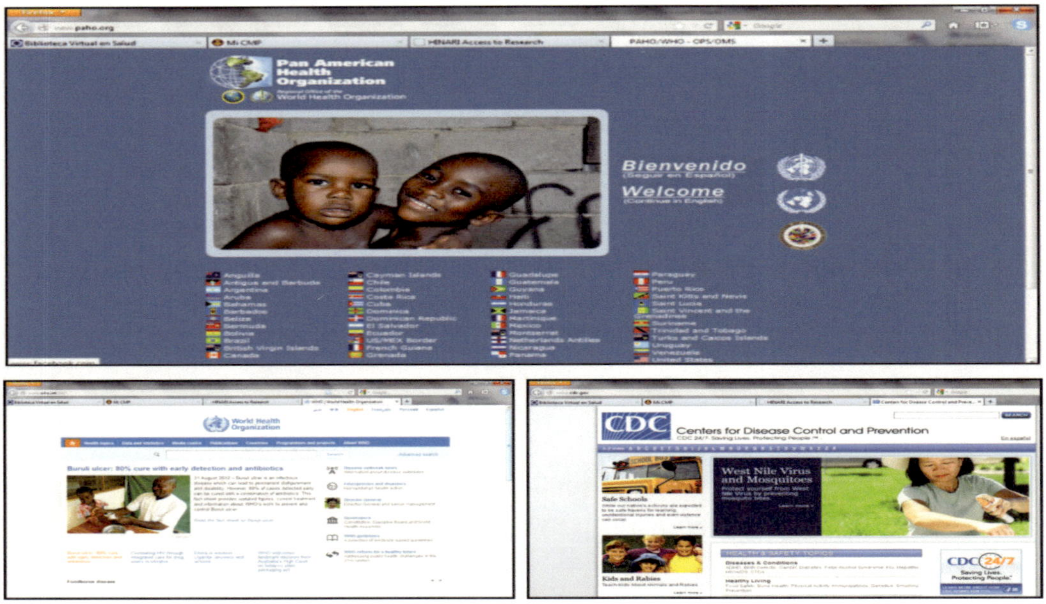

Figure 9. Panamerican Health Organization, World Health Organization, The Center for Disease Control and Prevention (CDC).

To access a consensus, the National Guideline Clearinghouse (http://www.guideline.gov/) (Figure 10) contains evidence-based clinical guidelines of the main medical societies in the USA and Canada, National Institute of Clinical Studies, National Institute of Health and Medical Research Council (NHMRC) which collects the CLG developed in Australia (http://www.clinicalguidelines.gov.au/) (Figure 10), National Institute for Health and Clinical Excellence (NICE), an independent agency of the UK's NHS in England and Wales (http://www.nice.org.uk) (Figure 10) or the Scottish Intercollegiate Guidelines Network (SIGN) which develops these products for the UK's NHS in Scotland (http://www.sign.ac.uk/) (Figure 10) [60].

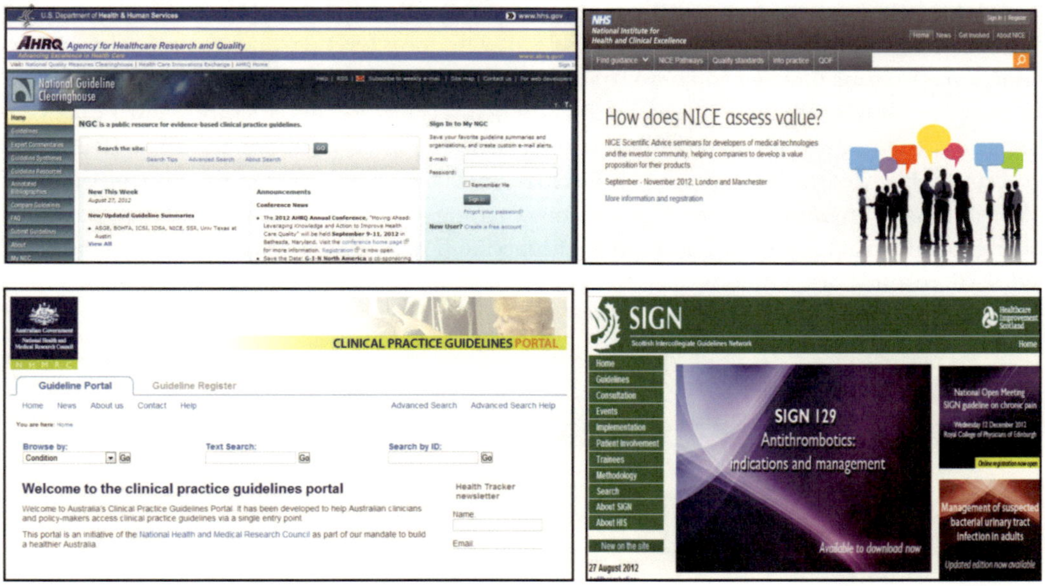

Figure 10. The Nacional Guideline Clearinghouse (AHRQ), National Institute of Clinical Studies (NHMRC), National Institute for Health and Clinical Excellence (NHS) y el Scottish Intercollegiate Guidelines Network (SIGN).

Other informatic applications for access to information on health, are represented by social networks, like Twitter, to promote research, disseminating scientific knowledge and funding opportunities, and being very useful for students, researchers and health professionals. [61,62]

4.2. Bibliographic reference managers

A bibliographic reference (BR) is a minimal group of data that allows the identification of a publication or a part of the same. There are as many types of BR as information sources. Among them, journal articles, electronic articles, books, chapters of books, thesis, norms, technical documents, videos, etc.

In turn, every BR is made up of diverse fields, some compulsory and other optional, which structure changes according to the BR format. However, in practice, every journal chooses its own format of citing and BR, being the most used: American Psychological Association (APA), Modern Language Association (MLA), National Library of Medicine (NLM), Vancouver style, among others.

Aiming to standardize the great diversity of formats available, in 1978, the Vancouver Group, later International Committee of Medical Journal Editors (ICMJE), requested the National Library of Medicine to estipulate the rules to write the BR [63], and in 1991, the NIH published the *NLM Recommended Formats for Bibliographic*, based on the *American National Standard for Bibliographic References* [64].

Taking into account the need to manage the BR in a more efficient and agile way, endless softwares have been made available for the management of BR, being the most socialized in the world the Endnote [65]. It is commercial software for references and images, whose main function is to store, manage and search bibliographic references in a personal reference library. Besides, it allows organizing images including graphics, tables, pictures and equations, assigning each image its own caption and keywords. However, there are other free access resources, like Zotero [66], which is a Firefox-Mozilla Add-on, created by the University of Washington as an improved and free version. This software will let us automatically store our search results from Pubmed, build our BR library, and cite everyone in direct communication with Microsoft Word, Outlook, etc.

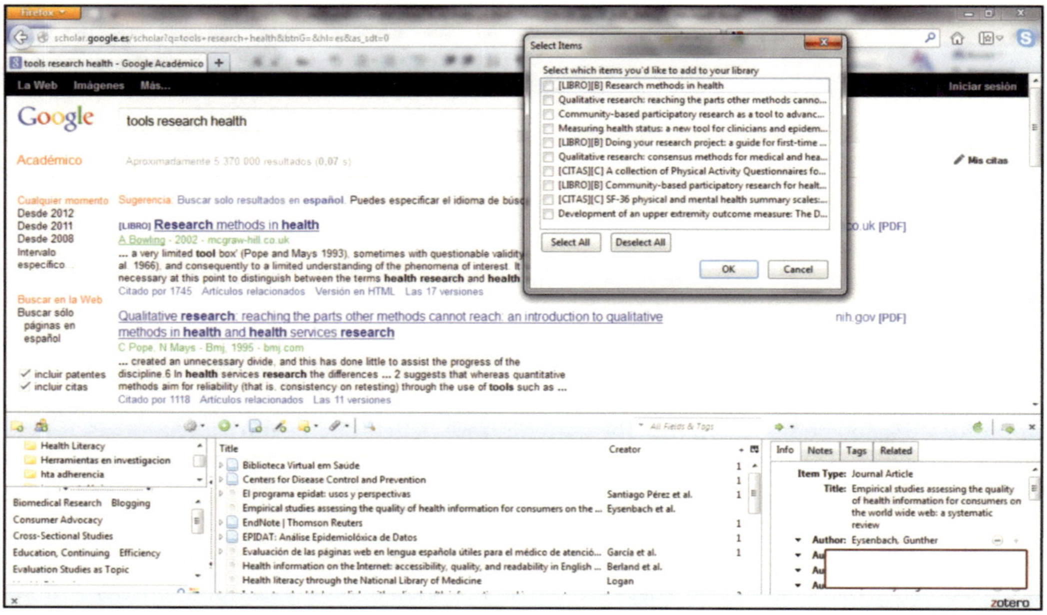

Figure 11. Applications of Zotero.

4.3. Statistic applications

A statistical package is a program or set of programs that allow sub applied to the same data file an unlimited set of statistical procedures in sync, without leaving the program. Among the statistical applications of special interest to the investigation, is the EPIDAT [67], which is a free program developed by public and led to epidemiologists and other health professionals to manage tabular data, allowing us to make a descriptive analysis, data filtering and imputation, sampling, parameters inference, contingency tables, matching and consistency, diagnostic tests, rates adjustment, demographics, logistic regression, survival analysis, probability distributions, Bayesian analysis, meta-analysis, monitoring public health, measuring health inequalities, economic evaluation methods, etc. [68].

One of the most popular and used statistical packages is the SPSS, which is a statistical analysis and data management in a graphical environment system, using descriptive menus and simple dialog boxes that do most of the work, consisting of a simple interface, a data editor, with features such as multidimensional pivot tables, high-resolution graphics, database access, data processing, electronic distribution, and online help. Other programs of great usefulness are Stata, R, among others [69]

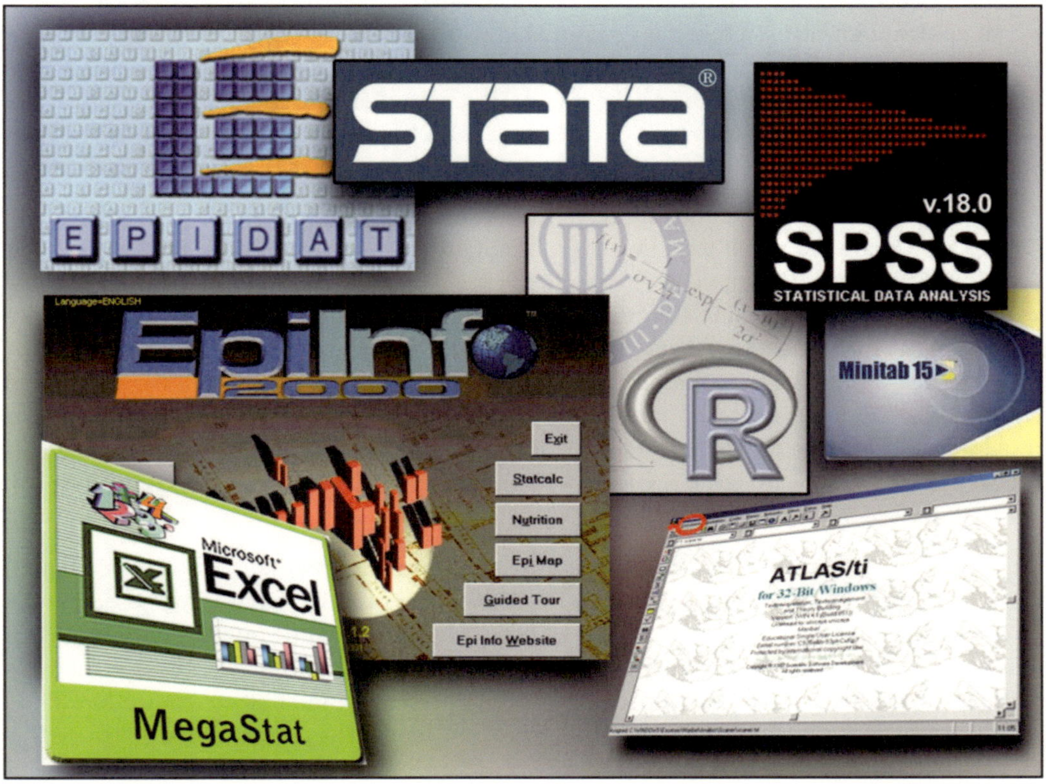

Figure 12. Software Statistics

5. Social epidemiology and the health inequities

5.1. Social epidemiology

Despite some theories, methodologies and tools currently used by social epidemiology date back to the 17th century, it hasn't been until the past century's last decades that it has consolidated as a scientific discipline. And, like any young discipline, it faced the questioning characteristic of its not well defined scope [8,9]. Some skeptics argued that the term 'social epidemiology' was redundant, because epidemiology is inherently a social term. However, the contributions made by Durkheim (1987), John Cassel (1976), Geoffrey Rose (1992) or Mervyn Susser (1994, 1996, 1998), to mention some of the most important; set the basis of the social determinants and health status of the population approach [9].

Social epidemiology is defined as the branch of epidemiology that studies the social distribution and social determinants of the health, implying that the purpose of its study is the identification of socio-environmental exposures that can be related to a wide range of physical and mental health problems [63]. To put it simpler, what distinguishes the action of a conventional epidemiologist from a social epidemiologist is the level of causal thinking. While the first one thinks: why does a person get sick?, identifying the best statistic tool to evaluate the association between a risk factor and the disease, the second one wonders: why is a society not healthy?, making out that factors which determine collective health are not individual, but that social determinants which have a direct impact on the health status of a population exist [8].

The concepts of social epidemiology have been evidenced since the findings of John Grant (1662), who identified social variations of mortality that was quantified on England chapels on the 17th century. Villerme (1830) and Virchow (1848) identified the social class and the working conditions as crucial determinants for sickness and health. Since then, these findings constitute the theoretic foundation necessary to try to resolve the persistency and even the recent increase in social inequities in health. While some communicable diseases have been eradicated, other have emerged or re-emerged. The epidemiologic transition has changed the disease profile to favor the chronic or non-communicable diseases, and the social inequities of health prevail [9]. This makes it necessary to incorporate social variables like direct determinants of disease or population disability [70].

This approach widens the need to use theories, and especially multidisciplinary techniques, to answer the new questions and rethink the answers to questions that were posed before. Theories like the social capital, particular of economy, can now be applied to resolve social epidemiology problems. Tools such as the multilevel analysis (multilevel regression models), first designed for social sciences (especially pedagogic research) and that were introduced into epidemiology in the beginning of the 80s, are now being spread as powerful analysis tools [71].

5.2. Differences between social epidemiology and field epidemiology

Even though field epidemiology and social epidemiology have the same epistemological, methodological and practical bases [4], in some situations they can be considered as the two extremes of a spectrum, between the practical application of the information for action on an individual territory and the usage of the information for the elaboration of theories about the macro-social economic and political determinants, with few or hard practical application [4]. It is necessary then, to highlight some differences over the practical development of these disciplines and the implications these carry.

Taking into account this duo action-reflection, we could say that on one hand, field epidemiology it is developed an individual analysis of the diseases risk factors, searching for its application in the field to control the outbreaks, aided by strategies such as epidemiologic vigilance. On the other hand, social epidemiology seeks to analyze social factors (considered social determinants) and their distribution in populations as aggregate variables that have are more distantly related but crucial in the behavior of diseases in population groups [4].

It is important to mention than the places where both disciplines take place are different. While the first one acts in confined environments, the second one tries to take on broader territories, in which the public politics' implementation and design are necessary for health management. Social epidemiology focuses its concerns in the generation of evidence, to avoid health inequities, and its effect in the socio-environment conditions that increase a population's risk of getting ill. Otherwise, field epidemiology centers its work in the search for recognizable risk factors on an individual and collective level, to attend immediate healthcare problems such as epidemic outbreaks. However, the limit between these two disciplines is diffuse, so the challenge for young professionals in epidemiology is exactly to strengthen an integral and multidisciplinary profile to guarantee the generation of the best evidence that will allow answering to diverse problems of public health in all the levels

5.3. Theoretical background of social epidemiology

The role of the theoretical background to guide the direction of addressing the main research question in general in epidemiology, and particularly in social epidemiology, is unquestionable. The main theories that have given base over time to the foundation of social epidemiology can be summarized in: the psychosocial theory, the theory of social production of a disease, and the ecosocial theory of disease and its multilevel dynamic perspectives [72]. These theories not only allow to define the social epidemiology and to draw work lines in its field, but also to direct the dynamic and connections between the individual-biologic levels, along with our social existence.

5.4. Methodological background of social epidemiology

Most efforts to generate new methodological paradigms in social epidemiology are based in the generation of models that seek for the best way to incorporate the social factor in biomedical research. The simplest and most common model to incorporate these social processes considers them as distal antecedents of the biological cause of disease [73]. This implies that the distal social factors are related with a disease through common causal paths. Then, for example, the educative levels (distal social factor) are related to an inadequate diet and this, in time, may be related to many diseases like cardiovascular disease or cancer. Despite this focus would contribute evidence for the prevention, adding these distal social factors would not be entirely necessary if we had an adequate knowledge of the biological factors, so we could indirectly eliminate the social gradient, taking part only the proximal factors.

A second model considers social factors as biological factors modifiers, in a way that these two would interact, generating biological processes that lead to disease. This model if genetic-environmental interaction implies that the presence of genetic factors is not enough to make a disease express itself, but that it depends of the environmental context in which it raises. Analogously, the influence of social factors depends on the underlying genetic conditions of the individual [73].

The third model considers social factors as an integral part of two biological systems, with the capacity to modify functional and structurally the biological aspects of individuals. This way, social experiences are able to generate direct changes in biological systems, being a fundamental piece on the understanding of these complex systems [73].

5.5. Social epidemiology and the analysis of health inequities

Currently, epidemiology constitutes an emerging field with an enormous potential to generate improvements in public heath, for it becomes evident that social factors and group dynamics affect the health status [74]. Understanding the biological phenomenon related to disease is necessary, but it is also vital to understand how society influences in biology, aiming to modify the illness risk. Social understanding is fundamental in the process of change and reduction of the burden of disease [75].

In the poor countries, people die unnecessarily. In rich countries, this also happens. This is explained by a social gradient that generates high mortality rates among those who have unfavorable socio-economic conditions, for which it is also considered unnecessary. The term inequity has a moral and ethical dimension: it means to differences that are unnecessary and avoidable, but also considered unfair and arbitrary. So, to be able to describe a specific situation as inequitable, the cause must be examined and judged as unfair in the context of what is happening to the rest of society. The crucial evidence to know if the resulting health differences are considered unfair seems to largely depend if the people chose the situation that caused the ill health or if that was basically out of their direct control [76]. Therefore, in the contexts where the fundamental and necessary execution of the autonomy and personal freedom is impossible, the health is powerfully affected, and it is the social conditions that determine the degree of these fundamental needs limits [75].

The health inequities analysis is based in the social epidemiology, to reinforce the important role of the environment as cause of the disease. A typical example is the modification of the disease profile that happens in migrant population when they change their resident environment [75]. And this environment is the own social context in which diverse factor interact to favor the development of diseases. The analysis and understanding of the dynamic that governs the interactions of individual and social factors would allow us to modify the inequities and improve the health. Besides, we must take into account some considerations: there is the need to act over the social gradient that limits the people's autonomy and freedom, to adopt healthy surroundings, but one must not focus the efforts only on the poorest sectors, but in the whole social gradient aspect [76]. This way we can generate health politics that will cover all the sectors in an integral way, with a proportionally bigger impact in the least favored sectors. This politics generation must be sustained in the systematic application of the best evidence, relating knowledge with action and opening new opportunities for the prevention [77].

6. Health inequities in Latin America and Peru

Latin America is considered the region with the largest inequities on the planet. It's the continent where, according to multiple studies, the polarizations are larger in diverse fields, and the access to opportunities is notably different for the different social sectors; and maybe where the difference is more notorious is in health, which belongs to the most basic human rights category [78].

There have been considerable progresses in the health matter in Latin America. However, there are serious problems that show the presence of an acute pattern of inequity. The national averages show progress, but when they are broken down to socioeconomic levels, regions, gender and ages, there can be observed wide sectors of the population with serious problems [78].

In this context, the clinical epidemiology has the commitment to measure the impact of the healthcare interventions, where the clinical trials rarely are reported by socioeconomic levels, given that the population's health and the clinical epidemiology support evaluating the efficacy, effectiveness and cost-effectiveness are very importan to define the impact of healthcare in health inequities [17].

In Peru, this type of analysis is being carried out more frequently since the beginning of the past decade. For example, in the year 2002, the Grupo de Análisis para el Desarrollo (Group of Analysis for the Development - GRADE), led by Dr. Martin Valdivia, did a study about the health inequities in Peru, using socio-economic indicators taken from socio-demographic national surveys and evaluating its strength to generalize the results [79].

The descriptive analysis establishes that the largest inequity is in the children's chronic malnutrition and the usage of health services in general. About 30% of the rural children of the poorest decile suffer from chronic malnutrition, but this rate is *just* 4% in the richest decile. This means that the poor/rich ratio is 7.8. In rural areas, this ratio is *just* 3.6, but this is the reflection of an even worse generalized condition where the malnutrition rate between the poorest children reaches 64%. On the other hand, medical attention during labor shows an inverse relation where the rich/poor ratio in rural areas reaches 17.2, and less than 4% of the poorest rural women have a doctor present at the moment of labor. This ratio decreases to 2 in urban zones, and almost 50% of the women of the poorest decile can access this type of healthcare. This results don't change with the socio-economic level indicator (ELI) used, except In the case of child mortality, where an astounding and disturbing result is that there is no finding of an overwhelming relation with the ELI of the home, especially in the rural areas [77]

7. Evidence based medicine in hospital practice and in public health

Currently, the tendency of science is focused in the generation of evidence to contribute in its development and has an impact on the patient's health. This approach of Evidence Based Medicine (EBM) is shown mainly in healthcare, related to drugs and medical devices. However, it is admitted that the community interventions through Public Health deserve to be recognized as transcendent elements that have had an impact in the population's health. In this way, it is necessary to recognize the existence of research that advocate to evidence the impact of Public Health's diverse activities.

The Evidence Based Public Health (EBPH) maintains a cause-effect logic, and allows to add the health determinants, like lifestyles, culture and environment, in a scientific context, because many times it's them who characterize the good or bad performance of a certain intervention. This way, EBPH is a new tendency that has been joining efforts to give the best information for the most efficient politics decisionmaking.

7.1. Evidence based medicine in the clinical environment

The practice of EBM in the hospital environment benefits doctors and students, for it collaborates in the obtaining of evidence selected for its quality, informatics value and relevance for the user (for example, the services produced by McMaster premium service literature [PLUS] as well as the ACP Journal Club Plus). One of the current benefits is that it allows concentrating opinions related to methodological quality and potential relevance for its use. This way, the McMaster University has developed the program 'McMaster Online Rating of Evidence' (MORE), in which it allows the professional to have literature of the most technical quality and relevance. This is through a classification given by professionals from diverse latitudes from around the world. Beside, these services present clear and relevant results, and offer to visualize comments or criticism, independently for the management of said information [76]. This information, according to the analogy used, tells us that 'the EBM and nuclear fission can be very powerful when they are appropriately used and dangerous if not', because the fact that EBM separates describing, the underlying quality of the evidence, the magnitude of the effects or the applicability of any of the results in the context, the values and the preferences of the patients should not be considered [80].

Therefore, there is no doubt that EBM has allowed to progress in the medical practice. However, the application in the Health System has been inconsistent, meaning that the EBM would improve the health of the population. The differences in the health systems, globally, on the healthcare of the population, limit the capacity to incorporate easily the progress of the EBM, or often to certain discriminating point by economic or politic limitations [81]. Nevertheless, it is important to point out that it has been found in primary healthcare a relation between the high knowledge of EBM and a better quality of healthcare [82]. Although, when evaluating EBM at workplace, as a method of formative performance evaluation, there is not much evidence that shows the impact on the education of the doctors and their performance [83].

In relation to the use of EBM, one can point out that the public hospitals there is a favorable attitude. Besides, it is recognized that doctors who practice the EBM show a more prone attitude to change information and counseling through mutual collaboration networks [84,85]. Doctors recognize also the gap that exists between the EBM applications to clinical practice, for it is difficult to avoid the clinical experience, colleague's opinions or some scientific studies, which are not EBM, in their decision making. The confidence in decision making based on clinical experience increases with the time of service. However, there are few doctors that inform that clinical experience should be the only one used. Most doctors estimated that EBM practice should be guided by local evidence collected from local practice, because it will allow to back up their actions in clinical practice [86]. Therefore, the fact of automanaging the evidence would help the patient's, for example, chronic diseases and to pay attention to the unhealthy factors of a community, which could be added in the EBM to create a wider paradigm [81].

Regarding this, it should be noted the experiences from Canadian family doctors (where the EBM was born) who report positive attitude toward EBM, recognizing that it improves patient's healthcare and considering that the research findings are useful in the management of everyday patients. However, in clinical practice, the decision making can be influenced by a demanding patient, that can call for some detection test (OR: 5.15; IC95%: 2.9-9.2). Though this relation was not kept regarding the therapeutic, it is important to value the preferences of the patient and the clinical context seems to reflect more precisely the clinical reality of EBM and primary healthcare doctors [87].

7.2. Evidence based medicine compared to evidence based public health

The EBM is a methodology to evaluate the published clinical research, and its use is starting to be considered as a referent for knowledge and in the clinical practice evaluation, Its methodology is mainly based in the usage of evidence, like systematic reviews and meta-analysis, through which it seeks to offer answers to concrete clinical questions, this answer being backed up by statistic evidence. The application of EBM has multiple benefits, but also has various difficulties in clinical practice for it is hard to hold it freely, without taking into account the cultural, academic and socio-economic environment of every latitude. Therefore, its correct use is a challenge for contemporary medicine [10]. This approach of EBM allows the health provider (health professional) to use it in favor of his clinical practice, like in the hospital environment. Athough it is not compulsory, its utilization serves in health teams committed to improve hospital healthcare.

This EBM approach, applied to the Public Health interventions, it is not adequately adjusted, because EBm uses as a gold standard the clinical trials, whose use in public health is of difficult extrapolation for when it is applied to the population, it demands other variables to be considered that may directly influence over the expected outcome [83]. To this situation, the EBPH approach collaborates to concentrate efforts to sustain evidence that backs up the health politics and community interventions, though there are known limitations of the EBPH's use of evidence for using observational studies that have been systematically underestimated by EBM as a reference. Currently, models of technical evaluation have been developed, serving as a filter for evidence and collaborating to improve the selection of more methodological stringency studies to be used in Public Health.

Among some of the evaluation models for effectiveness of the Public Health interventions, many maintain common aspects. However, there still isn't a global consensus regarding it. Some strategies can be noted, lie the TREND (Transparent Reporting of Evaluations with Non randomized Designs), which evaluates the severity of publications which inform of Public Health interventions. The MOOSE (Meta-analysis Of Observational Studies in Epidemiology), for the reading of observational studies meta-analysis, or the STROBE (STrenghtening the Reporting of OBservational studies in Epidemiology), for cohorts and case-control studies, can complement the ability to improve the systematization of information related to Public Health interventions [11].

In general, it can be said that the EBM and EBPH have a common origin, which is the use of epidemiology as a decisive tool for the selection, evaluation and recommendation of evidence for its use, whether in hospital clinical practice of the social environment, which is Public Health.

It can also be said that there are obstacles in the incorporation of research in the politics, apart from limited budgets. Although the politic makers could benefit of the EBM if they train in said approach, to help them identify and evaluate high quality information. This way, researchers and those who are designing health politics can make a synergy for the best decision making for the population and the country. This can be used as generation and intervention experience exchange networks for future health politics [88].

8. The cause-effect logic in the public health interventions

Epidemiology as such helps the health sciences to understand the diverse causal mechanisms where the cause-effect relation aids to evidence factors that determine health problems. This way, Public Health is one of the specialties that uses it as an essential tool to show reliable evidence that will help understand the diverse health problems that populations have. However, at the moment of structuring the causal map, in many of the public health causal factors it can be seen that they rely on social determinants. And, on the other hand, that the public health problematic is multifactorial. The analysis shows us that this is the epidemiology's challenge to obtain a critical causal path that collaborates to understand that the modification of an event sequence (factors) can be stimulated to generate the expected outcome in the health problems of a population, being this event sequence the critical causal path.

According to what it is stated, a group of steps that aid to develop this critical causal path will be explained, which will be used as an axis for the diverse approaches of the public health's interventions.

Step 1: Recognize the public health problem: The problem evaluation approach in public health can be obtained from different sources, primary or secondary. Primary sources are the most difficult to be obtained, because they demand resources and time to be able to get scientific studies that collect the divers health problematic. In general, given the technical and political

http://dx.doi.org/10.5772/54901

circumstances, it is more viable to use secondary sources, which collaborate to problematize the health status of a population. This way, one of the main management tools used according to the geographic space is the Health Situation Analysis (HAS), whose methodology allows to evaluate three important aspects: social determinants (socio-economic, cultural, lifestyle, commerce, environmental, etc. aspects), morbidity and mortality (Child mortality rate, Maternal death rate, main diseases and death causes, etc) and the social answer (health systems, health establishments, human resources in health, equipment, etc.) which, when analyzed in an integral way, can issue the main health problems of a certain geographic space, as well as its interaction with the intervention carried out by the Nation. At the end, it must be highlighted the health problem that must be taken in tis real context.

Step 2: Causal map with an evidence approach. It is the evidence systematic evaluation that explains the health problem related to its causes and the effects it can generate. When graphed in a causal map, it aids to show the cause-effect relation, and being back up by scientific evidence, it makes the health decision maker to have a wider spectrum of the multiple causality of the health problem. Then, it helps to maintain a multifactorial perspective of the public health problems. In the design of the causal map one should provide the most scientific evidence there exists, doing a bibliographic research using the informatics tools and main scientific portals, without putting aside the selection and evaluation of the articles with the methodological severity already noted in the EBPH.

As an example, it can be shown in Figure 13, the causal map of the health problema: "Chronic malnutrition in children under 5 years old from rural zones".

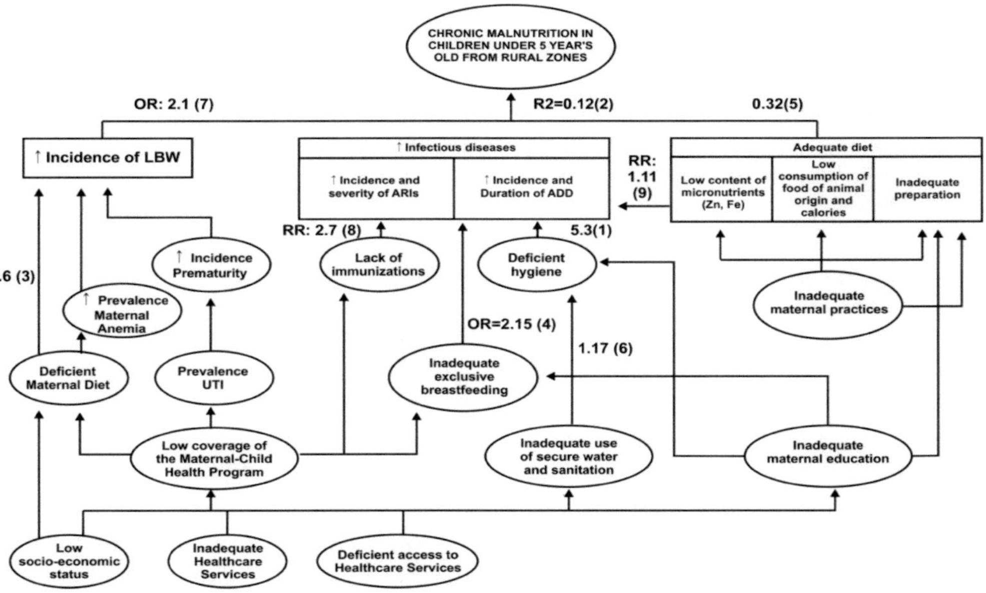

Figure 13. Causal map of chronic malnutrition in children under 5 years old from rural zones.

Evidence	Place	Type of Study	Interventions/Results	Evidence level	Quality of Evidence	Value
1.- N. Etilera, S. Velipasaoglub, M. Aktekinc. Risk factors for overall and persistent diarrhoea in infancy in Antalya, Turkey: a cohort study. Public Health (2004) 118, 62–69. (13)	Turkey	Cohort	Evaluation of lack of hygiene and increase of ADD.	II-2	3	RR : 5.3
2.- Peter G. Lunn. The impact of infection and nutrition on gut function and growth in childhood. Medical Research Council, Ke Peter.Lunn1@tesco.net CAB International PNS Proceedings of the Nutrition Society (P185©N4S N 9u9tr-i1ti1o6nC Slion cicieatly nutrition in childhood P. G. Lunn147 2000)© Nutrition Society 2000 59. (14)	Gambia	Review	Papers done in Gambia on the association between digestive infections and chronic malnutrition are evaluated.	II-3	4	R^2 : 0.12
3.- Maleta K, Virtanen S.M, Chilhood malnutriition and its predictor in rural Malawi. Paediatric & Perinatal Epidemilogy, volume 17, Number 4, October 2003, pp. 384-390. (15)	Malawi	Case-Control	Evaluates the association between deficient maternal diet and the increase in LBW.	II-2	3	RR: 2.6
4.- Alex K Anderson, Grace Damio, Sara Young, Donna Chapman. A Randomized Trial Assessing the Efficacy of Peer counseling on Exclusive Breastfeeding in a predominantly Latina Low income Community. Arch Pediatric Adolesc Med 2005; 159, 836-841. (16)	Latin communities	Randomized Clinical Trial	Association between breastfeeding and ADD	II-1	1	RR: 2.15
5.- Bhandari N, Mazumder S, Bahl R, Martines J, Black R and Bhan M. An Educational Intervention to Promote Appropriate Complementary Feeding Practices and Physical Growth in Infants and Young Children in Rural Haryana, India.J. Nutr. 134:2342-2348, September 2004 (17)	India	Cluster Clinical Trial	Evaluation of the educational intervention in feeding practices and malnutrition.	I-2	1	Difference in growth 0.32 cm and 0.5cm
6.- Merchant AT, Jones .C, Kiure A, Kupka R, Fitzmaurice G, Herrera MG, Fawzi WW. Water and sanitation associated with improved child growth European journal of clinical nutrition 2003 Dec57 12 1562-8 (18)	India	Observational	Association between inadequate water-drainage services and inadequate practices.	II-3	3	OR: 1.6
7.- Instituto Nacional de Estadística e Informática PRISMA – Dirección de Investigación. Determinantes de la desnutrición aguda y crónica en niños menores de 3 años. Un sub-análisis de la ENDES 1992 y 1996. (19)	Peru	Observational	Association between low birth weight and malnutrition.	II-3	3	OR: 2.1
8- Deb SK. Acute respiratory disease survey in Tripura in case of children below five years of age. J Indian Med Assoc. 1998 Apr;96(4):111-6. (20)	India	Cohort	Association between immunizations and ARIs.	II-2	3	RR: 2.7
9- Tarun Gera, H P S Sachdev. Effect of iron supplementation on incidence of infectious illness in children: systematic review. BMJ vol 325 16 Nov. 2002. (21)	-	Systematic Review	Effect of iron on infections in ADD.	I-1	1	RR: 1.11

Table 5. Evidence of the causal map of chronic malnutrition in children under 5 years old from rural zones.

Following the direction of the arrows in the causal map, the cause-effect logic can be defined, and the numbers attached to the arrows represent the scientific evidence that support said causal relation, which can be compiled in an evidence table as it is shown in Table 5.

So, showing the interaction of variables in relation to a health problem, the decision maker of health policy can see in the bottom of causal map, which it can fall on social determinants, such as low socio-economic status, and often it is not feasible his intervention from short to medium term. On the other hand, we can see that variables are likely to be modified, and that the modification of these stimulates the changing chain of whom it has direct causal association. Under this perspective the formulation of a critical causal pathway can be based.

Step 3: Build critical causal pathways: Many times in the search for evidence in Public Health to develop interventions that will reduce health problem, one must have clear interaction of the direct and indirect variables that are related to health problems, in order to provide technical support on what you want to modify. Thus the critical causal pathway contributes to show schematically the interaction of the direct and indirect variables to health problems and allows the decision maker to choose to evaluate the various critical paths that can be noted in health interventions. Regarding the causal map example of Figure 14, one can observe the causal pathway designed as an example of a way of assessing a probable health intervention, which pretends to check how the intervention with fortified food programs can collaborate to reduce chronic malnutrition in children under 5 years old

http://dx.doi.org/10.5772/54901

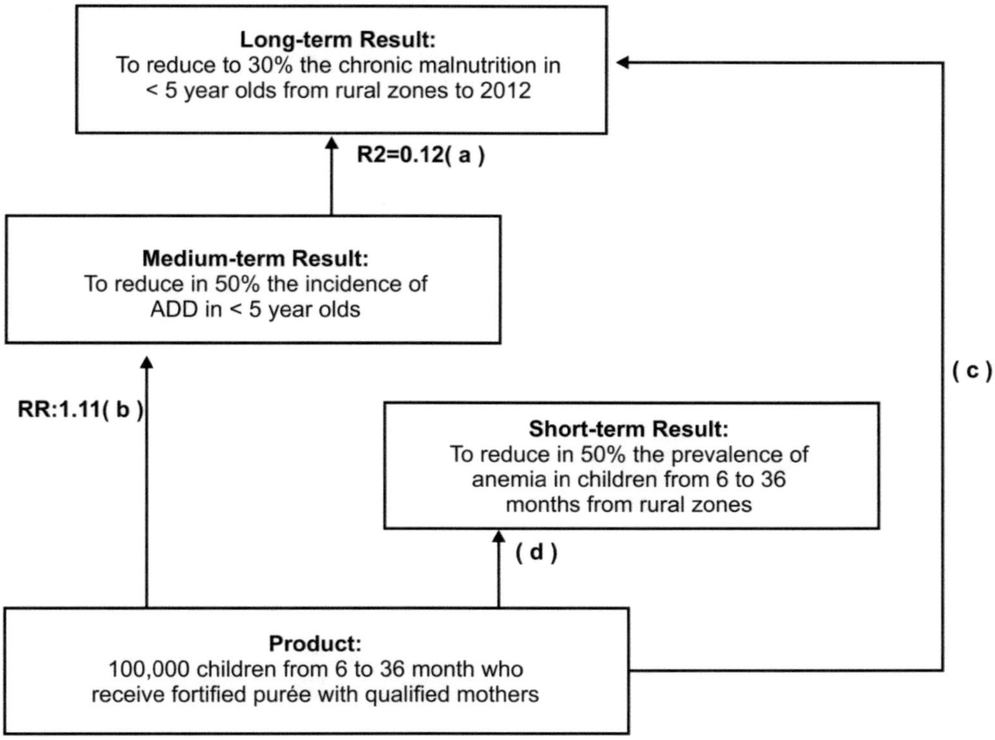

Figure 14. Critical causal chain of the fortified food program to reduce the chronic malnutrition in children under 5 years old from rural zones.

Author	Design	Outcome	Population	Effect	Degree of recommendation	Evidence level
Peter G (a)	Analytical	Chronic malnutrition	Children	Diarrhea increases chronic malnutrition (R2 : 0.12)	B	III
Tarun Gera (b)	Review	Diarrhea	Children	Iron supplement RR: 1.11	A	Ia
Apolaya M (c)	Review	Chronic malnutrition	6 to 36 months	Non conclusive	A	Ia
Assunção MCF (d)	Review	Anemia	Infants	Non conclusive	A	Ia

Table 6. Evidence that sustains the causality relationship

Furthermore, it is important to contextualize the propositions of health interventions with economic aspects of each one, and the methodologies, as economic assessments developed by each country. That brings us to rethink that one must recognize that the health problems or health interventions that are probable to be carried out are greatly influenced by socio-political considerations, but that despite the political and circumstances it is our desire, as technical authorities, to show, in the most objective, efficient and effective way in this task, with the support of scientific information through the MBE or SPBE (Table 6)

9. Conclusion

Clinical epidemiology and field epidemiology share the same methodology and tools, differing in individual application and the population respectively, but are complementary to public health.

The EBM is demanded by patients for a better diagnosis and treatment, in addition to recognizing the importance of clinical epidemiology in the development and promotion of research, progress that is driven by the software tools that facilitate the researchers' performance and in modern times it is essential to know and apply them.

Social epidemiology studies the social distribution and social determinants of health states ranging from individual levels (risk factors) to social phenomena (social determinants), seeking answers to the complex dynamics behind social distribution of health and in that context is EBPH an important tool to improve the analysis of public health interventions that can help to improve decision-making at the policy makers of a country's health.

Finally clinical epidemiology has enormous potential to generate real and positive changes in public health, becoming a challenge for new professionals in epidemiology and public health for their increasing and complex development

Acknowledgements

We acknowledge Víctor Calderón Chávez y Vannessa Elizabeth Sánchez Vélez, for their support in the review of the writing and to Agimiro Yangua Jaramillo for the elaboration of the manuscript figures.

Author details

Cristian Díaz-Vélez[1], Víctor Soto-Cáceres[2], Ricardo E. Peña-Sánchez[3], Moisés A. Apolaya Segura[4] and Edén Galán-Rodas[5]

http://dx.doi.org/10.5772/54901

1 Faculty of Medicine, University San Martín de Porres-Filial Norte. National Hospital Almanzor Agui, Perú

2 Faculty Medicine, National University Pedro Ruiz Gallo. Lambayeque, Peru

3 University San Martin de Porres-Filial Norte. Regional Health. Lambayeque, Peru

4 Japanese Peruvian Centennial Clinic, Health Directorate of the Fuerza Aerea del Peru, Lima, Peru

5 Social Security of Peru, EsSalud, Lima, Peru

References

[1] Field Epidemiologist Definition | eHow.com [Internet]. [citado 2012 ago 29]. Available a partir de: http://www.ehow.com/facts_5502586_field-epidemiologist-definition.html

[2] Medicina (Buenos Aires) - La Epidemiología Clínica hegemónica [Internet]. [citado 2012 ago 29]. Available a partir de: http://www.scielo.org.ar/scielo.php?script=sci_arttext&pid=S0025-76802006000300015

[3] Field Epidemiologist Definition | eHow.com [Internet]. [citado 2012 ago 29]. Available a partir de: http://www.ehow.com/facts_5502586_field-epidemiologist-definition.html

[4] Segura del Pozo J. Epidemiología de campo y epidemiología social. Gaceta Sanitaria. 2006;20(2):153–8.

[5] Trenti T. Evidence-based laboratory medicine as a tool for continuous professional improvement. Clinica chimica acta. 2003;333(2):155–67.

[6] Cabrera-Enriquez JA; Cruzado-Mendoza C; Purizaca-Rosillo N; López-Samanamú RO; CPC-SOCIMEP; Peña-Sanchez ER; Apolaya-Segura M; Díaz-Vélez C. Associated factors to the level of knowledge and attitudes towards research in students of the Peruvian Schools of Medicine. Rev Panam Salud Publica [en prensa]

[7] Le T, Stein ML. Medical education and the Internet: This changes everything. JAMA: The Journal of the American Medical Association. 2001;285(6):809–809.

[8] Kawachi I. Social epidemiology. Social Science & Medicine. 2002 jun;54(12):1739–41

[9] Berkman LF, Kawachi I. Social Epidemiology. Oxford University Press; 2000

[10] Durá JRR. Medicina basada en evidencias: beneficios, inconvenientes y riesgos de un nuevo dogma. Ginecol Obstet Mex. 2008;76(3):167–73.

[11] Morales Asencio JM, Gonzalo Jiménez E, Martín Santos FJ, Morilla Herrera JC. Salud pública basada en la evidencia: recursos sobre la efectividad de intervenciones en la comunidad. Revista española de salud pública. 2008;82(1):05–20.

[12] Rothman KJ, Greenland S, Lash TL. Modern epidemiology [Internet]. Lippincott Williams & Wilkins; 2008

[13] Home | TEPHINET [Internet]. [citado 2012 ago 30]. Available a partir de: http://www.tephinet.org/

[14] Oficina General de Epidemiología. Plan Curricular Programa Residentado de Campo (PREC). Lima 1989;

[15] Gregg MB, Dicker RC, Goodman RA. Epidemiología de Campo. 2º ed. New York: Oxford University Press; 2002.

[16] Thacker SB, Buffington J. Applied epidemiology for the 21st century. International journal of epidemiology. 2001;30(2):320–5.

[17] Anderson GM, Bronskill SE, Mustard CA, Culyer A, Alter DA, Manuel DG. Both clinical epidemiology and population health perspectives can define the role of health care in reducing health disparities. Journal of clinical epidemiology. 2005;58(8):757–62.

[18] clinical epidemiology - Definition [Internet]. [citado 2012 ago 29]. Available a partir de: http://www.mondofacto.com/facts/dictionary?clinical+epidemiology

[19] Clinical epidemiology reconstructed - Campbell - 2005 - Internal Medicine Journal - Wiley Online Library [Internet]. [citado 2012 ago 28]. Available a partir de: http://onlinelibrary.wiley.com/doi/10.1111/j.1445-5994.2005.00778.x/abstract

[20] Sackett DL. The fall of« clinical research» and the rise of« clinical-practice research». Clinical and Investigative Medicine. 2000;23(6):331–3.

[21] Braude HD. Clinical intuition versus statistics: different modes of tacit knowledge in clinical epidemiology and evidence-based medicine. Theoretical medicine and bioethics. 2009;30(3):181–98.

[22] [Hegemonic Clinical Epidemiology]. [Medicina (B Aires). 2006] - PubMed - NCBI [Internet]. [citado 2012 ago 28]. Available a partir de: http://www.ncbi.nlm.nih.gov/pubmed/16871919

[23] Sørensen HT. Clinical Epidemiology–a fast new way to publish important research. Clinical epidemiology. 2009;1:17.

[24] [Hegemonic clinical epidemiology]. [Medicina (B Aires). 2007] - PubMed - NCBI [Internet]. [citado 2012 ago 28]. Available a partir de: http://www.ncbi.nlm.nih.gov/pubmed/17593612

[25] Gray JA. Evidence based policy making. Bmj. 2004;329(7473):988–9.

[26] Hembroff L, Holmes-Rovner M, Wills C. Treatment decision-making and the form of risk communication: Results of a factorial survey. BMC Medical Informatics and Decision Making. 2004;4(1):20.

[27] Ahmadi-Abhari S, Soltani A, Hosseinpanah F. Knowledge and attitudes of trainee physicians regarding evidence-based medicine: a questionnaire survey in Tehran, Iran. Journal of evaluation in clinical practice. 2008;14(5):775–9.

[28] Guyatt G, Cook D, Haynes B. Evidence based medicine has come a long way. Bmj. 2004;329(7473):990–1.

[29] Akl EA, Oxman AD, Herrin J, Vist GE, Terrenato I, Sperati F, et al. Using alternative statistical formats for presenting risks and risk reductions. Cochrane Database of Systematic Reviews [Internet]. 2011 [citado 2012 ago 28];3. Available a partir de: http://apps.who.int/entity/rhl/reviews/langs/cd006776.pdf

[30] Heller RF, Sandars JE, Patterson L, McElduff P. GPs' and physicians' interpretation of risks, benefits and diagnostic test results. Family practice. 2004;21(2):155–9.

[31] Estellat C, Faisy C, Colombet I, Chatellier G, Burnand B, Durieux P. French academic physicians had a poor knowledge of terms used in clinical epidemiology. Journal of clinical epidemiology. 2006;59(9):1009–14.

[32] Straus SE, Green ML, Bell DS, Badgett R, Davis D, Gerrity M, et al. Evaluating the teaching of evidence based medicine: conceptual framework. BMJ. 2004;329(7473): 1029–32.

[33] Hatala R, Guyatt G. Evaluating the teaching of evidence-based medicine. JAMA: the journal of the American Medical Association. 2002;288(9):1110–2.

[34] Straus SE, Jones G. What has evidence based medicine done for us? Bmj. 2004;329(7473):987–8.

[35] Zea-Vera A, Liendo-Caro C, Luna-Carrillo L, Prevost-Ruiz Y, Castañeda-Guarderas A, Málaga G. Knowledge of epidemiological risk indicators used in clinical trials among medical students in advanced years and medical residents. Rev Peru Med Exp Salud Publica. 2012; 29(2):218-22.

[36] Rhodes M, Ashcroft R, Atun RA, Freeman GK, Jamrozik K. Teaching evidence-based medicine to undergraduate medical students: a course integrating ethics, audit, management and clinical epidemiology. Medical teacher. 2006;28(4):313–7.

[37] Dunn K, Wallace EZ, Leipzig RM. A dissemination model for teaching evidence-based medicine. Academic Medicine. 2000;75(5):525.

[38] Rucker L, Morrison E. The« EBM Rx»: An initial experience with an evidence-based learning prescription. Academic Medicine. 2000;75(5):527.

[39] Díaz-Vélez C, Manrique-González L, Galán-Rodas E, Apolaya-Segura M. Conocimientos, actitudes y prácticas en investigación de los estudiantes de pregrado de facultades de medicina del Perú. Acta Med Per. 2008;25(1):10.

[40] Díaz-Vélez C, León-Jiménez F, Peña-Sánchez R, Soto-Cáceres V, Galán-Rodas E, Málaga G. Simposio: importancia de la investigación científica en ciencias de la salud. Rev. cuerpo méd. HNAAA 2011. 4(2):107-114

[41] Reyes L, Aular J, Palencia J, Muñoz D. Una visión integradora de la investigación estudiantil en pregrado. Revista de Ciencias Sociales. 2010;16 (2):250-9.

[42] Kohlwes RJ, Shunk RL, Avins A, Garber J, Bent S, Shlipak MG. The PRIME curriculum. Journal of general internal medicine. 2006;21(5):506–9.

[43] Strom BL, Kelly TO, Norman SA, Farrar JT, Kimmel SE, Lautenbach E, et al. The master of science in clinical epidemiology degree program of the Perelman School of Medicine at the University of Pennsylvania: A model for clinical research training. Academic Medicine. 2012;87(1):74.

[44] Atallah AN. Essential clinical epidemiology in clinical education. Sao Paulo Med J. 1998 Jul-Aug;116(4):1745-6

[45] How can clinical epidemiology better support evidence-based guidelines and policies in low-income countries? | Collaboration for Evidence Based Health Care in Africa [Internet]. [citado 2012 ago 28]. Available a partir de: http://www.cebha.org/content/how-can-clinical-epidemiology-better-support-evidence-based-guidelines-and-policies-low-inco

[46] Berland GK, Elliott MN, Morales LS, Algazy JI, Kravitz RL, Broder MS, et al. Health information on the Internet: accessibility, quality, and readability in English and Spanish. JAMA. 2001 May 23;285(20):2612–21.

[47] García IR, Pendás JAR, Estébanez RV, Fayad MA, Pérez RD, García DÁ. Evaluación de las páginas web en lengua española útiles para el médico de atención primaria. Aten Primaria. 2003;31(9):575–84.

[48] Leung L. Internet embeddedness: links with online health information seeking, expectancy value/quality of health information websites, and Internet usage patterns. CyberPsychology & Behavior. 2008;11(5):565–9.

[49] Eysenbach G, Powell J, Kuss O, Sa E-R. Empirical studies assessing the quality of health information for consumers on the world wide web: a systematic review. JAMA. 2002 May 22;287(20):2691–700.

[50] Logan RA. Health literacy through the National Library of Medicine. Health Aff (Millwood). 2012 May;31(5):1128.

[51] Ospina EG, Reveiz Herault L, Cardona AF. Uso de bases de datos bibliográficas por investigadores biomédicos latinoamericanos hispanoparlantes: estudio transversal. Rev Panam Salud Pública. 2005;17(4):230–6

[52] PubMed - NCBI [Internet]. [cited 2012 Aug 27]. Available from: http://www.ncbi.nlm.nih.gov/pubmed

[53] LILACS [Internet]. [cited 2012 Aug 27]. Available from: http://lilacs.bvsalud.org/

[54] Biblioteca Virtual em Saúde [Internet]. [cited 2012 Aug 27]. Available from: http://regional.bvsalud.org/php/index.php?lang=pt

[55] SciELO - Scientific Electronic Library Online [Internet]. [cited 2012 Aug 27]. Available from: http://www.scielo.org/php/index.php

[56] OMS | Acerca de HINARI [Internet]. WHO. [cited 2012 Aug 27]. Available from: http://www.who.int/hinari/about/es/

[57] PAHO/WHO - OPS/OMS [Internet]. [cited 2012 Aug 27]. Available from: http://new.paho.org/

[58] WHO | World Health Organization [Internet]. WHO. [cited 2012 Aug 27]. Available from: http://www.who.int/en/

[59] Centers for Disease Control and Prevention [Internet]. [cited 2012 Aug 27]. Available from: http://www.cdc.gov/

[60] National Guideline Clearinghouse | Home [Internet]. [cited 2012 Aug 27]. Available from: http://www.guideline.gov/

[61] Chew C, Eysenbach G. Pandemics in the age of Twitter: content analysis of Tweets during the 2009 H1N1 outbreak. PLoS One. 2010;5(11):e14118.

[62] Curioso WH, Alvarado-Vásquez E, Calderón-Anyosa R. Using twitter to promote continuous educat ion and health research in Peru. Revista Peruana de Medicina Experimental y Salud Pública. 2011;28(1):163–4.

[63] García AM. Nueva versión de los «Requisitos de uniformidad para los manuscritos enviados a revistas biomédicas y de ciencias de la salud». Gaceta Sanitaria. 2004;18(3):163–5.

[64] Patreas K. Recommended Formats for Bibliographic Citation. National Library of Medicine, Reference Service, Bethesda, MD. 1991;

[65] EndNote | Thomson Reuters [Internet]. [cited 2012 Aug 27]. Available from: http://endnote.com/

[66] Zotero | Home [Internet]. [cited 2012 Aug 27]. Available from: http://www.zotero.org/

[67] EPIDAT: Análise Epidemiolóxica de Datos [Internet]. [cited 2012 Aug 27]. Available from: http://www.sergas.es/MostrarContidos_N3_T01.aspx?IdPaxina=62713

[68] Santiago Pérez MI, Hervada Vidal X, Naveira Barbeito G, Silva LC, Fariñas H, Vázquez E, et al. El programa epidat: usos y perspectivas. Revista Panamericana de Salud Pública. 2010;27(1):80–2.

[69] Siller AB, Tompkins L. The big four: analyzing complex sample survey data using SAS®, SPSS®, STATA®, and SUDAAN®. Proceedings of the Thirty-first Annual SAS® Users Group International Conference: 26-29 March 2006; San Francisco [Internet]. 2006 [cited 2012 Aug 31]. p. 172–31. Available from: http://www.bettycjung.net/Pdfs/Big4.pdf

[70] Krieger N. A glossary for social epidemiology. J Epidemiol Community Health. 2001 ene 10;55(10):693–700.

[71] Michel W. Research methods from social science can contribute much to the health sciences. Journal of Clinical Epidemiology. 2008 jun;61(6):519–20

[72] Krieger N. Teorias para la epidemiología social en el siglo XXI: una perspectiva ecosocial. International Journal of Epidemiology. 2001;30:668–77.

[73] Ana V. DR. Integrating Social and Biologic Factors in Health Research: A Systems View. Annals of Epidemiology. 2007 jul;17(7):569–74

[74] Oakes JM. Causal inference and the relevance of social epidemiology. Social Science & Medicine. 2004 may;58(10):1969–71.

[75] Marmot M. Health in an unequal world. The Lancet. 9;368(9552):2081–94.

[76] Whitehead M. The concepts and principles of equity and health. International journal of health services. 1992;22(3):429–45.

[77] Marmot M, Bell R. Fair society, healthy lives. Public Health [Internet]. [citado 2012 ago 29];(0). Available a partir de: http://www.sciencedirect.com/science/article/pii/S0033350612001862

[78] Kliksberg B. la inequidad en el campo de la salud pública en América Latina: una cuestion crucial. Economía y Sociedad [Internet]. 2002 [citado 2012 ago 30];(19). Available a partir de: http://www.revistas.una.ac.cr/index.php/economia/article/view/1188

[79] Valdivia M, para el Desarrollo GA. ACERCA DE LA INEQUIDAD EN SALUD EN EL PERÚ1. 2002 [citado 2012 ago 29]; Available a partir de: http://www.grade.org.pe/download/docs/MV-DT%20Inequidad%20en%20salud.PDF

[80] Montori VM, Guyatt GH. Progress in evidence-based medicine. JAMA: the journal of the American Medical Association. 2008;300(15):1814–6.

[81] Moskowitz D, Bodenheimer T. Moving from evidence-based medicine to evidence-based health. Journal of general internal medicine. 2011;26(6):658–60.

[82] Shuval K, Linn S, Brezis M, Shadmi E, Green ML, Reis S. Association between primary care physicians' evidence-based medicine knowledge and quality of care. International Journal for Quality in Health Care. 2010;22(1):16–23.

[83] Miller A, Archer J. Impact of workplace based assessment on doctors' education and performance: a systematic review. BMJ: British Medical Journal [Internet]. 2010 [citado 2012 ago 31];341. Available a partir de: http://www.ncbi.nlm.nih.gov/pmc/articles/PMC2945627/

[84] Mascia D, Cicchetti A, Fantini MP, Damiani G, Ricciardi W. Physicians' propensity to collaborate and their attitude towards EBM: A cross-sectional study. BMC health services research. 2011;11(1):172.

[85] De Vito C, Nobile CG, Furnari G, Pavia M, De Giusti M, Angelillo IF, et al. Physicians' knowledge, attitudes and professional use of RCTs and meta-analyses: A cross-sectional survey. The European Journal of Public Health. 2009;19(3):297–302.

[86] Hay MC, Weisner TS, Subramanian S, Duan N, Niedzinski EJ, Kravitz RL. Harnessing experience: exploring the gap between evidence-based medicine and clinical practice. Journal of evaluation in clinical practice. 2008;14(5):707–13.

[87] Tracy CS, Dantas GC, Moineddin R, Upshur REG. The nexus of evidence, context, and patient preferences in primary care: postal survey of Canadian family physicians. BMC Family Practice. 2003;4(1):13.

[88] Jewell CJ, Bero LA. «Developing Good Taste in Evidence»: Facilitators of and Hindrances to Evidence-Informed Health Policymaking in State Government. Milbank Quarterly. 2008;86(2):177–208.

Chapter 13

Evidence Based Public Health

Ajay K Parsaik and Balwinder Singh

Additional information is available at the end of the chapter

http://dx.doi.org/10.5772/52643

1. Introduction

Evidence based medicine includes asking clinical questions that can be answered by research, finding the best available evidence based on available research, judging whether the evidence is accurate and applicable to the patients, and applying this evidence in clinical practice [1]. The aim of evidence based medicine in "Public health" is to apply the current best knowledge from research in the prevention, detection, and care of health disorders [1]. The importance of use of scientific knowledge for policy making has grown over the last two-three decades. Systematic review of all the available research data are undertaken to limit bias in the systematic assembly, critical appraisal and pooled result synthesis [2]. The use of evidence based approach helps in distinguishing effective interventions from less effective interventions. Evidence based medicine has been systematized by several groups, especially the U.S. Preventive Services Task Forces and Cochrane Collaboration [3, 4]. The Task Force on "Community Preventive Services" was formed with an aim of synthesizing the scientific information on effectiveness of disease prevention and health promotion interventions [5], and has reviewed hundreds of related topics. Half of the interventions reviewed by task forces have been considered as insufficient evidence to determine the effectiveness, because of inadequate quality and/or inconsistent evaluation outcomes.

Evidence of effectiveness is the central part of public health, with rapidly growing demand for the recent and best evidence. Public health improvement plans look for the evidence of program effectiveness before considering intervention options, to meet the health goals. Evidence based strategies have been highly recommended to achieve the state and national objective of improved population health [6, 7].

Ideally, evidence based approach should always be used by public health practitioners while implementing programs, developing health policies and evaluating the progress [8, 9]. Evidence based services such as electronic databases, systematic reviews, and journals make accessing the current best evidence feasible, and easy in clinical settings. However, intervention decisions are often taken based on the short term applications in day-to-day clinical practice, lacking the evidence based systematic approach. Since scientific knowledge changes over time, it is necessary to make a decision based on the current scientific evidence. For that, public health providers and policy makers should be trained to synthesize conclusions based on the outcomes of interventions, including latest research in the concerned field. However, very few individuals in the public health practice have been trained to utilize the evidence based approach appropriately [10]. Many health care providers have difficulty finding, assessing, interpreting, and applying current best evidence[11]. Therefore, it would be of great interest to enumerate the importance of evidence based approaches in public health. Also, it is not always easy to implement evidence based approaches in public health due to various barriers like lack of relevant research, improper information systems, lack of leadership, incompetencies and political issues [11, 12]. Therefore, identification of barriers would help in making policies to overcome these obstacles, while applying evidence based medicine in public health sectors.

The objectives of this chapter are:

To define the evidence based medicine, evidence based public health, and enumerate the importance of evidence based medicine in public health.

To define the key analytical tools which could increase the adoption of evidence based medicine in clinical decision making in public health sector.

To enumerate the challenges and opportunities for implementing evidence based medicine in public health sector.

To describe the future issues of evidence based medicine in public health

1.1. Evidence based medicine & public health

Evidence includes the available body of facts or information which helps in defining whether a proposition is true or valid. Evidence for public health professional includes qualitative and quantitative data, programs results and policy evaluations, and the public health evidence is complex cycle of observation, theory and experiments [13, 14]. Three types of scientific evidence have been defined for public health practice, in literature [8, 15]. Type 1 evidence defines the severity and preventability of diseases and its risk factors, and suggests that something should be done about it. Type 2 evidence defines the impact of specific interventions on health improvement, and suggest that specifically this should be done [8]. Type 3 evidence informs, how something should be done as it define that under what conditions interventions were implemented, and how they were implemented and received [15].

There are many differences between evidence based approaches in medicine and public health. Pharmaceuticals and procedural medical studies rely on the results of randomized controlled trials, whereas public health interventions are based on cross-sectional and time series analysis, which sometime lack a comparison group unlike in clinical trials. Very few public health interventions have been performed over the last few decades compared to

http://dx.doi.org/10.5772/52643

randomized trials for medical treatments, as they are difficult to perform and are more costly [16, 17]. Population based studies require longer time to complete, and thus require more efforts and resources as compared to randomized clinical trials. In public health, intervention often involves combination of several interventions within the community, unlike randomized clinical trials where intervention is referred to one particular therapeutical, diagnostic or other measure.

In public health, there are limited academic credentials to certify the public health practitioners. Therefore, formal training is much more variable in public health sector as compared to other clinical disciplines, and only less than half of the workers of public health sectors have documented formal training in different disciplines like epidemiology, health educations etc. [18]. Public health is a heterogeneous sector where complex decisions making process involve multiple perspectives.

There are four groups of evidence based public health audience (Figure 1):

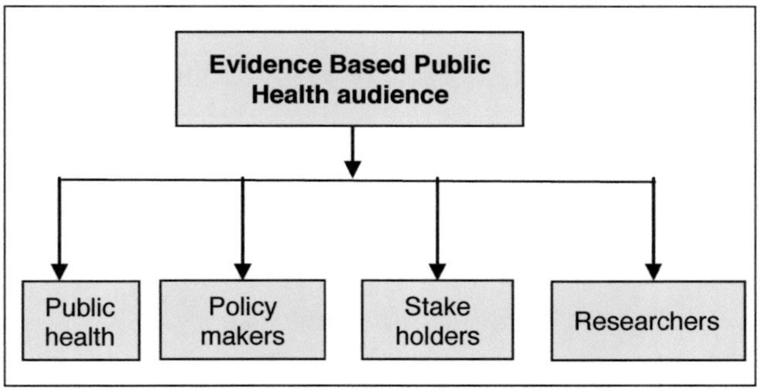

Figure 1. Audience of Evidence Based Public Health

1. Public health practitioners: This group has executive and managerial responsibilities. The public health practitioners want to know about the scope of alternative strategies and quality of evidence for such alternatives, however they have a narrow set of options. They should carefully review the evidence for alternative strategies to achieve the desired health goals in community.

2. Policy makers: The policy makers at local, regional, state, national and international levels have responsibility of allocating the public resources and making the policies on controversial public issues.

3. Stake holders: This includes the public and interest groups, who support or oppose the specific policies. This is the group which is affected by the interventions.

4. Researchers: The researchers evaluate the impact of any policy, program or intervention on population health.

Now it is a well known fact that practicing evidence based medicine improves patients' health, reduces complications, and help in saving more lives. In addition, increased focus of evidence based medicine has many other direct and indirect benefits. Evidence based medicine provide access to high quality information regarding different programs, policies and treatments plans with higher likelihood of success, with greater productivity [8, 11, 19]. It also helps in better usage of public and private resources in medicine.

To improve the evidence based approach in public health practice, we need to understand several concepts. First, we need detailed information on the policies and programs that will most likely be effective in promoting public health [8, 19, 20]. Then, we need to translate the science into practice. We also need to better define the different processes that lead to evidence based decision making in public health, for which we need to gather maximum possible relevant information from peer-reviewed literature [8, 21]. Finally, different effective interventions must occur consistently at local, state and national levels [22].

Dfferent qualitative and quantitative factors should be taken into account while making the public health policy decisions [23]. These factors are described below (Figure 2):

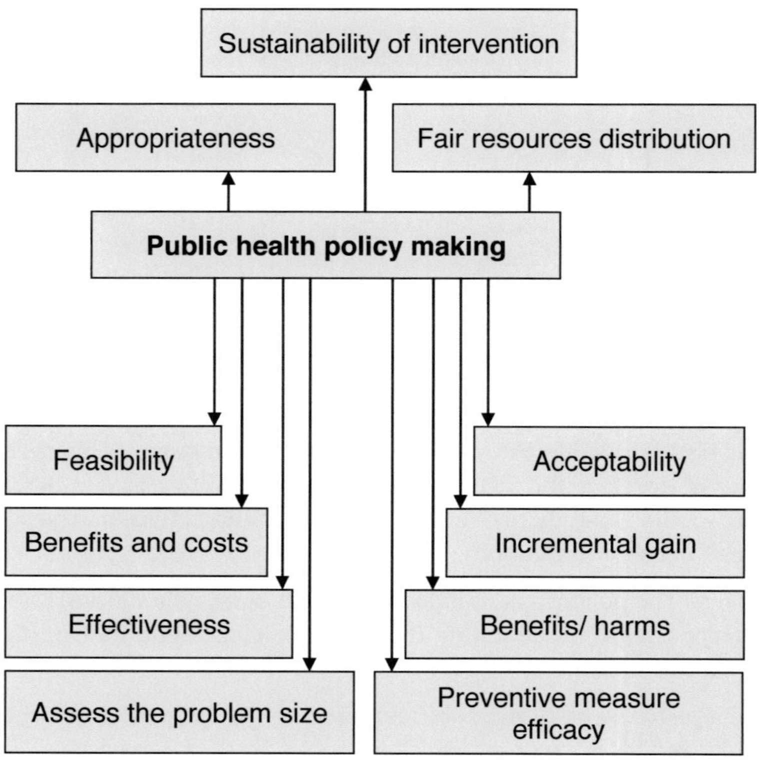

Figure 2. Factors necessary for making public health policy decisions

1. Size of problem: We should always evaluate the problem first, and make sure that it is an important issue with significant health burden.

http://dx.doi.org/10.5772/52643

2. Problem preventability: We should evaluate the efficacy and biological plausibility of the preventive measures before making any decisions.
3. Interventions effectiveness: We should evaluate the effectiveness and generalizability of intervention and make sure that it works in real world settings. We should also analyze the intervention in ideal settings and compare, how much less effective it would be? And, if there is better alternative intervention?
4. Benefits and harms: We should evaluate all the possible benefits and harms of intervention.
5. Comparison of benefits and costs: We should evaluate the total value of intervention and compare it with the possible alternative intervention.
6. Incremental gain: We should also evaluate if there is any additional cost and benefits associated with the intervention we are planning to implement.
7. Feasibility: Feasibility of intervention in prospect of money and time should also be assessed.
8. Acceptability: Acceptability of intervention by community culture and values, as well as by religious and political situations should be evaluated.
9. Appropriateness: Always analyze if the intervention is likely to work in particular settings and various populations?
10. Equitably: Intervention should distribute resources fairly.
11. Sustainability: Can intervention be maintained by available resources and incentives?

2. Analytical tools of evidence based public health

There are several analytical tools which can enhance the adoption of evidence based public health (Figure 3).

2.1. Public health surveillance

Public health surveillance is a very important tool for evidence based public health users. The public health surveillance involves timely and systematic collection, analysis and interpretation of data, and then dissemination of this data to the public health programs, who are responsible for preventing and controlling the disease [24]. To use this data effectively, public health surveillance system should regularly evaluate the effectiveness of disseminated data.

2.2. Systematic review and evidence-based guidelines

To get comprehensive information of any particular research topic, systematic-reviews are crucial, and can be efficient way to become familiar with any specific public health topic

[25-27]. Reviews done with systematic approach are a great source of reliable results, because of limited bias and chance effects. Such results can be used for making decisions in the public health. Guide to Community Preventive Services is one of the most useful sets of review regarding public health interventions, which provides overview of current scientific literature in well defined methods [28].

2.3. Economic evaluation

Another important tool of evidence based practice is economical evaluation, which provides the information about alternative expenditure on public health programs and interventions. Cost-effectiveness analysis compares health interventions with health impacts and outcomes, and can suggest the relative value of alternative interventions and policies [29]. In public health care sector, there is limited data available to support cost-effectiveness analysis for designing policies and programs [30].

2.4. Health impact assessment

Health impact assessment estimate the probable impact of non-health sector interventions on population health, and focus on involving stake holders in project development. Health impact assessment has now been accepted as a tool and is used to assess the potential effects of many health programs and policies on public health status and other outcomes [31, 32].

2.5. Participatory approach

Participatory approach engage communities in the evidence based public heath, by involving communities' members in research and intervention projects [33, 34]. This approach relies on stake-holder's inputs where practitioners and community members define the issues, develop intervention strategies and evaluate the outcomes [35]. Stake holders should include people who would potentially benefit from those particular interventions/policies. Three groups of stake holders are important: those involved in program operations like sponsors, administrators, staff etc.; those affected by the program\interventions like family members, clients, elected officials etc.; and users of the evaluation, including those who decide about the programs.

3. Implementation of evidence based public health and challenges

Implementation of evidence based public health is a process which involves several steps.

3.1. Generating evidence from the research

Biomedical research is the first step in implementation of evidence based public health. Initial testing of innovations occurs mostly in laboratories, from where products/processes with merit undergo field trials to assess the efficacy and toxicity. Those with merits further undergo definite testing in large controlled trials with important clinical endpoints.

http://dx.doi.org/10.5772/52643

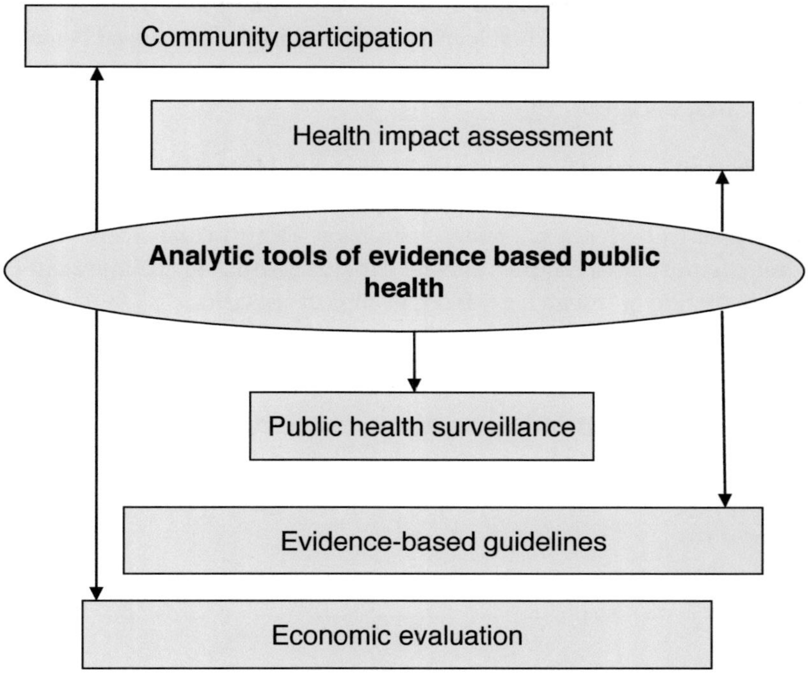

Figure 3. Analytic tools of evidence based public health

3.2. Synthesizing the evidence

Since most of the research results are published in large number of journals, readers are bound to be overwhelmed. Therefore, research results needs to be synthesized in compact format which is ready to be applied in clinical settings. Many services like Cochrane collaboration has taken the initiative to summarize the randomized controlled trials of healthcare interventions, and Cochrane library is a robust source of synthesized evidence [36]. Beside this, advances in information technologies and computerized decision support systems are making practice of evidence based health care system more feasible.

3.3. Developing policies based on evidence

Clinical policies should be both evidence based and clinically useful, therefore policies must balance between strengths and limitations of all the relevant research evidence with the practical reality of clinical settings. There are many non-evidence based factors like culture, religion, ideology etc. which are often considered by policy makers while making the national health care policies. Therefore, clinicians should balance research evidence with clinical circumstances, and should act a part of team planning for change.

3.4. Applying evidence based polices in practice

Once policies are ready, they should be applied at the right time, right place and right away. However certain local and individual level barriers need to be addressed before application.

3.5. Making clinical decisions

Final step in the implementation of evidence based public health is clinical decisions. Research evidence must be integrated with the patient's clinical circumstances, preferences, values and wishes to derive a meaningful decision about management. Evaluating a patient's clinical circumstances requires clinical expertise, which is an important factor for the correct implementation of research evidence in clinical scenarios.

4. Challenges in implementation of evidence based public health

While implementing the evidence based public heath, many challenges are faced as described below (Figure 4):

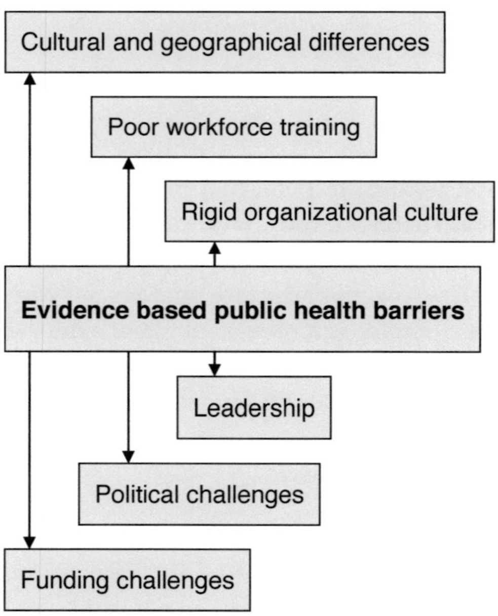
Cultural and geographical differences
Poor workforce training
Rigid organizational culture
Evidence based public health barriers
Leadership
Political challenges
Funding challenges

Figure 4. Barriers of evidence based public health

4.1. Organizational culture

Evidence based public health often relies on the evidence champions, who are willing to challenge the status quo and promote the new ways of decision making. For innovation, it is very important that organization support the changes [37]. Rigid personnel system is a barrier to the evidence based public heath, which make implementation of new programs and approaches difficult. The continuation of old practices requires less effort than working through the new programs. Therefore, persons who propose the new approaches may get opposed and threatened by colleagues and supervisors, who want to continue with the old approaches.

4.2. Leadership

Leaders of the public health system are important factors in determining the organizational culture and use of resources for evidence based approach. Attention of leadership toward science, quality and performance are important predictors of strong public health system [38]. However in public health, leaders have to face challenges in choosing and implementing the evidence based new approaches.

4.3. Political challenges

Political challenges are big barriers in the implementation of evidence based public health. Policy making often occur quickly on the generalized knowledge and demands from the stake holders, rather than being based on the evidence collected though experimental studies by the researchers [39, 40]. Stake holders often create obstacles for public health agencies in implementing the new evidence based interventions. Occasionally, politics want to implement an intervention before there is sufficient evidence to support it e.g. Drug Abuse Resistance Education.

4.4. Funding challenges

Adhering to the requirements of funding agencies is another barrier in the implementation of evidence based public health. Most of the public health funding is categorical and limits the flexible use of funds to implement the new evidence based programs.

4.5. Workforce training

Poor workforce training is common in public health sectors. Less than 50% of the workers in public health sectors have formal training in public health disciplines [41], and even lesser number have formal graduate training from a public health program. Principles of evidence based medicine are not uniformly taught in the public health sectors. However, competencies for effective public health practice are becoming clearer and many new evidence based public programs have been developed to increase the specific training in public health [10]. However for the success of such training programs, life-long learning by leadership and staff are required [42].

4.6. Cultural and geographical differences

There are large differences across the different continents in evidence based public health. Whereas evidence based public health has been mostly developed in western world, use of evidence based approach to meet the public health problems are limited in developing countries [43, 44]. Even in developed world, results published in journal might not be true representative of all the populations of interest.

5. Future perspectives of evidence based medicine in public health

Out of nearly $30 billion spent annually on health related research in United States, only a small proportion of it is spent on public health related research [45]. Translation from research to clinical practice requires long time [17, 46], which needs to be accelerated in future for the early adoption of evidence base interventions, to improve public health.

For early and effective adoption of research based evidence in public health will require intensive efforts in different fields, which include expansion of evidence based research and knowledge, engaging leadership, expanding skillful training in public heath sectors, enhancing the accountability for public expenditures and overcoming the disparities in evidence based public health across the nations, different races, and communities.

In summary, implementation of evidence based public health is a difficult task which requires immediate attention. Public health is both an art and science, which should balance between research based evidence and beneficial policy decisions. Different barriers should be identified successfully, and early efforts are required to overcome these barriers. At the same time, analytic tools of evidence based public health should be utilized properly. By applying these concepts, public health practice can be improved in near future, across the all nations.

Author details

Ajay K Parsaik[1] and Balwinder Singh[2]

1 Department of Neurology,Mayo Clinic College of Medicine, Rochester, Minnesota, USA

2 Division of Pulmonary & Critical Care Medicine, Mayo Clinic, Rochester, Minnesota, USA

References

[1] Sackett DL, Rosenberg WM, Gray JA, Haynes RB, Richardson WS: Evidence based medicine: what it is and what it isn't. BMJ 1996, 312(7023):71-72.

[2] Cook DJ, Sackett DL, Spitzer WO: Methodologic guidelines for systematic reviews of randomized control trials in health care from the Potsdam Consultation on Meta-Analysis. Journal of clinical epidemiology 1995, 48(1):167-171.

[3] The Cochrane Collaboration. The Cochrane Library. www.cochrane.org. Accessed June 4, 2012.

[4] U.S. Preventive Services Task Force. www.ahrq.gov/clinic/uspstfix.htm. Accessed June 3, 2012.

[5] Services TFoCP: The guide to community preventive services. What works to promote health? Oxford University Press, New York 2005, Also available at www.thecommunityguide.org Accessed June 4, 2012.

[6] Fielding JE, Briss PA: Promoting evidence-based public health policy: can we have better evidence and more action? Health affairs 2006, 25(4):969-978.

[7] R.C. Brownson EAB, T.L. Leet, K.N. Gillespie: Evidence-based public health. Oxford University Press, New York 2003.

[8] Brownson RC, Gurney JG, Land GH: Evidence-based decision making in public health. Journal of public health management and practice : JPHMP 1999, 5(5):86-97.

[9] McGinnis JM: Does proof matter? why strong evidence sometimes yields weak action. American journal of health promotion : AJHP 2001, 15(5):391-396.

[10] Dreisinger M, Leet TL, Baker EA, Gillespie KN, Haas B, Brownson RC: Improving the public health workforce: evaluation of a training course to enhance evidence-based decision making. Journal of public health management and practice : JPHMP 2008, 14(2):138-143.

[11] Haynes B, Haines A: Barriers and bridges to evidence based clinical practice. BMJ 1998, 317(7153):273-276.

[12] Baker EL, Potter MA, Jones DL, Mercer SL, Cioffi JP, Green LW, Halverson PK, Lichtveld MY, Fleming DW: The public health infrastructure and our nation's health. Annual review of public health 2005, 26:303-318.

[13] McQueen DV, Anderson LM: What counts as evidence: issues and debates. WHO Reg Publ Eur Ser 2001(92):63-81.

[14] Rimer BK, Glanz K, Rasband G: Searching for evidence about health education and health behavior interventions. Health Educ Behav 2001, 28(2):231-248.

[15] Rychetnik L, Hawe P, Waters E, Barratt A, Frommer M: A glossary for evidence based public health. J Epidemiol Community Health 2004, 58(7):538-545.

[16] Oldenburg BF, Sallis JF, Ffrench ML, Owen N: Health promotion research and the diffusion and institutionalization of interventions. Health Educ Res 1999, 14(1): 121-130.

[17] Brownson RC BE, Leet TL, Gillespie KN: Evidence-Based Public Health. New York: Oxford Univ Press 2003.

[18] Tilson H, Gebbie KM: The public health workforce. Annu Rev Public Health 2004, 25:341-356.

[19] Hausman AJ: Implications of evidence-based practice for community health. Am J Community Psychol 2002, 30(3):453-467.

[20] Black BL, Cowens-Alvarado R, Gershman S, Weir HK: Using data to motivate action: the need for high quality, an effective presentation, and an action context for decision-making. Cancer Causes Control 2005, 16 Suppl 1:15-25.

[21] Green LW: Public health asks of systems science: to advance our evidence-based practice, can you help us get more practice-based evidence? Am J Public Health 2006, 96(3):406-409.

[22] Kerner J, Rimer B, Emmons K: Introduction to the special section on dissemination: dissemination research and research dissemination: how can we close the gap? Health Psychol 2005, 24(5):443-446.

[23] Anderson LM, Brownson RC, Fullilove MT, Teutsch SM, Novick LF, Fielding J, Land GH: Evidence-based public health policy and practice: promises and limits. American journal of preventive medicine 2005, 28(5 Suppl):226-230.

[24] Thacker SB, Berkelman RL: Public health surveillance in the United States. Epidemiol Rev 1988, 10:164-190.

[25] Hutchison BG: Critical appraisal of review articles. Can Fam Physician 1993, 39:1097-1102.

[26] Milne R, Chambers L: Assessing the scientific quality of review articles. J Epidemiol Community Health 1993, 47(3):169-170.

[27] Mulrow CD: The medical review article: state of the science. Ann Intern Med 1987, 106(3):485-488.

[28] Zara S BP, Harris KW, eds: The Guide to Community Preventive Services: What Works to Promote Health? . New York: Oxford Univ Press 2005.

[29] Gold MR SJ, Russell LB, Weinstein MC: Cost-effectiveness in Health and Medicine. New York: Oxford Univ Press 1996.

[30] Brownson RC, Royer C, Ewing R, McBride TD: Researchers and policymakers: travelers in parallel universes. Am J Prev Med 2006, 30(2):164-172.

[31] Cole BL, Wilhelm M, Long PV, Fielding JE, Kominski G, Morgenstern H: Prospects for health impact assessment in the United States: new and improved environmental impact assessment or something different? J Health Polit Policy Law 2004, 29(6): 1153-1186.

[32] Mindell J, Sheridan L, Joffe M, Samson-Barry H, Atkinson S: Health impact assessment as an agent of policy change: improving the health impacts of the mayor of London's draft transport strategy. J Epidemiol Community Health 2004, 58(3): 169-174.

[33] Cargo M, Mercer SL: The value and challenges of participatory research: strengthening its practice. Annu Rev Public Health 2008, 29:325-350.

[34] Israel BA, Schulz AJ, Parker EA, Becker AB: Review of community-based research: assessing partnership approaches to improve public health. Annu Rev Public Health 1998, 19:173-202.

[35] Green LW, Mercer SL: Can public health researchers and agencies reconcile the push from funding bodies and the pull from communities? Am J Public Health 2001, 91(12):1926-1929.

[36] Library TC: Cochrane Collaboration. Oxford: Update Software 1996. Update quarterly.

[37] Simpson DD: A conceptual framework for transferring research to practice. J Subst Abuse Treat 2002, 22(4):171-182.

[38] Scutchfield FD, Knight EA, Kelly AV, Bhandari MW, Vasilescu IP: Local public health agency capacity and its relationship to public health system performance. J Public Health Manag Pract 2004, 10(3):204-215.

[39] Bero LA, Jadad AR: How consumers and policymakers can use systematic reviews for decision making. Ann Intern Med 1997, 127(1):37-42.

[40] Choi BC, Pang T, Lin V, Puska P, Sherman G, Goddard M, Ackland MJ, Sainsbury P, Stachenko S, Morrison H et al: Can scientists and policy makers work together? J Epidemiol Community Health 2005, 59(8):632-637.

[41] BJ T: Public Health: What It Is and How It Works. Gaithersburg, MD: Aspen 2001:354pp.

[42] Chambers LW: The new public health: do local public health agencies need a booster (or organizational "fix") to combat the diseases of disarray? Can J Public Health 1992, 83(5):326-328.

[43] McQueen DV: Strengthening the evidence base for health promotion. Health Promot Int 2001, 16(3):261-268.

[44] McQueen DV: The evidence debate. J Epidemiol Community Health 2002, 56(2): 83-84.

[45] Budget. OoMa: Budget: Department of Health and Human Services. Washington, DC: Exec Off Pres 2008.

[46] Balas EA: From appropriate care to evidence-based medicine. Pediatr Ann 1998, 27(9):581-584.

Section 4

Communicable Diseases in Public Health

Chapter 14

Public Health, Infection and Infectious Agents: The Etiology is Seemingly Always 'Clever'

Erasto Vitus Mbugi

Additional information is available at the end of the chapter

http://dx.doi.org/10.5772/52108

1. Introduction

While humans have been struggling to search for the best means to control infection to humans, infectious agents have been evolving with new means for evading efforts by the body immune defense to arrest infections. We know that infectious agents escape body defense mechanisms through evasion of the immune system or development of resistance to drugs intended to inhibit growth or activity of these organisms. Sometimes using host's resources to flourish and unfairly destroying the host and its resources! Malaria parasite for example, infects human red blood cells, produce clones of itself with different levels of resistance and immune evasion diversity. The virus e.g. retroviruses, use human genetic materials to reproduce their own nucleic acids (reverse transcription) within infected cells, altering planned activities, consequently damaging the host cells! This chapter explores step by step why we can regard infecting organisms as clever than us.

2. Viral infections

Host immune evasion

Existing belief indicates that from primordial soup in which life originated [1], viruses developed together with variety of their hosts. In these past millions of years, the hosts have developed a complex immune defense system against viral infections but the intelligent viruses have though developed strategies to evade these host defences and replicate themselves using host's resources. The host immune response is responsible for defence against viruses and their consequences. It consists of a complex interwoven series of chemical, cytokine and cellular interactions that work in synergy in an attempt to remove these invading viruses from the body. The outcome of viral infections in an animal is determined by a balance between the speed of viral replication and spread, as well as the immune response [2]. Yet, viruses are regarded as important natural means of transferring genes between different species, which increases genetic diversity while in seat to drive evolution [3].

The concern for infections and their evasion strategies arises from the fact that vast of infections and all poverty related infections are predominantly found in Africa, for example HIV/AIDS (Figure 1).

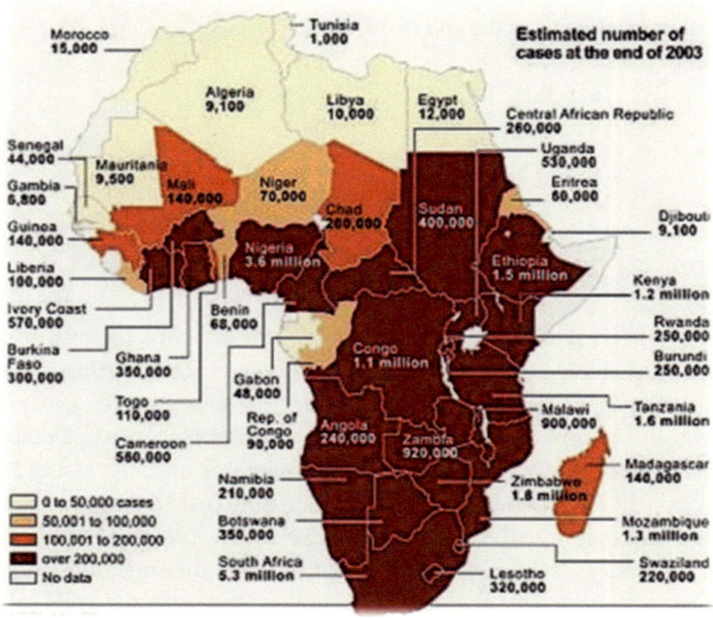

Figure 1. More than two-third of the estimated 39.4 million people living with HIV worldwide are found in Africa. (*Source: UNSAIDS*)

The host immunity consists of innate and adaptive immune responses geared at restraining the viral and other pathogen invasion to keep the host healthy. The innate immune responses comprise of effector cells that include macrophages, neutrophils, natural killer (NK) cells, mast cells, basophils and eosinophils. The humoral component of the innate immune response includes the complement cascade, interferon and a host of cytokines and chemokines associated with inflammation. These cytokines and chemokines interact to attract, activate and control the function of effector cells. NK cells are prime effector cells of the innate immune response to virally infected cells and they act by destroying infected cells through release of effector granules such as perforins and granzymes. Detection of virally infected cells and control of activation is achieved through the balance of activating and inhibitory receptors on the NK cells. All nucleated cells within the body express Major Histocompatibility Complex (MHC)-1 molecule on their surface. MHC-1 molecules bind to receptors (CD94/

NKG2A) on the surface of NK cells and act as inhibitors of NK cell activity. If these MHC-1 molecules are not present or reduced in number on a cell (such as virally infected cell), there is no inhibition of NK cell and the NK cell destroy the infected cell. To counter effect this action by NK cells, the virus cleverly evade this immune protective response through various ways namely: modification of expression of ligands on the surface of the infected cell either increased expression of inhibitory ligands, expression of viral mimics of inhibitory ligands or decreased expression of activating ligands, inhibition of cytokines such as Interferon-γ (IFN-γ) or IL-18, viral molecules that competitively bind IL-18 receptors or disruption of the release of effector molecules like perforins and granzymes. These potentially cleverly strategies enable viruses to escape punishment from host defence, including the complement system, antibodies, interferon, T-cells, cytokines, and programmed cell death, apoptosis [4,5]. Humans have been doing various researches in attempt to block these evasive mechanisms by the virus but the virus always plans different means as though fighting against invading viruses remains to be a vicious cycle.

The remarkable number and the complexities of the virus adaptations to suit the diverse immune response approach by the host poses a challenge to human intelligence on fighting infectious agents. It is said that through virus-host interactions at molecular level, interference occurs through gene regulation that consequently modulates a range of fundamental cellular processes [6]. While it is not surprising that the viruses develop strategies to overcome host defences, the great rapidity with which viruses adapt and replicate within host cells to survive the complex immune mechanisms with multiple adaptations has given the virus an evolutional complement. The virus genome is relatively small as compared to most of its hosts and many viruses produce proteins that act in multiple different ways on different portions of the immune system. This creates a challenge for which best approach should scientists use to counter effect these virus strategical intelligence.

Antiviral Resistance

Anti-viral resistance is an additional issue of concern. Like with other infections, drug resistance to anti-vials and clinical implication has been described [7]. Nevertheless, the management of this drug resistance is suggested to be through optimization of host factors and drug delivery, selection of alternative therapies based on knowledge of mechanisms of resistance, and the development of new antivirals. All these are subject to intelligence by the virus to counter effect, which may be rapid as well! For example, prolonged drug exposure is said to lead to the selection of resistant strains which normally develop via viral mutations necessitating a strategical approach to restraint viral infections [8] which may include testing for resistance to drugs before therapy begins [9]. Proposed ways for possible blockade of immune evasion domains on viruses has been suggested including the suitability of the therapeutic and vaccine efficacy potential [10] but the constantly dynamic and regularly changing strategies for evasion by pathogenic viruses remain a critical challenge. Prescriptions ranging from single to multiple 'cocktail' drugs have been currently been given to people with HIV in an attempt to make emergence of resistance less likely. In such situation, the idea is such that even if a strain evolves resistance to one of the drugs, it will still succumb to other drugs in the combination. However, the virus has been able to evolve resistance to more than one drug, some strains being resistant to all major classes of drugs used to combat the virus [11]. The virus which can develop resistant to reverse transcriptase (RT) inhibitors, protease inhibitors, fusion/entry inhibitors, integrase inhibitors as well as multidrug combinations fielding more than one class into a single product must be far clever than us! With the frequency of cross-resistance between drugs within a class said to be high, it further efforts to control viral replication more complicated [12-15]. This is because to combat virus strains from becoming resistant to specific antiretroviral drugs, healthcare providers have been recommending people infected with HIV to take a combination of highly active antiretroviral drugs therapy (HAART) to enable viruses resistant to single class of drugs not to have an escape route. In addition, some antiretroviral drugs have been combined into one pill, known as a 'fixed dose combination' to reduce the number of pills to be taken each day by the patient. Development of resistance to at least major classes of anti-retroviral drugs is a blow to the HAART strategy of combining drugs from at least two different antiretroviral drug classes for the purpose.

The major control in pathogen control is clearing of susceptible strains while maintaining spread of resistant strains. This is because once there is transmission of drug-resistant strains [16-18], it becomes difficult to contain the pathogen. Mutations in drug target markers is primarily important in development of drug resistance as indicated by Clavel and Hance [19] and genotyping for drug resistance markers by sequencing is a complex technology which presents a challenge for analysis, interpretation, and reporting [20]. This addresses the felt difficulties in containing infectious agents like viruses which are very minute with great survival strategies. The situation could be of substantial impact in sub-Saharan Africa where recent report on antiretroviral drugs indicates significant increase in prevalence resistance over time with possibility of spread of high levels of HIV-1 drug resistance in these resource-limited settings [21]. The findings also caution on possibility of the condition to potentially compromise the effectiveness of HIV treatment programs. An example of drugs and mechanisms of action and development of resistance is revealed in Table 1 with special attention on HIV virus.

Drugs	**Mechanisms of Action**	**Mechanisms of Resistance**
Nucleoside analogues Zidovudine Stavudine Lamivudine Didanosine Zalcitabine Abacavir	Analogues of normal nucleosides Active as triphosphate derivatives Incorporated into nascent viral DNA Prematurely terminate HIV DNA synthesis	Thymidine analogue mutations promote ATP-mediated and pyrophosphate-mediated excision of the incorporated terminator M184V or Q151M complex mutations impair incorporation of nucleoside analogues
Nucleotide analogues Tenofovir	Same as nucleoside analogues	K65R impairs incorporation of tenofovir into DNA

http://dx.doi.org/10.5772/52108

Drugs	Mechanisms of Action	Mechanisms of Resistance
		Thymidine analogue mutations often associated with cross-resistance to tenofovir
Nonnucleoside reverse-transcriptase inhibitors Nevirapine Efavirenz Delavirdine	Bind a hydrophobic pocket of HIV type 1 reverse transcriptase Block polymerization of viral DNA Inactive against HIV type 2	Mutations reduce affinity of the inhibitors for the enzyme Single mutations generally sufficient to induce high level of resistance
Protease inhibitors Saquinavir Ritonavir Indinavir Nelfinavir Amprenavir Lopinavir	Structure derived from natural peptidic substrates of the HIV type 1 protease Bind the active site of the protease	Mutations reduce affinity of the inhibitors for the enzyme High-level resistance requires accumulation of mutations
Fusion inhibitors Enfuvirtide	36-Amino-acid peptide derived from the HR2 domain of glycoprotein 41 Interferes with glycoprotein 41–dependent membrane fusion	Mutations affect HR1, a domain of glycoprotein 41 whose interaction with HR2 promotes membrane fusion

Table 1. Antiretroviral Agents Used in the Treatment of HIV InfectionSource: Clavel F, Hance [19].

3. Bacterial infections

Antigenic variation

One of the important characteristics of the host immune response is antigen-specificity through antibody production. In this context, once the host immune system is exposed to a certain pathogen, it develops a response that is memorable against that pathogen. Similar pathogen with similar proteins (immunologically called antigens) will be recognized as soon as the host encounters same infection. This ability by the host's immune response to remember previously encountered pathogen and act accordingly is termed immunological memory. This intelligence by the host's immune response is however not a big problem to bacterial pathogens. The surveillance by the immune response against invading infectious agents can still be escaped by the clever pathogen like bacteria. One way in which an infectious agent, particularly extracellular pathogens can evade immune surveillance is by altering its antigens against which the principal defence is the production of antibodies against their surface structures. This is called antigenic variation. Antigenic variation can be achieved through, existence in a wide variety of antigenic types by many infectious agents. Other means include antigenic drift (point mutations in the genes encoding for certain antigenic proteins) and programmed rearrangements in the DNA of some pathogens. For example

ability of the enteropathogenic Yersinia enterocolitica to survive and proliferate in host tissue is said to be favoured by suppression of cytokine response that significantly contributes to the evasion of antibacterial host defence against the pathogen [22]. We know that the immune system is highly diverse to counter effect the threats by various antigens from various pathogens but it seems that when we come to evolution, the pathogens evolve faster than the hosts! But why and how these pathogens look like they think ahead of higher organisms (their hosts)? It could mean that as the organism becomes complex the rate of evolution is slow as compared to lower organisms. It is known that the rate of evolutional change is governed by the life span of the species where, short-lived species are capable of changing faster compared to those with a longer life span [23]. On the other side of the coin floods of antigens per episode may probably confuse the stringent host's immune response. Bacterial pathogens for example, are said to dump more than 200 proteins into human macrophage cells, the 'effector proteins' [24]. In addition, these proteins are so similar to the human proteins enabling them to freely interfere with the body's immune response while protecting the pathogen. Despite the fact that even short-lived species such as bacteria, which have generation times measured in minutes, do not manifest noticeable evolutionary changes in a humans lifetime, in some cases, evolution rates can depend on mutation rates [23]. The changes that will definitely influence the survival strategy of the pathogen like bacteria in presence of host like humans and animals.

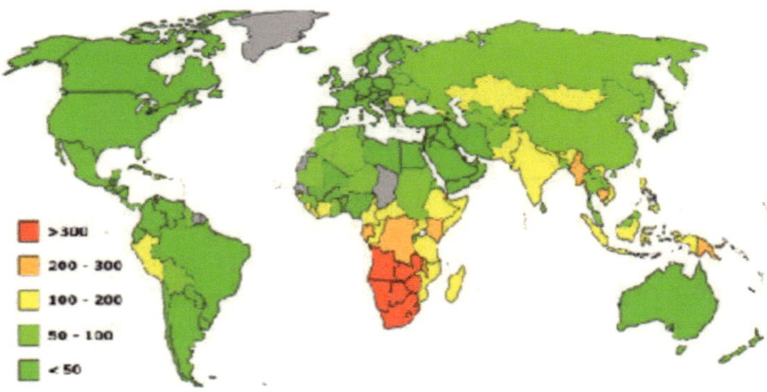

Figure 2. Global distribution of tuberculosis. In sub-Saharan Africa, TB remains the number one cause of death in HIV/Aids patients, and those infected with HIV show a much greater incidence of TB than those who are HIV-negative. WHO statistics do show, however, that HIV-positive adults receiving ARV treatment have substantially lower rates of TB infection than those who are not receiving treatment. This may not be the case following development of antiretroviral drug resistance!Source: http://myfundi.co.za/e/Global_distribution_of_diseases:_TB,_HIV/Aids,_cholera_and_malaria

Drug Resistance

Mimicry allows deadly bacteria to evade host's defense through continued sprouting of antibiotic resistance by simulating human proteins [24]. This process of "molecular mimicry" has led human bacterial pathogens which were at one time easily treatable with antibiotics to

http://dx.doi.org/10.5772/52108

recently re-emerge as highly infectious public health threats. This situation has drawn attention for increased preparedness for emerging and re-emerging diseases [25]. In this context, the suggested 'fit-for purpose' approaches such as the inter-discipline merging with a focus on 'one health' approach, use of participatory epidemiology and disease surveillance and mobile technologies may offer opportunity for optimal use of limited resources to improve early detection, diagnosis and response to disease events which could eventually reduce the impact of such diseases to animal and human populations.

Antibiotic resistance bears serious importance in public health. In both humans and animals, drug resistant bacteria have been a threat to health and economy due to costs incurred in an attempt to contain the disease situation which may finally not work out. This resistance may be natural or develop after antibiotic use. In bacteria, induction of changes in ability to become antibiotic resistant is influenced by mutations which could be evolutional. This is despite mutations seemingly not having major effects on limiting evolution as diversity in morphological evolution (evolution of physical characteristics) has been found not to correlate well with DNA mutation rates [23]. With mutations, bacteria which were once susceptible to certain antibiotics are currently no longer controlled or killed by those antibiotics, the bacteria being able to survive and even multiply in the presence of a respective antibiotic agent. We have observed this in chronic diseases such as tuberculosis, bovine mastitis and many other bacterial diseases. Genome sequencing has indicated a known family of kinases circulating in modern drug resistant pathogens reflecting the prevalence of resistance even in microbiomes isolated from human use of antibiotics [26]. Bacterial resistance to formally useful drugs occur in such ways as preventing the antibiotic from getting to its target through changing the cell permeability for the drug or use ATP to pump drugs outside the cell, thus reducing the chances that the drug will kill the bacteria. Other means incudes changing the structure of the target for the drug such that the antibiotic can no longer recognize or bind to it. In addition, bacteria may destroy the drug through production of say, beta-lactamases that directly neutralize penicillin. Acquisition of resistance by bacteria may be achieved through transformation, transposon and scavenging of DNA remnants from other degraded bacteria. These all are intelligence by the pathogen that needs no higher organisms (hosts like human and animals) assistance but own capabilities. One would wonder where these sorts of intelligence come from.

4. Parasitic infections

An example of well-studied tropical infectious parasite is the malaria parasite, Plasmodium falciparum. A lot of challenges have been posed to scientific community as regards immune evasion by the malaria parasite due to its ability to overwhelm the impact of host's immune response and through resistance to drugs of choice for the disease. Various researches in immunology have in principle shown parasite evasion of host immunity to be ubiquitous involving a wide range of molecular mechanisms [27]. Immune evasion generates a large spectrum of pathogenic effects, such as cytokine blows and inflammation. The relationships between the benefits of immune evasion and its pathogenic consequences could reflect evolutional and ecological host–parasite interactions. Such interactions have impacts on the dose, parasite virulence, immune defence strategies, immunopathology and host specificity [27]. Protective immunity to malaria for example is won by the parasite through its strategies used to evade host immunity, including antigen diversity/polymorphisms, antigen variation and total immune suppression [28].

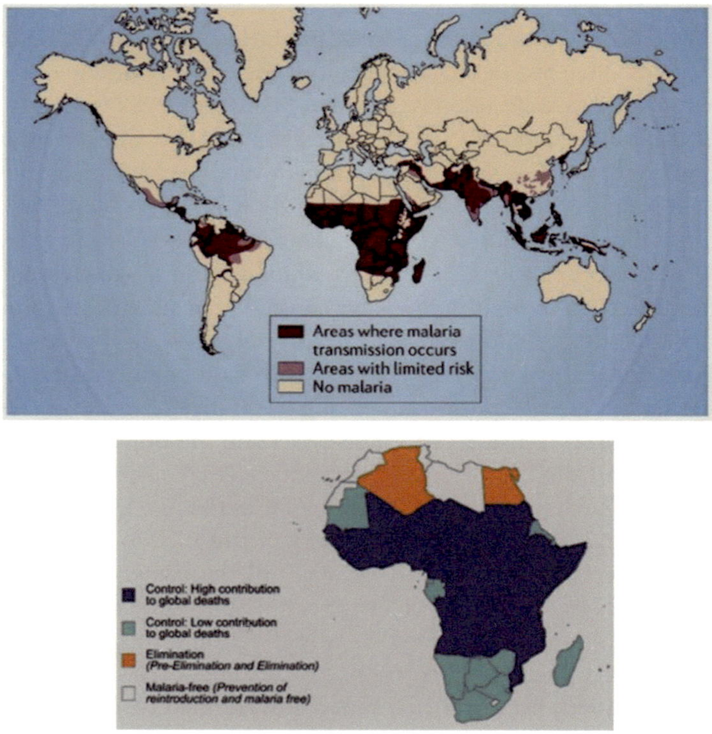

Figure 3. a:distribution of parasitic diseases, an example of malaria. See (figure above) the concentration of the disease insub-Saharan Africa. Source: http://www.nature.com/nrmicro/journal/v4/n9_supp/fig_tab/nrmicro1525_F2.html b:Despite the global distribution of malaria, high deaths are concentrated in Africa, south of Sahara where it also contributes to high deaths. This parasitic disease, despite antigen diversity, it is also resistant to most antimalarial drugs designed to restrain the disease. Consequently, the disease cause global economic and social burdens [29] particularly predominating in African countries. Source: http://www.nature.com/nrmicro/journal/v4/n9_supp/fig_tab/nrmicro1525_F2.html

Evidence from population genomics of the immune evasion (var) genes of Plasmodium falciparum [30] suggests recombination to play a key role in maintaining the extraordinary levels of polymorphism found in the immune evasion genes. Most malaria vaccine-candidate antigens have highly polymorphic surface proteins that elicit variant-specific immunity [31]. Nevertheless, this antigenic diversity is still beaten by an evasive malaria parasite as though no vaccine yet to arrest malaria troubles in endemic areas. Exploration on evolutional relationships for the design of vaccines based on ancestral sequences, with the potential for inducing

http://dx.doi.org/10.5772/52108

cross-protection against a wide range of antigenic variants [32] has been proposed, but the parasite always seems to be ahead of the scientific community. Thus, despite efforts for understanding the mechanisms and patterns of genetic recombination and sequence variation designing vaccines that represent the worldwide repertoire of polymorphic malarial surface antigens may be difficult due to dynamic continuum of antigenic variation in the parasite.

Drug resistance is another way apart from immune evasion that the parasite uses to win the battle against host efforts to fight parasitic infections. A range of drugs for example has been used for malaria treatment over decades but have ended disapprovingly through development of drug resistance. Similar strategies have been used by other parasites in animals as well as in humans. Drug resistance and genetic studies on P. falciparum have revealed a limited geographical genetic diversity in a genetically homogeneous parasite population [33]. Studies on competitive facilitation of drug-resistant Plasmodium falciparum malaria have indicated the most highly resistant parasites to out-compete less fit parasite populations [34]. Consequently, these resistant strains overgrow under drug pressure posing a great threat that at one moment there might be an existence of a parasite population which is highly resistant to drug use. Systematic mapping of genetic variation in Plasmodium falciparum to locate other loci that can facilitate parasite drug resistance [35] is important. However, all these efforts will be of value to the scientific community if we will finally be able to contain the parasite than it being always a hero.

5. Fungal infections

Under the kingdom of Fungi are many species with a wide spectrum of diseases that can infect humans and other animals most of which being accidentally originating from exogenous sources by inhalation (e.g. Aspergillus spp., Cryptococcus neoformans or endemic mycoses) but also as commensals of the gastrointestinal tract (e.g. Candida spp.) or reactivation of a latent infection [36]. Clinical manifestation and severity of fungal infections, including transition from potentially commensals to infections depends on the patient's immune response, the host-pathogen interaction and ability of the infecting pathogenic fungus to evade the host immune response [37-40]. Like other infections, the immunity to fungal infections comprises of both innate and adaptive responses. These host defence mechanisms require induction and activation after infection through invariant molecular structures shared by large groups of pathogens (collectively called pathogen-associated molecular patterns, PAMPs) which are recognized by a set of pattern recognition receptors (PRRs) in the host immune defence cells, including Toll-like receptors (TLRs) [41]. However, intelligent is the host's defence, the fungus can defend better! Thus the fungus has developed a variety of evasive mechanisms to escape host defence while nourishing themselves within host's resources.

Immune evasion in fungal infections is not uncommon phenomenon. A pathogen with a variety of strategies enabling its effective survival within the host while able to evade immune detection to overcome the smart host immune response is said to be successful. The well-known strategies employed by fungal pathogens to evade host defense mechanisms includes shielding of stimulatory PAMPs, modulation of inflammatory signals, shedding of distraction components, persistence in intracellular environments and complement evasion [42]. Among evasion mechanisms to overcome both innate and adaptive immunity by some fungal infections is phase transition through expression of yeast-phase specific genes and alteration of cell wall components [43]. In Candida albicans infection, specific enzyme is secreted to degrade and deactivate a host antimicrobial peptide involved in the protection of the oral mucosa against the fungus thus enhancing its transition from commensal to pathogen [44].

Similar to other infections, fungal immune evasion when coupled with resistance to potential antifungal drugs poses a setback towards arresting diseases; their clinical and pathological consequences. Further, we have to admit diagnosis, epidemiology and mechanisms of antifungal drug resistance [45] to be a challenge in control of fungal infections. A recent study [46] for instance, has revealed geographic variations in fungal species and antifungal resistance rates distribution among isolates pointing out a focused surveillance on emerging resistance patterns in Candida infection (see Table 2). The study does not cover African continent but should be taken as a warning alarm for the potential risks developing countries like those in Africa may similarly be facing. Antifungal resistance has also been surveyed in Aspergillus species using molecular tools showing resistance potential for multiple antifungal drugs [47]. In the same study, new species were in addition, identified which could reflect emergence of new fungal species potentially resistant to drugs. Importantly, it is a reflection that screening using advanced tools may help to restrain disease transmission through procedures such as transplantation and blood transfusion. Surveillance networks that incorporate sequence-based identification of clinical isolates to determine the species distribution, the clinical disease and outcome of patients with invasive fungal species have been suggested [48]. Factors driving fungal composition are primarily global and indoor fungal composition is again said to be geographically patterned with more diversity observed in temperate zones than in the tropics [49]. But the proposition should be viewed with special precaution not to rule out the situation to similarly occur in the tropics. This is particularly critical as fungi are ubiquitous components of indoor human environments, with most contact between humans and microbes probable thus raising the possibility of contribution to spread of resistant strains during disease transmission. The idea is that application of antifungal drugs will definitely kill susceptible strains leaving resistant strains to prevail and circulate in the community of hosts they infect.

Available reports indicate a change in epidemiology of systemic fungal infections citing the key elements in selection of appropriate antifungal agent which include; the type of patient (solid-organ or stem-cell transplant), severity of immunosuppression, history of prolonged exposure to antifungal drugs, and knowledge of the genera and species of the infecting pathogen and its typical susceptibility pattern [50]. Canonn et al. [51] pointed out on efflux-mediated antifungal drug resistance with a list of antifungal drugs, their targets and possible resistance mechanisms. The authors finally, suggest among other approaches that scientists can deploy to identify and possibly design multifunctional drugs that inhibit conventional targets as well as the transcription factors responsible for the overexpression of efflux pumps and the pumps themselves. This idea was also previously addressed by Monk

http://dx.doi.org/10.5772/52108

and Goffeau [52]. But we should bear in mind that despite these all efforts, the microbes, having no laboratories for designing and formulating mechanisms for survival in the host, can still generate resistance markers through genetic mutations and other gene rearrangements. Concerns regarding the development of resistance to even the available few antifungal drugs have been raised [53] and new diagnostic tools for rapid, sensitive, and specific detection of fungi in clinical material has been proposed to be a mandatory for effective discovery and designing of appropriate drugs [54]. But how fast and quick are we ahead of the 'microbe thinking'? I always think that, if it was learning, then the microbes have been learning faster than human beings! Who amongst us can agree this view? It is through surveillance on infections, immunity, chemotherapeutics, evolutional characteristics and differences between lower and higher organisms that we can get answers.

Species	**% of isolates by species and geographic region (n[b])**				
	Asia-Pacific (51)	**Latin America (348)**	**Europe (750)**	**North America (936)**	**Total (2,085)**
C. albicans	56.9	43.6	55.2	43.4	48.41
C. glabrata	13.7	5.2	15.7	23.5	18.0
C. parapsilosis	13.7	25.6	13.7	17.1	17.2
C. tropicalis	11.7	17.0	7.3	10.5	10.5
C. krusei	2.0	1.4	2.5	1.6	1.9
C. lusitaniae	0.0	0.9	1.2	2.2	1.6
C. dubliniensis	0.0	0.3	0.8	1.0	0.8
C. guilliermondii	0.0	1.7	0.1	0.1	0.4
Misc.[a]	2.0	1.6	1.7	0.6	1.2

Table 2. Species distribution of Candida bloodstream infection isolates across geographic regions out of African continentsSpecies distribution of Candida bloodstream infection isolates across geographic regions: SENTRY Surveillance Program, 2008 to 2009. [a]Miscellaneous species including 6 isolates of C. kefyr, 2 each of C. rugosa, C. sake, and C. pelliculosa, 3 each of C. famata and C. lipolytica, and 1 each of C. lambica, C. utilis, C. haemulonii, C. norvegensis, and C. inconspicua.n[b]: number tested.Source: Pfaller et al. [46].

6. Summary

This chapter has discussed in brief, the human infectious agents, host immune response, immune evasion and drug resistance to various anti-pathogen drugs. The chapter highlighted how smart is the host's immune defence mechanisms against infectious agents and how the pathogens device mechanisms for escape and survival within host's territory. The net balance between host defence and pathogen defence evasion is the one which determines the fate of infection to either resolve or develop to clinical disease plus its pathological consequences. In most cases it seems the pathogen wins the battle due to its always far ahead 'thinking' for counter strategies. It remains a question as to whether the pathogens are clever than their hosts, including humans or is just a miss by human efforts to capture relevant pathogenic factors without which the infecting organisms would be harmless. The scientific community is highly acknowledged for the efforts and a synergistic multi-disciplinary approach to control striking infections, particularly those with cross-transmission to animals other than human beings (zoonotic infections). The concern is that with time, the selected resistant or immune evasive strains will remain in circulation within human and animal population making control extremely difficult. Consequently, it raises a worry that probably higher organisms have fewer chances for successful life in presence of lower organisms. Several efforts in research including experimental, clinical and immunological potential impact of improved nutrition to specific infections have been in place [54-69]. Despite these efforts, however, vaccine and drug developments have been made difficult by the tricky survival strategies by pathogens making improvement in health focusing in nutrition not as good as might be if the pathogens were not that clever. The remaining challenge is how to bring together willing interested partners (stakeholders) for joint efforts in control of diseases. Attention should also be directed to zoonotic infections such as tuberculosis whose resistance may develop in one species and be detrimental to other species for instance drug resistant Mycobacterium bovis from cattle infecting humans. The 'one health' concept in such circumstances will stand a greater chance of playing a role in limiting transmission of the diseases across species.

Acknowledgements

Muhimbili University of Health and Allied sciences (MUHAS), my employer is acknowledged for granting time and support to prepare this chapter.

Author details

Erasto Vitus Mbugi*

Address all correspondence to: rerasto@yahoo.com

Biochemistry Department, School of Medicine, Muhimbili University of health and Allied Sciences, P.O. Box 65001, Dar es Salaam, Tanzania

References

[1] Strauss, E. G., Strauss, J. H., & Levine, A. J. (1996). Virus evolution. *Fields BN, Knipe DM, and Howley PM. (ed.) Fundamental virology, 3rd ed. New York: Raven Press*, 141-159.

[2] Diamond, M. S. (2003). Evasion of innate and adaptive immunity by flaviviruses. *Immunology and Cell Biology*, 81, 196-206.

[3] Canchaya, C., Fournous, G., Chibani-Chennoufi, S., Dillmann, M. L., & Brüssow, H. (2003). Phage as agents of lateral gene transfer. *Current. Opinion in Microbiology*, 6(4), 417-24.

[4] Alcami, A., & Koszinowski, U. H. (2000). Viral mechanisms of immune evasion. *Immunology Today*, 21, 447-455.

[5] Tortorella, D., Gewurz, B. E., Furman, M. H., Schust, D. J., & Ploegh, H. L. (2000). Viral subversion of the immune system. *Annual Review of Immunology*, 18, 861-926.

[6] Skalsky, R. L., & Cullen, B. R. (2010). Viruses, microRNAs, and Host Interactions. *Annual Review of Microbiology*, 64(1), 123-141.

[7] Strasfeld, L., & Chou, S. (2010). Antiviral Drug Resistance: Mechanisms and Clinical Implications. *Infectious Disease Clinics of North America*, 24(2), 413-437.

[8] Gammon, D. B., Snoeck, R., Fiten, P., Krecmerova, M., Holy, A., De Clercq, E., Opdenakker, G., Evans, D. H., & Andrei, G. (2008). Mechanism of Antiviral Drug Resistance of Vaccinia Virus: Identification of Residues in the Viral DNA Polymerase Conferring Differential Resistance to Antipoxvirus Drugs. *Journal of Virology*, 82(24), 12520-12534.

[9] Little, S. J., Holte, S., Routy-P, J., Daar, E. S., Markowitz, M., Collier, A. C., Koup, R. A., Mellors, J. W., Connick, E., Conway, B., Kilby, M., Wang, L., Whitcomb, J. M., Hellmann, N. S., & Richman, D. D. (2002). Antiretroviral-Drug Resistance among Patients Recently Infected with HIV. *New England Journal of Medicine*, 347(6), 385-394.

[10] Judson, K. A., Lubinski, J. M., Jiang, M., Chang, Y., Eisenberg, R. J., Cohen, G. H., & Friedman, H. M. (2003). Blocking Immune Evasion as a Novel Approach for Prevention and Treatment of Herpes Simplex Virus Infection. *Journal of Virology*, 77(23), 12639-12645.

[11] Shafer, R. W., Winters, MA, Palmer, S., & Merigan, T. C. (1998). Multiple concurrent reverse transcriptase and protease mutations and multidrug resistance of HIV-1 isolates from heavily treated patients. *Annals of Internal Medicine*, 128, 906-911.

[12] Hertogs, K., Bloor, S., Kemp, S. D., Van den, Eynde. C., Alcorn, T. M., Pauwels, R., Van Houtte, M., Staszewski, S., Miller, V., & Larder, AA. (2000). Phenotypic and genotypic analysis of clinical HIV-1 isolates reveals extensive protease inhibitor cross-resistance: a survey of over 6000 samples. *AIDS*, 14, 1203-1210.

[13] Richman, D. D. (1990). Susceptibility to nucleoside analogues of zidovudine-resistant isolates of human immunodeficiency virus. *American Journal of Medicine*, 88, 8S-10S.

[14] Miller, V., & Larder, BA. (2001). Mutational patterns in the HIV genome and cross-resistance following nucleoside and nucleotide analogue drug exposure. *Antiviral therapy*, 6(3), 25-44.

[15] Race, E., Dam, E., Obry, V., Paulous, S., & Clavel, F. (1999). Analysis of HIV cross-resistance to protease inhibitors using a rapid single-cycle recombinant virus assay for patients failing on combination therapies. *AIDS*, 13, 2061-8.

[16] Yerly, S., Kaiser, L., Race, E., Bru, J. P., Clavel, F., & Perrin, L. (1999). Transmission of antiretroviraldrug-resistant HIV-1 variants. *Lancet*, 354, 729-733.

[17] Little, S. J., Holte, S., Routy-P, J., Daar, E. S., Markowitz, M., Collier, A. C., Koup, R. A., Mellors, J. W., Connick, E., Conway, B., Kilby, M., Wang, L., Whitcomb, J. M., Hellmann, N. S., & Richman, D. D. (2002). Antiretroviral-drug resistance among patients recently infected with HIV. *New England Journal of Medicine*, 347(6), 385-394.

[18] Grant, R. M., Hecht, F. M., Warmerdam, M., Liu, L., Liegler, T., Petropoulos, C. J., Hellmann, N. S., Chesney, M., Busch, M. P., & Kahn, J. O. (2002). Time trends in primary HIV-1 drug resistance among recently infected persons. *The Journal of the American Medical Association*, 288, 181-188.

[19] Clavel, F., & Hance, A. J. (2004). HIV Drug Resistance. *New England Journal of Medicine*, 350, 1023-1035.

[20] Erali, E., Page, S., Reimer, L. G., & Hillyard, D. R. (2001). Human Immunodeficiency Virus Type 1 Drug Resistance Testing: a Comparison of Three Sequence-Based Methods. *Journal of Clinical Microbiology*, 39(6), 2157-2165.

[21] Gupta, R. K., Jordan, M. R., Sultan, B. J., Hill, A., Davis, D. H. J., Gregson, J., Sawyer, A. W., Hamers, R. L., Ndembi, N., Pillay, D., & Bertagnolio, S. (2012). Global trends in antiretroviral resistance in treatment-naive individuals with HIV after rollout of antiretroviral treatment in resource-limited settings: a global collaborative study and meta-regression analysis. *The Lancet*, 10.1016/S0140-6736(12)61038-1.

[22] Beuscher, H. U., Rödel, F., Forsberg, A., & Röllinghoff, M. (1995). Bacterial evasion of host immune defense: Yersinia enterocolitica encodes a suppressor for tumor necrosis factor alpha expression. *Infection and Immunity*, 63(4), 1270-1277.

[23] http://science.jrank.org/pages/2612/Evolutionary-Change-Rate.html, first accessed 24 January 2012.

[24] Champion, M. (2011). http://www.news-medical.net/news/20110603/Mimicry-allows-bacteria-to-evade-hosts-defense-responses.aspx.

[25] Karimuribo, E., Mboera, L. E. G., Mbugi, E., Simba, A., Kivaria, F. M., Mmbuji, P., & Rweyemamu, MM. (2012). Are we prepared for emerging and re-emerging diseases? Experience and lessons from epidemics that occurred in Tanzania during the last five decades. *Tanzania Journal of Health Research*, 13(1), 1-14.

[26] Bhullar, K., Waglechner, N., Pawlowski, A., Koteva, K., Banks, E. D., Johnston, M. D., Barton, H. A., & Wright, G. D. (2012). Antibiotic Resistance Is Prevalent in an Isolated Cave Microbiome. *PLoS ONE*, 7(4), e34953.

[27] Schmid-Hempel, P. (2009). Immune defence, parasite evasion strategies and their relevance for 'macroscopic phenomena' such as virulence. *Philosophical Transactions of the Royal Society B*, 364, 85-98.

[28] Hisaeda, H., Yasutomo, K., & Himeno, K. (2005). Malaria: immune evasion by parasites. *The International Journal of Biochemistry and Cell Biology*, 37(4), 700-706.

[29] Sachs, J., & Malaney, P. (2002). The economic and social burden of malaria. *Nature*, 415, 680-685.

[30] Barry, A. E., Leliwa-Sytek, A., Tavul, L., Imrie, H., Migot-Nabias, F., Brown, S. M., Mc Vean, G. A. V., & Day, K. P. (2007). Population Genomics of the Immune Evasion (var) Genes of Plasmodium falciparum. *PLoS Pathogens*, 3(3), e34.

[31] Ferreira, M. U., Nunes, MD, & Wunderlich, G. (2004). Antigenic diversity and immune evasion by malaria parasites. *Clinical and Diagnostic Laboratory Immunology*, 11(6), 987-995.

[32] Gaschen, B., Taylor, J., Yusim, K., Foley, B., Gao, F., Lang, D., Novitsky, V., Haynes, B., Hahn, B. H., Bhattacharya, T., & Korber, B. (2002). Diversity considerations in HIV-1 vaccine selection. *Science*, 296, 2354-2360.

[33] Peek, R., Van Gool, T., Panchoe, D., Greve, S., Bus, E., & Resida, L. (2005). Drug resistance and genetic diversity of Plasmodium falciparum parasites from suriname. *American Journal of Tropical Medicine and Hygiene*, 73(5), 833-838.

[34] Harrington, W. E., Mutabingwa, T. K., Muehlenbachs, A., Sorensen, B., Bolla, M. C., Fried, M., & Duffy, P. E. (2009). Competitive facilitation of drug-resistant Plasmodium falciparum malaria parasites in pregnant women who receive preventive treatment. *Proceedings of the National Academy of Sciences*, 106(22), 9027-9032.

[35] Kidgell, C., Volkman, S. K., Daily, J., Borevitz, J. O., Plouffe, D., Zhou, Y., Johnson, J. R., Le Roch, K., Sarr, O., Ndir, O., Mboup, S., Batalov, S., Wirth, D. F., & Winzeler, E. A. (2006). A systematic map of genetic variation in Plasmodium falciparum. *PLoS Pathogens*, 2(6), e57.

[36] Romani, L. (2001). Overview of the fungal pathogens. *Kaufmann SHE, Sher A, Ahmed R. (eds.). Washington DC: ASM Press*, 25-37.

[37] Romani, L. (2004). Immunity to fungal infections. *Nature Reviews Immunology*, 4(1), 1-23.

[38] Marr, K. A., Patterson, T., & Denning, D. (2002). Aspergillosis: Pathogenesis, clinical manifestations, and therapy. *Infectious Disease Clinics of North America*, 16, 875-894.

[39] Fidel, P. L. Jr, & Sobel, JD. (1994). The role of cell-mediated immunity in candidiasis. *Trends in Microbiology*, 2, 202-206.

[40] Puccetti, P., Romani, L., & Bistoni, F. (1995). A Th1-Th2-like switch in candidiasis: new perspectives for therapy. *Trends Microbiol*, 3, 237-240.

[41] Abbas, A. K., & Lichtman, A. H. (2003). Cellular and Molecular Immunology. *Fifth Edition edn. Philadephia: Elsevier Science (USA).*

[42] Chai, L. Y. A., Netea, M. G., Vonk, A. G., & Kulliberg-J, B. (2009). Fungal strategies for overcoming host innate immune response. *Medical Mycology*, 47, 227-236.

[43] Gauthier, G., & Klein, BS. (2008). Insights into Fungal Morphogenesis and Immune Evasion: Fungal conidia, when situated in mammalian lungs, may switch from mold to pathogenic yeasts or spore-forming spherules. *Microbe Washington DC*, 3(9), 416-423.

[44] Meiller, T. F., Hube, B., Schild, L., Shirtliff, M. E., Scheper, M. A., Winkler, R., Ton, A., & Jabra-Rizk, M. A. (2009). A Novel Immune Evasion Strategy of Candida albicans: Proteolytic cleavage of a salivary antimicrobial peptide. *PLoS ONE*, 4(4), e5039.

[45] Chamilos, G., & Kontoyiannis, D. P. (2005). Update on antifungal drug resistance mechanisms of Aspergillus fumigatus. *Drug Resistance Updates*, 8(6), 344-58.

[46] Pfaller, M. A., Moet, G. J., Messer, S. A., Jones, R. N., & Castanheira, M. (2011). Geographic Variations in Species Distribution and Echinocandin and Azole Antifungal Resistance Rates among Candida Bloodstream Infection Isolates: Report from the SENTRY Antimicrobial Surveillance Program (2008 to 2009). *Journal of Clinical Microbiology*, 49(1), 396-399.

[47] Balajee, S. A., Kano, R., Baddley, J. W., Moser, S. A., Marr, K. A., Alexander, B. D., Andes, D., Kontoyiannis, D. P., Perrone, G., Peterson, S., Brandt, M. E., Pappas, P. G., & Chiller, T. (2009). Molecular Identification of Aspergillus Species Collected for the Transplant-Associated Infection Surveillance Network. *Journal of Clinical Microbiology*, 47(10), 3138-3141.

[48] van der Linden, J. W. M., Warris, A., & Verweij, P. E. (2011). Aspergillus species intrinsically resistant to antifungal agents. *Medical Mycologyl*, 49(1), S82-S89.

[49] Amend, AS, Seifert, K. A., Samson, R., & Bruns, T. D. (2010). Indoor fungal composition is geographically patterned and more diverse in temperate zones than in the tropics. *Proceedings of the National Academy of Sciences*, 107(31), 13748-13753.

[50] Richardson, M., & Lass-Flörl, C. (2008). Changing epidemiology of systemic fungal infections. *Clinical Microbiology and Infection*, 14(4), 5-24.

[51] Cannon, R. D., Lamping, E., Holmes, A. R., Niimi, K., Baret, P. V., Keniya, M. V., Tanabe, K., Niimi, M., Goffeau, A., & Monk, B. C. (2009). Efflux-mediated antifungal drug resistance. *Clinical Microbiology Review*, 22(2), 291-321.

[52] Monk, B. C., & Goffeau, A. (2008). Outwitting multidrug resistance to antifungals. *Science*, 321, 367-369.

[53] Loeffler, L., & Stevens, D. A. (2003). Antifungal drug resistance. *Clinical Infectious Diseases*, 36(1), S31-41.

http://dx.doi.org/10.5772/52108

[54] Stevens, D. A., & Holmberg, K. (1999). Resistance to antifungal drugs: current status and clinical implications. *Current opinion in anti-infective investigational drugs*, 1, 306-317.

[55] Prasad, A. S. (1998). Zinc in human health: An update. *The Journal of Trace Elements in Experimental Medicine*, 11(2-3), 63-87.

[56] Prasad, A. S. (1998). Zinc and immunity. *Molecular and Cellular Biochemistry*, 188(1-2), 63-69.

[57] Prasad, A. S. (2008). Zinc in Human Health: Effect of Zinc on Immune Cells. *Molecular Medicine*, 14(5-6), 353-357.

[58] Mbugi, E. V., Meijerink, M., Veenemans, J., Jeurink, P. V., Mc Call, M., Olomi, R. M., Shao, J. F., Verhoef, H., & Savelkoul, H. F. J. (2010). Alterations in early cytokine-mediated immune responses to Plasmodium falciparum infection in Tanzanian children with mineral element deficiencies: a cross-sectional survey. *Malaria Journal*, 9(1), 130.

[59] Mbugi, E. V., Meijerink, M., Veenemans, J., Jeurink, P. V., Mc Call, M., Olomi, R. M., Shao, Chilongola. J. O., Verhoef, H., & Savelkoul, H. F. J. (2010). Effect of nutrient deficiencies on in vitro Th1 and Th2 cytokine response of peripheral blood mononuclear cells to Plasmodium falciparum infection. *Malaria Journal*, 9(1), 162.

[60] Savino, W., & Dardenne, M. (2010). Micronutrients and the immune system Nutritional imbalances and infections affect the thymus: consequences on T-cell-mediated immune responses. *Proceedings of the Nutrition Society*, 69, 636-643.

[61] Shvetsov, Y. B., Hernandez, B. Y., Wilkens, L. R., Thompson, P. J., Franke, AA, Zhu, X., & Goodman, M. T. (2010). Plasma Micronutrients and the Acquisition and Clearance of Anal Human Papillomavirus Infection: The Hawaii HPV Cohort Study. *Cancer Research*, 70(23), 9787-9797.

[62] Alexander, S., Maike, W., & Andreas, H. (2011). Micronutrients at the Interface Between Inflammation and Infection Ascorbic Acid and Calciferol. Part 1: General Overview with a Focus on Ascorbic Acid. *Inflammation and Allergy- Drug Targets*, 10(1), 54-63.

[63] Liu, Y., Jing, H., Wang, J., Zhang, R., Zhang, Y., Zhang, Y., Xu, Q., Yu, X., & Xue, C. (2011). Micronutrients decrease incidence of common infections in type 2 diabetes outpatients. *Asia Pacific Journal of Clinical Nutrition*, 20(3), 375-382.

[64] Taylor, C. E., & Camargo, C. A. Jr. (2011). Impact of micronutrients on respiratory infections. *Nutrition Reviews*, 69(5), 259-269.

[65] Veenemans, J., Mank, T., Ottenhof, M., Baidjoe, A., Mbugi, E. V., Demir, A. Y., Wielders, J. P. M., Savelkoul, H. F. J., & Verhoef, H. (2011). Protection against Diarrhea Associated with Giardia intestinalis Is Lost with Multi-Nutrient Supplementation: A Study in Tanzanian Children. *PLoS Neglected Tropical Diseases*, 5(6), e1158.

[66] Veenemans, J., Milligan, P., Prentice, A. M., Schouten, L. R., Inja, N., van der Heijden, A. C., De Boer, L. C., Jansen, E. J., Koopmans, A. E., Enthoven, W. T., Kraaijenhagen, R. J., Demir, A. Y., Uges, D. R., Mbugi, E. V., Savelkoul, H., & Verhoef, H. (2011). Effects of zinc and other micronutrients on malaria in Tanzanian children: a randomised trial. *PLoS Medicine*, 8(11), e1001125.

[67] Dekker, L. H., Fijnvandraat, K., Brabin, B. J., & van Hensbroek, M. B. (2012). Micronutrients and sickle cell disease, effects on growth, infection and vaso-occlusive crisis: A systematic review. *Pediatric Blood and Cancer*, 59(2), 211-215.

[68] Lahner, E., Persechino, S., & Annibale, B. (2012). Micronutrients (Other than iron) and Helicobacter pylori Infection: A Systematic Review. *Helicobacter*, 17(1), 1-15.

[69] Reilly, L., Nausch, N., Midzi, N., Mduluza, T., & Mutapi, F. (2012). Association between Micronutrients (Vitamin A, D, Iron) and Schistosome-Specific Cytokine Responses in Zimbabweans Exposed to Schistosoma haematobium. *Journal of Parasitology Research*, 2012, 1-9.

Chapter 15

Epidemiological Burden of Tuberculosis in Developing Countries

Diana M. Castañeda-Hernández and
Alfonso J. Rodriguez-Morales

Additional information is available at the end of the chapter

http://dx.doi.org/10.5772/53363

1. Introduction

Tuberculosis (TB) is an infectious disease caused by different species of the genus *Mycobacteria*. Together with human immunodeficiency virus infection (HIV)/Acquired Immunodeficiency Syndrome (AIDS) and malaria, tuberculosis is one of the biggest killers in the Word (Rodríguez-Morales AJ et al 2008, Murcia-Aranguren MI et al 2001). Human disease is usually caused by *Mycobacterium tuberculosis*, also know as the Koch's bacilli (Figure 1), which can affect any organ or tissue in the body, and in some cases due to *M. bovis* (Castañeda-Hernández DM & Rodríguez-Morales AJ 2012a). Although this, pulmonary disease, with their particular hallmarks such as occurrence of cough with expectoration lasting more than 15 days, is the main corporal area affected by this mainly tropical pathogen (Rodríguez-Morales AJ et al 2008; Castañeda-Hernández DM & Rodríguez-Morales AJ 2012). In such cases, previous to a microbiological diagnosis, individuals in such state are so-called respiratory symptomatic.

Besides those symptoms/signs, disease can be manifested with hemoptisis, fever, night sweating, general malaise, thoracic pain, anorexia and weight lost. This disease is still a significant public health problem due to is highly transmissibility, but is highly potentially preventable and treatable condition (Curto et al. 2010, Dim et al. 2011, Orcau et al. 2011, Marais & Schaaf 2010, Glaziou et al. 2009). Even more, in the context of HIV and newer immunosuppressive conditions mycobacterial diseases emerge as public health threat in the World (Vargas et al. 2005).

Tuberculosis is a human threat and still a significant public health problem in the World, but particularly in developing countries. Today, together with the burden of infection due to

Human Immunodeficiency Virus (HIV), this coinfection drives most of the tuberculosis morbidity and mortality in many regions (e.g. Africa) and makes more complicated its control and reduction in many terms. According to the World Health Organization (WHO) Global Tuberculosis Control Report 2011 (the most important and official document regard the epidemiology and other aspects of TB worldwide), in 2010, there were 8.8 million (range, 8.5–9.2 million) incident cases of TB, 1.1 million (range, 0.9–1.2 million) deaths from TB among HIV-negative people and an additional 0.35 million (range, 0.32–0.39 million) deaths from HIV-associated TB (World Health Organization 2011). Important new findings at the global level are: a) the absolute number of TB cases has been falling since 2006 (rather than rising slowly as indicated in previous global reports); b) TB incidence rates have been falling since 2002 (two years earlier than previously suggested); c) Estimates of the number of deaths from TB each year have been revised downwards; d) In 2009 there were almost 10 million children who were orphans as a result of parental deaths caused by TB (World Health Organization 2011).

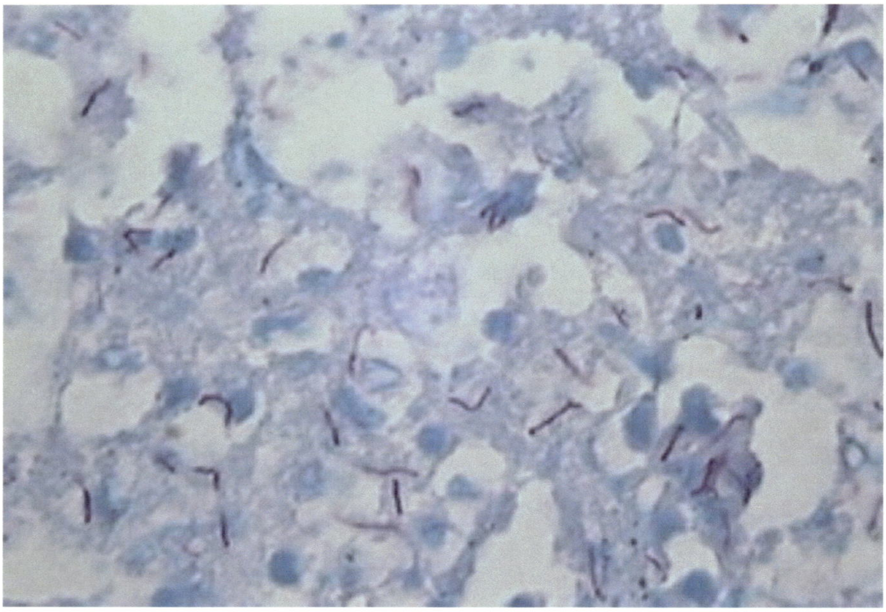

Figure 1. Acid fast-bacilli in a Ziehl-Neelsen stain from a sample of a patient with pulmonary TB (400 X) (Fernández M & Dickson González SM 2007).

Epidemiology of tuberculosis can be influenced by multiple not only clinical factors, but also demographical, geographical and social aspects at local or national levels, as the development of the country (Rodríguez-Morales AJ & Castañeda-Hernández DM 2012), currently measured by indicators such as the Human Development Index (HDI). Finding there, that negative relationships between both morbidity and mortality due to tuberculosis and HDI exist, with better HDI levels lower morbidity and mortality due TB is found (Rodríguez-Mo-

http://dx.doi.org/10.5772/53363

rales AJ & Castañeda-Hernández DM 2012). As has been reported with other diseases with high prevalence in developing countries, burden of diseases such as TB can be an impediment in achieving the Millennium Development Goals (Franco-Paredes et al 2007b). Then strategies to reduce its impact and improving the health of populations, most of the times neglected, should be implemented (Franco-Paredes et al 2007a).

In developing countries another aspect influencing this is the limited research on tuberculosis that usually is made (Castañeda-Hernández DM et al 2012a). For example scientific production on TB in Colombia is low, not just comparing it with developed countries (USA, 4.08 articles/100,000 hab.) but also with others in Latin America with even lower TB incidence such as Chile (19 cases/100,000 hab.) but with a better productivity 2.19 times higher (1.09 articles/100,000 hab.). A higher promotion of research, beginning in undergraduate studies, better interaction between public and private organizations, as well more academic and international cooperation, would allow to decrease those gaps, increase scientific publication and let that the application of that generated knowledge in the same country contribute to improve the TB epidemiology and different aspects of disease (Castañeda-Hernández DM & Rodríguez-Morales AJ 2012a).

Beyond its epidemiology, particularly mostly due to pulmonary disease (Figure 2), other important forms of disease represent also a significant burden in the World. When the infection affects organ other than the lung is called extrapulmonary TB. The most common form of this disease is at the pleura, followed by the lymphatic nodes. Extrapulmonary TB includes various manifestations according to the affected organ. Prognosis and time to develop disease also can vary according to the affected organ (Castañeda-Hernández DM & Rodríguez-Morales AJ 2012a).

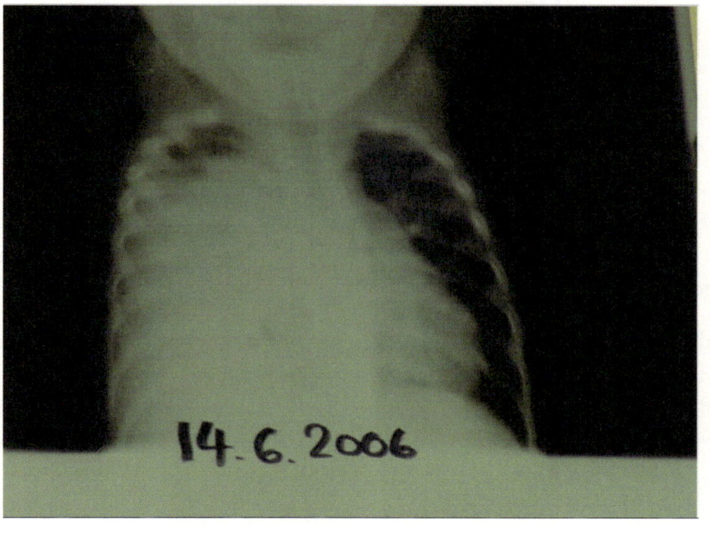

Figure 2. Pulmonary TB in a very young child from Tanzania, Africa (taken by Rodriguez-Morales AJ).

Disease can ranges a spectrum that can begin from a latent infection or reactivation slowly evolving into a focal or whole spread and involvement of multiple organs, which makes it difficult to diagnosis by clinicians and health care workers, who many times could not identify it timely. One of the most severe forms of extrapulmonary TB is the meningitis (TB meningitis), which occurs as a result of hematogenous spread of bacilli into the subarachnoid space. This is known as a complication of primary TB and may occur years later as an endogenous reactivation of a latent tuberculosis or as a result of exogenous reinfection (Glaziou et al. 2009, Hoek et al. 2011, Galimi 2011, Garcia-Rodriguez et al. 2011). Currently in the case of latent TB developing countries usually counts only with the PPD to diagnose this condition. However, recently new alternatives have risen for the diagnosis in these cases, using IFNγ release assays (IGRAs) to diagnose latent TB infection (LTBI). This is actually proposed for public health purposes in developing countries (Castañeda-Hernández DM et al 2012d).

Tuberculosis is a complex disease in terms of the multiple factors that are involved in its occurrence and persistence in the human societies. In first place there are factors associated with the bacillus (viability, transmissibility and virulence), with the host as a biological individual (immune status, genetic susceptibility, duration and intensity of exposure) as well, at the bacillus-host interaction (place of affection, severity of illness) (Castañeda-Hernández DM & Rodríguez-Morales AJ 2012a).

At a second, clinical level, the occurrence of pulmonary tuberculosis undiagnosed or untreated, overcrowding, malnutrition, immunosuppresion from any cause (HIV infection, use of immunosuppressive drugs, diabetes, cancer, chronic renal failure, silicosis, alcoholism and drug addiction), are also important factors (Castañeda-Hernández DM & Rodríguez-Morales AJ 2012a). In developing countries there are also multiple epidemiological contexts where TB can be highly prevalent in comparison with general population, such as in prisons, among homeless persons and indigenous individuals (Castañeda-Hernández DM et al 2012b, Castañeda-Hernández DM & Rodríguez-Morales AJ, 2012b).

At community public health interventional level, protective factors include the BCG (Bacille Calmette Guerin) vaccine, applied in developing countries, which provides protection before exposure and prevent severe infection forms, especially in infants and young children, reaching up to 80% of protection against the development of forms of the disease such as meningeal and miliary TB (Garcia-Rodriguez et al. 2011, Garg 2010, Black et al. 2003, Francis et al. 2002, Arbelaez et al. 2000, Ginsberg 2000).

Additional to those clinical implications, changes in the susceptibility of the etiological agent to the therapy used drugs has imposed more challenges in the management of TB. The magnitude of problem with TB now lies in the fact that one third of the world population is infected by *Mycobacterium tuberculosis*. Even in the 21st century, TB kills more people than any other infective agent. This, then, occurs in part as a result of a progressive decrease in its susceptibility to anti-TB drugs or resistance emergence. Cases of resistant TB, defined by the recommendations of the World Health Organization (WHO) as primary, initial, acquired multidrug resistant (MDR-TB) or extensively drug resistant TB (XDR-TB) are emerging in different areas of the World (Torres et al. 2011, Solari et al. 2011, Chadha et al. 2011, Arenas-Suarez et al. 2010, Ferro et al. 2011, Martins 2011, Robledo et al 2008).

The development of resistance in TB may result from the administration of mono-therapy or inadequate combinations of anti-TB drugs. A possible role of health care workers in the development of multi drug-resistant TB is very important. Actually, multi drug-resistant TB is a direct consequence of mistakes in prescribing chemotherapy, provision of anti-tuberculosis drugs, surveillance of the patient and decision-making regarding further treatment as well as in a wrong way of administration of anti-TB drugs. The problem of XDR-TB in the world has become very alarming. Only adequate treatment according to directly supervised short regiment for correctly categorized cases of TB can stop the escalation of MDR-TB or XDR-TB, which is actually, in large magnitude, a global threat in the 21st century (Torres et al. 2011, Solari et al. 2011, Chadha et al. 2011, Arenas-Suarez et al. 2010, Ferro et al. 2011, Martins 2011, Robledo et al 2008).

Another important issue in TB is the social component, related to a complex background and multiple interacting factors that internally and externally affect individuals affected by the disease, which still represents a significant stigma in many communities in the World. Given this setting, TB approach is complex and requires not only medical but also psychological and especially sociological approaches in order to improve its management from a collective medicine perspective as well better acceptability by non-affected people surrounding infected individuals at their communities or neighborhoods. In this way, programs approaching taking all these considerations in count will benefit with better strategies that allow good interactions between social actors involve in the complex social matrix in which sometimes TB can be present at societies. Taking advantage from this, regular activities, such as proper diagnosis and treatment would be achieve in a more efficient way (Murray et al. 2011, Santin & Navas 2011, Juniarti & Evans 2011).

One challenge in the current context of TB particularly in developing countries is the access to reliable diagnostic tests (Castañeda-Hernández DM et al 2012d), particularly those than allow to confirm species diagnostics as well to identify those isolates that are not fully susceptible to antimicobacterial first line drugs. However, today many diagnostic tests have been developed, but many of them are only used routinely in developed countries (e.g. IGRAs and molecular biology-based tests) (Castañeda-Hernández DM et al 2012d). Although is clear that DOTS (directly observed treatment strategy, short-course) programmes have contributed in the successful treatment of TB, particularly because this strategy includes six major components that are: (i) pursue high-quality DOTS expansion and enhancement; (ii) address TB/HIV, MDR-TB (multi-drug resistant TB), and the needs of poor and vulnerable populations; (iii) contribute to health-system strengthening based on primary health care; (iv) engage all care providers; (v) empower people with TB, and communities through partnership; and (vi) enable and promote research; it is necessary to increase its coverage and usefulness particularly in those highly TB prevalent countries in the developing World in order to achieve the goals that have been established for 2015 in the Global Plan to Stop TB (2011-2015) of the World Health Organization and the Stop TB Partnership (Castañeda-Hernández DM & Rodriguez-Morales AJ. 2012a). The epidemiological burden of

TB in developing countries can be measured directly from different global and national indicators and estimators, however, those mainly to be addressed should be incidence, prevalence, mortality, MDR-TB incidence, XDR-TB (extensively drug-resistant TB) incidence, case notifications, treatment outcomes and case detection rates. In this chapter, such topics are furtherly revised and prepared in the setting of highest available evidence (evidenced-based public health) and epidemiological data, including a detailed analysis according to some highly endemic countries sources in different developing regions, suggesting also new strategies for control as well providing updated information on epidemiological tools relevant for TB in developing countries. Relevant new epidemiological settings will be also discussed, such as the importance of TB in homeless, indigenous, migrated and prison populations as has been suggested.

2. Tuberculosis in developing countries

Tuberculosis is a disease present, due the raise of HIV coinfection in most countries in the World. Until two to three decades ago, TB was decreasing in importance in the World and was predominantly endemic in developing countries. However after the origin of the AIDS pandemic in June 1981, TB has been increasing again in importance not only in these countries but also in those developed in North America and Europe. Besides this, the multiple problems that countries with a high burden of TB have to face are major in developing countries in Africa, Asia and Latin America, especially when this is also associated to other conditions and diseases, such as HIV, comorbidities, poverty and when living in resource-constrained areas where diagnosis and treatment is not prompt as in other areas.

In order to know the real burden of disease in developing countries is necessary that these make things well in epidemiology and public health regard TB. Recording and reporting of data is a fundamental component of care of patients with tuberculosis (TB) and control of the disease. Data recording and reporting is necessary to monitor trends in the TB epidemic at global, national and subnational levels; to monitor progress in the treatment of individual patients and groups (cohorts) of patients and ensure continuity of care when patients are referred between healthcare facilities; and to plan, raise funds for, implement and evaluate programmatic efforts to control TB, including forecasting the numbers of cases and the associated requirements for staffing, medicines and laboratory supplies; and analysing treatment outcomes (World Health Organization 2012).

Global burden of TB in the World is estimated in 8.8 million (range, 8.5–9.2 million) incident cases of TB (Table 1) for rates ranging 123.7 to 133.9 cases/100,000 pop. (Table 1); however this can be very different among the WHO Regions in the World, being higher in Africa where those estimates can reach 250.9 to 298.7 cases/100,000 pop. (Table 1). Rates of incidence are important because can show the real populational problem of the disease. For example in South East Asia there are more crude number of cases of TB, estimated in 3.5 million (range, 3.2–3.7 million) incident cases, however the incidence rates are quite lower than in Africa, reaching 177.0 to 204.7 cases/100,000 pop. (Table 1) (Figure 4).

http://dx.doi.org/10.5772/53363

			Incidence (cases)		Incidence rates (cases/ 100,000pop)		
Region	**Population**	**Best**	**Low**	**High**	**Best**	**Low**	**High**
Global burden	6,869,573,000	8,800,000	8,500,000	9,200,000	128.1	123.7	133.9
WHO African Region	836,970,000	2,300,000	2,100,000	2,500,000	274.8	250.9	298.7
WHO South-East Asia Region	1,807,594,000	3,500,000	3,200,000	3,700,000	193.6	177.0	204.7
WHO Eastern Mediterranean Region	596,747,000	650,000	580,000	730,000	108.9	97.2	122.3
WHO Western Pacific Region	1,798,335,000	1,700,000	1,500,000	1,800,000	94.5	83.4	100.1
WHO European Region	896,480,000	420,000	390,000	450,000	46.8	43.5	50.2
WHO Region of the Americas	933,447,000	270,000	250,000	280,000	28.9	26.8	30.0

Table 1. Estimated epidemiological burden of incident TB, according regions by the WHO in 2010 (World Health Organization 2011). Incidence rates were calculated for this chapter.

Regard the prevalence of TB, which for some countries is still difficult to estimate and in many cases even are not reported and/or analyzed. According the WHO, for 2010 the prevalence was estimated in 12.0 million (range, 11.0–14.0 million) prevalent cases of TB (Table 2) for rates ranging 160.1 to 203.8 cases/100,000 pop. (Table 2); however this can be very different among the WHO Regions in the World, being higher in Africa where those estimates can reach 274.8 to 394.3 cases/100,000 pop. (Table 2).

			Prevalence (cases)		Prevalence rates (cases/ 100,000pop)		
Region	**Population**	**Best**	**Low**	**High**	**Best**	**Low**	**High**
Global burden	6,869,573,000	12,000,000	11,000,000	14,000,000	174.7	160.1	203.8
WHO African Region	836,970,000	2,800,000	2,300,000	3,300,000	334.5	274.8	394.3
WHO European Region	896,480,000	2,500,000	2,200,000	2,800,000	278.9	245.4	312.3
WHO Western Pacific Region	1,798,335,000	5,000,000	3,700,000	6,500,000	278.0	205.7	361.4
WHO Eastern Mediterranean Region	596,747,000	1,000,000	670,000	1,500,000	167.6	112.3	251.4
WHO Region of the Americas	933,447,000	330,000	260,000	410,000	35.4	27.9	43.9
WHO South-East Asia Region	1,807,594,000	560,000	430,000	720,000	31.0	23.8	39.8

Table 2. Estimated epidemiological burden of prevalent TB, according regions by the WHO in 2010 (World Health Organization 2011). Prevalence rates were calculated for this chapter.

Regard the deaths, WHO estimates indicate that around 1.1 million (range, 0.9–1.2 million) deaths from TB among HIV-negative people occurred and an additional 0.35 million (range,

0.32–0.39 million) deaths from HIV-associated TB were also reported (World Health Organization 2011) (Table 3). Higher mortality rates are reported in Africa, ranging 26.3 to 33.5 deaths/100,000 pop. (Table 3), but very close to those reported by South East Asia, ranging 20.5 to 35.4 deaths/100,000 pop. (Table 3).

		Mortality (deaths)			Mortality rates (deaths/ 100,000pop)		
Region	**Population**	**Best**	**Low**	**High**	**Best**	**Low**	**High**
Global burden	6,869,573,000	1,100,000	920,000	1,200,000	16.0	13.4	17.5
WHO African Region	836,970,000	250,000	220,000	280,000	29.9	26.3	33.5
WHO South-East Asia Region	1,807,594,000	500,000	370,000	640,000	27.7	20.5	35.4
WHO Eastern Mediterranean Region	596,747,000	95,000	74,000	120,000	15.9	12.4	20.1
WHO Western Pacifi c Region	1,798,335,000	130,000	120,000	150,000	7.2	6.7	8.3
WHO European Region	896,480,000	61,000	48,000	75,000	6.8	5.4	8.4
WHO Region of the Americas	933,447,000	20,000	17,000	23,000	2.1	1.8	2.5

Table 3. Estimated epidemiological burden of mortality due to TB, according regions by the WHO in 2010 (World Health Organization 2011) (excluding HIV positive deaths). Mortality rates were calculated for this chapter.

Tuberculosis incidence in HIV-patients is a very relevant indicator worldwide for TB epidemiology and burden (Table 4). Africa presented the highest rates for HIV-Positive Incident TB cases, ranging from 98.0 to 117.1 cases/100,000pop. (Table 4).

		HIV-Positive Incident TB Cases			Rates (Cases/100,000pop)		
Region	**Population**	**Best**	**Low**	**High**	**Best**	**Low**	**High**
Global burden	6,869,573,000	1,100,000	1,000,000	1,200,000	16.0	14.6	17.5
WHO African Region	836,970,000	900,000	820,000	980,000	107.5	98.0	117.1
WHO South-East Asia Region	1,807,594,000	190,000	140,000	230,000	10.5	7.7	12.7
WHO Region of the Americas	933,447,000	35,000	31,000	38,000	3.7	3.3	4.1
WHO European Region	896,480,000	20,000	19,000	22,000	2.2	2.1	2.5
WHO Eastern Mediterranean Region	596,747,000	12,000	9,800	15,000	2.0	1.6	2.5
WHO Western Pacifi c Region	1,798,335,000	35,000	26,000	45,000	1.9	1.4	2.5

Table 4. Estimated epidemiological burden of mortality due to TB, according regions by the WHO in 2010 (World Health Organization 2011) (excluding HIV positive deaths). Mortality rates were calculated for this chapter.

Even more, difference in all these aspect can differ among countries and be higher. For example in Colombia, TB is still a significant public health problem. Figure 3 shows the WHO profile for TB in Colombia for 2010.

http://dx.doi.org/10.5772/53363

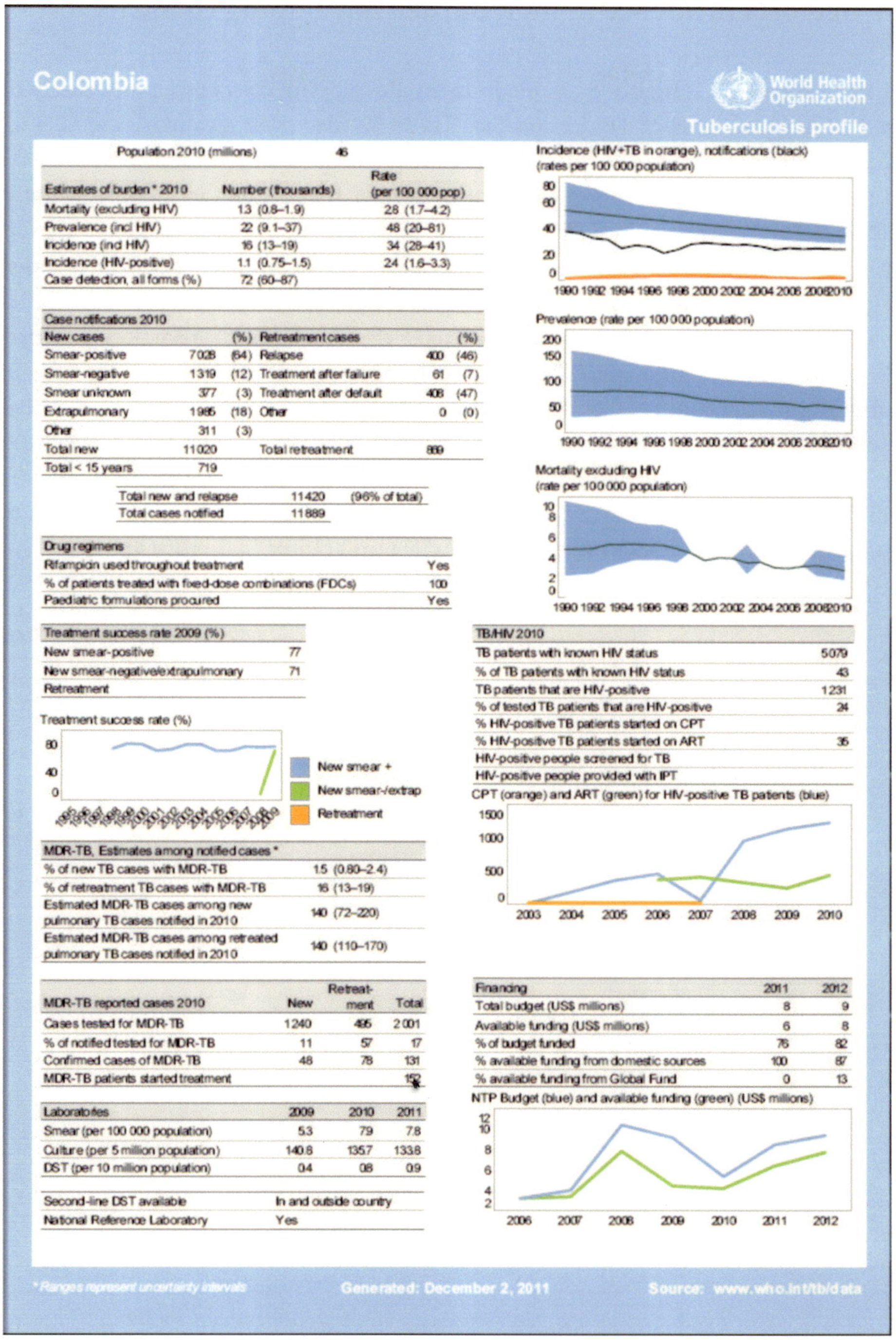

Colombia

World Health Organization

Tuberculosis profile

Population 2010 (millions) 46

Estimates of burden * 2010	Number (thousands)	Rate (per 100 000 pop)
Mortality (excluding HIV)	1.3 (0.8–1.9)	2.8 (1.7–4.2)
Prevalence (incl HIV)	22 (9.1–37)	48 (20–81)
Incidence (incl HIV)	16 (13–19)	34 (28–41)
Incidence (HIV-positive)	1.1 (0.75–1.5)	2.4 (1.6–3.3)
Case detection, all forms (%)	72 (60–87)	

Case notifications 2010					
New cases		(%)	Retreatment cases		(%)
Smear-positive	7028	(64)	Relapse	400	(46)
Smear-negative	1319	(12)	Treatment after failure	61	(7)
Smear unknown	377	(3)	Treatment after default	408	(47)
Extrapulmonary	1985	(18)	Other	0	(0)
Other	311	(3)			
Total new	11020		Total retreatment	869	
Total < 15 years	719				

Total new and relapse	11420	(96% of total)
Total cases notified	11889	

Drug regimens	
Rifampicin used throughout treatment	Yes
% of patients treated with fixed-dose combinations (FDCs)	100
Paediatric formulations procured	Yes

Treatment success rate 2009 (%)	
New smear-positive	77
New smear-negative/extrapulmonary	71
Retreatment	

Treatment success rate (%)

New smear +
New smear-/extrap
Retreatment

MDR-TB, Estimates among notified cases *	
% of new TB cases with MDR-TB	1.5 (0.80–2.4)
% of retreatment TB cases with MDR-TB	16 (13–19)
Estimated MDR-TB cases among new pulmonary TB cases notified in 2010	140 (72–220)
Estimated MDR-TB cases among retreated pulmonary TB cases notified in 2010	140 (110–170)

MDR-TB reported cases 2010	New	Retreat-ment	Total
Cases tested for MDR-TB	1240	495	2001
% of notified tested for MDR-TB	11	57	17
Confirmed cases of MDR-TB	48	78	131
MDR-TB patients started treatment			152

Laboratories	2009	2010	2011
Smear (per 100 000 population)	5.3	7.9	7.8
Culture (per 5 million population)	140.8	135.7	133.8
DST (per 10 million population)	0.4	0.8	0.9

Second-line DST available	In and outside country
National Reference Laboratory	Yes

Incidence (HIV+TB in orange), notifications (black) (rates per 100 000 population)

Prevalence (rate per 100 000 population)

Mortality excluding HIV (rate per 100 000 population)

TB/HIV 2010	
TB patients with known HIV status	5079
% of TB patients with known HIV status	43
TB patients that are HIV-positive	1231
% of tested TB patients that are HIV-positive	24
% HIV-positive TB patients started on CPT	
% HIV-positive TB patients started on ART	35
HIV-positive people screened for TB	
HIV-positive people provided with IPT	

CPT (orange) and ART (green) for HIV-positive TB patients (blue)

Financing	2011	2012
Total budget (US$ millions)	8	9
Available funding (US$ millions)	6	8
% of budget funded	76	82
% available funding from domestic sources	100	87
% available funding from Global Fund	0	13

NTP Budget (blue) and available funding (green) (US$ millions)

* Ranges represent uncertainty intervals

Generated: December 2, 2011

Source: www.who.int/tb/data

Figure 3. Tuberculosis epidemiological profile for Colombia according to the World Health Organization, 2010.

3. Tuberculosis incidence in high burden developing countries

As has been stated TB is highly endemic in many developing countries, particularly of Africa and Asia highest rates of TB are located. These 22 countries, summarizing 62.9% of the World population (4,321,966,000 pop) concentrated 81.5% of the incident cases of TB in the World (7,169,000 cases), reaching mean incidence rates higher than in the rest of the World, 165.9 cases/100,000pop. (Table 5). However in many of these countries those numbers are higher. India (although considered not official data) in 2010 reported 2,300,000 incident cases (ranging from 2,000,000 to 2,500,000 cases) (Table 5), followed by China with 1,000,000 incident cases (ranging from 910,000 to 1,200,000 cases) (Table 5) and South Africa with 490,000 incident cases (ranging 400,000 to 590,000 cases) (Table 5). Although that, again rates are higher in this last country, South Africa, where for the same year were reported between 797.9 to 1176.9 cases/100,000 pop. (7.9 to 11.8 cases/1,000 pop or 0.8 to 1.2 cases/100 pop) (Table 5). For Asia the country with highest rates is Cambodia (374.9 to 509.3 cases/100,000 pop.) (Table 5). For Latin America the country with highest rates (and the only from that region in this list) is Brazil (35.9 to 51.3 cases/100,000 pop.) (Table 5) (Figure 4).

		Incidence (cases)			Incidence rates (cases/100,000pop)		
Countries	**Population**	**Best**	**Low**	**High**	**Best**	**Low**	**High**
South Africa	50,133,000	490,000	400,000	590,000	977.4	797.9	1176.9
Zimbabwe	12,571,000	80,000	61,000	100,000	636.4	485.2	795.5
Mozambique	23,391,000	130,000	87,000	170,000	555.8	371.9	726.8
Cambodia	14,138,000	62,000	53,000	72,000	438.5	374.9	509.3
Myanmar	47,963,000	180,000	160,000	210,000	375.3	333.6	437.8
DR Congo	65,966,000	220,000	190,000	250,000	333.5	288.0	379.0
Kenya	40,513,000	120,000	120,000	130,000	296.2	296.2	320.9
Philippines	93,261,000	260,000	210,000	310,000	278.8	225.2	332.4
Ethiopia	82,950,000	220,000	20,000	230,000	265.2	24.1	277.3
Pakistan	173,593,000	400,000	330,000	480,000	230.4	190.1	276.5
Bangladesh	148,692,000	330,000	270,000	400,000	221.9	181.6	269.0
Uganda	33,425,000	70,000	56,000	85,000	209.4	167.5	254.3
Vietnam	87,848,000	180,000	130,000	220,000	204.9	148.0	250.4
Afghanistan	31,412,000	59,000	49,000	71,000	187.8	156.0	226.0
India	1,224,614,000	2,300,000	2,000,000	2,500,000	187.8	163.3	204.1
Indonesia	239,871,000	450,000	370,000	540,000	187.6	154.2	225.1
UR Tanzania	44,841,000	79,000	75,000	85,000	176.2	167.3	189.6
Thailand	69,122,000	94,000	78,000	110,000	136.0	112.8	159.1
Nigeria	158,423,000	210,000	99,000	360,000	132.6	62.5	227.2
Russian Federation	142,958,000	150,000	130,000	180,000	104.9	90.9	125.9
China	1,341,335,000	1,000,000	910,000	1,200,000	74.6	67.8	89.5
Brazil	194,946,000	85,000	70,000	100,000	43.6	35.9	51.3
Subtotal	4,321,966,000	7,169,000	5,868,000	8,393,000	165.9	135.8	194.2
% from global burden	62.9	81.5	69.0	91.2	-	-	-
Global burden	6,869,573,000	8,800,000	8,500,000	9,200,000	128.1	123.7	133.9

Table 5. Estimated epidemiological burden of TB incidence in the countries with the considered higher burden of TB, according WHO in 2010 (World Health Organization 2011). Incidence rates were calculated for this chapter.

http://dx.doi.org/10.5772/53363

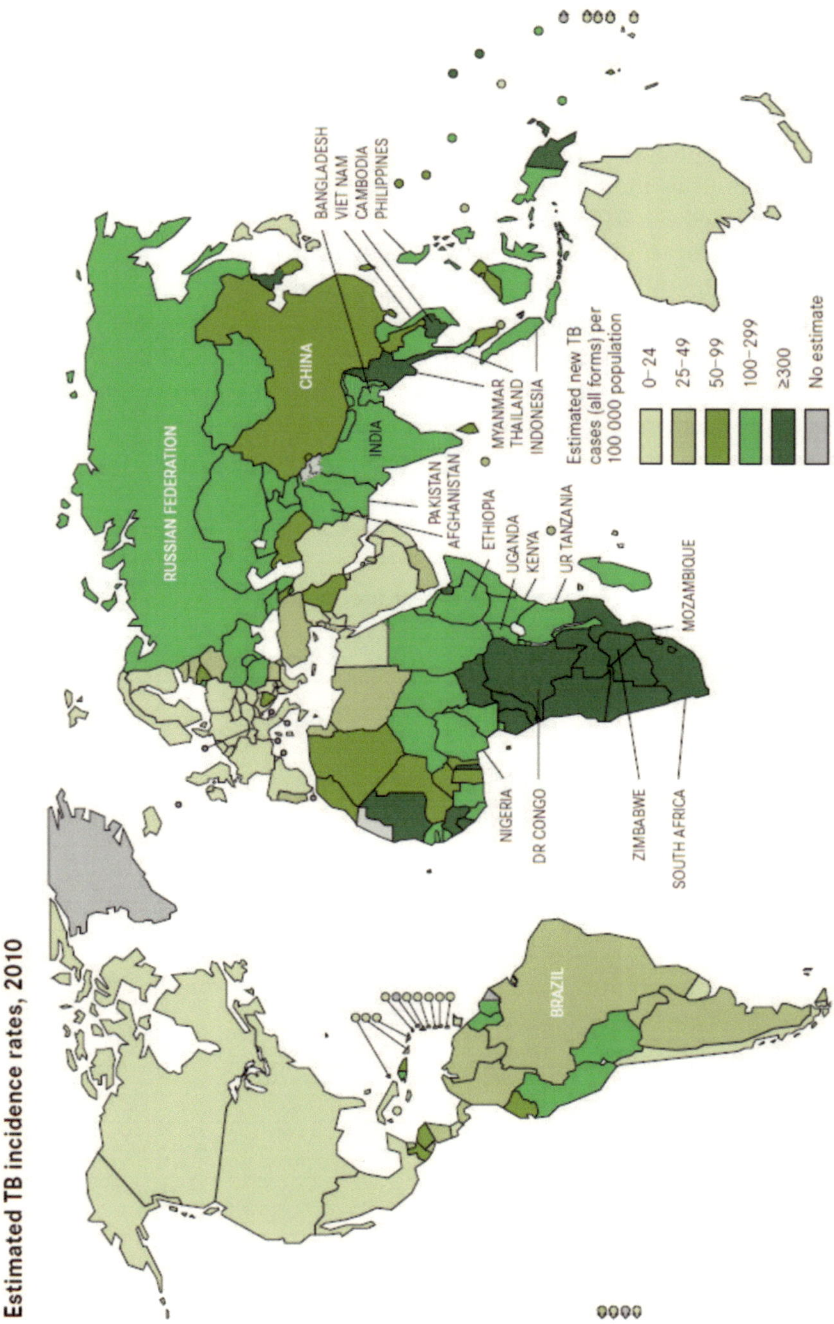

Figure 4. Map of the World with the Tuberculosis incidence rates classified according to the World Health Organization, 2010.

4. Tuberculosis prevalence in high burden developing countries

For prevalence a similar epidemiological situation is seen. These 22 countries, concentrated 83.1% of the prevalent cases of TB in the World (9,972,000 cases), reaching mean prevalence rates higher than in the rest of the World, 230.7 cases/100,000pop. (Table 6). However in many of these countries those numbers are higher. India (although considered not official data) in 2010 reported 3,100,000 prevalent cases (ranging from 2,000,000 to 4,600,000 cases) (Table 6), followed by China with 1,500,000 prevalent cases (ranging from 1,300,000 to 1,700,000 cases) (Table 6) and Indonesia with 690,000 prevalent cases (ranging 300,000 to 1,200,000 cases) (Table 6). Although that, again rates are higher in other countries, such as South Africa, where for the same year were reported between 359.0 to 1256.7 cases/100,000 pop. (3.6 to 12.6 cases/1,000 pop or 0.4 to 1.3 cases/100 pop) (Table 6). For Asia the country with highest prevalence rates is Cambodia (297.1 to 1061.0 cases/100,000 pop.) (Table 6). For Latin America the country with highest rates (and the only from that region in this list) is Brazil (17.4 to 82.1 cases/100,000 pop.) (Table 6).

		Prevalence (cases)			Prevalence rates (cases/ 100,000pop)		
Countries	**Population**	**Best**	**Low**	**High**	**Best**	**Low**	**High**
South Africa	50,133,000	400,000	180,000	630,000	797.9	359.0	1256.7
Cambodia	14,138,000	93,000	42,000	150,000	657.8	297.1	1061.0
DR Congo	65,966,000	350,000	160,000	560,000	530.6	242.5	848.9
Myanmar	47,963,000	250,000	180,000	310,000	521.2	375.3	646.3
Philippines	93,261,000	470,000	410,000	530,000	504.0	439.6	568.3
Mozambique	23,391,000	110,000	54,000	200,000	470.3	230.9	855.0
Bangladesh	148,692,000	610,000	280,000	1,000,000	410.2	188.3	672.5
Zimbabwe	12,571,000	51,000	23,000	80,000	405.7	183.0	636.4
Ethiopia	82,950,000	330,000	140,000	520,000	397.8	168.8	626.9
Pakistan	173,593,000	630,000	270,000	1,100,000	362.9	155.5	633.7
Afghanistan	31,412,000	110,000	51,000	180,000	350.2	162.4	573.0
Viet Nam	87,848,000	290,000	130,000	510,000	330.1	148.0	580.5
Indonesia	239,871,000	690,000	300,000	1,200,000	287.7	125.1	500.3
Kenya	40,513,000	110,000	49,000	180,000	271.5	120.9	444.3
India	1,224,614,000	3,100,000	2,000,000	4,600,000	253.1	163.3	375.6
Nigeria	158,423,000	320,000	110,000	690,000	202.0	69.4	435.5
Uganda	33,425,000	64,000	32,000	100,000	191.5	95.7	299.2
Thailand	69,122,000	130,000	55,000	210,000	188.1	79.6	303.8
UR Tanzania	44,841,000	82,000	39,000	130,000	182.9	87.0	289.9
Russian Federation	142,958,000	190,000	70,000	330,000	132.9	49.0	230.8
China	1,341,335,000	1,500,000	1,300,000	1,700,000	111.8	96.9	126.7
Brazil	194,946,000	92,000	34,000	160,000	47.2	17.4	82.1
Subtotal	4,321,966,000	9,972,000	5,909,000	15,070,000	230.7	136.7	348.7
% from global burden	62.9	83.1	53.7	107.6	-	-	-
Global burden	6,869,573,000	12,000,000	11,000,000	14,000,000	174.7	160.1	203.8

Table 6. Estimated epidemiological burden of TB prevalence in the countries with the considered higher burden of TB, according WHO in 2010 (World Health Organization 2011). Prevalence rates were calculated for this chapter.

http://dx.doi.org/10.5772/53363

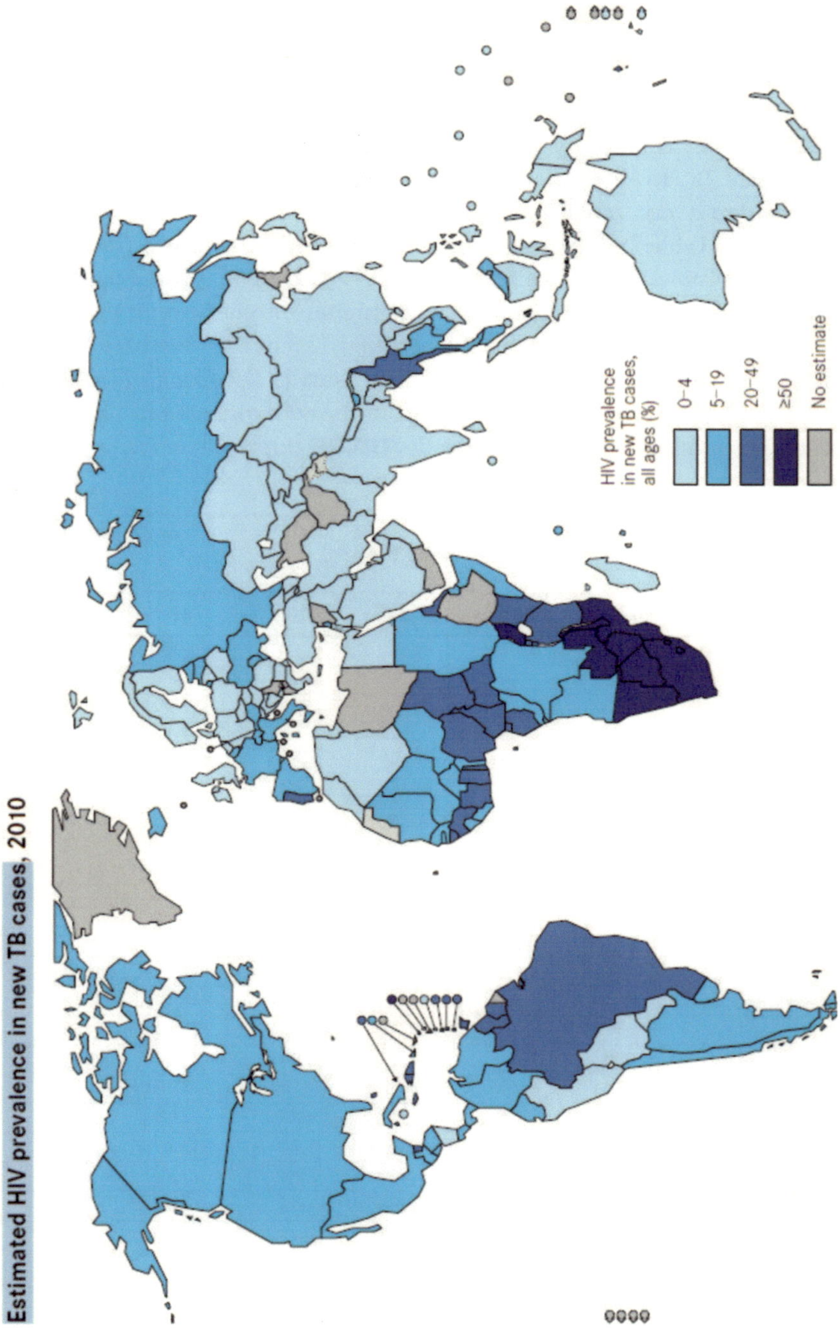

Figure 5. Map of the World with the estimated HIV prevalence in new TB cases classified according to the World Health Organization, 2010.

5. Tuberculosis mortality in high burden developing countries

For mortality a similar epidemiological situation is seen. These 22 countries, concentrated 78.0% of the deaths due to TB in the World (857,800 deaths, ranging 581,900 to 1,229,000 deaths), reaching mean mortality rates higher than in the rest of the World, 19.8 deaths/ 100,000pop. (Table 7). However in many of these countries those numbers are higher. India (although considered not official data) in 2010 reported 320,000 deaths (ranging from 210,000 to 470,000) (Table 7), followed by Indonesia with 64,000 deaths (ranging from 42,000 to 91,000 deaths) (Table 7) and Bangladesh with 64,000 deaths (ranging 47,000 to 85,000 deaths) (Table 7). Although that, again rates are higher in other countries, such as Cambodia, where for the same year were reported between 43.9 to 84.9 deaths/100,000 pop. (Table 7). For Africa the country with highest mortality rates is DR Congo (40.9 to 68.2 deaths/ 100,000 pop.) (Table 7). For Latin America the country with highest rates (and the only from that region in this list) is Brazil (1.6 to 4.3 deaths/100,000 pop.) (Table 7).

		Mortality (deaths)			Mortality rates (deaths/ 100,000pop)		
Countries	**Population**	**Best**	**Low**	**High**	**Best**	**Low**	**High**
Cambodia	14,138,000	8,600	6,200	12,000	60.8	43.9	84.9
DR Congo	65,966,000	36,000	27,000	45,000	54.6	40.9	68.2
South Africa	50,133,000	25,000	16,000	38,000	49.9	31.9	75.8
Mozambique	23,391,000	11,000	7,000	17,000	47.0	29.9	72.7
Bangladesh	148,692,000	64,000	47,000	85,000	43.0	31.6	57.2
Myanmar	47,963,000	20,000	12,000	31,000	41.7	25.0	64.6
Afghanistan	31,412,000	12,000	8,600	16,000	38.2	27.4	50.9
Ethiopia	82,950,000	29,000	23,000	35,000	35.0	27.7	42.2
Pakistan	173,593,000	58,000	39,000	84,000	33.4	22.5	48.4
Philippines	93,261,000	31,000	21,000	43,000	33.2	22.5	46.1
Viet Nam	87,848,000	29,000	19,000	43,000	33.0	21.6	48.9
Zimbabwe	12,571,000	3,400	2,100	5,100	27.0	16.7	40.6
Indonesia	239,871,000	64,000	42,000	91,000	26.7	17.5	37.9
India	1,224,614,000	320,000	210,000	470,000	26.1	17.1	38.4
Nigeria	158,423,000	33,000	11,000	68,000	20.8	6.9	42.9
Russian Federation	142,958,000	26,000	16,000	42,000	18.2	11.2	29.4
Kenya	40,513,000	6,900	4,900	9,400	17.0	12.1	23.2
Thailand	69,122,000	11,000	7,000	16,000	15.9	10.1	23.1
Uganda	33,425,000	5,100	3,300	7,300	15.3	9.9	21.8
UR Tanzania	44,841,000	5,800	4,700	6,900	12.9	10.5	15.4
China	1,341,335,000	54,000	52,000	56,000	4.0	3.9	4.2
Brazil	194,946,000	5,000	3,100	8,300	2.6	1.6	4.3
Subtotal	4,321,966,000	857,800	581,900	1,229,000	19.8	13.5	28.4
% from global burden	62.9	78.0	63.3	102.4	-	-	-
Global burden	6,869,573,000	1,100,000	920,000	1,200,000	16.0	13.4	17.5

Table 7. Estimated epidemiological burden of TB mortality in the countries with the considered higher burden of TB, according WHO in 2010 (World Health Organization 2011). Mortality rates were calculated for this chapter.

http://dx.doi.org/10.5772/53363

6. Tuberculosis-HIV incidence in high burden developing countries

Coinfection in high burden developing countries is one the main problems those countries should face in the public health threat that TB represents. These 20 countries, concentrated 78.1% of the cases of TB-HIV in the World (859,600 cases, ranging 636,200 to 1,128,900 cases), reaching mean TB-HIV rates higher than in the rest of the World, 20.4/100,000pop. (Table 8). However in many of these countries those numbers are higher. Africa in 2010 reported 300,000 cases TB-HIV (ranging 240,000 to 350,000) followed by India (although considered not official data) in 2010 reported 110,000 cases TB-HIV (ranging from 75,000 to 160,000) (Table 8), and Mozambique with 77,000 cases (ranging 53,000 to 110,000) (Table 8). Although that, again rates are higher in other countries. South Africa is the country with highest rates of TB-HIV, 478.7 to 698.1 cases/100,000 pop. (Table 8). For Asia the country with highest TB-HIV rates is Myanmar (43.8 to 118.8 cases/100,000 pop.) (Table 8). For Latin America the country with highest rates (and the only from that region in this list) is Brazil (5.1 to 14.4 cases/100,000 pop.) (Table 8) (Figure 5).

		HIV-positive incident TB cases			HIV-TB rates (cases/100,000 pop)		
Countries	**Population**	**Best**	**Low**	**High**	**Best**	**Low**	**High**
South Africa	50,133,000	300,000	240,000	350,000	598.4	478.7	698.1
Zimbabwe	12,571,000	60,000	47,000	76,000	477.3	373.9	604.6
Mozambique	23,391,000	77,000	53,000	110,000	329.2	226.6	470.3
Kenya	40,513,000	50,000	45,000	55,000	123.4	111.1	135.8
Uganda	33,425,000	38,000	30,000	46,000	113.7	89.8	137.6
Myanmar	47,963,000	37,000	21,000	57,000	77.1	43.8	118.8
UR Tanzania	44,841,000	30,000	28,000	31,000	66.9	62.4	69.1
Nigeria	158,423,000	51,000	25,000	87,000	32.2	15.8	54.9
Cambodia	14,138,000	4,000	3,400	4,700	28.3	24.0	33.2
DR Congo	65,966,000	18,000	13,000	24,000	27.3	19.7	36.4
Thailand	69,122,000	12,000	13,000	18,000	17.4	18.8	26.0
Brazil	194,946,000	18,000	10,000	28,000	9.2	5.1	14.4
India	1,224,614,000	110,000	75,000	160,000	9.0	6.1	13.1
Viet Nam	87,848,000	7,600	4,600	11,000	8.7	5.2	12.5
Indonesia	239,871,000	18,000	9,900	29,000	7.5	4.1	12.1
Russian Federation	142,958,000	8,100	6,800	9,400	5.7	4.8	6.6
China	1,341,335,000	18,000	10,000	28,000	1.3	0.7	2.1
Philippines	93,261,000	1,000	500	1,800	1.1	0.5	1.9
Pakistan	173,593,000	1,200	700	1,900	0.7	0.4	1.1
Bangladesh	148,692,000	700	300	1,100	0.5	0.2	0.7
Subtotal	4,207,604,000	859,600	636,200	1,128,900	20.4	15.1	26.8
% from global burden	61.2	78.1	63.6	94.1	-	-	-
Global burden	6,869,573,000	1,100,000	1,000,000	1,200,000	16.0	14.6	17.5

Table 8. Estimated epidemiological burden of TB-HIV in the countries with the considered higher burden of TB, according WHO in 2010 (World Health Organization 2011). Rates were calculated for this chapter.

7. Multidrug resistant tuberculosis in high burden developing countries

Multidrug resistant (MDR) tuberculosis is a public health problem (Gotuzzo E 2011, Tamaru et al 2012). Its burden particularly in developing countries is a relevant issue to be addressed. In some countries, proportions as high as 26% of the new TB cases can be MDR-TB (Figure 6).

MDR strains arose over the past 30 years as a variety of antituberculosis drugs were introduced in medicine, and they largely discount the results of chemotherapy for tuberculosis. The most dangerous of them are strains with extensive drug resistance (XDR), which are resistant to four or five different drugs on average. The molecular mechanisms that make a strain resistant are considered. XDR and MDR strains result from successive and usually independent resistance mutations, which arise in various regions of the mycobacterial genome. In addition, the formation of resistant strains is affected by the phenomenon of tolerance and mycobacterial latency in infected tissues (Prozorov AA et al 2012).

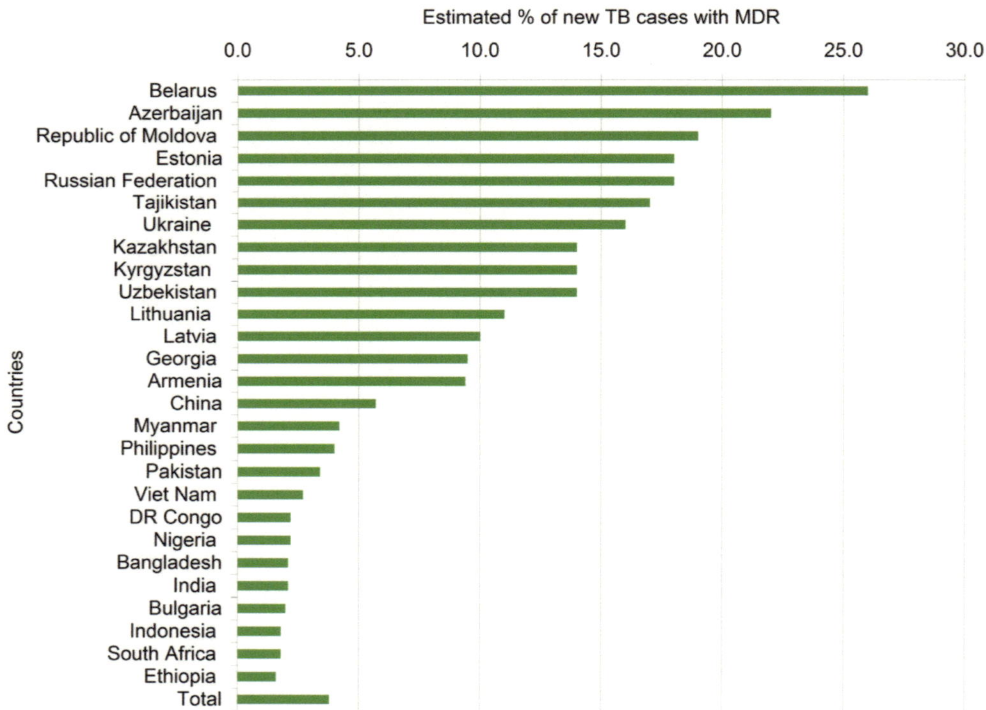

Figure 6. Estimated proportion of TB cases that have MDR-TB.

The increasing emergence of multidrug-resistant (MDR) and extensively drug-resistant (XDR) tuberculosis (TB) in the era of human immunodeficiency virus (HIV) infection presents a major threat to effective control of TB. Drug resistance in *Mycobacterium tuberculo-*

http://dx.doi.org/10.5772/53363

sis arises from spontaneous chromosomal mutations at low frequency. Clinical drug-resistant TB largely occurs as a result of man-made selection during disease treatment of these genetic alterations through erratic drug supply, suboptimal physician prescription and poor patient adherence. Molecular mechanisms of drug resistance have been elucidated for the major first- and second-line drugs rifampicin, isoniazid, pyrazinamide, ethambutol, the aminoglycosides and the fluoroquinolones. The relationship between drug resistance in *M. tuberculosis* strains and their virulence/transmissibility needs to be further investigated. Understanding the mechanisms of drug resistance in *M. tuberculosis* would enable the development of rapid molecular diagnostic tools and furnish possible insights into new drug development for the treatment of TB (Zhang Y & Yew WW, 2009).

8. Tuberculosis in Colombia and in a city of the country: Pereira

In Colombia for 2010 incident cases were 16,000 cases (ranging 13,000 to 19,000 cases) for a rate of 34 cases/100,000 pop (28 to 41 cases/100,000 pop). Prevalence was estimated in 22,000 cases (9,100 to 37,000 cases) for a rate of 48 cases/100,000 pop (ranging 20 to 81 cases/100,000 pop.). Mortality was estimated in 1,300 deaths (ranging 800 to 1,900 deaths) for a mortality rate of 2.8 deaths/100,000 pop. (1.7 to 4.2 deaths/100,000 pop.). All these figures are excluding HIV cases. TB incidence in HIV positive patients is 1,100 cases (ranging 750 to 1,500 cases) for a rate of 2.4 cases/100,000 pop. (ranging from 1.6 to 3.3 cases/100,000 pop.).

As an example of place where the burden of TB is high, Pereira, a city in Colombia can be presented. Pereira is the capital municipality of the Department of Risaralda (Figure 7). It stands in the center of the western region of the country, located in a small valley that descends from a part of the western Andes mountain chain. Its strategic location in the coffee producing area makes the city an urban center in Colombia, as does its proximity to Bogotá, Cali and Medellín.

For 2011, Pereira municipality has an estimated population of 459,690. Official reported records for TB in Risaralda registered a disease incidence for 2010 of 25 cases per 100,000 pop (which is above the national average rate of 24 cases per 100,000 pop). Pereira is divided into 19 urban submunicipalities: Ferrocarril, Olímpica, San Joaquín, Cuba, Del Café, El Oso, Perla del Otún, Consota, El Rocío, El poblado, El Jardín, San Nicolás, Centro, Río Otún, Boston, Universidad, Villavicencio, Oriente and Villasantana. Additionally also has rural townships which include Altagracia, Arabia, Caimalito, Cerritos, La Florida, Puerto Caldas, Combia Alta, Combia Baja, La Bella, Estrella, La Palmilla, Morelia and Tribunas. The municipality of Pereira has a diversified economy: the primary sector accounts for 5.7% of domestic product, the secondary sector shows a relative weight of 26.2%, while the tertiary sector is the most representative with a 68.1%. The GDP of Pereira grew by 3.7% in 2004. For 2010, Pereira reported 301 cases of TB (incidence rate of 65.85 cases per 100,000pop). In Pereira, previously reported interventions have been developed and working intersectorially with the academia in order to increase the impact of activities in TB control (Castañeda-Hernández DM et al. 2012c, Castañeda-Hernández DM & Rodríguez-Morales AJ 2012a).

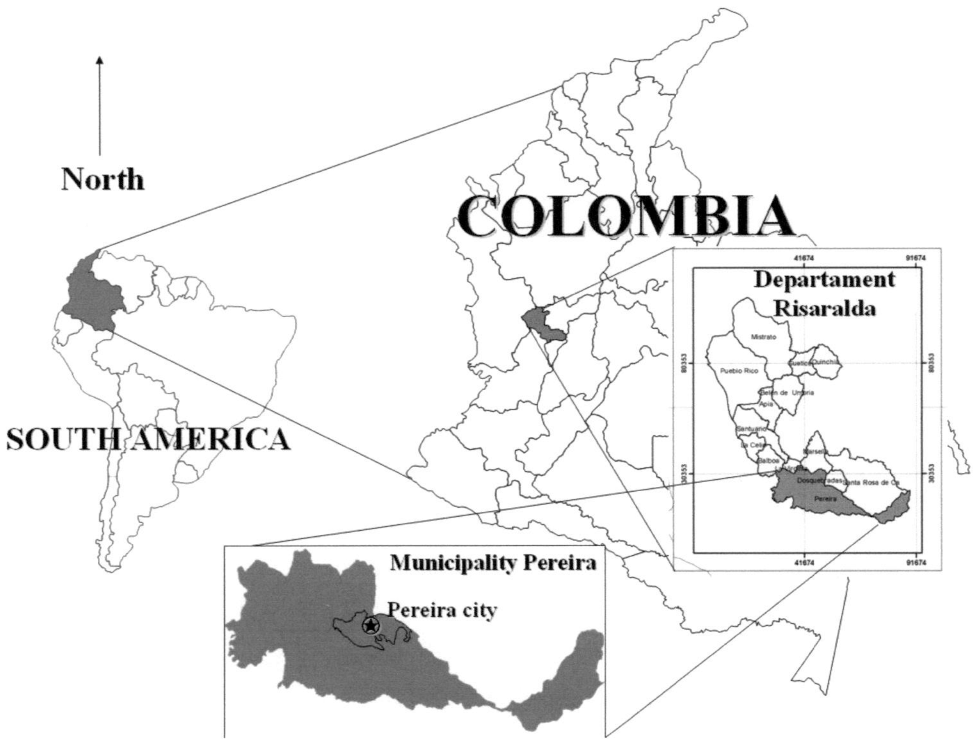

Figure 7. Relative location of Pereira, Risaralda, Colombia, South America.

In the country, the strategic plan "*Colombia Libre de Tuberculosis para la Expansión y Fortalecimiento de la Estrategia Alto a la TB, 2010-2015*" (Colombia Free of TB for the Expansion and Enhancement of the Strategy Stop TB, 2010-2015), define as goal the achievement of notifications of new positive baciloscopy cases in more than 70% and a curation rate of at least 85%. In this context the routine surveillance allow to follow management and measurement of the impact of the realized actions by the control programs at municipal, departmental and national level, in order to generate interventions that contribute to achievement of the established goals to stop the advance of TB in the country.

In Pereira, control of TB among homeless have found that between 2007 and 2010, 74 homeless persons with TB were evaluated, from a total of 1,470 registered homeless persons (from the Social Development Secretary of Pereira) (cumulated incidence=50.3 cases/ 1,000pop., range 5.44 to 22.44; year 2010=16.32). Outcome condition was in 43.2% treatment self-withdrawal (range 36.4%-55.6%), therapeutical failure, 4.1%(0.0-9.1%), deaths, 2.7%(0.0%-8.3%), cured, 39.2%(33.3%-42.4%) and finished treatments, 10.8%(4.2%-25.0%). Comparing the 2010 TB incidence among homeless persons with that of the general population (0.6585/1,000pop.) that is 76.45 times higher in that risk population. In the same way, case fatality rate in 2010 was 2.5 times higher than in the general population (3.3%). These results have important implications in public health as well in the management and evolution of TB in these individuals, persistence of infection, drug-resistance and potential transmission to those that can be around these populations (Castañeda-Hernández DM & Rodríguez-Morales AJ, 2012b).

Also, as part of the integrative control of TB in special populations, surveillance have included control in a prison. Evaluating TB among prisoners between 2010 and 2012, seven prisoners with TB (AFB+), from a total of 1,508 registered prisoners at the penitentiary were diagnosed (cumulated incidence=4.64 cases/1,000pop., 2.99 in 2010 and 2.13 in 2011). Mean age was 40.5 y-old (100% males), all were pulmonary disease. All of them received voluntary counseling and testing for HIV, one of them was HIV+. Three of them are under anti-TB treatment, 2 were transferred, 1 finished treatments and 1 was a therapeutical failure. Comparing the 2011 TB incidence among prisoners with that of the general population (0.67/1,000pop.) that was 3.19 times higher in that risk population. In 2010 in Pereira was 0.66/1,000pop., then being 4.55 times higher in prisoners (Castañeda-Hernández DM et al 2012b). These results have important implications in public health as well in the management and evolution of TB in these individuals, persistence of infection, drug-resistance and potential transmission to those that can be around these prisoners. This is in agreement with recent data indicating that TB incidence rates among prisoners can be as higher as approximately 5 to 50 times higher them than in general population. In Brazil this has been reported as high as 61.8 times higher for latent TB and 36.08 for active TB. Prisoners are at risk rapidly progress to a latent TB or have an active TB posterior a recent infection or reactivation due to latent coexisting pathologies, particularly HIV infection, IV drug use and poor nutritional status. It has been shown that workers in such facilities as well the community, are at risk. For these reasons strategies oriented to bring an integral, social, epidemiological, clinical, diagnostic and therapeutic management, are proposed and for the Americas, the Pan-American Health Organization (PAHO) guideline for the TB control in population in prisons should be followed (OPS 2008).

9. Conclusions

Tuberculosis control in the XXI century requires new approaches and interventions, particularly those based in education and prevention with a community-based orientation to continuously progress in the achieved reduction of burden of disease in the region of the Americas, including in countries such as Colombia. Different approach programs such the development of social networks for control program, as has been developed in Pereira, Colombia (Castañeda-Hernández DM & Rodríguez-Morales AJ 2012a), should performed in other highly endemic places. As the WHO recommends to pursue the ACMS (advocacy, communication and social mobilization), strategies as the social network allow to enhance particularly the communication and social mobilization components. Unfortunately at many national plans of TB control, how translate the ACMS in specific actions is not well defined in most occasions.

As has been previously stated, in the establishment of a social network for TB, previous diagnosis, including geo-referenced characterization, it is necessary to select the areas where the nodes will be established, taking also in consideration the suitability as the willingness of the potential participants of the network in each area and node. Finally, with the mining of the activities described, but also beginning with the idea of raise the awareness about the disease, taking in consideration a high level of diversity on the activities, as has been stated in order to warrant the continuous interest and participation of the network members on it.

In the future, in order to enhance the function and structure of the whole social network, further meetings between the nodes are expected. As now, only nodes interact internally, but the idea for the future activities in this setting is increase the links internally, but also between the main nodes in order to potentially increase the participation in the whole network.

Activities such as the development of social network of TB in Pereira will enhance the prevention, education and surveillance in the community, allowing a better integrated approach to the TB control in these scenarios and increasing the health profile in the community decreasing the lost opportunities for diagnosis and treatment of TB cases, finally leading to an improvement of the TB prevention and control.

Integrating additionally control in populations were TB is highly prevalent such as in prisons and homeless persons (Figure 8) (Castañeda-Hernández DM et al 2012b, Castañeda-Hernández DM & Rodríguez-Morales AJ, 2012b), an integrative control of disease can be achieved and finally control and reduce the burden of disease in a developing country.

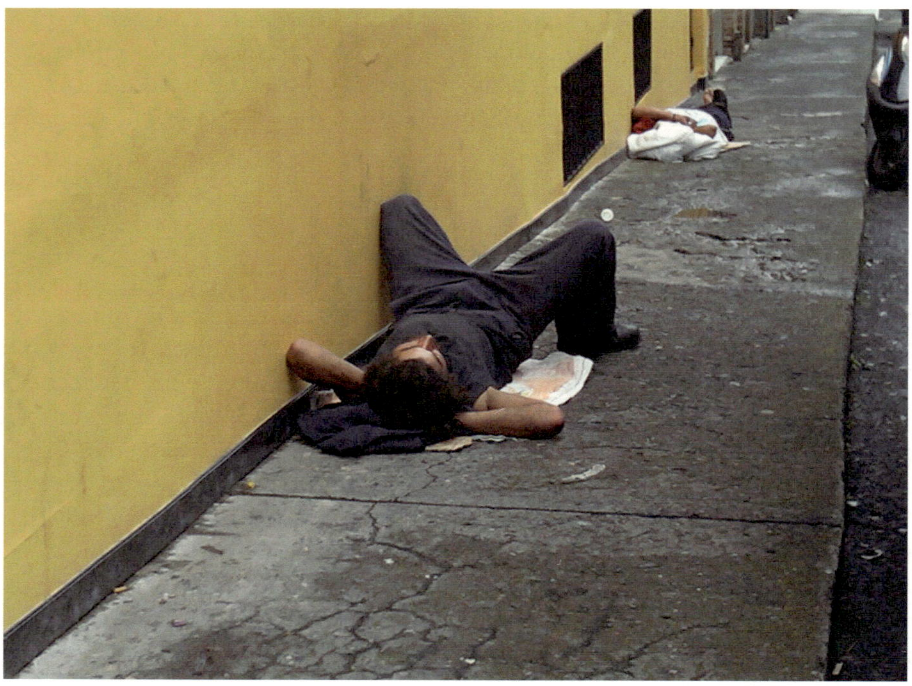

Figure 8. Homeless persons in the center of Pereira, Colombia (taken by Rodriguez-Morales AJ).

Author details

Diana M. Castañeda-Hernández[1] and Alfonso J. Rodriguez-Morales[2,3]

1 Tuberculosis Control Program, Health and Social Security Secretary, Pereira and Fundación Universitaria del Área Andina, Pereira; Committee on Tuberculosis, Asociación Colombiana de Infectología (ACIN), Bogotá, Colombia

2 Department of Community Medicine, Faculty of Health Sciences, Universidad Tecnológica de Pereira, Pereira; Office of Scientific, Research, Cooperativa de Entidades de Salud de Risaralda (COODESURIS), Pereira; Postgraduate in Epidemiology, Fundación Universitaria del Área Andina, Pereira, Colombia

3 Instituto José Witremundo Torrealba, Universidad de Los Andes, Trujillo, Venezuela

References

[1] Arbelaez MP, Nelson KE, Munoz A. 2000. BCG vaccine effectiveness in preventing tuberculosis and its interaction with human immunodeficiency virus infection. Int. J Epidemiol. 29(6):1085-91.

[2] Arenas-Suárez NE, García-Gutiérrez AM, Coronado-Ríos SM, Beltrán-Bocanegra CA, Acosta-Botero SM, Gómez-Marín JE, Quintero-Álvarez L. 2010. Prevalence of childhood tuberculosis in Armenia, Colombia. Rev Salud Publica (Bogota) 12(6):1000-9.

[3] Black GF, Weir RE, Chaguluka SD, Warndorff D, Crampin AC et al. 2003. Gamma interferon responses induced by a panel of recombinant and purified mycobacterial antigens in healthy, non-mycobacterium bovis BCG-vaccinated Malawian young adults. Clin. Diagn. Lab Immunol. 10(4):602-11.

[4] Castañeda-Hernández DM, Bolívar-Mejía A, Rodríguez-Morales AJ. 2012a. Scientific research in tuberculosis: bibliometric assesment of the colombian contributions to the literature. Infectio 16(S1):33.

[5] Castañeda-Hernández DM, Martínez-Ramírez JE, Rodríguez-Morales AJ. 2012b. Tuberculosis en una prisión de risaralda: epidemiología e implicaciones para el programa de control. Infectio 16(S1):66.

[6] Castañeda-Hernández DM, Mondragón-Cardona A, Canapo Betancourth CF, Tobón-García D, Alzate-Carvajal V, Jiménez Canizales CE, Rodríguez-Morales AJ. 2012c. Impacto de una Actividad Formativa en los Conocimientos, Actitudes y Percepciones (CAP) sobre Tuberculosis (TB) de Estudiantes de Medicina de una Universidad de Risaralda, Colombia. Gaceta Médica de Caracas 120(1):40-47.

[7] Castañeda-Hernández DM, Rodríguez-Morales AJ. 2012a. Social Networking in Tuberculosis: Experience in Colombia. In: Rodriguez-Morales AJ. (Editor). Current Top-

ics in Tropical Medicine. ISBN 978-953-51-0274-8. InTech, Croatia, March. Chapter 5: 67-80.

[8] Castañeda-Hernández DM, Rodríguez-Morales AJ. 2012b. Epidemiología de la tuberculosis en habitantes de calle, municipio Pereira, Risaralda, 2007-2010 y propuesta de un proyecto para mejorar su abordaje y evolución. Infectio 16(S1):33-34.

[9] Castañeda-Hernández DM, Rodríguez-Morales AJ, Sepulveda-Arias JC. 2012d. Importancia del uso de pruebas de medición de la liberación de interferon-gamma en la vigilancia epidemiológica de la tuberculosis. Rev Med Chile 140(1):128-129.

[10] Chadha SS, Sharath BN, Reddy K, Jaju J, Vishnu PH, Rao S, Parmar M, Satyanarayana S, Sachdeva KS, Wilson N, Harries AD. 2011. Operational challenges in diagnosing multi-drug resistant TB and initiating treatment in Andhra Pradesh, India. PLoS One 6(11):e26659.

[11] Curto M, Scatena LM, de Paula Andrade RL, Palha PF, de Assis EG et al. 2010. Tuberculosis control: patient perception regarding orientation for the community and community participation. Rev. Lat. Am. Enfermagem. 18(5):983-9.

[12] Dim CC, Dim NR, Morkve O. 2011. Tuberculosis: a review of current concepts and control programme in Nigeria. Niger. J Med 20(2):200-6.

[13] Fernández M & Dickson González SM. 2007. Coloraciones especiales e impregnaciones argénticas. Rev Soc Med Quir Hosp Emerg Perez de Leon 38(1):8-10.

[14] Ferro BE, Nieto LM, Rozo JC, Forero L, van Soolingen D. 2011. Multidrug-resistant Mycobacterium tuberculosis, Southwestern Colombia. Emerg Infect Dis 17(7): 1259-62.

[15] Francis J, Reed A, Yohannes F, Dodard M, Fournier AM. 2002. Screening for tuberculosis among orphans in a developing country. Am. J Prev. Med 22(2):117-9.

[16] Franco-Paredes C, Jones D, Rodriguez-Morales AJ, Santos-Preciado JI. 2007a. Commentary: improving the health of neglected populations in Latin America. BMC Public Health 7:11.

[17] Franco-Paredes C, Von A, Hidron A, Rodriguez-Morales AJ, Tellez I et al. 2007b. Chagas disease: an impediment in achieving the Millennium Development Goals in Latin America. BMC Int. Health Hum. Rights 7:7.

[18] Galimi R. 2011. Extrapulmonary tuberculosis: tuberculous meningitis new developments. Eur. Rev Med Pharmacol. Sci 15(4):365-86.

[19] Garcia-Rodriguez JF, Alvarez-Diaz H, Lorenzo-Garcia MV, Marino-Callejo A, Fernandez-Rial A, Sesma-Sanchez P. 2011. Extrapulmonary tuberculosis: epidemiology and risk factors. Enferm. Infecc. Microbiol. Clin. 29(7):502-9.

[20] Garg RK. 2010. Tuberculous meningitis. Acta Neurol. Scand. 122(2):75-90.

[21] Ginsberg AM. 2000. A proposed national strategy for tuberculosis vaccine development. Clin. Infect Dis. 30 Suppl 3:S233-S242.

[22] Glaziou P, Floyd K, Raviglione M. 2009. Global burden and epidemiology of tuberculosis. Clin. Chest Med 30(4):621-36, vii.

[23] Gotuzzo E. 2011. Xpert MTB/RIF for diagnosis of pulmonary tuberculosis. Lancet Infect Dis 11(11):802-3.

[24] Hoek KG, Van RA, van Helden PD, Warren RM, Victor TC. 2011. Detecting drug-resistant tuberculosis: the importance of rapid testing. Mol. Diagn. Ther. 15(4):189-94.

[25] Marais BJ, Schaaf HS. 2010. Childhood tuberculosis: an emerging and previously neglected problem. Infect Dis. Clin. North Am. 24(3):727-49.

[26] Murcia-Aranguren MI, Gómez-Marin JE, Alvarado FS, Bustillo JG, de Mendivelson E, Gómez B, León CI, Triana WA, Vargas EA, Rodríguez E. 2001. Frequency of tuberculous and non-tuberculous mycobacteria in HIV infected patients from Bogota, Colombia. BMC Infect Dis 1:21.

[27] Organización Panamericana de la Salud. 2008. "Guía para el control de la tuberculosis en poblaciones privadas de libertad de América Latina y el Caribe". Washington, D.C.: OPS.

[28] Orcau A, Cayla JA, Martinez JA. 2011. Present epidemiology of tuberculosis. Prevention and control programs. Enferm. Infecc. Microbiol. Clin. 29 Suppl 1:2-7.

[29] Prozorov AA, Zaĭchikova MV, Danilenko VN. 2012. *Mycobacterium tuberculosis* mutants with multidrug resistance: history of origin, genetic and molecular mechanisms of resistance, and emerging challenges. Genetika 48(1):5-20.

[30] Robledo J, Mejia GI, Paniagua L, Martin A, Guzmán A. 2008. Rapid detection of rifampicin and isoniazid resistance in Mycobacterium tuberculosis by the direct thin-layer agar method. Int J Tuberc Lung Dis 12(12):1482-4.

[31] Rodríguez-Morales AJ, Lorizio W, Vargas J, Fernández L, Durán B, Husband G, Rondón A, Vargas K, Barbella RA, Dickson SM. 2008. Malaria, Tuberculosis, VIH/SIDA e Influenza Aviar: ¿Asesinos de la Humanidad? Rev Soc Med Quir Hosp Emerg Perez de Leon 39(1):52-76.

[32] Rodríguez-Morales AJ, Castañeda-Hernández DM. 2012. Relationships Between Morbidity and Mortality from Tuberculosis and the Human Development Index (HDI) in Venezuela, 1998-2008. Int J Infect Dis 16(9):e704-e705.

[33] Solari L, Gutiérrez A, Suárez C, Jave O, Castillo E, Yale G, Ascencios L, Quispe N, Valencia E, Suárez V. 2011. Cost analysis of rapid methods for diagnosis of multidrug resistant tuberculosis in different epidemiologic groups in Perú. Rev Peru Med Exp Salud Publica 28(3):426-31.

[34] Tamaru A, Nakajima C, Wada T, Wang Y, Inoue M, Kawahara R, Maekura R, Ozeki Y, Ogura H, Kobayashi K, Suzuki Y, Matsumoto S. 2012. Dominant Incidence of Mul-

tidrug and Extensively Drug-Resistant Specific *Mycobacterium tuberculosis* Clones in Osaka Prefecture, Japan. PLoS One 7(8):e42505.

[35] Torres J, Sardón V, Soto MG, Anicama R, Arroyo-Hernández H, Munayco CV. 2011. Cluster of multidrug-resistant tuberculosis cases in a school of the district of Ica, Peru. Rev Peru Med Exp Salud Publica 28(3):497-502.

[36] Vargas J, Gamboa C, Negrin D, Correa M, Sandoval C et al. 2005. Disseminated Mycobacterium mucogenicum infection in a patient with idiopathic CD4+ T lymphocytopenia manifesting as fever of unknown origin. Clin. Infect Dis. 41(5):759-60.

[37] World Health Organization. 2011. 2011 Global Tuberculosis Control, Geneva: WHO.

[38] World Health Organization. 2012. Electronic recording and reporting for tuberculosis care and control, Geneva: WHO.

[39] Zhang Y, Yew WW. 2009. Mechanisms of drug resistance in *Mycobacterium tuberculosis*. Int J Tuberc Lung Dis 13(11):1320-30.

Chapter 16

Beating Cervical Cancer in the Developed Countries: A Dream or a Reality?

Mosiur Rahman, Abdur R. Mia,
Syed Emdadul Haque, Mostofa Golam,
Nowsheen Sharmin Purabi and S. A. R. Choudhury

Additional information is available at the end of the chapter

http://dx.doi.org/10.5772/52881

1. Introduction

Cervical cancer is the third most commonly diagnosed cancer and the fourth leading cause of cancer death in women worldwide, with an estimated 529,000 new cases and 275,000 deaths expected to occur in 2008, of which about 80% occurred in developing countries (Ferlay et al., 2010). Western countries have experienced dramatic reductions in the incidence of and mortality from invasive cervical cancer (Day, 1984; Hristova & Hakama, 1997; Duguid, Duncan, & Currie, 1985; Taylor et al., 2001). In developed countries, incidence rates of cervical cancer are generally low and accounts for only 3.6% (Bray et al., 2005). The disproportionate burden of cervical cancer in developing countries and elsewhere in medically underserved populations is mainly due to lack of effective screening program (Hristova & Hakama, 1997; Duguid, Duncan, & Currie, 1985; Taylor et al., 2001).

Cervical cancer is almost completely preventable, because unlike many cancers, which are caused by a number of physical, genetic, lifestyle and environmental factors, almost all cervical cancer is caused by a sexually transmitted virus, the human papillomavirus (HPV) (Kari & Mark, 2008). Over the past decades, scientists, public health researchers, clinicians, policymakers, women's health and cancer advocates and private sector partners have worked tirelessly to raise global awareness of cervical cancer. They have identified and developed high-impact low-cost solutions to prevent this devastating disease. Today, there are a combination of new and affordable high-tech tools and effective simple solutions.

The purpose of this chapter is to explore the opportunities to limit the epidemic by (a) examining the causes, signs and symptoms and complications of cervical cancer (b) reviewing the epidemiology of cervical cancer in the developed region, and (c) prevention of cervical cancer strategy in the developed countries.

2. Disease issues

2.1. Risk factors of cervical cancer

Basically every woman who has ever been sexually active can develop cancer of the cervix. A vast 99% of cervical cancers are caused by HPV (Kari & Mark, 2008). Of the more than 100 types of HPV, most are benign and resolve without intervention. Visible lesions or warts, known as condylomata acuminate, may be seen. High-risk HPV types tend to persist and are associated with development of precancerous lesions and cervical cancer. Although cervical cancer is associated with about 15 high-risk HPV types, invasive cervical cancer is predominantly caused by HPV 16 and 18 (Tiffen & Mahon 2006).

2.1.1. Other factors thought to be associated with cancer of the cervix

2.1.1.1. Marital and sexual factors

The epidemiologists have noted that risk of cervical cancer is strongly influenced by sexual behavior. This has led to discovery of the role of HPV infection. Studies have shown increased risk due to marriage at young age, onset of regular sex at an early age <20yrs, multiple lifetime number of sexual partners (Karlsson et al., 1995). These risk factors remain significant especially among those women without apparent human papilloma virus infection (HPV). Frequency of intercourse has not been found to be a risk factor after accounting for the effects of number of sexual partners.

2.1.1.2. The role of the male sexual partner

In most studies, the husbands of the cervical cancer patients were found to report more sexual partners, history of various genital infections like venereal warts, gonorrhea and herpes simplex genitalis compared to husbands of control subjects. Frequent use of condoms was associated with a lower risk for cancer of the cervix (Miller, Blumenthal & Blanchard, 2004).

2.1.1.3. Gynecological and obstetric events

Multiparity with short intervals between pregnancies (<2 yrs) has been consistently shown to increase the risk of cervical cancer (Hsieh et al., 1999). There is little evidence to show that the risk of cervical cancer is affected by age at menarche and menopause, characteristics of menses or personal hygiene (Smith et al., 2003).

http://dx.doi.org/10.5772/52881

2.1.1.4. Contraceptive methods

Recent research is showing that long-term users of oral contraceptives are at excess risk for cervical cancer, even after adjusting for sexual and social factors. The risk may be stronger for adenocarcinoma than squamous cell neoplasm (Smith et al., 2003).

2.1.1.5. Genetic factors

Although some reports suggest that a familial tendency does exist, but there is still little attention to it (Horng et al., 2004). Whether this tendency reflects environmental or genetic factors is unknown.

2.1.1.6. Dietary factors

Micronutrients (e.g. carotenoids, vitamin C and folate) are thought to have a protective effect to cervical cancer by promoting the regression of low grade squamous intra-epithelial lesion (SIL). Some components of fruits and vegetables have been suggested to be protective too (Hermandez et al., 2003).

2.1.1.7. Smoking

Some case control studies and a cohort investigation have demonstrated increased risk of cervical cancer and SIL among smokers even after controlling for most other risk factors. However, the smoking effect is restricted to squamous cell carcinoma and not among other histological types (Clifford et al., 2005). Smoking is strongly associated with high risk of cervical HPV infection because of correlation between smoking and sexual behavior (Clifford et al., 2005).Therefore, HPV status can confound studies of smoking and cervical cancer.

2.2. Infections other than HPV

HPV may not be the only agent involved in causation of cervical cancer. Of the other agents examined, most attention has been focused on herpes simplex virus type 2 (HSV-2) and Chlamydia which have been shown to increase the risk (Smith et al., 2002). One of the studies conducted in Uganda showed an increased risk of cervical cancer with multiple and concurrent infections, thus addressing the hypothesis that chronic cervico vaginal infection may increase the risk of HPV leading to cancer of the cervix (Schmauz et al., 1989). HIV infection is another viral infection which has been found to increase the risk of high grade lesions of the cervix and thus increasing risk of cancer of the cervix too. The effect is much higher among patients with both HIV and HPV (possible interaction). This may explain why the younger women are reporting with advanced cancer of the cervix.

2.3. Signs and symptoms

Symptoms usually do not appear until abnormal cervical cells become cancerous and invade nearby tissue. When this happens, the most common symptom is abnormal vaginal bleeding. Bleeding may start and stop between regular menstrual periods, or it may occur after sexual intercourse, douching, or a pelvic exam (Kumar et al., 2007). Menstrual bleeding may last longer and be heavier than usual. Bleeding after menopause or increased vaginal discharge may also be symptoms of cervical cancer.

2.4. Complications of cancer of the cervix

The common ones include: severe anemia as a result of severe or chronic on and off bleeding from the cervix; kidney complications and later kidney failure (renal failure with hydronephrosis) due to obstruction of the ureters by the infiltrating cancer which continues to spread to the pelvic walls; vesico vaginal fistula (communication between the urinary bladder and vagina) and rectal vaginal fistula (communication between rectum and vagina); and severe pain as a result of infiltration of the sacral nerves (Canavan & Doshi, 2000). Mortality is commonly due to anemia and Uremia (due to kidney failure).

3. Epidemiological issues

3.1. Cervical cancer: Burden of disease in the developed regions

Estimated incidence and mortality of cervical cancers in 2008 varied widely between countries in each developed regions (Table 1). Highest incidence rates for this cancer within the European region were recorded for Hungry (16.6/100, 00) followed by Czech Republic (13.8/100,000), and Poland (12.3/100,000), with lowest incidence rates in Finland, Greece, and Switzerland and Greece. Death rates due to cervical cancer are highest in Poland (6.2/100, 00) and lowest in Finland and Switzerland within the developed countries of European region (Table 1).

The lowest incidence (1.7/100,000) and mortality rate (5.7/100,000) from cervical cancer was registered in United States, while Canada had the highest incidence (6.6/100,000) and mortality rate (1.9/100,000), within the North America region (Table 1). Within the South America and Middle East region, Brazil and Israel had the highest incidence and mortality rate due to cervical cancer. A wide variation of cervical cancer incidence and mortality rate is observed among countries from the developed countries of Asia and the Pacific, whre highest incidence (10.8/100,000) and mortality rate (2.7/100,000) was registered in Republic of Korea (South Korea), while Australia had the lowest incidence (4.9/100,000) and mortality rate (1.4/100,000) (Table 1).

Region/Country	Annual incidence rates per 100,000	Annual cervical cancer deaths per 100,000
	Europe	
Belgium	9.4	2.7
Czech Republic	13.8	4.2
Denmark	11.0	2.5

Region/Country	Annual incidence rates per 100,000	Annual cervical cancer deaths per 100,000
Finland	3.7	0.9
France	7.1	1.8
Germany	6.9	2.3
Hungry	16.6	5.8
Iceland	6.3	1.6
Ireland	10.9	3.1
Italy	6.7	1.5
Luxemburg	6.3	1.9
Netherlands	5.4	1.5
Norway	9.3	2.3
Poland	12.3	6.2
Portugal	12.2	3.6
Spain	6.3	1.9
Sweden	7.4	1.8
Switzerland	4.0	0.9
United kingdom	7.2	2.0
	North America	
Canada	6.6	1.9
United States	5.7	1.7
	South America	
Brazil	24.5	10.9
Uruguay	16.5	6.8
	Middle East	
Israel	5.6	2.1
Saudi Arabia	2.1	0.8
Turkey	4.2	1.6
	Asia/Pacific	
Australia	4.9	1.4
Japan	9.8+	2.6
Republic of Korea	10.8	2.7
New Zealand	5.5	1.6

Source: Globocan 2008, International Agency for Research on Cancer

Table 1. Age-adjusted cervical cancer incidence and mortality rates for 2008 for 31 developed countries

3.2. Cervical cancer incidence in United Kingdom

Cervical cancer is the 9th most common cancer in the UK in 2009, accounting for 1% of all new cases and it is the11th most common cancer among women in the UK, accounting for around 2% of all new cases of cancer in females (Cancer Statistics Registrations, England, 2011). In 2009, there were 3,378 new cases of cervical cancer in the UK (Table 2). The crude incidence rate shows that there are around 11 new cervical cancer cases for every 100,000 females in the UK. The European age-standardized incidence rates (AS rates) of cervical cancer are significantly higher in Northern Ireland compared with England (Table 2). However, the rates do not differ significantly between the other countries.

	England	Wales	Scotland	Northern Ireland	United Kingdom
Cases	2,747	186	326	119	3,378
Crude rate	10.4	12.1	12.2	13.1	10.8
AS rate	9.8	11.4	11.2	12.9	10.1
AS rate-95% LCL*	9.4	9.8	10.0	10.6	9.8
AS rate-95% UCL**	10.2	13.0	12.4	15.2	10.5

** 95% LCL and 95% UCL are the 95% lower and upper confidence limits around the age standardized rate (AS rate)

Source: Cancer Research, United Kingdom

Table 2. Cervical Cancer, Number of New Cases, Crude and European Age-Standardized (AS) Incidence Rates per 100,000 Population, Females, UK, 2009

3.2.1. Trends of cervical cancer incidence in the United Kingdom over time

Cervical cancer incidence rates decreased dramatically since the late 1980s following the introduction of the national NHS cervical screening programs around the UK in 1988. Rates then reached a plateau in the early 2000s (shown for Great Britain in Figure 1). Rates decreased by 49% in Great Britain from their peak in 1985-1987 (at 16.3 per 100,000 women) to the lowest rate in 2002-2004 (at 8.4 per 100,000 women). This is because cervical screening detects and treats abnormal cells, and so can help prevent many cases of cervical cancer from ever developing (Thompson et al., 2010).

http://dx.doi.org/10.5772/52881

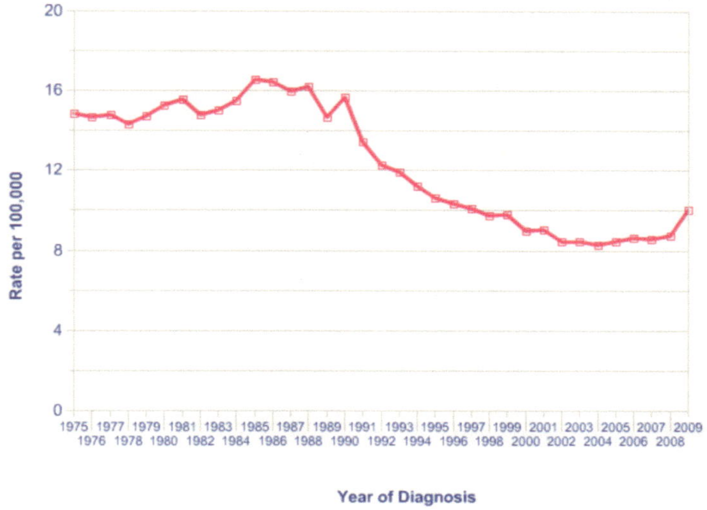

Figure 1. Cervical cancer: European age-standardized incidence rates, females, Great Britain, 1975-2009. Source: Cancer Research, UK

The age-standardized incidence rate for the UK initially shows a similar downward trend from 1993 onwards (Figure 2). However, since 2002-2004, the incidence rate has been increasing by more than 9% (from 8.4 in 2002-2004 to 9.2 in 2007-2009). Between 2008 and 2009 there was an increase in the age specific incidence rate of 14% for all ages in the UK (Figure 2).

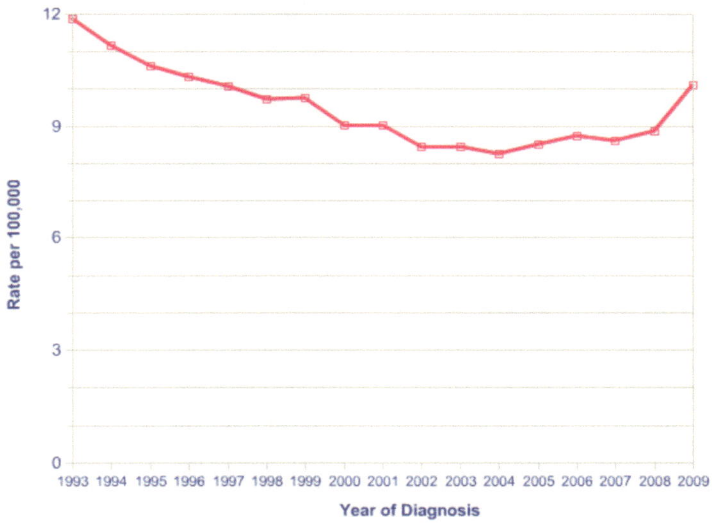

Figure 2. Cervical cancer: European age-standardized incidence rates, females, UK, 1993-2009. Source: Cancer Research, UK

3.3. Cervical cancer incidence in United States

Cervical cancer used to be the leading cause of cancer death for women in the United States. However, in the past 40 years, the number of cases of cervical cancer and the number of deaths from cervical cancer have decreased significantly. This decline largely is the result of many women getting regular Pap tests, which can find cervical pre cancer before it turns into cancer. It is estimated that 12,170 women will be diagnosed with and 4,220 women will die of cancer of the cervix uteri in 2012.

Although cervical cancer incidence and mortality rates have declined approximately 50% in the United States over the past three decades, the disease remains a serious health threat. There are large differences in the rates of new cases of and deaths from cervical cancer among women from different racial and ethnic groups in the United States. Death rates of cervical cancer for older Black women are nearly three times greater than those for White women of the same age group (Figure 3). Older Hispanic women, Asian women and American Indian/Alaska Native women also have much higher death rates from cervical cancer than do White women.

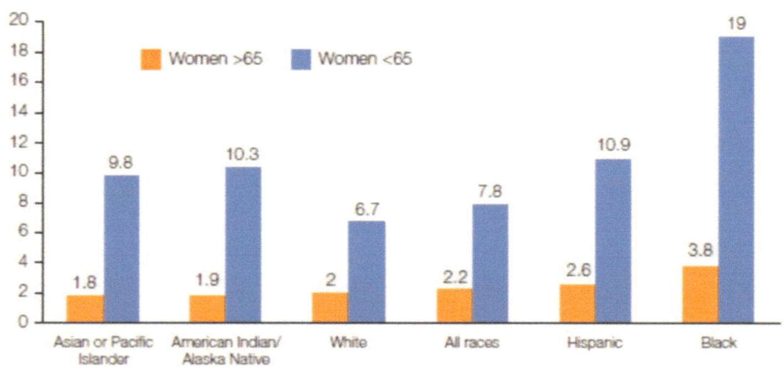

Figure 3. Mortality rate due to cervical cancer by race and age in United States. Source: National Cancer Institute, SEER data: Cancer Statistics Branch, released April 2006.

4. Prevention of cervical cancer

Cervical cancer is one of the most preventable types of cancer. The following preventive measures can be undertaken to help cross- out the cervical cancer: primary prevention and secondary prevention

4.1. Vaccines as primary prevention

By 2007 two prophylactic vaccines, both highly effective against oncogenic HPV types 16 and 18, available in industrialized countries. Between June and October 2006, a quadrivalent

http://dx.doi.org/10.5772/52881

HPV vaccine protective against HPV types 6, 11, 16 and 18 (Gardasil®, Merck) was licensed for use first by the US regulatory authorities and then by the European Commission (EC). EC approval for a bivalent vaccine protective against HPV types 16 and 18 (Cervarix®, GlaxoSmithKline Biologicals) is expected to follow (Harper et al., 2004; Villar et al., 2005) Clinical trial data to date suggest a minimum of four to five years' efficacy of close to 100% in preventing persistent infection and precancerous cervical abnormalities (cervical dysplasia) caused by type-specific disease. However, the vaccines are given in a series of three 0.5 ml intramuscular injections over a six month period, and duration of response is only available for the complete series (Harper et al., 2006).

In addition, women vaccinated with the bivalent vaccine had a 94% reduction in new infections with two other oncogenic HPV types, while those vaccinated with the quadrivalent formulation showed a measurable antibody response to those same additional types, giving evidence of cross-protection (Harper et al., 2006; Smith et al., 2006). One model suggests that a vaccine with 98% efficacy against HPV-16 and 18 could, within 40 to 50 years, reduce cervical cancer incidence by 51% if all adolescent girls were vaccinated before initiation of sexual activity (Goldie et al., 2003). The actual impact of the vaccine will be highly dependent on country-specific parameters, including the capacity to deliver current vaccines that require three consecutive doses, cold chain management and a possible booster dose year later (Lowndes, & Gill, 2005).

The new vaccine is designed to prevent cervical cancer by stimulating the body's immune system to make antibodies that will prevent the virus from infecting the woman. Unlike many vaccines that may contain live or killed virus particles, the HPV vaccine does not contain any genetic material responsible for creating warts, dysplasia or cancer (Anne-Sophie et al., 2011). Instead, the HPV virus is made up of the outer protein coat (cover) of the HPV virus. This cover tricks the immune system and causes it to make antibodies that protect the patient from infection. Because the vaccine contains none of the harmful viral genetic material, the vaccine is quite safe to administer to patients. While the vaccine is a huge step in fighting a preventable and treatable cancer, it is not the end-all be-all in cervical cancer care. There are over 30 types of HPV and the vaccines only protect against two or four strains, respectively. There are still other strains of HPV that cause cancer, and it is possible that a woman could already be infected by HPV when she was vaccinated. As a result, even with vaccination routine Pap tests or other cervical cancer screening tests are still necessary.

4.1.1. Vaccine implementation in the developed countries

In developed countries, the widespread use of cervical "Pap smear" screening programs has reduced the incidence of invasive cervical cancer by 50% or more. Current preventive vaccines reduce, but do not eliminate the chance of getting cervical cancer. Therefore, experts recommend that women combine the benefits of both programs by seeking regular Pap smear screening, even after vaccination.

Country	Vaccine implementation
Australia	Commencing in 2007 The Australian federal government began funding a voluntary program to make Gardasil available free of charge to women aged 12–26 for a period of two years, with an ongoing vaccination program for 12- and 13-year-olds as part of the pre-existing high school vaccination program. The Australian government and the Pharmaceutical Benefits Scheme (PBS) have approved the vaccine for use, and in 2007 began a nationwide vaccination program free of charge to schoolgirls in years 7 to 12. Australia also approved Gardasil for boys 9–15 years old, but Australia is not providing government funding for vaccinating boys.
Canada	Canada has approved use of Gardasil. Free vaccinations to protect women against HPV were slated to begin in September 2007 and will be offered to girls ages 11–14.
Denmark	Introduced in Denmark from 1 January 2009 as part of the Danish Childhood Vaccination program.
France	On July 17, 2007, France issued a directive authorizing state-aided voluntary vaccination for girls aged 14–23 years who have not yet become sexually active, or have been sexually active for less than a year.
Germany and Italy	On March 26, 2007, early approval for Gardasil vaccinations was granted in both Germany and Italy.
Greece	On February 12, 2007, Greece made HPV vaccination mandatory for girls entering gymnasion (7th grade). All vaccines including hepatitis B are mandatory and are supplied free to everyone in Greece, with parents being allowed to opt out of vaccinating their kids. Cervarix and Gardasil are supplied free to all girls and women between the ages of 12 and 26.
Norway	In Norway, starting from the fall of 2009, HPV vaccination was introduced into the national immunization program, for girls aged 12–13. In March 2010, 57% of all girls born in 1997 had received the first dose of the vaccine
South Korea	On July 27, 2007, South Korean government approved Gardasil for use in girls and women aged 9 to 26 and boys aged 9 to 15.Approval for use in boys was based on safety and immunogenicity but not efficacy.
Sweden	In Sweden, starting January 1, 2010, girls born in 1999 or later and in the ages 10 to 12 can receive a free HPV vaccine.
United Kingdom	In the UK the vaccine is licensed for girls aged 9 to 15, for women aged 16 to 26, and for boys aged 9–15.HPV vaccination with cervarix was introduced into the national immunization program in September 2008, for girls aged 12–13 across the UK. A two-year catch up campaign started in Autumn 2009 to vaccinate all girls up to 18 years of age. Catch up vaccination will be offered to: girls aged between 16 and 18 from autumn 2009, and girls aged between 15 and 17 from autumn 2010.By the end of the catch up campaign, all girls under 18 will have been offered the HPV vaccine.
United States	According to the US Centers for Disease Control and Prevention (CDC), getting as many girls vaccinated as early and as quickly as possible will reduce the cases of cervical cancer among middle-aged women in 30 to 40 years and reduce the transmission of this highly communicable infection.

Source: European Cervical Cancer Association; American Cancer Society

Table 3. Vaccine implementation by various developed countries

4.2. Cervical cancer screening: Secondary prevention

The objective of cervical cancer screening is to reduce both incidence and mortality. A successful screening program detects early, pre invasive lesions during the preclinical detectable phase and is able to reduce deaths by preventing the occurrence of invasive cancer. Diagnostic assessment requires colposcopy examination, with assessment of morphological features of the cervix as well as histological evaluation. Over the past five decades, widespread access to cervical screening and early treatment has been a cornerstone of basic reproductive health services for women in wealthy countries. The Papanicolaou test or "Pap smear" has significantly reduced the burden of cervical cancer in developed countries program (Hristova & Hakama, 1997; Duguid, Duncan, & Currie, 1985; Taylor et al., 2001).

In resource-rich settings, women are usually able to make repeated visits to seek screening, diagnosis and treatment in clinics. The health system is equipped with skilled lab technicians, referral systems and clinicians capable of effectively managing this disease. It is estimated that regular screening reduces the risk of cancer by 80% to 98% (Olesen, 1988; WHO 1986). Organized screening programs for cervical cancer using Pap smears have been shown to be more effective than opportunistic or non-organized screening. Opportunistic screening typically misses the women at greatest risk (Anttila et al., 2004). Studies show that if a woman is screened only once in her lifetime between the ages of 30 to 40 it would reduce her lifetime risk of cervical cancer between 25-36%.

In Finland, the population-based cervical cancer screening program which began in 1963 achieved a 60% reduction in the incidence of cancer at 10 years (Nieminen, Kallio & Hakama, 1995). In Norway, a population-based nationwide cervical cancer screening program was introduced in 1995. Two years later the incidence of invasive cancer was 22% lower (Nygard, Skare & Thoresen, 2002). In the United Kingdom the incidence of cervical cancer in women aged 20-69 years fell by 33% between 1991-1993 and 1998-2000; mortality fell by 36% over the same period (Canfell, Sitas & Beral, 2006). In Sweden, for example, the overall incidence of cervical cancer declined by 67% over a 40-year period, from 20 cases per 100 000 women (world standard rate) in 1965 to 6.6 cases per 100 000 women in 2005. Conversely, the incidence of invasive cancer increased in an area of Denmark where organized screening had been discontinued (Lynge, 1998). Other screening methods include direct visualization of the cervix, liquidbased cytology and HPV screening.

A number of National guidelines are currently moving towards less frequent smear tests (once every 3-5 years) since the cervical lesions develop fairly slowly after several years. Women with high grade lesions of the cervix are further evaluated using colposcopy, biopsy and subsequent treatment of confirmed lesions. The women with low grade lesions are generally advised to return for routine follow up smears. Organized programs with systematic call recall and follow up showed greatest effect in Finland and Iceland using fewer resources compared to USA where they are successful but more resources used (Sankaranarayanan, Budukh, & Rajkumar, 2001). Since progression to cervical cancer occurs after several years and the low grade lesions tend to regress spontaneously or may not progress, high frequency of screening would help in detection of previously missed high-grade lesion of the cervix.

Current procedures that involve screening women once every 1-5yrs have considerable cost and resource implications.

4.2.1. Status of cervical screening in the European Union

Almost all EU countries have a screening policy for cervical cancer. However, there are major variations in how the screening is organized, the type of screening activities, the targeted age range and the recommended screening interval, as well as payment strategies. A review in 2004 (Mackay et al, 2006) showed that national screening programs were in place in the Nordic countries, the United Kingdom, Latvia, Slovenia, the Netherlands and Hungary. Regional screening programs were operational in Spain, Portugal, Italy, Romania, Czech Republic, Austria and Belgium. Pilot programs existed in France, Greece, Ireland and Estonia. No population-based screening program was in place in Germany, although there was a screening policy.

The recommended screening interval ranges between three and five years in most EU countries for which information is available. Some countries or regions recommend an excessive number of smears, with consequent potential for over diagnosis and overtreatment. Similarly, the population covered by the screening programs varied between 30% in Slovenia and 100% in the Nordic countries and Italy (Anttila et al., 2004).EU recommendations state that cervical cancer screening should be offered on a population basis in organized screening programs. Pap smear screening for cervical abnormalities should start by the age of 30 (at the latest) and definitely not before the age of 20 (Council of the European Union, 2003). Detailed European guidelines on quality assurance screening programmes have been developed (European Cancer Network, 2007). Centralized data systems are essential for monitoring and evaluating the effectiveness of such programs.

4.2.2. Status of cervical screening in the US

The United States Preventive Services Task Force supports screening every 5 years in those who are between 30 and 65 years when cytology is used in combination with HPV testing. The American Cancer Society recommends these screening guidelines for most adults: (i) cervical cancer screening (testing) should begin at age 21; (ii) women under age 21 should not be tested;(iii) women between ages 21 and 29 should have a Pap test every 3 years. Now there is also a test called the HPV test. HPV testing should not be used in this age group unless it is needed after an abnormal Pap test result; (iv) women between the ages of 30 and 65 should have a Pap test plus an HPV test (called "co-testing") every 5 years; (v) women over age 65 who have had regular cervical cancer testing with normal results should not be tested for cervical cancer. Once testing is stopped, it should not be started again; (vi) women with a history of a serious cervical pre-cancer should continue to be tested for at least 20 years after that diagnosis, even if testing continues past age 65; (vii) a woman who has had her uterus removed (and also her cervix) for reasons not related to cervical cancer and who has no history of cervical cancer or serious pre-cancer should not be tested; (viii) a woman who has been vaccinated against HPV should still follow the screening recommendations

http://dx.doi.org/10.5772/52881

for her age group. Some women – because of their history – may need to have a different screening schedule for cervical cancer.

5. Conclusions

Cervical cancer is a unique public health challenge. It is gender-specific, caused by a sexually transmitted virus, and its primary and secondary prevention strategies target opposite ends of a wide age spectrum. The natural history of cervical cancer is well studied, and screening programs that identify pre-cancers early have been successful at significantly reducing disease, albeit at significant financial cost. Primary prevention through HPV vaccination will most likely be one of the most remarkable medical advances of this century. Together, secondary prevention through screening and early treatment and primary prevention through early adolescent vaccination could provide a comprehensive strategy for a long-term vision to eliminate cervical cancer. Thanks to the effectiveness of national screening programs, the incidence and mortality rates for cervical cancer have declined dramatically in developed countries. Vaccination against HPV infection could reduce the risk of infection and, most importantly, decrease the incidence of cervical cancer. Therefore, beating cervical cancer in the developed countries is not a dream in the far future, it is happening today.

Author details

Mosiur Rahman[1*], Abdur R. Mia[2], Syed Emdadul Haque[3], Mostofa Golam[4], Nowsheen Sharmin Purabi[5] and S. A. R. Choudhury[6]

*Address all correspondence to: swaponru_2000@yahoo.com

1 Department of International Health, Division of Public Health, Graduate School of Tokyo Medical and Dental University, Tokyo, Japan

2 Senior Assistant Secretary, Ministry of Establishment, Government of Bangladesh, Bangladesh

3 University of Chicago Research Bangladesh LTD, Mohakhali, Dhaka, Bangladesh

4 Department of Population Science and Human Resource Development, University of Rajshahi, Rajshahi, Bangladesh

5 Register Gynecology and Obstetrics, Anwar Khan Modern Medical College, Bangladesh

6 Department of Pharmacology, Bangubandhu Sheikh Mujib Medical University (BSMMU), Shahabagh, Dhaka, Bangladesh

References

[1] Anne-Sophie, B., Andrew, K., Ian, H.F., & Deepak, M. (2011). New approaches to immunotherapy for HPV associated cancers. Cancers, 3, 3461-3495.

[2] Anttila, A., Ronco, G., Clifford, G., Bray, F., Hakama, M., Arbyn, M., & Weiderpass, E.. (2004). Cervical cancer screening programs and policies in 18 European countries. Br J Cancer, 91(5),935-941.

[3] Bray, F., Wibe, A., & Dorum, L.M. (2005). Global cancer statistics, 2002. CA Cancer J Clin, 74, 74-108.

[4] Canavan, T.P., & Doshi, N.R. (2000). "Cervical cancer". Am Fam Physician, 61 (5), 1369–76.

[5] Cancer Statistics Registrations, England. (2011). Cervical cancer incidence statistics. Available at: http://www.ons.gov.uk/ons/rel/vsob1/cancer-statistics-registrations--england--series-mb1-/index.html.

[6] Canfell, K., Sitas, F., & Beral, V. (2006). Cervical cancer in Australia and the United Kingdom: comparison of screening policy and uptake, and cancer incidence and mortality. Med J Aust, 185(9), 482-486.

[7] Clifford, G.M., Polesel, J., Rickenbach, M., Dal Maso, L., Keiser, O., Kofler, A.,. et al. (2005). Cancer risk in the Swiss HIV Cohort study: associations with immunodeficiency, smoking and highly active antiretroviral therapy. J Natl Cancer Inst, 97(6), 425-32.

[8] Council of the European Union (2003). Council recommendation of 2 December 2003 on cancer screening, Official Journal of the European Union (2003/878/EC, L327/34-38).

[9] Day, N.E. (1984). Effect of cervical cancer screening in Scandinavia. Obstet Gynecol, 63,714–8.

[10] Duguid, H.L., Duncan, I.D., & Currie, J. (1985). Screening for cervical intraepithelial neoplasia in Dundee and Angus 1962–81 and its relation with invasive cervical cancer. Lancet, 2, 1053–6.

[11] European Cancer Network. (2007). European Guidelines for Quality Assurance in Cervical Cancer Screening. (available at:http://www.cancernetwork.de/cervical/cerv_guidelines.htm, accessed 28 November 2007).

[12] Ferlay, J., Shin, H.R., Bray, F., Forman, D., Mathers, C., & Parkin, D.M. (2010). Cancer incidence and mortality worldwide: IARC Cancer Base No. 10 [Internet]. Lyon (France): IARC; 2010, Available from: http://globocan.iarc.fr.

[13] Goldie, S.J., Grima, D., Kohli, M., Wright, T.C., Weinstein, M., & Franco, E. (2003). A comprehensive natural history model of HPV infection and cervical cancer to esti-

mate the clinical impact of a prophylactic HPV 16/18 vaccine. Int J Cancer, 106, 896–904.

[14] Harper, D.M., Franco, E.L., Wheeler, C., Ferris, D.G., Jenkins, D., Schuind ,A., et al. (2004). Efficacy of a bivalent L1 virus-like particle vaccine in prevention of infection with human papilloma virus types 16 and 18 in young women: a randomized controlled trial. Lancet, 364, 1757–1765.

[15] Harper, D.M., Franco, E.L., Wheeler, C.M., Moscicki, A.B., Romanowski, B., Roteli-Martins, C.M. et al. (2006). Sustained efficacy up to 4-5 years of a bivalent L1 virus-like particle vaccine against human papillomavirus types 16 and 18: follow-up from a randomised control trial. Lancet, 367(9518),1247-1255.

[16] Hermandez, B.Y., McDuffie, K., Wilkens, L.R., Kamemoto, L., Goodman, M.T. (2003). Diet and pre-malignant lesions of the cervix: Evidence of a protective role for folate, riboflavin, thiamin and vitamin B12.Cancer Causes Control, 14(9), 859-70.

[17] Horng, J.T., Hu, K.C., Wu, L.C., Huang, H.D., Lin, F.M., Huang, S.L., et al. (2004). Identifying the combination of genetic factors that determine susceptibility to cervical cancer. IEEE Trans inf Technol Biomed, 8(1), 59-66.

[18] Hristova, L., & Hakama, M. (1997). Effect of screening for cancer in the Nordic countries on deaths, cost and quality of life up to the year 2017. Acta Oncol, 36(Suppl 9),1–60.

[19] Hsieh, C.Y., You, S.L, Kao, C.L., & Chen, C.J. (1999). Reproductive and infectious risk factors for invasive cervical cancer in Taiwan. Anticancer Res, 19(5C), 4495-500.

[20] Kari, P.B., & Marc, R.L. (2008). Human Papillomavirus (HPV), HPV-Related Disease, and the HPV Vaccine . Rev Obstet Gynecol, 1(1), 2–10.

[21] Karlsson, R., Jonsson, M., Edlund, K., Evander, M., Gustavasson, A., Boden, E, et al. (1995). Life time number of partners as the only independent risk factor for human papillomavirus infection: a population based study. Sex Transm Dis, 22(2), 119.

[22] Kumar, V., Abbas, A.K., Fausto, N., & Mitchell, R.N. (2007). Robbins Basic Pathology ((8th ed.) ed.). Saunders Elsevier. pp. 718–721.

[23] Lowndes, C.M., & Gill, O.N. (2005). Cervical cancer, human papillomavirus, and vaccination. Brit Med J, 331(7522), 915–916.

[24] Lynge, E. (1998). Mammography screening for breast cancer in Copenhagen April 1991-March 1997. Mammography Screening Evaluation Group, APMIS Suppl, 83:1-44.

[25] Mackay, J., Jemal, A., Lee, N.C., & Parkin, D.M. (eds) (2006). The Cancer Atlas. Atlanta, Ga. American Cancer Society, 2006:70-71

[26] (available at: http://www.cancer.org/downloads/AA/CancerAtlas22. pdf, accessed on 28 November 2007)

[27] Miller, K., Blumenthal, P., & Blanchard, K. (2004). Oral contraceptives and cervical cancer: Critique of a recent review. Contraception, 69(5), 347-51.

[28] Nieminen, P., Kallio, M., Hakama, M. (1995). The effect of mass screening on incidence and mortality of squamous and adenocarcinoma of cervix uteri. Obstet Gynecol, 85(6):1017-1021.

[29] Nygard, J.F., Skare, G.B., Thoresen, S.O. (2002). The cervical cancer screening programme in Norway, 1992-2000: changes in Pap smear coverage and incidence of cervical cancer. J Med Screen, 9(2), 86-91.

[30] Olesen, F. (1988). A case-control study of cervical cytology before diagnosis of cervical cancer in Denmark. Int J Epidemiol 17,501-508.

[31] Sankaranarayanan, R., Budukh, A.M., & Rajkumar, R. (2001). Effective screening programmes for cervical cancer in low- and middle-income developing countries. Bull World Health Organ, 79(10), 954-62.

[32] Schmauz, R., Okong, P., de Villiers, E.M., Dennin, R., Brade, L., Lwanga, S.K., et al. (1989). Owor r. Multiple infections in cases of cervical cancer from a high incidence area in tropical Africa. Int J Cancer, 43(5), 805-9.

[33] Smith, J.S., Green, J., de Gonzalez A, et al. (2003). Cervical cancer and use of hormonal contraceptives. a systematic review. Lancet, 361, 1159-67.

[34] Smith, J.S., Herrero, R., Bosetti, C., Bosch, F.X., Eluf-Neto, J., Castellsague, X., et al. (2002). International Agency for research on Cancer (IARC). Multi Centric Cervical cancer study Group. Herpes simplex virus-2 as a human papillomavirus cofactor in the etiology of invasive cervical cancer J Natl Cancer.Inst, 94(21), 1604-13.

[35] Smith, J.F., Brownlow, M.K., Brown, M.J., Esser,. M.T., Ruiz, W., Brown, D.R. (2006). Gardasil antibodies cross-neutralize pseudovirion infection of vaccine-related HPV types. Presented at the 23rd International Papillomavirus Conference and Clinical Workshop. Prague

[36] Taylor, R.J., Morrell, S.L., Mamoon, H.A., & Wain, G.V. (2001). Effects of screening on cervical cancer incidence and mortality in New South Wales implied by influences of period of diagnosis and birth cohort. J Epidemiol Community Health, 55(11), 782–8.

[37] Tiffen, J., & Mahon, S.M. (2006). Cervical cancer: What should we tell women about screening? Clinical Journal of Oncology Nursing, 10(4), 527-531.

[38] Thomson, C.S., Woolnough , S., Wickenden, M., Hiom, S., & Twelves, C.J. (2010). Sunbed use in children aged 11-17 in England: face to face quota sampling surveys in the National Prevalence Study and Six Cities Study. BMJ, 340, c877.

[39] Villa,, L.L., Costa, R.L., Petta, C.A., Andrade, R.P., Ault, K.A., Giuliano, A.R. et al. (2005). Prophylactic quadrivalent human papillomavirus (types 6, 11, 16, 18) L1 vi-

rus-like particle vaccine in young women: A randomized double-blind placebo-controlled multicentre phase II efficacy trial. Lancet, 6, 271–278.

[40] WHO (1986). Screening for cancer of the uterine cervix, 1ARC. Geneva, World Health Organization.

Chapter 17

Burden of Human Papillomavirus Infection in Latin America

Juan Carlos Sepúlveda-Arias and
Adalucy Álvarez-Aldana

Additional information is available at the end of the chapter

http://dx.doi.org/10.5772/53662

1. Introduction

Human papillomavirus (HPV)-associated disease is an important public health problem worldwide. HPV is not only associated with 530,000 new cases of cervical cancer and 275,000 cervical cancer deaths worldwide each year but also causes vulvar, vaginal, anal, and penile cancers as well as cervical and vulvar/vaginal precancerous lesions, genital warts, and respiratory papillomatosis. Most individuals are not aware that they are infected with HPV because of its subclinical or asymptomatic presentation, and thus, the virus can be spread easily and unknowingly during sexual foreplay or sexual intercourse [1].

Cervical HPV infection is the most prevalent sexually transmitted disease [2]. HPV is so common that more than half of all sexually active adults will be infected in their lifetime, although young, sexually active women bear the brunt of both infection and clinical complications. The Centers for Disease Control estimates that at least half of all sexually active individuals will acquire HPV at some point in their lives, and at least 80% of women will acquire an HPV infection by age 50 [3]. At least 50% of men will acquire a genital HPV infection during their lifetime [1].

In 1995, the International Agency for Research on Cancer (IARC) first classified HPV types 16 and 18 as carcinogenic to humans, but based on more recent evidence, the list of carcinogenic HPV types has been expanded to include a total of 13 genital mucosotropic HPV types as being definite or probable carcinogens (grade 1 or 2a) based on their frequent association with invasive cervical cancer (ICC) (4). The causal role of HPV in all cancers of the uterine cervix has been firmly established biologically and epidemiologically. The proteins of the early genes E6 and E7 of the high-risk HPV types act as oncoproteins and play a key role in carcinogenesis [5]. HPV-16 and -18 account for approximately 70% of cancers of the cervix, vagina, and anus and approximately 30–40% of cancers of the vulva, penis, and oropharynx. Other cancers that are causally linked to HPV include non-melanoma skin cancer and cancer of the conjunctiva. Although HR-HPV infection is a necessary cause of cervical cancer, it is not a sufficient cause [6].

For the vast majority of people, these infections will be asymptomatic and will clear within 1–2 years [7-12]; however, a substantial increase in the risk for cervical cancer exists for women who develop persistent infection with HR-HPV [13-16]. Infection with low oncogenic risk HPV types (LR-HPV) is also responsible for considerable morbidity associated with benign lesions known as condyloma acuminata (genital warts) and a proportion of low-grade squamous intraepithelial cervical lesions [17-19].

Because cervical cancer affects relatively young women, it represents the single biggest cause of years of life lost (YLL) from cancer in the developing world, contributing more to this burden of disease measure than tuberculosis, maternal conditions or acquired immunodeficiency syndrome (AIDS). In developed countries, Papanicolaou (PAP) smear test screening has decreased the incidence of cervical cancer by approximately 70% in recent decades; however, cervical cancer still represents a major public health issue in Latin America because of the failure of prevention programs [20].

Cervical cancer is the third most common malignancy in women worldwide and the second most common malignancy in women living in developing countries. More than 85% of the global burden occurs in developing countries. Cervical cancer accounts for 13% of all female cancers, and South America is a high-risk region (2.5%); approximately 88% of deaths occur in developing countries. These differences between countries are believed to reflect protection through screening, differences in exposure to HPV and other cofactors. HPV is associated with 68,220 new cases of cervical cancer and 31,712 associated cervical cancer deaths in Latin America each year [21]. Cervical cancer is a major public health problem in Latin America, which has some of the highest incidence and mortality rates worldwide. Information on HPV prevalence and type distribution in several countries in Latin America is crucial to predict the future impact of HPV16/18 vaccines and screening programs and to establish appropriate post-vaccine virological surveillance.

The discovery of HPV infection as a necessary cause of cervical cancer has created many new paths for prevention. The most promising strategies include screening for infection with HR-HPV types and immunization to prevent infection with HR-HPV types. Unfortunately, many developing countries that have invested in screening programs have yet to witness a substantial reduction in cervical cancer [22]. HPV DNA testing has been suggested as an alternative to primary screening; HPV DNA testing is less dependent on the quality of personnel training [23-26]. Prophylactic HPV vaccination, which currently protects against the most common LR-HPV types (HPVs 6 and 11) and HR-HPV types (HPVs 16 and 18), offers the greatest potential to reduce the burden of ICC and other HPV-related diseases [1]. In many of the nations where the burden of HPV and cervical cancer is the highest, vaccination and HPV testing remain too expensive.

In this chapter, we will discuss HPV infection and provide data on HPV prevalence and genotype distribution, risk factors for HPV infection, co-factors associated with HSIL or ICC progression, the burden of cervical cancer and prevention strategies. All of these topics will be discussed in the context of Latin America. We hope that this chapter will provide researchers with important up-to-date information concerning the problem of HPV infection and HPV-associated cancers in Latin America.

2. HPV prevalence and genotype distribution

The establishment of the etiologic role of HPV on cervical cancer and the development of proposals for preventive and clinical applications have prompted considerable interest in exploring the epidemiological characteristics of HPV infection in different populations.

Worldwide, there are important variations in the prevalence of HPV in different age groups. Although in the United States, Europe, and some Asian countries, HPV prevalence declines with age [27-30], in Latin American countries, the majority of studies with age-specific HPV prevalence data have shown a slight U-shaped curve [31]. Overall, HPV prevalence in the Latin American and Caribbean (LAC) population has been found to be 2-fold higher than the average worldwide prevalence [32]. Different studies from countries in Latin America have assessed the prevalence of HPV infection and types in healthy women [33] and patients with pre-neoplastic and neoplastic cervical lesions (HSIL, ICC) [20]. These studies showed prevalence rates of HPV infection of 16.1%, 82% and 89% in NC, HSIL and ICC, respectively. The most prevalent HPV types were the following: NC (HPV-16, 31, 18, 58, and 6), HSIL (HPV-16, 18, 58, 31, and 33), and ICC (HPV-16, 18, 31, 45, and 33). See Tables 1 and 2.

Country	More prevalent HPV types	Cyto-histological diagnosis	HPV prevalence (%)	References
Argentina	16,18,6,11,31,58	NC LSIL HSIL ICC	26 - 43 33.1 - 96 71.4 - 100 100	[34 - 39]
Bolivia	6,11,26, 52,66,39	NC LSIL HSIL ICC	5.9 NR NR NR	[40]

Country	More prevalent HPV types	Cyto-histological diagnosis	HPV prevalence (%)	References
Brazil	16,18,33,6,11,58	NC LSIL HSIL ICC	12 - 25 26.4 - 90.4 57 - 100 41.8 - 93	[41 - 50]
Chile	16,18,31,33,45,52	NC LSIL HSIL ICC	11.2 - 40 61.2 - 100 55.9 - 100 71 - 95	[51 - 58]
Colombia	16,18,31,58,33,45	NC LSIL HSIL ICC	10.5 - 39.1 46.9 - 83.9 53.8 – 91.8 70 - 100	[10, 59 - 64]
Ecuador	16,31,18,6,52,56	NC LSIL HSIL ICC	20 - 20.6 44.8 - 76.9 50 - 100 81	[65 - 68]
Paraguay	16,18,33,31,45, 52	NC LSIL HSIL ICC	25 68 78 97	[69 - 71]
Perú	16,18,31,35,45,52	NC LSIL HSIL ICC	13.4 - 17.7 NR NR 92 - 95.3	[72, 73]
Venezuela	16,18,33,45,52,58	NC LSIL HSIL ICC	NR 68 92.8 - 95.3 98.7 - 98.9	[74, 75]

Table 1. HPV prevalence and more frequent HPV types in South America.

Country	More prevalent HPV types	Cyto-histological diagnosis	HPV prevalence (%)	References
Costa Rica	16,18,58,31,33	NC	11 - 22.4	[76, 77]
		LSIL	73 - 80.9	
		HSIL	87.5 - 89	
		ICC	88 - 97.1	
Cuba	16,31,52,66,18	NC	NR	[78]
		LSIL	33.3	
		HSIL	55.6	
		ICC	NR	
Guatemala	16,18,56,66,35	NC	33.6 - 59	[79]
		LSIL	NR	
		HSIL	NR	
		ICC	82.6 – 95.2	
Honduras	16,18,31,58,45,11,51	NC	39.5 - 51	[80 - 83]
		LSIL	47.7 - 81	
		HSIL	66.7 - 97	
		ICC	80 - 93	
Mexico	16,18,31,58,45,59	NC	8.8 - 40.9	[28, 84 - 91]
		LSIL	24 - 94.5	
		HSIL	29.4 - 93.7	
		ICC	84.6 - 100	
Nicaragua	16,58,31,52,51	NC	48.1	[92]
		LSIL	67.5	
		HSIL	86.8	
		ICC	94.7	
Panama	16[a]	NC	NR	[93]
		LSIL	NR	
		HSIL	NR	
		ICC	70	

Table 2. HPV prevalence and more frequent HPV types in Central America and Mexico.

[a] Only HPV 16 was detected.

3. Risk factors for HPV infection and co-factors associated with HSIL or ICC progression

Epidemiological studies investigating risk factors for HPV infection have clearly and consistently shown that sexual behavior patterns influence the acquisition of HPV because the primary mode of transmission of HPV is sexual. Sexual behavior patterns include early age at first sexual intercourse, the number of sexual partners, and the sexual behavior of male partners [32].

Almost all cases of cervical cancer are attributable to persistent HPV infections, leading to the conclusion that HPV infection is a necessary cause of the disease [94]. Follow-up studies of women with and without cervical abnormalities have indicated that the continuous presence of HR-HPV is necessary for the development, maintenance and progression of cervical intraepithelial neoplasia (CIN) [9-13]. However, only a small fraction of women with cervical HPV infection develop ICC, suggesting that other co-factors in addition to HPV are necessary to cause cancer progression. High parity, the long-term use of oral contraceptives, cigarette smoking, and co-infection with human immunodeficiency virus (HIV) have been described [32].

Tables 3 and 4 describe the co-factors associated with HPV infection and co-factors associated with HSIL or ICC progression in several studies from Central and South America, respectively.

Country	Co-factors	Reference
Argentina	Number of sexual partners, *C. trachomatis* infection or history of previous sexually transmitted diseases, early age at first intercourse, early age at first pregnancy.	[35, 36, 38, 95]
Brazil	Marital status, age under 30, number of sexual partners, sexually transmitted diseases, alcohol abuse, sexual behavior.	[49,96]
Colombia	Number of sexual partners, indigenous ethnicity, no history of previous pregnancies, nulliparity, early age at first intercourse, *C. trachomatis* infection, high parity.	[97 - 99]
Costa Rica	High vaginal pH, *C. trachomatis* infection, number of sexual partners.	[77, 100]
Cuba	Parity, early age at first sexual intercourse.	[78]
Ecuador	Number of sexual partners.	[66]
Guatemala	Occasional partner during the last 6 months and smoking habit.	[79]
Honduras	Sexual behavior, smoking, exposure to wood smoke and low socioeconomic status, single female.	[82, 83, 101, 102]
Mexico	Age, marital status, number of sexual partners, infection with *C. trachomatis*, progesterone-based contraceptives, history of sexually transmitted diseases and use of emergency contraceptive pill.	[28, 103, 104]
Peru	Early age at first sexual intercourse and number of sexual partners.	[105]

Table 3. Co-factors associated with HPV infection in Latin America.

http://dx.doi.org/10.5772/53662

Country	Co-factors	Reference
Brazil	Age[a], ethnicity[b], early age at first sexual intercourse[c], number of sexual partners[d], history of sexually transmitted diseases or concurrent sexually transmitted disease[e], smoking habit[f], *C. trachomatis* infection[g].	[41, 44, 106, 107]
Colombia	Parity[h], exposure to wood smoke[i], viral load[j].	[61, 108]
Costa Rica	Number of live births[k], use of oral contraceptives[l] and smoking habit[f].	[109]
Honduras	Number of sexual partners[d], parity[h], early age at first sexual intercourse[c], exposure to wood smoke[i], low socioeconomic status[m], absence of Pap smear screening[n].	[80, 82]
Mexico	Age[a], early age at first sexual intercourse[c], number of sexual partners, parity[h], viral load[j].	[84, 88, 110]
Panama	Early age at first sexual intercourse[c], parity[h], absence of Pap smear controls[n], smoking habit[f].	[93]
Paraguay	Parity[h], early age at first intercourse[c], no schooling[o], number of sexual partner[d] and absence of Pap smear screening[n].	[69]
Peru	Parity[h], age[a], no schooling[o], lack of good-quality screening and of adequate follow-up care[p], long-term use of oral contraceptives[q] and smoking habit[f].	[72, 105]

Measures of risk (OR or RR) and their corresponding 95% CI and reference.

[a] OR 231 [25,48-2108,63] Ref 41; OR 2,1 [1,1-4,1] Ref 110.

[b] OR 5,77 [2,76-12,09] Ref 41.

[c] OR 6,83 [1,46-32,02] Ref 41; OR 1,26 [0,76-2,08] Ref 82; OR 2,11 [1,2-3,6] Ref 110; OR 8,5 [4,4-16,8] Ref 84; OR 1,91 [1,2-3] Ref 93; OR 7,8 [3,4-17,7] Ref 69.

[d] OR 5,43 [2,58-11,40] Ref 41; OR 2,25 [1,32-3,82] Ref 82; OR 7,4 [3,8-14,5] Ref 69.

[e] OR 13 [1,9-56,3] Ref 44, 106.

[f] OR 11,24 [5,09-24,83] Ref 41; RR 2,7 [1,1-6,7] Ref 109; OR 1,86 [1,1-3,1] Ref 93.

[g] OR 2,1 [1,1-4] Ref 107.

[h] OR 4,1 [1,6-10,6] Ref 108; OR 6,3 [1,36-2,98] Ref 80; OR 10,9 [2,6-46,5] Ref 84; OR 1,87 [1,2-3] Ref 93; OR 9,3 [3,6-23,9] Ref 69; OR 8,3 [1-65,6] Ref 105; OR 6,5 [1,1-6,93] Ref 72.

[i] OR 7,3 [3-19,4] Ref 108; OR 4,89 [0,51-47,1] Ref 80.

[j] OR 13,4 [2,4-74] Ref 61; OR 3,51 [2,2-5,6] Ref 110; OR 365,8 [94,7-1412] Ref 88.

[k] RR 3,7 [1,8-7,4] Ref 109.

[l] RR 1,6 [0,89-2,9] Ref 109.

[m] OR 1,8 [1,2-2,5] Ref 82.

[n] OR 2,31 [1,16-4,63] Ref 82; OR 2,88 [1,8-4,5] Ref 93; OR 23,9 [10,4-54,9] Ref 69.

[o] OR 27,7 [9,6-79,9] Ref 69; OR 3,2 [1,3-8,3] Ref 105.

[p] OR 29,4 [3,6-240,1] Ref 105.

[q] OR 2,6 [0,9-7,6] Ref 72.

Table 4. Co-factors associated with HSIL or ICC progression in Latin America.

4. Burden of cervical cancer

After breast and colorectal cancer, cervical cancer is the third leading cancer site worldwide, and it is second among women. The incidence of cervical cancer in Latin America is among the highest in the world. Cervical cancer incidence and mortality are a significant public health problem. In total, 85% of the global burden of cervical cancer occurs in developing countries, where it accounts for 13% of all female cancers. South America is a region of high risk. In 2008, cervical cancer was responsible for 275,000 deaths, 31,400 in Latin America and the Caribbean [21].

In Latin American countries, the incidence and mortality of ICC ranges from 14.4 to 39.9 and 6.8 to 20.6 cases per 100,000 women, respectively, with the highest incidence and mortality rates in Nicaragua (39.9 and 20.6, respectively, Table 5). The data were taken fron Globocan (http://globocan.iarc.fr/factsheets/cancers/cervix.asp). These differences between countries are most likely a reflection of screening programs and differences in exposure to HPV and other cofactors.

5. Prevention strategies

Cervical cancer caused by HPV is a major public health problem that can be prevented with cervical cancer screening programs. Public health programs for cervical cancer screening with cytology and the effective treatment of early pre-cancers and cancers have resulted in a major reduction in mortality from cervical cancer. Unfortunately, cervical cancer screening programs have not yet been successful in most developing countries [111], despite the highest burden of cervical cancer in these countries [21].

In Colombia, supply problems are found in cervical cancer in therms of structure, processes and results [112]. The follow-up for women with abnormal cytology has not been carried out, information systems are insufficient, and problems in the quality of cytology readings have been reported ([112, 113]. These deficiencies explain, in part, the low impact that screening has had on cervical cancer in Colombia, and the national screening and diagnostic services offered are not organized into a structured program [112].

Country	Incidence rate (per 100,000 women)	Mortality rate (per 100,000 women)
Argentina	17.5	7.4
Bolivia	36.4	16.7
Brazil	24.5	10.9
Chile	14.4	6.6
Colombia	21.5	10.0
Costa Rica	17.5	6.7
Cuba	23.1	8.9
Ecuador	27.1	13.3
Guatemala	30.5	15.2
Honduras	37.8	19.7
Nicaragua	39.9	20.6
Panama	25.3	12.6
Paraguay	35.0	16.6
Peru	34.5	16.3
Uruguay	16.5	6.8
Venezuela	31.4	14.4

Table 5. Incidence and mortality rates for ICC in Latin America.

To screen successfully in LAC, the screening programs must follow the requirements of low-resource settings: screening, diagnosis and treatment provided on-site or in clinics accessible to the majority of at-risk women; a low-cost, low-technology screening test that can lead to the immediate treatment of abnormalities; wide coverage of at-risk women; appropriate educational programs directed toward health workers and women to ensure correct implementation and high participation; and a built-in mechanism for evaluation of the screening program [22].

With the advent of newer technology, such as HPV vaccines and HPV tests, followed by simple well-known techniques, such as Pap, VIA and cryotherapy, cervical cancer rates may start to decrease worldwide. Prophylactic HPV vaccines containing oncogenic types HPV-16 and 18 can prevent up to 65–70% of cervical cancer deaths. However, they have yet to become accessible to poorer countries, where the greatest burden of disease exists. The price per dose is expensive for use in most countries in LAC. This situation is extremely disappointing because the experience of resource-poor countries in LAC has demonstrated that vaccination programs have been very effective. The results from different countries in Latin America have indicated that HPV testing has a greater sensitivity to detect CIN 2/3 and ICC than the Pap test [114-116], and HPV typing is an inexpensive and effective method for identifying cervical neoplasia and women at risk of developing cervical neoplasia; HPV typing improves quality control for both false-negative and false-positive cytology results [117].

The screening guidelines of the American College of Obstetricians and Gynecologists indicate that if HPV testing is used in combination with Pap smears, women who are negative for both tests should return to be tested in three years [35]. This strategy minimizes unnecessary follow-up visits and invasive procedures without compromising the detection of disease. This scheme is more appropriate for communities with limited access to public health services, such as countries in Latin America.

Different studies in countries in Latin America have described recommendations for successful screening programs, such as greater HPV education of the public and health care practitioners [118]; educational interventions for physicians in screening and management norms [119]; the implementation of sex education in schools and the promotion of condom use and an organized screening program to prevent cervical cancer in young women [120]; a screening program with high follow-up rates, not only high coverage [121]; and behavioral measures, including delaying sexual intercourse and the regular use of latex condoms [66]. HPV information is complex, and many women remain confused after reading educational materials; thus, it is important to ensure that HPV information is accessible to people at all levels [23].

The Regional Strategy for Comprehensive Cervical Cancer Prevention and Control proposes to improve country capacity for the sustained implementation of comprehensive cervical cancer prevention and control programs, with the goal of reducing incidence and mortality. It promotes an integrated package of services for health information and education; screening of asymptomatic women and pre-cancer treatment (improving the quality of screening tests; considering introducing HPV DNA testing to triage HPV-positive women for further testing; increasing the screening coverage of women in the at-risk age group (>30 years); and increasing the proportion of timely and appropriate follow-up care for women with abnormal screening test results); invasive cervical cancer treatment and palliative care; and evidence-based policy decisions on whether and how to introduce HPV vaccines [122].

http://dx.doi.org/10.5772/53662

6. Conclusion

Cervical HPV infection is the most prevalent sexually transmitted disease. HPV is so common that more than half of all sexually active adults will be infected in their lifetime, although young, sexually active women bear the brunt of both infection and clinical complications. The Centers for Disease Control estimates that at least half of all sexually active individuals will acquire HPV at some point in their lives, whereas at least 80% of women will acquire an HPV infection by age 50. At least 50% of men will acquire a genital HPV infection during their lifetime. In developed countries, PAP smear test screening has decreased the incidence of cervical cancer by approximately 70% in recent decades; however, cervical cancer still represents a major public health issue in Latin America and the Caribbean because of the failure of prevention programs.

Cervical cancer is a major public health problem in Latin America, which has some of the highest incidence and mortality rates worldwide. Information on HPV prevalence and type distribution in several countries in Latin America is crucial to predict the future impact of HPV16/18 vaccines and screening programs and to establish appropriate post-vaccine virological surveillance, primarily with the information obtained from high-grade cervical lesions and invasive cervical cancer.

Ultimately, the integration of screening with prophylactic HPV vaccination, which currently protects against the most common LR-HPV types (HPVs 6 and 11) and HR-HPV types (HPVs 16 and 18), offers the greatest potential to reduce the burden of ICC and other HPV-related diseases. Unfortunately, for many of the nations where the burden of HPV and cervical cancer is the highest, vaccination and HPV testing remain too expensive. Fortunately, the Pan American Health Organization Revolving Fund for vaccine purchase will allow vaccine prices to be reduced, and the vaccine would be available for free in most Latin American countries. The implementation of HPV vaccination will have a great impact on the reduction of the incidence and mortality of HPV-associated cancers.

Acknowledgement

The authors gratefully acknowledge financial support from COLCIENCIAS (Contrato 371-2008) and Vicerrectoría de Investigaciones, Innovación y Extensión, Universidad Tecnológica de Pereira. The author(s) declare that they have no conflict of interest.

Nomenclature

CIN - Cervical intraepithelial neoplasia.

LSIL- Low-grade intraepithelial lesions.

HSIL – High-grade intraepithelial lesions.

NC- Normal cytology.

ICC Invasive cancer cervical

Author details

Juan Carlos Sepúlveda-Arias* and Adalucy Álvarez-Aldana

*Address all correspondence to: jcsepulv@utp.edu.co

Faculty of Health Sciences, Department of Basic Sciences, Grupo Infección e Inmunidad, Universidad Tecnológica de Pereira, Pereira, Colombia

References

[1] Paavonen J. Human papillomavirus infection and the development of cervical cancer and related genital neoplasias. Int J Infect Dis. 2007 Nov 11; Suppl 2:S3-9.

[2] Jamison JH, Kaplan DW, Hamman R, Eagar R, Beach R, Douglas JM, Jr. Spectrum of genital human papillomavirus infection in a female adolescent population. Sex Transm Dis. 1995 Jul-Aug;22(4):236-43.

[3] Ault KA. Epidemiology and natural history of human papillomavirus infections in the female genital tract. Infect Dis Obstet Gynecol. 2006; Suppl:40470.

[4] Bouvard V, Baan R, Straif K, Grosse Y, Secretan B, El Ghissassi F, et al. A review of human carcinogens--Part B: biological agents. Lancet Oncol. 2009 Apr;10(4):321-2.

[5] Álvarez-Aldana A, Sepúlveda-Arias JC, Siller López F. Human papillomavirus-induced carcinogenesis. Investigaciones Andina. 2012;14(24):438 - 56.

[6] Munoz N, Castellsague X, de Gonzalez AB, Gissmann L. Chapter 1: HPV in the etiology of human cancer. Vaccine. 2006 Aug 31;24 Suppl 3:1-10.

[7] Franco EL, Villa LL, Sobrinho JP, Prado JM, Rousseau MC, Desy M, et al. Epidemiology of acquisition and clearance of cervical human papillomavirus infection in women from a high-risk area for cervical cancer. J Infect Dis. 1999 Nov;180(5):1415-23.

[8] Hildesheim A, Schiffman MH, Gravitt PE, Glass AG, Greer CE, Zhang T, et al. Persistence of type-specific human papillomavirus infection among cytologically normal women. J Infect Dis. 1994 Feb;169(2):235-40.

[9] Ho GY, Bierman R, Beardsley L, Chang CJ, Burk RD. Natural history of cervicovaginal papillomavirus infection in young women. N Engl J Med. 1998 Feb 12;338(7): 423-8.

[10] Molano M, Van den Brule A, Plummer M, Weiderpass E, Posso H, Arslan A, et al. Determinants of clearance of human papillomavirus infections in Colombian women with normal cytology: a population-based, 5-year follow-up study. Am J Epidemiol. 2003 Sep 1;158(5):486-94.

[11] Moscicki AB, Shiboski S, Broering J, Powell K, Clayton L, Jay N, et al. The natural history of human papillomavirus infection as measured by repeated DNA testing in adolescent and young women. J Pediatr. 1998 Feb;132(2):277-84.

[12] Richardson H, Kelsall G, Tellier P, Voyer H, Abrahamowicz M, Ferenczy A, et al. The natural history of type-specific human papillomavirus infections in female university students. Cancer Epidemiol Biomarkers Prev. 2003 Jun;12(6):485-90.

[13] Ho GY, Burk RD, Klein S, Kadish AS, Chang CJ, Palan P, et al. Persistent genital human papillomavirus infection as a risk factor for persistent cervical dysplasia. J Natl Cancer Inst. 1995 Sep 20;87(18):1365-71.

[14] Liaw KL, Glass AG, Manos MM, Greer CE, Scott DR, Sherman M, et al. Detection of human papillomavirus DNA in cytologically normal women and subsequent cervical squamous intraepithelial lesions. J Natl Cancer Inst. 1999 Jun 2;91(11):954-60.

[15] Remmink AJ, Walboomers JM, Helmerhorst TJ, Voorhorst FJ, Rozendaal L, Risse EK, et al. The presence of persistent high-risk HPV genotypes in dysplastic cervical lesions is associated with progressive disease: natural history up to 36 months. Int J Cancer. 1995 May 4;61(3):306-11.

[16] Ylitalo N, Josefsson A, Melbye M, Sorensen P, Frisch M, Andersen PK, et al. A prospective study showing long-term infection with human papillomavirus 16 before the development of cervical carcinoma in situ. Cancer Res. 2000 Nov 1;60(21):6027-32.

[17] Chapman R, Soldan K, Jit M. Modelling borderline and mild dysplasia associated with HPV 6 and 11 infection. Vaccine. 2011 Apr 5;29(16):2881-6.

[18] Nielsen A, Iftner T, Norgaard M, Munk C, Junge J, Kjaer SK. The importance of low-risk HPV infection for the risk of abnormal cervical cytology/histology in more than 40 000 Danish women. Sex Transm Infect. 2012 Jul 6.

[19] Woodhall SC, Jit M, Soldan K, Kinghorn G, Gilson R, Nathan M, et al. The impact of genital warts: loss of quality of life and cost of treatment in eight sexual health clinics in the UK. Sex Transm Infect. 2011 Oct;87(6):458-63.

[20] Ciapponi A, Bardach A, Glujovsky D, Gibbons L, Picconi MA. Type-specific HPV prevalence in cervical cancer and high-grade lesions in Latin America and the Caribbean: systematic review and meta-analysis. PLoS One. 2011;6(10):e25493.

[21] Ferlay J, Shin HR, Bray F, Forman D, Mathers C, Parkin DM. Estimates of worldwide burden of cancer in 2008: GLOBOCAN 2008. Int J Cancer. 2010 Dec 15;127(12): 2893-917.

[22] Denny L, Quinn M, Sankaranarayanan R. Chapter 8: Screening for cervical cancer in developing countries. Vaccine. 2006 Aug 31;24 Suppl 3: 71-7.

[23] Cuzick J, Arbyn M, Sankaranarayanan R, Tsu V, Ronco G, Mayrand MH, et al. Overview of human papillomavirus-based and other novel options for cervical cancer screening in developed and developing countries. Vaccine. 2008 Aug 19;26 Suppl 10:K29-41.

[24] Naucler P, Ryd W, Tornberg S, Strand A, Wadell G, Elfgren K, et al. Efficacy of HPV DNA testing with cytology triage and/or repeat HPV DNA testing in primary cervical cancer screening. J Natl Cancer Inst. 2009 Jan 21;101(2):88-99.

[25] Prasad SR. Management strategies and cost effectiveness in the prevention of cervical cancer. Clinicoecon Outcomes Res. 2009;1:17-23.

[26] Schiffman M, Herrero R, Hildesheim A, Sherman ME, Bratti M, Wacholder S, et al. HPV DNA testing in cervical cancer screening: results from women in a high-risk province of Costa Rica. JAMA. 2000 Jan 5;283(1):87-93.

[27] Burk RD, Kelly P, Feldman J, Bromberg J, Vermund SH, DeHovitz JA, et al. Declining prevalence of cervicovaginal human papillomavirus infection with age is independent of other risk factors. Sex Transm Dis. 1996 Jul-Aug;23(4):333-41.

[28] Giuliano AR, Papenfuss M, Abrahamsen M, Denman C, de Zapien JG, Henze JL, et al. Human papillomavirus infection at the United States-Mexico border: implications for cervical cancer prevention and control. Cancer Epidemiol Biomarkers Prev. 2001 Nov;10(11):1129-36.

[29] Kjaer SK, van den Brule AJ, Bock JE, Poll PA, Engholm G, Sherman ME, et al. Determinants for genital human papillomavirus (HPV) infection in 1000 randomly chosen young Danish women with normal Pap smear: are there different risk profiles for oncogenic and nononcogenic HPV types? Cancer Epidemiol Biomarkers Prev. 1997 Oct; 6(10):799-805.

[30] Peto J, Gilham C, Deacon J, Taylor C, Evans C, Binns W, et al. Cervical HPV infection and neoplasia in a large population-based prospective study: the Manchester cohort. Br J Cancer. 2004 Aug 31;91(5):942-53.

[31] Smith JS, Gilbert PA, Melendy A, Rana RK, Pimenta JM. Age-Specific Prevalence of Infection with Human Papillomavirus in Females: A Global Review. J Adolesc Health. 2011 Jun;48(6):540-52

[32] Almonte M, Albero G, Molano M, Carcamo C, Garcia PJ, Perez G. Risk factors for human papillomavirus exposure and co-factors for cervical cancer in Latin America and the Caribbean. Vaccine. 2008 Aug 19;26 Suppl 11:L16-36.

[33] Bruni L, Diaz M, Castellsague X, Ferrer E, Bosch FX, de Sanjose S. Cervical human papillomavirus prevalence in 5 continents: meta-analysis of 1 million women with normal cytological findings. J Infect Dis. 2010 Dec 15;202(12):1789-99.

[34] Venezuela RF, Kiguen AX, Frutos MC, Cuffini CG. Circulation of human papillomavirus (HPV) genotypes in women from Cordoba, Argentina, with squamous intraepithelial lesions. Rev Inst Med Trop Sao Paulo. 2012 Jan-Feb;54(1):11-6.

[35] Badano I, Pedrozo RW, Ruiz Diaz LS, Galuppo JA, Picconi MA, Campos RH, et al. Human papillomavirus (HPV) detection and Papanicolaou cytology in low-resource women in Posadas city, Misiones, Argentina. Rev Argent Microbiol. 2011 Oct-Dec; 43(4):263-7.

[36] Deluca GD, Basiletti J, Schelover E, Vasquez ND, Alonso JM, Marin HM, et al. Chlamydia trachomatis as a probable cofactor in human papillomavirus infection in aboriginal women from northeastern Argentina. Braz J Infect Dis. 2011 Dec;15(6):567-72.

[37] Sijvarger CC, Gonzalez JV, Prieto A, Messmer AG, Mallimaci MC, Alonio VL, et al. [Cervical infection epidemiology of human papillomavirus in Ushuaia, Argentina]. Rev Argent Microbiol. 2006 Jan-Mar;38(1):19-24.

[38] Tonon SA, Picconi MA, Zinovich JB, Liotta DJ, Bos PD, Galuppo JA, et al. Human papillomavirus cervical infection and associated risk factors in a region of Argentina with a high incidence of cervical carcinoma. Infect Dis Obstet Gynecol. 1999;7(5): 237-43.

[39] Tonon SA, Picconi MA, Zinovich JB, Nardari W, Mampaey M, Badano I, et al. Human papillomavirus cervical infection in Guarani Indians from the rainforest of Misiones, Argentina. Int J Infect Dis. 2004 Jan;8(1):13-9.

[40] Cervantes J, Lema C, Hurtado L, Andrade R, Quiroga G, Garcia G, et al. Prevalence of human papillomavirus infection in rural villages of the Bolivian Amazon. Rev Inst Med Trop Sao Paulo. 2003 May-Jun;45(3):131-5.

[41] Fernandes JV, Meissner Rde V, Carvalho MG, Fernandes TA, Azevedo PR, de Azevedo JW, et al. Human papillomavirus prevalence in women with normal cytology and with cervical cancer in Natal, Brazil. Mol Med Report. 2011 Nov-Dec;4(6):1321-6.

[42] Camara GN, Cerqueira DM, Oliveira AP, Silva EO, Carvalho LG, Martins CR. Prevalence of human papillomavirus types in women with pre-neoplastic and neoplastic cervical lesions in the Federal District of Brazil. Mem Inst Oswaldo Cruz. 2003 Oct; 98(7):879-83.

[43] Carvalho MO, Carestiato FN, Perdigao PH, Xavier MP, Silva K, Botelho MO, et al. Human papillomavirus infection in Rio de Janeiro, Brazil: a retrospective study. Braz J Infect Dis. 2005 Oct;9(5):398-404.

[44] Cavalcanti SM, Zardo LG, Passos MR, Oliveira LH. Epidemiological aspects of human papillomavirus infection and cervical cancer in Brazil. J Infect. 2000 Jan;40(1): 80-7.

[45] Cavalcanti SM, Frugulhetti IC, Passos MR, Fonseca ME, Oliveira LH. Prevalence of human papillomavirus DNA in female cervical lesions from Rio de Janeiro, Brazil. Mem Inst Oswaldo Cruz. 1994 Oct-Dec;89(4):575-80.

[46] Fernandes JV, Meissner RV, Carvalho MG, Fernandes TA, Azevedo PR, Sobrinho JS, et al. Prevalence of human papillomavirus in archival samples obtained from patients with cervical pre-malignant and malignant lesions from Northeast Brazil. BMC Res Notes. 2010;3(1):96.

[47] Oliveira LH, Rosa ML, Pereira CR, Vasconcelos GA, Silva RA, Barrese TZ, et al. Human papillomavirus status and cervical abnormalities in women from public and private health care in Rio de Janeiro State, Brazil. Rev Inst Med Trop Sao Paulo. 2006 Sep-Oct;48(5):279-85.

[48] Rabelo-Santos SH, Zeferino L, Villa LL, Sobrinho JP, Amaral RG, Magalhaes AV. Human papillomavirus prevalence among women with cervical intraepithelial neoplasia III and invasive cervical cancer from Goiania, Brazil. Mem Inst Oswaldo Cruz. 2003 Mar;98(2):181-4.

[49] Silva KC, Rosa ML, Moyse N, Afonso LA, Oliveira LH, Cavalcanti SM. Risk factors associated with human papillomavirus infection in two populations from Rio de Janeiro, Brazil. Mem Inst Oswaldo Cruz. 2009 Sep;104(6):885-91.

[50] Ayres AR, Silva GA. Cervical HPV infection in Brazil: systematic review. Rev Saude Publica. 2010 Oct;44(5):963-74.

[51] Valdivia LI, Aguayo GF, Pruyas AM, Snijders PJ, Corvalan RA, Ferreccio RC. [Human papillomavirus (HPV) genotypes in cervix uterine cancer patients in a public hospital and private clinic from Santiago, Chile]. Rev Chilena Infectol. 2010 Feb;27(1):11-6.

[52] Ferreccio C, Prado RB, Luzoro AV, Ampuero SL, Snijders PJ, Meijer CJ, et al. Population-based prevalence and age distribution of human papillomavirus among women in Santiago, Chile. Cancer Epidemiol Biomarkers Prev. 2004 Dec;13(12):2271-6.

[53] Melo A, Garcia P, Capurro I, Guzman P, Brebi P, Ili C, et al. [Human papillomavirus genotyping in cervical adenocarcinoma in the Region of La Araucania-Chile]. Rev Chilena Infectol. 2010 Aug;27(4):297-301.

[54] Lopez MJ, Ili GC, Brebi MP, Garcia MP, Capurro VI, Guzman GP, et al. [Human papillomavirus genotyping of cervical uterine preneoplastic lesions in a high risk area]. Rev Med Chil. 2010 Nov;138(11):1343-50.

[55] Brebi MP, Ili GC, Lopez MJ, Garcia MP, Melo AA, Montenegro HS, et al. [Detection and genotyping of human papillomavirus in biopsies of uterine cervical adenocarcinoma]. Rev Med Chil. 2009 Mar;137(3):377-82.

[56] Melo A, Montenegro S, Hooper T, Capurro I, Roa JC, Roa I. [Human papilloma virus (HPV) typing in preneoplastic and neoplastic lesions of the uterine cervix in the IX region-Chile]. Rev Med Chil. 2003 Dec;131(12):1382-90.

[57] Aedo AS, Melo AA, Garcia P, Guzman GP, Capurro VI, Roa SJ. [Detection and typification of human papilloma virus in pre cancerous cervical lesions]. Rev Med Chil. 2007 Feb;135(2):167-73.

[58] Roa JC, Garcia P, Gomez J, Fernandez W, Gaete F, Espinoza A, et al. HPV genotyping from invasive cervical cancer in Chile. Int J Gynaecol Obstet. 2009 May;105(2):150-3.

[59] Murillo R, Molano M, Martinez G, Mejia JC, Gamboa O. HPV prevalence in Colombian women with cervical cancer: implications for vaccination in a developing country. Infect Dis Obstet Gynecol. 2009 Dec;653598.

[60] Camargo M, Soto-De Leon S, Sanchez R, Munoz M, Vega E, Beltran M, et al. Detection by PCR of human papillomavirus in Colombia: Comparison of GP5+/6+ and MY09/11 primer sets. J Virol Methods. 2011 Dec;178(1-2):68-74.

[61] Bosch FX, Munoz N, de Sanjose S, Navarro C, Moreo P, Ascunce N, et al. Human papillomavirus and cervical intraepithelial neoplasia grade III/carcinoma in situ: a case-control study in Spain and Colombia. Cancer Epidemiol Biomarkers Prev. 1993 Sep-Oct;2(5):415-22.

[62] Garcia DA, Cid-Arregui A, Schmitt M, Castillo M, Briceno I, Aristizabal FA. Highly Sensitive Detection and Genotyping of HPV by PCR Multiplex and Luminex Technology in a Cohort of Colombian Women with Abnormal Cytology. Open Virol J. 2011;5:70-9.

[63] Sepúlveda-Arias JC, Henao J, Mantilla LE, Porras GL, Beltrán L. Detección del virus del papiloma humano (VPH) en pacientes con citología anormal: un estudio preliminar. Rev Med Risaralda. 2006;12(2):14-21.

[64] Molano M, van den Brule AJ, Posso H, Weiderpass E, Ronderos M, Franceschi S, et al. Low grade squamous intra-epithelial lesions and human papillomavirus infection in Colombian women. Br J Cancer. 2002 Dec 2;87(12):1417-21.

[65] Paez C, Konno R, Yaegashi N, Matsunaga G, Araujo I, Corral F, et al. Prevalence of HPV DNA in cervical lesions in patients from Ecuador and Japan. Tohoku J Exp Med. 1996 Nov;180(3):261-72.

[66] Brown CR, Leon ML, Munoz K, Fagioni A, Amador LG, Frain B, et al. Human papillomavirus infection and its association with cervical dysplasia in Ecuadorian women attending a private cancer screening clinic. Braz J Med Biol Res. 2009 Jul;42(7):629-36.

[67] Tornesello ML, Buonaguro L, Izzo S, Lopez G, Vega X, Maldonado Reyes CF, et al. A pilot study on the distribution of human papillomavirus genotypes and HPV-16 variants in cervical neoplastic lesions from Ecuadorian women. J Med Virol. 2008 Nov; 80(11):1959-65.

[68] Gonzalez-Andrade F, Sanchez D. HPV genotyping in anogenital abnormal samples of Ecuadorian women. Cancer Biomark. 2009;5(4):225-32.

[69] Rolon PA, Smith JS, Munoz N, Klug SJ, Herrero R, Bosch X, et al. Human papillomavirus infection and invasive cervical cancer in Paraguay. Int J Cancer. 2000 Feb 15;85(4):486-91.

[70] Kasamatsu E, Cubilla AL, Alemany L, Chaux A, Tous S, Mendoza L, et al. Type-specific human papillomavirus distribution in invasive cervical carcinomas in Paraguay. A study of 432 cases. J Med Virol. 2012 Oct;84(10):1628-35.

[71] Torres LM, Paez M, Insaurralde A, Rodriguez MI, Castro A, Kasamatsu E. Detection of high risk human papillomavirus cervical infections by the hybrid capture in Asuncion, Paraguay. Braz J Infect Dis. 2009 Jun;13(3):203-6.

[72] Santos C, Munoz N, Klug S, Almonte M, Guerrero I, Alvarez M, et al. HPV types and cofactors causing cervical cancer in Peru. Br J Cancer. 2001 Sep 28;85(7):966-71.

[73] Klug SJ, Wilmotte R, Santos C, Almonte M, Herrero R, Guerrero I, et al. TP53 polymorphism, HPV infection, and risk of cervical cancer. Cancer Epidemiol Biomarkers Prev. 2001 Sep;10(9):1009-12.

[74] Correnti M, Medina F, Cavazza ME, Rennola A, Avila M, Fernandes A. Human papillomavirus (HPV) type distribution in cervical carcinoma, low-grade, and high-grade squamous intraepithelial lesions in Venezuelan women. Gynecol Oncol. 2011 Jun 1;121(3):527-31.

[75] Sanchez-Lander J, Cortinas P, Loureiro CL, Pujol FH, Medina F, Capote-Negrin L, et al. Human papillomavirus in invasive cervical cancer and cervical intraepithelial neoplasia 2 and 3 in Venezuela: A cross-sectional study. Cancer Epidemiol. 2012 May 16.

[76] Herrero R, Hildesheim A, Bratti C, Sherman ME, Hutchinson M, Morales J, et al. Population-based study of human papillomavirus infection and cervical neoplasia in rural Costa Rica. J Natl Cancer Inst. 2000 Mar 15;92(6):464-74.

[77] Herrero R, Castle PE, Schiffman M, Bratti MC, Hildesheim A, Morales J, et al. Epidemiologic profile of type-specific human papillomavirus infection and cervical neoplasia in Guanacaste, Costa Rica. J Infect Dis. 2005 Jun 1;191(11):1796-807.

[78] Soto Y, Mune M, Morales E, Goicolea A, Mora J, Sanchez L, et al. Human Papillomavirus infections in Cuban women with cervical intraepithelial neoplasia. Sex Transm Dis. 2007 Dec;34(12):974-6.

[79] Valles X, Murga GB, Hernandez G, Sabido M, Chuy A, Lloveras B, et al. High prevalence of human papillomavirus infection in the female population of Guatemala. Int J Cancer. 2009 Sep 1;125(5):1161-7.

[80] Velema JP, Ferrera A, Figueroa M, Bulnes R, Toro LA, de Barahona O, et al. Burning wood in the kitchen increases the risk of cervical neoplasia in HPV-infected women in Honduras. Int J Cancer. 2002 Feb 1;97(4):536-41.

[81] Ferrera A, Olivo A, Alaez C, Melchers WJ, Gorodezky C. HLA DOA1 and DOB1 loci in Honduran women with cervical dysplasia and invasive cervical carcinoma and their relationship to human papillomavirus infection. Hum Biol. 1999 Jun;71(3): 367-79.

[82] Tabora N, Bulnes R, Toro LA, Claros JM, Massuger LF, Quint WG, et al. Human papillomavirus infection in Honduran women with cervical intraepithelial neoplasia or cervical cancer. J Low Genit Tract Dis. 2011 Jan;15(1):48-53.

[83] Tabora N, Bakkers JM, Quint WG, Massuger LF, Matute JA, Melchers WJ, et al. Human papillomavirus infection in Honduran women with normal cytology. Cancer Causes Control. 2009 Nov;20(9):1663-70.

[84] Illades-Aguiar B, Cortes-Malagon EM, Antonio-Vejar V, Zamudio-Lopez N, Alarcon-Romero Ldel C, Fernandez-Tilapa G, et al. Cervical carcinoma in Southern Mexico: Human papillomavirus and cofactors. Cancer Detect Prev. 2009;32(4):300-7.

[85] Illades-Aguiar B, Alarcon-Romero Ldel C, Antonio-Vejar V, Zamudio-Lopez N, Sales-Linares N, Flores-Alfaro E, et al. Prevalence and distribution of human papillomavirus types in cervical cancer, squamous intraepithelial lesions, and with no intraepithelial lesions in women from Southern Mexico. Gynecol Oncol. 2010 May;117(2): 291-6.

[86] Velazquez-Marquez N, Paredes-Tello MA, Perez-Terron H, Santos-Lopez G, Reyes-Leyva J, Vallejo-Ruiz V. Prevalence of human papillomavirus genotypes in women from a rural region of Puebla, Mexico. Int J Infect Dis. 2009 Nov;13(6):690-5.

[87] Gonzalez-Losa Mdel R, Rosado-Lopez I, Valdez-Gonzalez N, Puerto-Solis M. High prevalence of human papillomavirus type 58 in Mexican colposcopy patients. J Clin Virol. 2004 Mar;29(3):202-5.

[88] Hernandez-Hernandez DM, Ornelas-Bernal L, Guido-Jimenez M, Apresa-Garcia T, Alvarado-Cabrero I, Salcedo-Vargas M, et al. Association between high-risk human papillomavirus DNA load and precursor lesions of cervical cancer in Mexican women. Gynecol Oncol. 2003 Aug;90(2):310-7.

[89] Pina-Sanchez P, Hernandez-Hernandez DM, Lopez-Romero R, Vazquez-Ortiz G, Perez-Plasencia C, Lizano-Soberon M, et al. Human papillomavirus-specific viral types are common in Mexican women affected by cervical lesions. Int J Gynecol Cancer. 2006 May-Jun;16(3):1041-7.

[90] Torroella-Kouri M, Morsberger S, Carrillo A, Mohar A, Meneses A, Ibarra M, et al. HPV prevalence among Mexican women with neoplastic and normal cervixes. Gynecol Oncol. 1998 Jul;70(1):115-20.

[91] Montoya-Fuentes H, Suarez Rincon AE, Ramirez-Munoz MP, Arevalo-Lagunas I, Moran Moguel MC, Gallegos Arreola MP, et al. [The detection of human papillomavirus 16, 18, 35 and 58 in cervical-uterine cancer and advanced degree of squamous intraepithelial lesions in Western Mexico: clinical-molecular correlation]. Ginecol Obstet Mex. 2001 Apr;69:137-42.

[92] Hindryckx P, Garcia A, Claeys P, Gonzalez C, Velasquez R, Bogers J, et al. Prevalence of high risk human papillomavirus types among Nicaraguan women with histologi-

cal proved pre-neoplastic and neoplastic lesions of the cervix. Sex Transm Infect. 2006 Aug;82(4):334-6.

[93] Acs J, Hildesheim A, Reeves WC, Brenes M, Brinton L, Lavery C, et al. Regional distribution of human papillomavirus DNA and other risk factors for invasive cervical cancer in Panama. Cancer Res. 1989 Oct 15;49(20):5725-9.

[94] Muñoz N, Hernandez-Suarez G, Mendez F, Molano M, Posso H, Moreno V, et al. Persistence of HPV infection and risk of high-grade cervical intraepithelial neoplasia in a cohort of Colombian women. Br J Cancer. 2009 Apr 7;100(7):1184-90.

[95] Matos E, Loria D, Amestoy GM, Herrera L, Prince MA, Moreno J, et al. Prevalence of human papillomavirus infection among women in Concordia, Argentina: a population-based study. Sex Transm Dis. 2003 Aug;30(8):593-9.

[96] Girianelli VR, Thuler LC, e Silva GA. [Prevalence of HPV infection among women covered by the family health program in the Baixada Fluminense, Rio de Janeiro, Brazil]. Rev Bras Ginecol Obstet. 2010 Jan;32(1):39-46.

[97] Camargo M, Soto-De Leon SC, Sanchez R, Perez-Prados A, Patarroyo ME, Patarroyo MA. Frequency of human papillomavirus infection, coinfection, and association with different risk factors in Colombia. Ann Epidemiol. 2011 Mar;21(3):204-13.

[98] Soto-De Leon SC, Camargo M, Sanchez R, Leon S, Urquiza M, Acosta J, et al. Prevalence of infection with high-risk human papillomavirus in women in Colombia. Clin Microbiol Infect. 2009 Jan;15(1):100-2.

[99] Munoz N, Bosch FX, de Sanjose S, Vergara A, del Moral A, Munoz MT, et al. Risk factors for cervical intraepithelial neoplasia grade III/carcinoma in situ in Spain and Colombia. Cancer Epidemiol Biomarkers Prev. 1993 Sep-Oct;2(5):423-31.

[100] Clarke MA, Rodriguez AC, Gage JC, Herrero R, Hildesheim A, Wacholder S, et al. A large, population-based study of age-related associations between vaginal pH and human papillomavirus infection. BMC Infect Dis. 2012;12:33.

[101] Ferrera A, Tabora N, Flores Y, Zelaya A, Massuger L, Melchers WJ. Assessment of HPV infection among female university students in Honduras via Roche linear array. Int J Gynaecol Obstet. 2011 May;113(2):96-9.

[102] Tabora N, Zelaya A, Bakkers J, Melchers WJ, Ferrera A. Chlamydia trachomatis and genital human papillomavirus infections in female university students in Honduras. Am J Trop Med Hyg. 2005 Jul;73(1):50-3.

[103] Lopez Rivera MG, Flores MO, Villalba Magdaleno JD, Sanchez Monroy V. Prevalence of human papillomavirus in women from Mexico city. Infect Dis Obstet Gynecol. 2012;2012:384758.

[104] Sanchez-Aleman MA, Uribe-Salas FJ, Lazcano-Ponce EC, Conde-Glez CJ. Human papillomavirus incidence and risk factors among Mexican female college students. Sex Transm Dis. 2011 Apr;38(4):275-8.

[105] Almonte M, Ferreccio C, Gonzales M, Delgado JM, Buckley CH, Luciani S, et al. Risk factors for high-risk human papillomavirus infection and cofactors for high-grade cervical disease in Peru. Int J Gynecol Cancer. 2011 Dec;21(9):1654-63.

[106] Cavalcanti SM, Deus FC, Zardo LG, Frugulhetti IC, Oliveira LH. Human papillomavirus infection and cervical cancer in Brazil: a retrospective study. Mem Inst Oswaldo Cruz. 1996 Jul-Aug;91(4):433-40.

[107] Smith JS, Munoz N, Herrero R, Eluf-Neto J, Ngelangel C, Franceschi S, et al. Evidence for Chlamydia trachomatis as a human papillomavirus cofactor in the etiology of invasive cervical cancer in Brazil and the Philippines. J Infect Dis. 2002 Feb 1;185(3):324-31.

[108] Sierra-Torres CH, Acosta-Aragon MP, Orejuela-Aristizabal L. [Papillomavirus and factors associated with high-risk, cervical intraepithelial neoplasia in Cauca, Colombia]. Rev Salud Publica (Bogota). 2006 May;8 Suppl 1:47-58.

[109] Hildesheim A, Herrero R, Castle PE, Wacholder S, Bratti MC, Sherman ME, et al. HPV co-factors related to the development of cervical cancer: results from a population-based study in Costa Rica. Br J Cancer. 2001 May 4;84(9):1219-26.

[110] Flores YN, Bishai DM, Shah KV, Lazcano-Ponce E, Lorincz A, Hernandez M, et al. Risk factors for cervical cancer among HPV positive women in Mexico. Salud Publica Mex. 2008 Jan-Feb;50(1):49-58.

[111] Murillo R, Almonte M, Pereira A, Ferrer E, Gamboa OA, Jeronimo J, et al. Cervical cancer screening programs in Latin America and the Caribbean. Vaccine. 2008 Aug 19;26 Suppl 11:L37-48.

[112] Wiesner C, Tovar S, Piñeros M, Cendales R, Murillo R. La oferta de servicios para tamización de cáncer de cuello uterino en Colombia. Rev Colomb Cancerol. 2009;13(3): 134 - 44.

[113] Cendales R, Wiesner C, Murillo RH, Pineros M, Tovar S, Mejia JC. [Quality of vaginal smear for cervical cancer screening: a concordance study]. Biomedica. 2010 Jan-Mar; 30(1):107-15.

[114] Ferreccio C, Barriga MI, Lagos M, Ibanez C, Poggi H, Gonzalez F, et al. Screening trial of human papillomavirus for early detection of cervical cancer in Santiago, Chile. Int J Cancer. 2012 Jun 9.

[115] Flores Y, Bishai D, Lazcano E, Shah K, Lorincz A, Hernandez M, et al. Improving cervical cancer screening in Mexico: results from the Morelos HPV Study. Salud Publica Mex. 2003;45 Suppl 3:S388-98.

[116] Flores YN, Bishai DM, Lorincz A, Shah KV, Lazcano-Ponce E, Hernandez M, et al. HPV testing for cervical cancer screening appears more cost-effective than Papanicolau cytology in Mexico. Cancer Causes Control. 2011 Feb;22(2):261-72.

[117] Lorenzato F, Ho L, Terry G, Singer A, Santos LC, De Lucena Batista R, et al. The use of human papillomavirus typing in detection of cervical neoplasia in Recife (Brazil). Int J Gynecol Cancer. 2000 Mar;10(2):143-50.

[118] Moreira ED, Jr., Oliveira BG, Ferraz FM, Costa S, Costa Filho JO, Karic G. Knowledge and attitudes about human papillomavirus, Pap smears, and cervical cancer among young women in Brazil: implications for health education and prevention. Int J Gynecol Cancer. 2006 Mar-Apr;16(2):599-603.

[119] Aldrich T, Landis S, Garcia SG, Becker D, Sanhueza P, Higuera A. Cervical cancer and the HPV link: identifying areas for education in Mexico City's public hospitals. Salud Publica Mex. 2006 May-Jun;48(3):236-43.

[120] Oliveira LH, Ferreira MD, Augusto EF, Melgaco FG, Santos LS, Cavalcanti SM, et al. Human papillomavirus genotypes in asymptomatic young women from public schools in Rio de Janeiro, Brazil. Rev Soc Bras Med Trop. 2010 Jan-Feb;43(1):4-8.

[121] Andres-Gamboa O, Chicaiza L, Garcia-Molina M, Diaz J, Gonzalez M, Murillo R, et al. Cost-effectiveness of conventional cytology and HPV DNA testing for cervical cancer screening in Colombia. Salud Publica Mex. 2008 Jul-Aug;50(4):276-85.

[122] Luciani S, Andrus JK. A Pan American Health Organization strategy for cervical cancer prevention and control in Latin America and the Caribbean. Reprod Health Matters. 2008 Nov;16(32):59-66.

Chapter 18

Haemorrhagic Fevers Transmitted by Vectors in the Neotropics

Salim Mattar, Nelson Alvis and Marco Gonzalez

Additional information is available at the end of the chapter

http://dx.doi.org/10.5772/55420

1. Introduction

During the past 20 years there has been a dramatic emergence and re-emergence of epidemic of haemorrhagic vector-borne-disease (VBD) that have been caused by viruses believed to be under control such as dengue, yellow fever, Venezuelan equine encephalitis, Saint Louis Virus, Arenavirus, hantavirus or viruses that have extended their geographic distribution such as West Nile and Rift Valley fever. Bacteria like *Leptospira* and *Rickettsia* have also re-emerged.

Many reports have demonstrated the changing global and tropics epidemiology. The population growth, urbanization, human activities, and even climate variability all help to a continual fluctuation in the epidemiology of several haemorrhagic fevers transmitted by vectors in the tropics.

Haemorrhagic fevers produced by bacterial or virus share many general features. Those infectious agents are arthropod-borne cause many haemorrhagic fevers. For some viral haemorrhagic fevers, person-to-person transmission may occur through direct contact with infected blood or secretions. Infectious agents are transmitted by arthropod like mosquitoes and ticks. Animal reservoirs are usually wild rodents, however, pets, domestic livestock, urban mice, monkeys, and other primates may also provide as intermediate hosts.

The term viral hemorrhagic fever describes a potentially fatal clinical syndrome characterized by an insidious onset of nonspecific signs followed by bleeding manifestations and shock. The haemorrhagic fever syndrome is also characterized by a combination of a capillary leak syndrome and bleeding diathesis. The clinical manifestations and even histopathological findings are pretty similar and difficult to make a differential diagnosis

(Table 1, Figure1). In the tropics where endemic haemorrhagic fevers are frequent that is a big concern.

This chapter gives an overview of the epidemiology and ecology of haemorrhagic fevers transmitted by vector taking place exclusively in the neotropics, hence it shows the principal clinical syndromes associated to vectors.

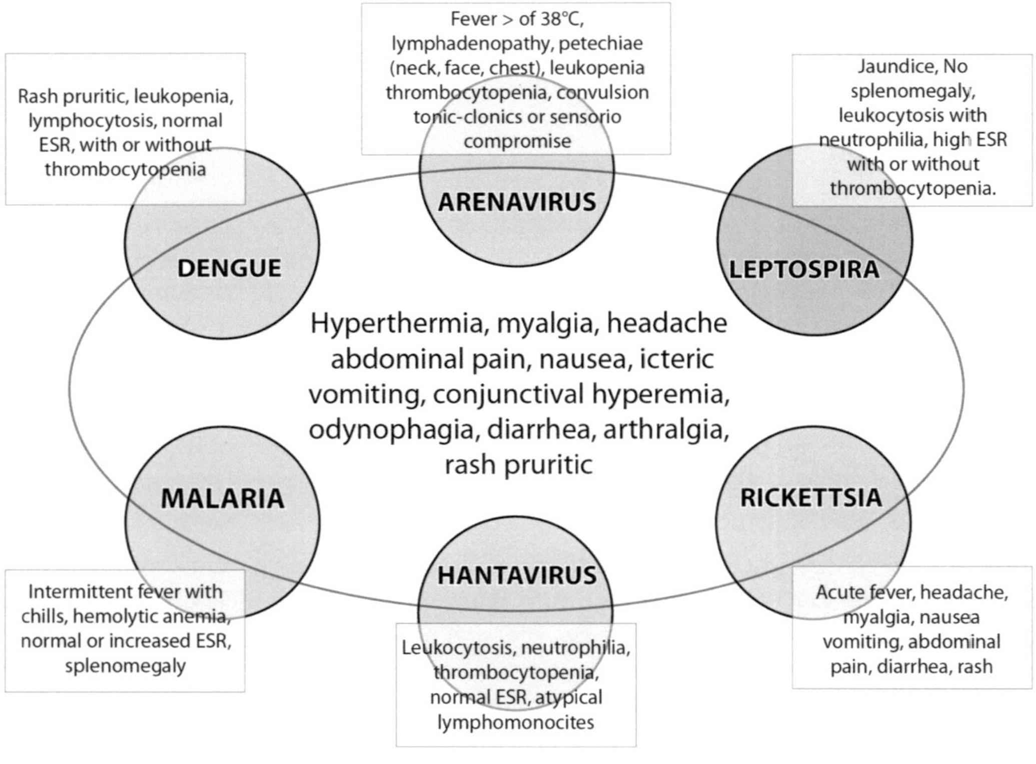

Figure 1. Clinical diagnostic challenges of the haemorrhagic fevers in the tropics

http://dx.doi.org/10.5772/55420

Disease	Leptospirosis	Dengue Fever	Enteric fever	Yellow fever	Severe *P. vivax* malaria	Acute viral hepatitis	Hantavirus	Rocky Mountain spotted fever
Infectious agent	*Leptospira* sp.	Dengue virus	*Salmonella typhi* and *S. paratyphi*	Yellow fever virus	*P. vivax*	Hepatitis E virus, A, B	Hantavirus (different species)	*Rickettsia rickettsii*
Incubation period	(2 – 26) Average 10	7–10 days	7–14 days (range, 3–60 days)	incubation period of 3 to 6 days,	14 days (10 to 30) (occasionally months)	15 to 60 days, 45 to 180 (HBV)	14 to 17 days (range 9 to 33)	7 days (range, 2 to 14 days)
Clinical presentation	Abrupt onset of fever, rigors	Acute febrile disease	Non-specific febrile illness, often with an insidious onset.	Acute febrile disease	Abrupt onset of fever, rigors	Non-specific febrile illness, often with an insidious onset.	Fever, chills and myalgias, which can be severe in many cases	Acute febrile disease
Headache	Yes	Yes	Yes	Yes	Yes	Yes	Yes	Yes
Musculoskeletal pain	Yes	Yes	Yes	Yes	Yes	Yes	Yes	Yes
Nausea - vomiting	Yes	Yes	Yes	Yes	Yes	Yes	Yes	Yes
Abdominal pain	Occasionally	Occasionally	Yes	Yes	Rare	Yes	Yes	Yes
Diarrhea	No	Occasionally	Occasionally, antecedent of diarrhea at infection time	No	rare	Occasionally	Occasionally	yes
Cough	No	No	No	No	No	No	Occasionally	No
Physical examination								
Rash	Rare	yes after the third day of illness	Yes, rose spots	No	No	Occasionally (urticarial rash)	No	Yes after the fifth day of illness
Jaundice	Yes	rare	rare	yes	yes	Yes, cas definition	No	Yes
Hepatomegaly	Yes	Only in severe ill patient	yes	occasionally	rare	Yes	Only in severe ill patient	Only in severe ill patient
Splenomegaly	Yes	No	Yes	No	Yes	Rare	No	no
Ocular involvement	Yes, conjuntival suffusion	No	No	Conjunctivitis	No	No	No	conjunctivitis
Muscle tenderness	Yes	Yes	No	No	Rare	Occasionally	No	Only in severe ill patient
Hemorrhagic manifestations, such as petechiae, purpura	Only in severe ill patient	Yes	Only in severe ill patient	Only in severe ill patient	Only in severe ill patient	Only in severe ill patient	Only in severe ill patient	Only in severe ill patient
Abdominal pain	Yes	Only in severe ill patient	Yes	Yes	Yes	Yes	Yes	Yes
Other findings								Unlike other tickborne rickettsial diseases, the presence of inoculation eschar is rare in RMSF

Disease	Leptospirosis	Dengue Fever	Enteric fever	Yellow fever	Severe *P. vivax* malaria	Acute viral hepatitis	Hantavirus	Rocky Mountain spotted fever
Laboratory findings								
Hemogram	normal	normal	normal	normal	Yes, also severe anaemia < 70 g/dl	normal	normal	Normal
White blood cell (WBC)	counts are generally less than 10, 000/mm3 but may range between 3, 000 and 26, 000/microL; a shift to the left is seen in about two-thirds of patients	leukopenia with lymphopenia,	either leukopenia or leukocytosis; leukocytosis is more common in children	Leukopenia with a relative neutropenia,	Usually normal	Neutropenia, lymphopenia and atypical lymphocytes may occasionally be observed	Leukocytosis (as high as 90, 000 cells/microL) and the appearance of immunoblasts are more pronounced in those patients with severe forms of illness	may be low, normal, or elevated
Thrombocytopenia	Only in severe ill patient	Yes	Rare	Yes	Frequent	Rare	Rapid decline in the platelet count	yes
Blood chemistry								
Liver function tests	High bilirubin level despite minimal to moderate elevations of hepatic transaminases (usually <200 IU/L)	Moderate elevation of hepatic transaminases	Moderate elevation of hepatic transaminases	Important liver necrosis with high transaminases and bilirubin	High bilirubin level despite minimal to moderate elevations of hepatic transaminases (usually <200 IU/L)	Peak levels of ALT vary from 1000 U/L to 2000 U/L at the onset	Increase in serum levels of LDH, which often occurs early, and elevations in hepatocellular enzymes and lactate	Jaundice, only in severe ill patients
Hypoalbuminemia-albuminuria	Uncommon	Uncommon	Uncommon	Yes	frequent		Uncommon	Uncommon
Renal function test	Acute renal failure in 16 – 40 % of severe ill patients	ARF uncommon	ARF uncommon	ARF is frequent with albuminuria	Acute renal failure and hemoglobinuria	Only in severe ill patients	Only in severe ill patients	ARF in < 20% of caes
Creatine kinase	Elevation is found in approximately 50 percent of patients	Normal	Occasionally elevated	Occasionally elevated	Frequently elevated	Normal	Normal	Normal
Coagulation analyses	Normal	Normal	Normal	Prolonged clotting, and increased prothrombin time are common.	normal	Prolonged clotting	Coagulopathy with hemorrhage common in infections due to Andes virus	

http://dx.doi.org/10.5772/55420

Disease	Leptospirosis	Dengue Fever	Enteric fever	Yellow fever	Severe *P. vivax* malaria	Acute viral hepatitis	Hantavirus	Rocky Mountain spotted fever
Imaging								
Chest radiographs	May show small nodular densities, which can progress to confluent consolidation or a ground glass appearance	No contributive sometimes pleural effusion	No contributive	No contributive, sometimes pleural effusion	compatible with acute lung injury and non cardiogenic pulmonary edema	No contributory	Radiologic changes such as bilateral interstitial infiltrates compatible with acute lung injury and non cardiogenic pulmonary edema	Radiologic changes such as alveolar infiltrates, interstitial pneumonia, and pleural effusion occurs only in severe disease
Diagnosis								
Serologic test	Gold standard MAT (microscopic agglutination test) a single titer of >1:800 is strong evidence of current or recent infection with leptospira in a endemic area >1:200 in a non endemic area Serology may be insensitive, particularly in early acute-phase specimens. Delayed seroconversions are common, with up to 10% of patients failing to seroconvert within 30 days of the clinical onset	The most commonly used test for the diagnosis of dengue is the IgM capture ELISA, but this test is negative early in the course of the disease, should be performed only four to five days after the onset of symptoms, and gives only a probable diagnosis	Diagnosis of enteric fever requires the isolation of *S. typhi* or *S. paratyphi* from blood, bone marrow. The sensitivity of blood culture is only 40% to 80%, probably because of high rates of antibimicrobial use in endemic areas and the small quantities of *S. typhi*	ELISA IgM The assay is more than 95% sensitive when serum specimens obtained between 7 and 10 days after the onset are tested	Gold standard: Detection of parasites on Giemsa-stained blood smears by light microscopy	Gold standard ELISA IgM	By the time symptoms are evident, patients uniformly have antiviral antibodies of the IgM class In the United States, those state health departments that offer hantavirus diagnostic testing use IgG and mu-capture IgM ELISAs developed and distributed by the CDC	indirect fluorescent antibody (IFA) test Antibodies typically appear 7 to 10 days after the onset of the illness

Disease	Leptospirosis	Dengue Fever	Enteric fever	Yellow fever	Severe *P. vivax* malaria	Acute viral hepatitis	Hantavirus	Rocky Mountain spotted fever
Severe forms								
Hepatic involvement	Frequently, but is not associated with hepatocellular necrosis, and liver function returns to normal after recovery	Serum aminotransaminases are increased in most cases (60%–80%) and can be accompanied by symptoms of acute hepatitis including right upper quadrant pain, hepatomegaly, and jaundice.	Only, moderate elevation of hepatic transaminases	Frequently, with severe hepatocellular necrosis	Jaundice (high levels of bilirubin direct and indirect), in infrequently hepatocellular necrosis	Liver failure	No	Only, moderate elevation of hepatic transaminases
Renal involvement	Intrinsic renal failure (interstitial nephritis)	Only pre –renal failure	Glomerulonephritis (rare)	Intrinsic renal failure with characterized by oliguria, azotemia, and very high levels of protein in the urine	Acute renal failure (acute tubular necrosis)	Rare	Rare, associated with Oran virus	rare
Pulmonary involvement	Severe pulmonary hemorrhage syndrome	Only pleural effusion	No	No	ARDS, acute noncardiogenic pulmonary edema	Rare	ARDS, acute noncardiogenic pulmonary edema	Occasionally, interstitial pneumonia, pulmonary non cardiogenic edema
CNS involvement	Rare, meningoencephalitis	Rare, encephalitis	Rare, meningitis	Metabolic encephalopathy by hepatic dysfunction	Cerebral malaria: coma, multiple convulsions (more than two episodes in 24 h)	Hepatic encephalopathy	No	Frequently Meningoencephalitis
Hemorrhagic manifestations	Rare	Frequently, case definition DHF	Rare, CID	Frequently, hepatic-induced coagulopathy, with gastrointestinal bleeding	Rare, only in severe ill patients	Only in severe ill patients	Coagulopathy with hemorrhage common in infections due to Andes virus	Rare

http://dx.doi.org/10.5772/55420

Disease	Leptospirosis	Dengue Fever	Enteric fever	Yellow fever	Severe *P. vivax* malaria	Acute viral hepatitis	Hantavirus	Rocky Mountain spotted fever
Other	Uveitis, myocarditis		Intestinal perforation, gastrointestinal bleeding		hypoglycaemia (blood glucose <2.2 mmol/l or <40 mg/dl) metabolic acidosis (plasma bicarbonate <15 mmol/l) Spontaneous splenic rupture		Lactic acidosis associated with poor prognosis. Marked reduction of left ventricular ejection fraction at ecocardiography	Gangrene, Hyponatremia
Treatment								
	For hospitalized adults with severe disease, we suggest intravenous therapy with penicillin (6 million units daily), doxycycline (100 mg twice daily), ceftriaxone (1 g every 24 hours), or cefotaxime (1 g every six hours)	A rise in the hematocrit of 20 percent indicates considerable plasma loss, and patients with this condition require intensive care with intravenous replacement of fluids with cristaloids	For treatment of drug-susceptible typhoid fever, fluoroquinolones are the most effective class of agents Ceftriaxone, cefotaxime, and oral cefixime are effective agents for treatment of multidrug-resistant enteric fever	Ideally a severely ill patient is admitted to the intensive care unit (ICU) and provided with vasoactive medications, fluid resuscitation, and ventilator support.	Intravenous (IV) artesunate should be used in preference to quinine for the treatment of severe malaria in adults	Supportive, severe cases liver transplantation	Ideally a severely ill patient is admitted to the intensive care unit (ICU) and provided with vasoactive medications, fluid resuscitation, and ventilator support. The use of ribavirin off protocol cannot be recommended for established HCPS	Doxycycline is currently considered the drug of choice for nearly all patients with RMSF, including young children

Table 1. Clinical characteristics of some tropical infections with hemorrhagic manifestations presents in tropical South America

2. Common VBD in the tropics transmitted by arthropods and rodents

Etiological agents of HF affect humans on all continents. Most but not all agents causing HF are arboviruses, with transmission to humans resulting from an arthropod bite. However, animal reservoirs are generally rats and mice, but domestic livestock, monkeys, bats and other primates may also serve as intermediate hosts. Population growth, urbanization, human activities, and even climate change all contribute to a continual flux in the epidemiology of many HF transmitted by vectors arboviruses.

Haemorrhagic fevers share many clinical common features. Infectious agents that are arthropod-borne (usually mosquitoes and ticks) cause many viral hemorrhagic fevers. Some viral hemorrhagic fevers, person-to-person transmission may occur through direct contact with infected patients, their blood, or their secretions and excretions.

3. Flaviviral hemorrhagic fevers

Dengue is the mainly significant arboviral disease of humans with over half of the world's population existing in areas of risk. The occurrence and scale of epidemic dengue have augmented considerably in the last 40 years as the viruses and the mosquito vectors have both extended geographically in the tropical regions of the world in particular across South-east Asia, Africa, Western Pacific and tropics areas of the Americas, (Figure 2).

Dengue and Yellow fever are the prototype virus of the *Flaviviridae*, Dengue is a mosquito-transmitted viral disease very common in tropical areas of South America. The virus is transmitted mainly by *Aedes aegypti*, this mosquito is peridomestic and breeds in artificial containers around human settlements. The vector has a great preference feed for humans, which is a reason for the success disease; Dengue mainly is an urban disease and has no social class preferences. Dengue has two clinical presentations: dengue fever and hemorrhagic dengue. There are four dengue serotypes classified as 1, 2, 3, 4.

Dengue fever is supposed to generate about 230 million infections worldwide every year, of which 25,000 are lethal. Worldwide incidence has increasing swiftly in new decades with some 3.6 billion people, over half of the world's population, currently at risk, primarily in cities and villages centres of the tropics and subtropics. Demographic and community changes, in particular urbanization, globalization, and augmented worldwide journey, are most important contributors to the get higher incidence and geographic extension of dengue infections.

In modern lifetimes, the proliferate of unprepared urbanization, with related unsatisfactory housing, overcapacity and weakening in water, sewage and waste management systems, has produced model circumstances for enlarged diffusion of the dengue virus in tropical urban areas. Age frequency of dengue has been distributed in a broad ages either in adolescents or adults. In addition, the advance of tourism in the tropics has led to a boost in the number of tourists who become infected, mainly adults.

http://dx.doi.org/10.5772/55420

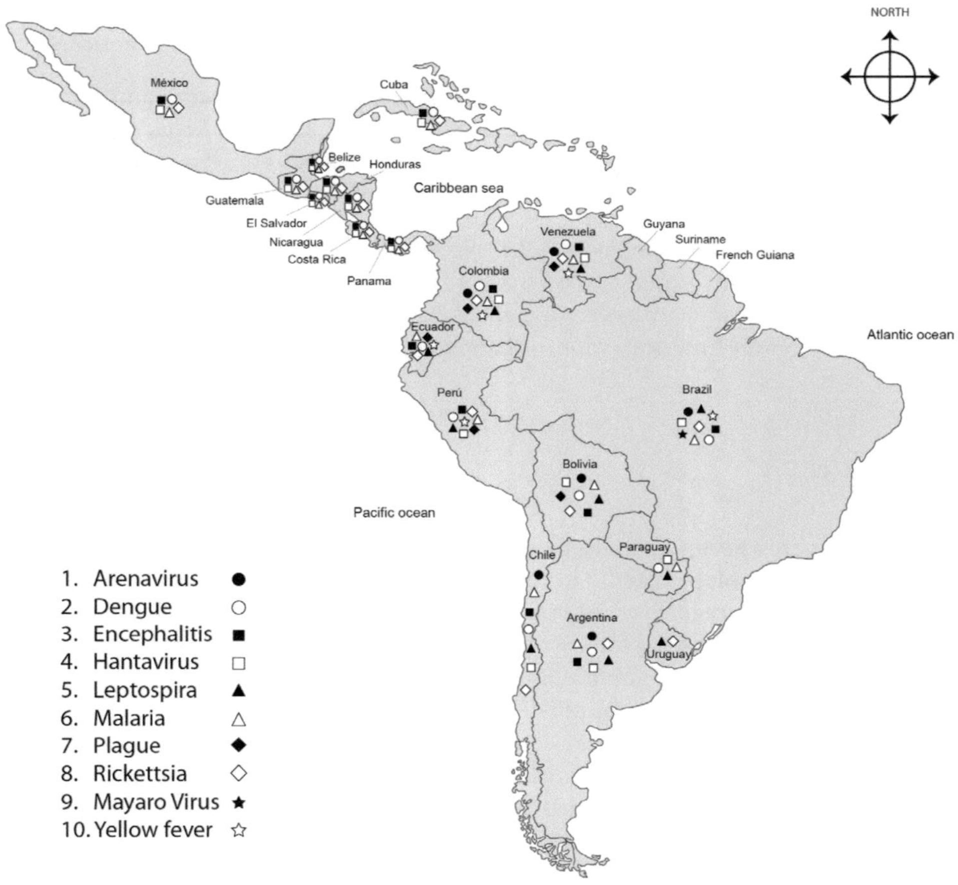

Figure 2. Distribution of several hemorrhagic fevers in Latin America

Symptoms and risk factors for dengue haemorrhagic fever (DHF) and severe dengue differ between children and adults, with co-morbidities and incidence in more elderly patients associated with greater risk of mortality. Treatment options for DF and DHF in adults, as for children, centre round fluid replacement (either orally or intravenously, depending on severity) and antipyretics. Further data are still needed on the optimal treatment of adult patients.

Because Dengue is endemic in the most tropical countries, the disease is overdiagnosed, therefore, many other hemorrhagic fevers as leptospirosis, hantavirus, arenavirus, rickettsiosis, Venezuelan equine encephalitis, chikungunya virus and malaria are erroneously diagnosed as dengue. Those diseases are clinically indistinguishable from dengue and other vector borne diseases and confirmatory diagnosis needs the employ of proficient laboratory tests that are difficult to pay for developing countries. Consequently, the endemic diseases above mentioned in developing countries remains mostly unidentified. Recent surveillance suggests that Venezuelan equine encephalitis, it may represent up to 10% of the dengue burden in neotropical cities, or tens-of-thousands of cases per year throughout Latin America.

On the other hand, yellow fever remains an important cause of mortality and morbidity in several South American countries like Colombia, Venezuela, Guyana, Ecuador, Peru, Bolivia and Brazil (Figure 2). The mosquitoes of *Haemagogus* and *Sabethes* are the main vectors in the rain forest, in contrast, *Aedes aegypti* in the urban areas cause YF.

YF has two different cycles: one endemic or sylvan cycle involving monkeys and epidemic urban cycle rare in South America. The frequented endemic sylvan YF constitutes to great source for introducing into urban environment. Despite the serious public health that YF represents, many South American countries abruptly discontinued YF campaigns.

4. Hantavirus

The hantaviruses are a group of emerging rodent-borne pathogens (family *Bunyaviridae;* Genus *Hantavirus)* that are etiologic agents for hemorrhagic fever with renal syndrome (HFRS) in Europe and Asia and hantavirus cardiopulmonary syndrome (HCPS) in the Americas. HFRS is associated with rodents of the family *Muridae,* subfamilies *Murinae* and *Arvicolinae*; HPS is associated with rodents of the subfamily *Sigmodontinae*. Since the identification of HCPS in USA in 1993, a huge number of cases of HPS and an rising number of hantaviruses and rodent reservoir hosts have been identified in Central and South America (Figure 2). Epidemiologic studies have demonstrated important differences in frequency of infection with hantaviruses in both human and rodent host populations. Antibody prevalences in rodent and human populations may vary from less than 1% to more than 40%. Currently, more than 1500 cases of HCPS have been reported and more than 15 genetically distinct variants of hantaviruses, all associated with sigmodontine rodents, have been identified throughout the Americas. Hantaviruses have been documented in South America from Argentina, Chile, Paraguay, Uruguay, Bolivia, Brazil, Peru, and Venezuela, and in Central America from Costa Rica and Panama.

Patients with HCPS typically present a short febrile prodrome of 3-5 days. In addition to fever and myalgias, early symptoms include headache, chills, dizziness, non-productive cough, nausea, vomiting, and other gastrointestinal symptoms. Malaise, diarrhoea, and lightheadedness are reported by approximately half of all patients, with less frequent reports of arthralgias, back pain, and abdominal pain. The mean duration of symptoms before hospitalization is 5.4 days. Remarkable hematologic result included a high white-cell count with augmented neutrophils, myeloid precursors, and atypical lymphocytes.

Several characteristics distinguish Latin American HCPS cases from the classical HCPS described for the first time in the USA. These include a variation in severity of disease from moderate and self-limiting to severe, the demonstration of person-to-person transmission, and a somewhat higher incidence of extrapulmonary clinical manifestations in the South American form of HCPS. Nevertheless, hantaviruses in the Americas is still far from complete knowl-

http://dx.doi.org/10.5772/55420

odgement. The factors involved in the dynamics of these viruses in nature, their establishment and transmission within host populations and from hosts to humans, and the variable pathology of these viruses in humans are complex. It is likely that more hantaviruses will be described in the future, and much more data will be required in order to describe the diversity and evolution of this group of pathogens. Latin America, as the centre of diversity for *Sigmodontine* rodents and their hantaviruses is presented with the unique opportunity as well as the challenge of being center stage for continued studies of the dynamics of hantaviruses in natural host populations and the links of host and virus to human populations.

5. Arenavirus

The *Arenaviridae* is a miscellaneous RNA viruses and contains the etiologic agents of some emerging zoonoses that are characterized by high case-fatality rates. Rats and mice (murids) are the main reservoirs of the arenaviruses. So far, six arenaviruses are reported to produce human disease: Guanarito (causes Venezuelan hemorrhagic fever), Junin (Argentine hemorrhagic fever), lymphocytic choriomeningitis (lymphocytic choriomeningitis), Lassa (Lassa fever), Machupo (Bolivian hemorrhagic fever), and Sabiá (human disease from Brazil).

The recognized arenaviruses in the Americas are hosted by rodents of the family *Cricetidae;* with the exception may be hosted by a bat (genus *Artibeus,* family *Phyllostomidae).* Pichindé virus, hosted by Oryzomys *albigularis,* was described from animals in the Pichindé Valley near Cali, Colombia, Guanarito virus, is also hosted by *Zygodontomys brevicauda,* the short-tailed cane mouse, causes Venezuelan hemorrhagic fever in the Venezuelan state of Portuguesa. This state borders on Colombia, and *Z. brevicauda* is a common species in Caribbean Colombia.

6. South American hemorrhagic viruses

Four members of the Tacaribe complex produce acute disease in humans: Junin, Machupo, Guanarito, and Sabiá viruses. Junin virus, the mainly considerably studied of the South American hemorrhagic fever viruses, is the agent of Argentine hemorrhagic fever. The disease disproportionately affect men, probably because of the job-related risk linked with agricultural work. The mouse *Calomys musculinus* is recognized the primary host of Junin virus.

Guanarito virus, the agent of Venezuelan hemorrhagic fever, mainly affects rural populations and has a restricted geographic circulation. Venezuelan hemorrhagic fever has been described close to the Portuguesa province in northwestern Venezuela, an intensively agricultural area. In 1989, previous to its detection as a dissimilar an hemorrhagic disease, irregular cases of Venezuelan hemorrhagic fever were probably mistaken diagnosed as dengue fever. Remarkably, deforestation and human intrusion into rodent environment may have resulted in augmented human contact to infected rodents and a concurrent enhance in human illnesses. The reservoir of Guanarito virus is a short-tailed rodent called *Zygodontomys brevicauda* and Sigmodon *alstoni.*

Regarding Bolivian hemorrhagic fever, Machupo virus is considered the etiology agent, which it was discovered in 1962 during an outbreak of viral hemorrhagic fever. Outbreaks of Bolivian hemorrhagic fever have occurred in cities and towns, probably connected to factors that privileged the invasion of human dwellings by rodents. Good practices control of outbreaks was capable through execution of intensive rodent trapping and education programs. The reservoir of Machupo virus is a sunset mouse *Calomys callosus*.

Regarding Brazilian hemorrhagic fever, Sabiá virus, is recognized as the etiologic agent. Sabiá virus was detected in 1994 from a Brazilian patient who was originally believed to have yellow fever, at that moment, a viral hemorrhagic fever was diagnosed. After that, no cases of acquired human disease caused by Sabiá virus have been reported. The reservoir of this virus is unknown, but is assumed to be a South American rodent. Sporadic cases of infections with Sabiá virus was been reported among laboratory workers in Brazil and the United States.

Arenavirus cases in Colombia have not been reported yet. However, we collected and tested 210 sigmodontine rodents of 3 species: 181 *Z. brevicauda*, 28 *Oligoryzomys fulvescens*, and 1 *Oecomys concolor*. Eleven serum samples, 10 from *Z. brevicauda* and 1 from *O. fulvescens*, had detectable arenavirus antibody. Three *Z. brevicauda* samples had antibody reactive to both Pichindé and Guanarito virus, and 7 more were positive for either Pichindé or Guanarito arenaviruses. The results demonstrated the presence of >1 arenaviruses circulating among common rodent hosts in Caribbean Colombia. We emphasize that many New World arena-viruses are likely cross-reactive to the antigens we used; recovery and sequencing of viral RNA will be essential to fully characterize these viruses. Hemorrhagic fever of arenaviral origin should be included in the differential diagnosis of tropical fevers, at least in studied region. As the human population of the rural Department of Córdoba and adjacent areas of the tropical Caribbean coast.

Besides the hemorrhagic South American virus described above, the principal old world arenavirus are the Lymphocytic choriomeningitis virus (LCMV) and Lassa virus. LCMV has a global spreading, which coincides with the geographic dispersion of its major host, the ever-present house mouse (*Mus musculus).* LCMV is a cause of acute aseptic meningoencephalitis and congenital malformations of the CNS and eye. People with a decreased immune system and women in the first or second trimester of pregnancy are at enlarged probability of developing severe disease. Mainly inhabitants are most likely to be infected by rodents in their homes; because population of *Mus musculus* are much larger in tropical countries, infections with LCMV in humans, may be frequent. Hence, deprived sanitation and other natural conditions facilitate mice incursion of human settlements.

In Europe and USA, peaks in the summer and fall are likely because more mice are entering homes. It is really unknown the incidence of infection in humans in different countries with lymphocytic choriomeningitis virus, but mainly experts believe the disease is not well known or underrecognized or underreported. The seroprevalence of lymphocytic choriomeningitis in different countries is between 0% and 60%. Vague clinical signs, demanding diagnostic problems, because require of knowledge on physicians and public health workers to put together recognition of lymphocytic choriomeningitis virus infections and its role diseases in humans.

http://dx.doi.org/10.5772/55420

Regarding Lassa fever is a significant cause of febrile disease in West Africa; it is projected about 100,000 to 300,000 cases and numerous deaths linked to Lassa virus. The cases are primarily reported from hyperendemic or endemic foci in the West African countries of Guinea, Liberia, Nigeria, and Sierra Leone.

7. Leptospirosis

It is a bacterial zoonotic disease that affects both humans and animals. Humans become infected through direct contact with the urine of infected animals or with a urine-contaminated environment. *Leptopira* is the bacteria belong to *Spirochetaceae* family transmitted directly or indirectly from animals to humans, who can suffer severe hemorrhagic, hepatic/renal and pulmonary disease. The bacteria enter the body through cuts or abrasions on the skin, or through the mucous membranes of the mouth, nose and eyes. Person-to-person transmission is rare. In the early stages of the disease, symptoms include high fever, severe headache, muscle pain, chills, redness of the eyes, abdominal pain, jaundice, haemorrhages in the skin and mucous membranes, vomiting, diarrhoea, and rash.

There are 20 known *Leptospira* species and hundreds of serovars, some of which belong to different species. Because there are pathogenic and non-pathogenic leptospira, it is basic to identify the pathogenic serovars of leptospires and their potential reservoirs to focus control strategies.

Pathogenic *Leptospira* spp are chronically maintained in renal tubules of a wide range of wild and domestic mammals and enzootic cycles are maintained by direct contact with infected urine or indirect contact with contaminated soil or water. More than 260 pathogenic serovars have been serologically identified and grouped in to 24 serogroups which have adapted to different animal species. Although some animal species may act as maintenance host for some serovars, they can also be incidental hosts from other serovars which may result in a range of clinical symptoms which is dependent upon the infecting strain, the geographical location and the hosts' immune response. Leptospirosis is a rural and occupational disease, which is considered to be an emerging zoonotic disease. In tropical and subtropical areas the transmission of leptospires is increased during heavy rainfall resulting in flooding, as well as poor sanitation and high host biodiversities, and has therefore become a major public health problem in these areas.

Outdoor and agricultural workers (rice-paddy and sugarcane workers for example) are particularly at risk but it is also a recreational hazard to those who swim or wade in contaminated waters. In endemic areas the number of leptospirosis cases may peak during the rainy season and even may reach epidemic proportions in case of flooding because the floods cause rodents to move into the city.

Prevention strategies of human leptospirosis include wearing protective clothing for people at job-related risk and evading of swimming in water that can be polluted. Leptospirosis control in animals dependent on the serovar and animal species, the management infection can be done by vaccination and rodent controls (24, 26).

8. Rickettsiosis

The genus *Rickettsia* includes bacteria Gram- negative in obligate association with eukaryote cells. A number of species have been identified in various terrestrial arthropods, and more recently in leeches and amoeba. Usually, pathogenic rickettsiae were classified into two groups: the typhus group (TG), composed of *Rickettsia prowazekii* and *Rickettsia typhi,* vectored by lice and fleas, respectively; and the spotted fever group (SFG), composed of more than 20 species mostly vectored by ticks. Other rickettsiae have shown antigenic and genetic particularities that preclude their inclusion in either the TG or SFG, such as *Rickettsia bellii* and *Rickettsia canadensis,* reported in ticks from the american continent.

Many *Rickettsia* species cause diseases in humans and animals, to which they are vectored by lice, fleas, ticks, or mites. Most of the recognized pathogenic *Rickettsia* species are classified into the SFG, which includes agents of spotted fever rickettsioses in humans in different parts of the world, vectored by ticks. During the last decades, there has been an increasing number of new *Rickettsia* species of unknown pathogenicity, mostly isolated from ticks. Some of them, previously considered non-pathogenic, were recently shown to be pathogenic to humans, such as the SFG *Rickettsia slovaca, Rickettsia aeschlimannii, Rickettsia massiliae,* and *Rickettsia monacensis* in Europe. In addition, *R. parkeri,* an 'old' SFG organism first reported in ticks in the 1939 was shown to be pathogenic 65 years later. These facts indicate that any novel described *Rickettsia* from invertebrate hosts, especially ticks, should be regarded as potentially pathogenic for humans.

In Latin America, several *Rickettsia* species (belonging mostly to the spotted fever group) pathogenic for humans or with unknown pathogenicity have been reported. *Rickettsia rickettsii,* the etiological agent of the most severe spotted fever in the world, has been reported in *Amblyomma cajennense* ticks in Brazil, Colombia, Panama, and Mexico and in *Amblyomma aureolatum* ticks in Brazil, (Figure 2).

In Colombia, Rocky Mountain Spotted Fever (RMSF) was first reported in 1937 by Patino. It was named Tobia fever because of the village where these cases occurred. The disease remained forgotten until 2003, when two fatal cases were identified and reported in Villeta, a locality next to Tobia. More recently, three outbreaks of RMSF have occurred in Colombia: in 2006 among military personnel in Necocli (Antioquia), in 2007 in a township of Los Cordobas (Colombia) and in 2008 in Altos de Mulatos (Antioquia). These reports defined the reemergence of the disease in Colombia and alerted the systems of surveillance across the country.

Eight *Rickettsia* species have been associated with human diseases in Latin America and Caribbean: *R. rickettsii* causing rocky mountain spotted fever in Mexico, Costa Rica, Panama, Colombia, Brazil and Argentina; *R. prowazekii* causing epidemic typhus in Argentina, Bolivia, Chile, Ecuador, Guatemala, Mexico, and Peru; *R. typhus* causing endemic typhus in Brazil, Colombia, Guatemala, Mexico, Panama, and Puerto Rico; *R. felis* causing flea spotted fever in Mexico and Brazil; *R. parkeri* causing spotted fever in Brazil, Uruguay, and Argentina; *R. africae* causing African tick bite fever in the Caribbean islands; *R. akari* causing

http://dx.doi.org/10.5772/55420

rickettsial pox in Costa Rica and Mexico; and *R. massiliae* causing spotted fever in Argentina. *R. massiliae* case was reported in a Spanish traveler presumed to have acquired the infection in Argentina, but suffered the disease after her return to Spain. The distribution of *R. felis*-infected fleas included seven countries (Costa Rica, Panama, Caribbean islands, Peru, Argentina, Chile, and Uruguay) where no human cases of infection have been reported so far.

A total of 10 *Rickettsia* species have been reported in both Spain and Portugal: *R. conorii, R. helvetica, R. monacensis, R. felis, R. slovaca, R. raoultii, R. sibirica, R. aeschlimannii, R. typhi,* and *R. prowazekii*. In addition, *R. rioja* has been reported in Spain, and *R. massiliae* has been reported to occur in Portugal. Amongst these *Rickettsia* species reported in Portugal and Spain, only *R. prowazekii, R. typhi, R. felis,* and *R. massiliae* have also been reported in Latin America.

9. Malaria

The etiologic agent of malaria is a parasite denominated *Plasmodium*, which is transmitted by means of the bites of infected *Anopheles* mosquitoes. The genus *Plasmodium* includes species of *malaria, vivax, falciparum*. Malaria is may be a main cause of morbidity and mortality in the tropics with *Plasmodium falciparum* responsible for the common of the disease burden and *P. vivax* being geographically most broadly circulated cause of malaria.

In the human body, the parasites reproduce in the liver, and then infect red blood cells. Symptoms of malaria consist of fever, headache, and vomiting, and usually show between 10 and 15 days after the mosquito bite. If not treated, malaria can rapidly turn into life-threatening by disturbing the blood provide to vital organs (30). In Africa and Latin America, the parasites have showed resistance to a several of malaria medicines. Means interventions to control malaria include: prompt and effective drug treatment; apply of insecticidal nets by people at risk; indoor residual spraying with insecticide to manage the vector mosquitoes, transgenic mosquitoes manipulated for resistance to malaria parasites and biological control of mosquitoes.

Malaria remains one of the world's serious health problems with 1.5 to 2.7 million deaths yearly; these deaths are mainly among children and pregnant women in sub-Saharan Africa. Of connotation, more people are dying from malaria today than 30 years ago. It seems to be the vector, the female anopheline mosquito is changing its behaviour or adapting to human activity such as creating new mosquito breeding sites. Hence, the impact of augmented population, and people displaced by violence can boost the incidence and proliferation of malaria. Furthermore, the difficulty of drug resistance by the parasites to almost all currently available antimalarial drugs.

Finally, most of the hemorrhagic tropical diseases describe above, can be also classified as neglected tropical diseases. Those represent some of the most common infections of the poorest people living in developing countries. Because they primarily affect the marginalized poor as well as preferred indigenous populations and people of African descent, the tropical hemorrhagic diseases in the Latin American and African countries are predominantly ignored diseases.

There is also misdiagnosis of hemorrhagic diseases in the tropics, mainly because the weak epidemiology and public health system in developing countries. The maximum disease problem of hemorrhagic diseases, such as leptospirosis, rickettsiosis, malaria and hantavirus infections, have first require scale-up of accessible funds or the advance of new measures instruments in order to accomplish control (32). The total elimination is implausible in the tropics, for that reason require and inter-disciplines efforts as social services, community education and environmental interventions.

10. Conclusions

The tropical hemorraghic fevers in the neotropics is a group of debilitating viral, bacterial and parasitic infections, that are very common aetiology of illness of the poorest people living in developing countries as Latin America. During the past 20 years there has been an intense emergence and re-emergence of epidemic of haemorrhagic vector-borne-disease (VBD) that have been produced by viruses supposed to be under control such as dengue, yellow fever, Venezuelan equine encephalitis, Saint Louis Virus, Arenavirus, hantavirus or viruses that have prolonged their geographic distribution such as West Nile and Rift Valley fever. Bacteria like *Leptospira* and *Rickettsia* have also re-emerged. Haemorrhagic fevers produced by bacterial or virus share many general features. Those infectious agents are arthropod-borne cause many haemorrhagic fevers. For some viral haemorrhagic fevers, person-to-person transmission may occur through direct contact with infected blood or secretions. Infectious agents are transmitted by arthropod like mosquitoes and ticks. Animal reservoirs are usually wild rodents, however, pets, domestic livestock, urban mice, monkeys, and other primates may also provide as intermediate hosts. Disease difficulties following from infection by these agents are common; the most tremendous manifestations include circulatory instability, augmented vascular permeability, and diffuse haemorrhages among them. Thus, the clinical manifestations and even histopathological findings are extremely comparable and challenging to make a differential diagnosis. Finally, in the Latin American the etiologic agents described in this chapter are disseminated in almost all countries, with exception of Uruguay.

Acknowledgements

To Dr. Juan Carlos Lozano, MD, for the cooperation and helpful in the design of Table 1.

http://dx.doi.org/10.5772/55420

Author details

Salim Mattar[1,2], Nelson Alvis[3,4] and Marco Gonzalez[1,2]

1 University of Cordoba, Monteria, Colombia

2 Institute for Tropical Biological Research, School of Veterinary Medicine, Colombia

3 University of Cartagena, Faculty of Economical Sciences, Research Group of Economics on Health, Cartagena, Colombia

4 University children's hospital Napoleon Franco, Research and teaching division. Cartagena, Colombia

References

[1] Gubler, D. J. The economic burden of dengue. The American journal of tropical medicine and hygiene. 2012; Epub (2012). , 86(5), 743-4.

[2] Hotez, P. J, Remme, J. H, Buss, P, Alleyne, G, Morel, C, & Breman, J. G. Combating tropical infectious diseases: report of the Disease Control Priorities in Developing Countries Project. Clinical infectious diseases: an official publication of the Infectious Diseases Society of America. 2004; Epub (2004). , 38(6), 871-8.

[3] Wilder-smith, A, Renhorn, K. E, & Tissera, H. Abu Bakar S, Alphey L, Kittayapong P, et al. DengueTools: innovative tools and strategies for the surveillance and control of dengue. Global health action. (2012). Epub 2012/03/28.

[4] Gubler, D. J. Dengue, Urbanization and Globalization: The Unholy Trinity of the 21(st) Century. Tropical medicine and health. 2011;39(4 Suppl): Epub (2012). , 3-11.

[5] Hotez PJ, Bottazzi ME, Franco-Paredes C, Ault SK, Periago MR. The neglected tropical diseases of Latin America and the Caribbean: a review of disease burden and distribution and a roadmap for control and elimination. PLoS neglected tropical diseases. 2008;2(9):e300. Epub 2008/09/30.

[6] Meltzer E. Arboviruses and viral hemorrhagic fevers (VHF). Infectious disease clinics of North America. 2012;26(2):479-96. Epub 2012/05/29.

[7] Aguilar PV, Estrada-Franco JG, Navarro-Lopez R, Ferro C, Haddow AD, Weaver SC. Endemic Venezuelan equine encephalitis in the Americas: hidden under the dengue umbrella. Future virology. 2011;6(6):721-40. Epub 2011/07/19.

[8] Tesh RB. Viral hemorrhagic fevers of South America. Biomedica: revista del Instituto Nacional de Salud. 2002;22(3):287-95. Epub 2002/10/31.

[9] Kibsgaard L, Lindberg J, Villumsen S, Larsen CS. [Rickettsiosis should be considered as a differential diagnosis in patients having fever related to travelling]. Ugeskrift for laeger. 2012;174(22):1525-8. Epub 2012/06/07. Rickettsiose som differentialdiagnostisk overvejelse ved rejserelateret feber.

[10] Tomashek KM, Gregory CJ, Rivera Sanchez A, Bartek MA, Garcia Rivera EJ, Hunsperger E, et al. Dengue deaths in Puerto Rico: lessons learned from the 2007 epidemic. PLoS neglected tropical diseases. 2012;6(4):e1614. Epub 2012/04/25.

[11] Adalja AA, Sell TK, Bouri N, Franco C. Lessons learned during dengue outbreaks in the United States, 2001-2011. Emerging infectious diseases. 2012;18(4):608-14. Epub 2012/04/04.

[12] Notes from the field: investigation of leptospirosis underreporting - Puerto Rico, 2010. MMWR Morbidity and mortality weekly report. 2012;61(22):421. Epub 2012/06/08.

[13] Chen LH, Wilson ME. Dengue and chikungunya in travelers: recent updates. Current opinion in infectious diseases. 2012;25(5):523-9. Epub 2012/07/25.

[14] Jonsson CB, Figueiredo LT, Vapalahti O. A global perspective on hantavirus ecology, epidemiology, and disease. Clinical microbiology reviews. 2010;23(2):412-41. Epub 2010/04/09.

[15] Ferreira MS, Nishioka S, Santos TL, Santos RP, Santos PS, Rocha A. Hantavirus pulmonary syndrome in Brazil: clinical aspects of three new cases. Revista do Instituto de Medicina Tropical de Sao Paulo. 2000;42(1):41-6. Epub 2000/04/01.

[16] Mattar S, Parra M. Serologic evidence of hantavirus infection in humans, Colombia. Emerging infectious diseases. 2004;10(12):2263-4. Epub 2005/01/28.

[17] Mir MA. Hantaviruses. Clinics in laboratory medicine. 2010;30(1):67-91. Epub 2010/06/02.

[18] Puerta H, Cantillo C, Mills J, Hjelle B, Salazar-Bravo J, Mattar S. [The new-world hantaviruses. Ecology and epidemiology of an emerging virus in Latin America]. Medicina. 2006;66(4):343-56. Epub 2006/09/19. Hantavirus del Nuevo Mundo. Ecologia y epidemiologia de un virus emergente en Latinoamerica.

[19] Phillips RS. Current status of malaria and potential for control. Clinical microbiology reviews. 2001;14(1):208-26. Epub 2001/01/09.

[20] Jay MT, Glaser C, Fulhorst CF. The arenaviruses. Journal of the American Veterinary Medical Association. 2005;227(6):904-15. Epub 2005/09/30.

[21] Mattar S, Guzman C, Arrazola J, Soto E, Barrios J, Pini N, et al. Antibody to arenaviruses in rodents, Caribbean Colombia. Emerging infectious diseases. 2011;17(7): 1315-7. Epub 2011/07/19.

[22] Mattar S, Miranda J, Rios R. Zoonosis. emergentes y reemeregentes, 2007; Universidad de Cordoba, ISBN-978-958-44-1148-5, Editorial Graficas del Caribe, Monteria, Cordoba, Colombia.

[23] WHO. Leptospirosis. Worl Health Organization; 2012 [cited 2012]; Available from: http://www.who.int/topics/leptospirosis/en/.

[24] Najera S, Alvis N, Babilonia D, Alvarez L, Mattar S. [Occupational leptospirosis in a Colombian Caribbean area]. Salud publica de Mexico. 2005;47(3):240-4. Epub 2005/08/18. Leptospirosis ocupacional en una region del Caribe colombiano.

[25] Labruna MB, Mattar V S, Nava S, Bermudez S, Venzal JM, Dolz G, et al. Rickettsioses in Latin America, Caribbean, Spain and Portugal. Revista MVZ Córdoba. 2011;16:2435-57.

[26] Paddock CD, Sumner JW, Comer JA, Zaki SR, Goldsmith CS, Goddard J, et al. Rickettsia parkeri: a newly recognized cause of spotted fever rickettsiosis in the United States. Clinical infectious diseases : an official publication of the Infectious Diseases Society of America. 2004;38(6):805-11. Epub 2004/03/05.

[27] Miranda J, Portillo A, Oteo JA, Mattar S. Rickettsia sp. strain colombianensi (Rickettsiales: Rickettsiaceae): a new proposed Rickettsia detected in Amblyomma dissimile (Acari: Ixodidae) from iguanas and free-living larvae ticks from vegetation. Journal of medical entomology. 2012;49(4):960-5. Epub 2012/08/18.

[28] WHO. Malaria. Worl Health Organization; 2012 [cited 2012]; Available from: http://www.who.int/topics/malaria/en/.

[29] Bousema T, Drakeley C. Epidemiology and infectivity of Plasmodium falciparum and Plasmodium vivax gametocytes in relation to malaria control and elimination. Clinical microbiology reviews. 2011;24(2):377-410. Epub 2011/04/13.

Section 5

Non-Communicable Diseases in Public Health

Chapter 19

Burden of Cardiovascular Disease in Colombia

Adrián Bolívar-Mejía and Boris E. Vesga-Angarita

Additional information is available at the end of the chapter

http://dx.doi.org/10.5772/53280

1. Introduction

Cardiovascular Diseases (CVD) is the first cause of mortality in the world. According to the World Health Statistics issued by the World Health Organization (WHO) in 2012, noncommunicable diseases (NCDs) caused 63% (36 millions) of 57 million of deaths that occurred in the world during 2008 [1]. Also, in the same period of time, CVD were the first cause of death by NCDs with 17 million of deaths (48% of the total deaths caused by NCDs). In 2010, this number reached to 18.1 million and it is estimated that will rise to 25 million by 2030. [1,2]. Likewise, it is calculated in That year, the number of deaths caused by NCDs in the world will reach to 55 million [1].

The outlook previously exposed at beginning worsen when it is consider that 80% of the deaths caused by NCDs have place in low and medium income countries, where the percentage of deaths in people under 70 years (48%) is greater than high income countries (26%). In fact, reports indicate that each year eight million people die prematurely in low and medium income countries due to NCDs, situation that produces a greater impact in terms of healthy life years lost and greater economic lose caused by no productivity in populations, that due to deficitary socioeconomic conditions are less able to face the burden that generates this growing public health problem [1,3]. In Latin America, according to the report about the health situation in the Americas issued by the Pan American Health Organization in 2011, between 2007 - 2009 the NCDs caused 76% of deaths reported, and 69% took place in medium and low income countries [4].

In Colombia similar to world statistics, NCDs are the main cause of death. According to the paper "Noncommunicable diseases country profiles 2011", issued by WHO, it is estimated that during 2008, NCDs caused 66% of total deaths, and CVD were the first cause of death from NCDs, causing 28% of all deaths, with a mortality rate of 205.9 and 166.7 by each 100,000 inhabitants in men and women, respectively (Figure 1) [5].

Colombia

2010 total population: 46 294 841
Income group: Upper middle

NCD mortality		
2008 estimates	***males***	***females***
Total NCD deaths (000s)	66.3	68.2
NCD deaths under age 60 (percent of all NCD deaths)	30.7	26.8
Age-standardized death rate per 100 000		
All NCDs	437.6	351.3
Cancers	112.9	92.1
Chronic respiratory diseases	43.0	29.9
Cardiovascular diseases and diabetes	205.9	166.7

Behavioural risk factors			
2008 estimated prevalence (%)	***males***	***females***	***total***
Current daily tobacco smoking	...	...	...
Physical inactivity	38.1	47.1	42.7

Metabolic risk factors			
2008 estimated prevalence (%)	***males***	***females***	***total***
Raised blood pressure	40.4	33.8	37.0
Raised blood glucose	6.0	5.7	5.9
Overweight	43.5	52.7	48.3
Obesity	11.3	22.9	17.3
Raised cholesterol	40.8	41.8	41.4

Proportional mortality (% of total deaths, all ages)

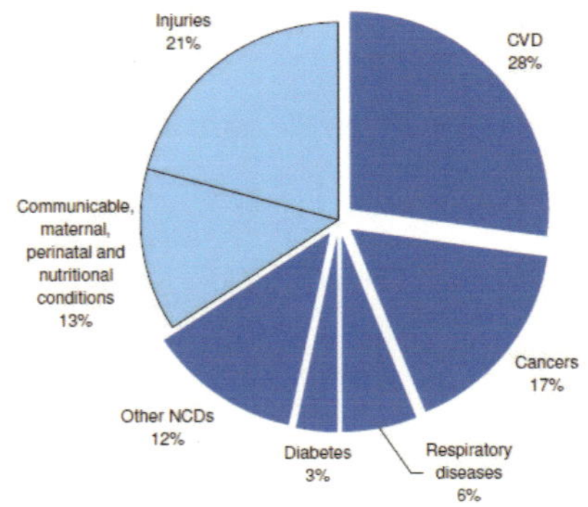

NCDs are estimated to account for 66% of all deaths.

Metabolic risk factor trends

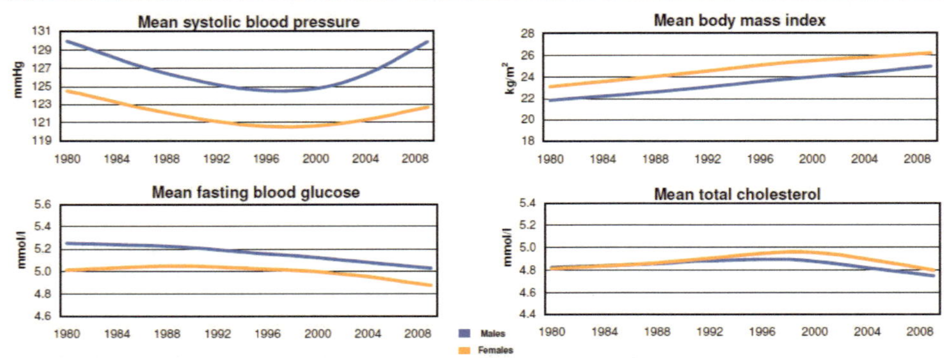

Country capacity to address and respond to NCDs	
Has a Unit / Branch / Dept in MOH with responsibility for NCDs	ND
There is funding available for:	
NCD treatment and control	ND
NCD prevention and health promotion	ND
NCD surveillance, monitoring and evaluation	ND
National health reporting system includes:	
NCD cause-specific mortality	ND
NCD morbidity	ND
NCD risk factors	ND
Has a national, population-based cancer registry	ND
Has an integrated or topic-specific policy / programme / action plan which is currently operational for:	
Cardiovascular diseases	ND
Cancer	ND
Chronic respiratory diseases	ND
Diabetes	ND
Alcohol	ND
Unhealthy diet / Overweight / Obesity	ND
Physical inactivity	ND
Tobacco	ND
Number of tobacco (m)POWER measures implemented at the highest level of achievement	2/5

... = no data available
ND = Country did not respond to country capacity survey

Figure 1. Noncommunicable diseases: epidemiological profile for Colombia, according to World Health Organization, 2011 [5].

Historically, coronary atherosclerotic disease represented a great burden in terms of mortality, which rises significantly after sixth decade of life. In Colombia, reports from late twentieth century, between 1998 and 2000, the mortality rate of coronary disease in men and women was 93.4 and 60.9 by each 100.000 inhabitants, respectively [6], nevertheless, between 2007 and 2009, the mortality rate was 124.7 for males and 88.3 for females by each 100.000 inhabitants, with a global rate of 104.5 by each 100,000 inhabitants [4]. This increase in mortality is probably associated to the demographic changes that have been taking place during the last decades, which are characterized by an increase in life expectancy at birth and a continued ageing of population. In Colombia, in the last 50 years, life expectancy at birth increased from 50 to 72 years-old, added to an increase in population older than 60 years from six to eight per cent, from 600,000 in 1950 to three million in 2001, and it is estimated that will reach 15.5 million in 2050 [7,8]. Such changes increased the population in which CVD are more prevalent, so it is expected that as the population continues ageing, the burden of CVD will continue showing a steady increase.

Stroke represents also a great social and economic burden, it is the second cause of death in the world, and the first cause of acquired disability in whole population [2]. Several reports show that the cerebrovascular disease is responsible of 55% of the total disability-adjusted life years (DALYs) produced by the neurological diseases in the world, estimating that in 2005 produced a total of 788.4 years of DALYs by each 100,000 inhabitants, representing 3.45% of the total DALYs worldwide [9]. It is estimated that in 2005, stroke caused a 9.9% of total deaths worldwide, according to estimations, it will rise up to 10.19% in 2015 and up to 10.63% in 2030 [9].

In Colombia, a study performed in 1997 in a northwestern town called Sabaneta (Figure 2), the annual incidence of cerebrovascular disease was calculated in 88.9 by each 100,000 inhabitants, with a greater incidence in men (118.7/100,000 inhabitants) versus women (61.8/100,000 inhabitants) [10]. Nevertheless, there are not national data available about the incidence of stroke.

Neuroepidemiological studies performed in different areas of Colombia, reported different prevalence of sequels of cerebrovascular disease according to the study area, data varied between 1.42 to 19.9 by each 1,000 inhabitants. Nevertheless, the results of these studies vary significantly due to some differences between the study populations, cultural habits, implementation of promotion and prevention strategies and ethnic factors. The most recent study, conducted in 2002 in Piedecuesta, Santander, northeastern Colombia, reported a prevalence of 5.7 by each 1,000 inhabitants [11-14].

In the State of Santander, Colombia, the analysis of mortality causes during 2007, reported that CVD were responsible of 32.07% of all deaths, with a mortality rate of 159.7 by each 100,000 inhabitants [15]. In the group of CVD, the ischemic heart disease produced 47.9% of deaths, followed by stroke (23.3%) and heart failure (9.6%) [15].

It is evident the growing problem that exists in the national and international context, where NCDs and specially CVD have become a great burden for populations, producing a great amount of deaths, that in low and medium income countries (included Colombia) occurred in an early way, affecting the life of their inhabitants at the time they are more productive economically. Therefore, the study of the CVD burden, as well as the design of intersectoral strategies to reduce the impact related to this burden, should be taken as a national and international priority, looking for mitigate and control this epidemic disease.

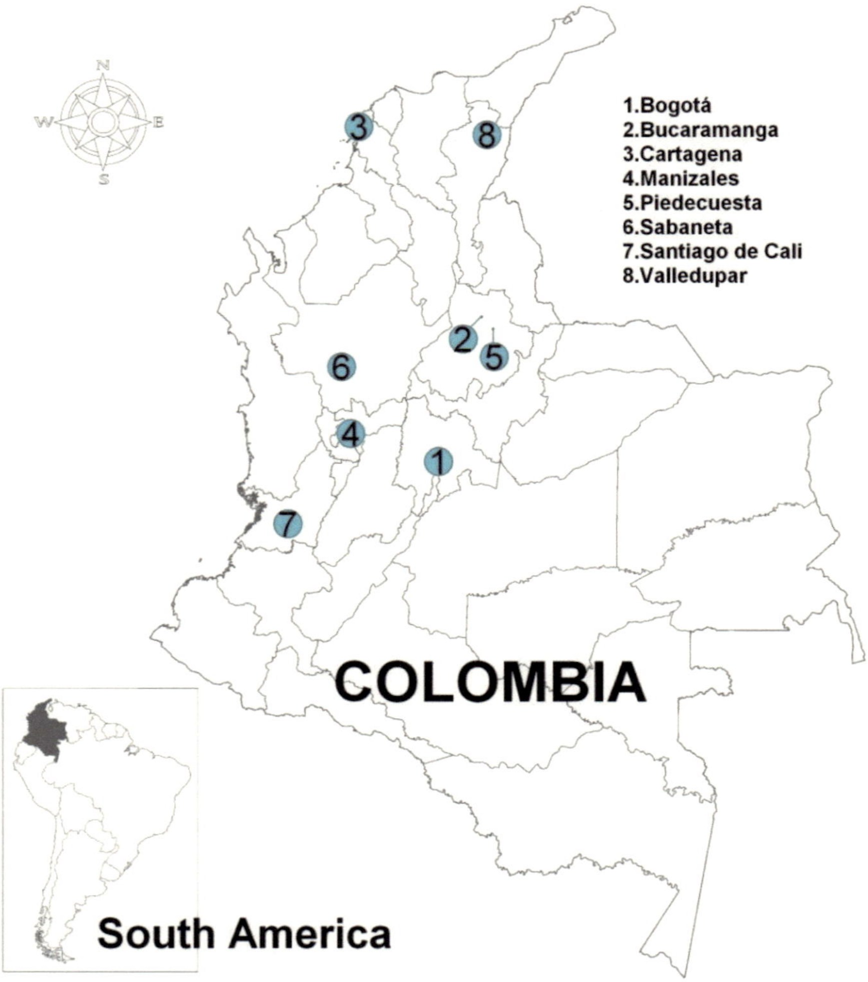

Figure 2. Geographic location of the Colombian cities mentioned on this paper.

2. Burden of CVD in Colombia according to DALYs

The DALYs are used as an indicator that estimates the global burden of a disease and the effectiveness of the health interventions aimed to diminish this burden, considering both, the years lived with disability and those lost by premature death [16,17]. Thus, when determining the burden of a disease through this indicator, we can observe the gap that exists between the real conditions of morbidity and mortality of a population and the ideals that this could reach if it was free from a particular disease [17].

According to the last study about Burden of Disease in Colombia, published in the 2005, the CVD (hypertensive heart disease, ischemic heart disease and cerebrovascular disease) are found to be in the first 10 causes of DALYs for both, disability and mortality in the adult population [17].

The hypertensive heart disease is the main cause of DALYs by disability in both gender, in the age groups of 30-44 years old (55.2 DALYs/1,000 inhabitants), 45-59 years old (78.5 DALYs/1,000 inhabitants) and 60-69 years old (75.6 DALYs/1,000 inhabitants). So, in a concerning way was observed that this disease was the second cause of DALYs by disability in both gender in the age group of 15-29 years-old (104.5 DALYs/1.000 inhabitants) and the fifth cause of DALYs in the age group of 5-14 years-old (2,9 DALYs/1,000 inhabitants) [17].

Meanwhile, ischemic heart disease is the main cause of DALYs by disability in people older than 70 years-old, with a total of 48.2 by each 1,000 inhabitants in the age group 70-79 years-old and 42.9 by each 1,000 inhabitants in the age group of 80 years-old or more. In the same way, this disease is the third cause of DALYs by disability in both gender in the age group 60-69 years old (31.8/1,000 inhabitants) and the sixth cause of DALYs by disability in the age group of 45-59 years old (12.9/1,000 inhabitants) [17].

When assessing the number of DALYs produced by mortality in both gender, it was found that ischemic heart disease was the first cause in group of 45-59 years-old (12.2/1,000 inhabitants), 60-69 years-old (29.5/1,000 inhabitants), 70-79 years (45.9/1,000 inhabitants) and 80 years-old or more (41.3/1,000 inhabitants). Stroke was the second cause of DALYs for mortality in both gender, in groups of 60-69 years old (11.8/1,000 inhabitants), 70-79 years old (21.8/1,000 inhabitants) and 80 years old or more (19.2/1,000 inhabitants) [17].

Finally, hypertensive heart disease was found as disease that more DALYs produces in the Colombian population, with a total of 52.5 DALYs by each 1,000 inhabitants when adding those produced by disability and mortality, accounting for 19% of the total DALYs [17].

The above results reveal that the CVD are the main cause of death in Colombia, but also represent a great burden for the population in what concerns to DALYs. It is surprisingly how CVD, besides producing a great proportion of the DALYs in the older population, also produce a great burden disease in the young adult population. These data are consistent with recent informs in where there is estimated that in lower and medium income countries the 29% of deaths by NCDs are produced in the population under 60 years-old. In contrast, the high-income countries only the 26% and 13% of deaths by NCDs are produce in the population under 70 and 60 years-old, respectively [1,18]. Additionally, it has been estimated that CVD are the main cause of death by NCDs in people under 70 years-old because, they produce the 39% of the total death in group, followed by cancer (27%) and chronic respiratory diseases [18].

Therefore, an important amount of the promotion and prevention strategies that emerge with the purpose of fighting the continuous increase of the CVD should be directed to sensitize the young people about the importance of adopting healthy life habits, in order to diminish the negative impact that CVD produce in the Colombian population.

3. The burden of the risk factors for CVD in Colombia

The risk factors more highly related with CVD include physical inactivity, smoking, alcohol drinking, unhealthy diet, overweight, obesity, hypertension, and high blood levels of cholesterol and glucose [2,19]. It is estimated that implementing effective prevention strategies based on the knowledge about the control of these risk factors, could prevent up to 70% of ischemic heart disease events and stroke and increase the life expectancy of the population in at least five years [2.20], in addition to reducing the risk for other diseases that share some risk factors with CVD such as cancer, respiratory chronic disease and diabetes [19]. Hence the importance of coordinating the implementation of promotion and prevention strategies in which it is linked the general population and the health personnel, in order to improve the risk profile for CVD of a particular community.

Even though, CVD continue being the main cause of mortality in the world, it has been documented in high-income countries that during the last two decades the mortality rates by CVD have diminished in a significant. While part of this decline is product of the improvements that have been presented during the treatment of the acute cardiovascular events, there is evidence that supports that the primary prevention strategies directed to the control of the main risk factors have contributed significantly to this decline [19,21]. In England and Gales, it is estimated that the mortality rate by coronary disease diminish from 1981 - 2000 to 65% in men and 45% in women between 25 - 84 years-old, which resulted in a decrease of approximately 68,230 deaths by the 2000 year, become interesting that such reduction in mortality was attributed in 58% to population control of risk factors for CVD, which empathizes the importance of knowing and identifying the more prevalent risk factors, in order to implement promotion strategies aimed to diminish their impact [21].

4. Tobacco consumption

It is estimated that tobacco consumption is responsible of 10% of the CVD deaths worldwide [19,20]. Despite the current knowledge about the consequences that tobacco produces in the human health and educational campaigns directed to the population in order to reduce its consumption, it is estimated that tobacco consumption causes approximately six million death each year, being responsible of six per cent of all deaths in women and 12% in men [19,20].

WHO considers tobacco consumption as a completely avoidable risk factor. Its association with CVD has been ratified in different studies, as also has been the benefits of its interruption. The INTERHEART study, in which Colombia participated, showed an odds ratio for acute myocardial infarction of 2.87 in smokers [22]. In a cohort of British doctors followed during 50 years was observed when comparing the mortality during the following in smokers versus nonsmokers and the ones who stop smoking, it was observed that those that stop smoking before the fourth decade can reach a similar life expectancy to those that have been never smoked [23]. Nevertheless, even after this age, the interruption of tobacco consumption brings significant benefits, so, life expectancy can be increase in 9 years if interruption of tobacco consumption is done around the age of 40, in 6 years if interruption is done at the age of 50 and still it can be increase in 3 years if interruption of tobacco consumption is done by the age of 60, when comparing with those that keep smoking. Therefore, it is emphasizing the tobacco interruption is justified almost in any moment of life [23].

In Latin America, the CARMELA study conducted between 2003 and 2005 in seven cities (Barquisimeto, Venezuela; Bogota, capital of Colombia; Buenos Aires, Argentina; Lima, Peru; Mexico City, Mexico; Quito, Ecuador; and Santiago de Chile), which sought to evaluate the prevalence of tobacco consumption in adult between 25 and 64 years old, the study found a prevalence between 21.8% and 45.4%. The ages where the consumption was highest were between 25 and 44 years old. In this study, Bogota showed a global prevalence of 22.2% with a confidence interval of 95% (CI 95%) of 19.1-25.2, being the consumption more prevalent in men (31.3, CI 95%: 27.1-35.5) than in women (15.0 CI 95% 11.1-18.9) [24].

In Colombia, as part of the *Tobacco-Free Initiative* developed in association with the WHO, the United Nations Children's Fund (UNICEF), the Center for Disease Control (CDC), and the Office on Smoking and Health (OSH) with the purpose of giving the countries the knowledge about the burden of tobacco consumption, the Global Youth Tobacco Survey (GYTS) was applied in Bogota city in 3,599 youths between 11 and 17 years old belonging to 231 official schools [25, 26]. In a concerning way, this study reported that the 62% of students have tasted at least once the tobacco, without finding significant differences between men and women [26]. From the total, 29.8% have consumed some tobacco derivatives in the last month, being the cigarette the most frequent (94.4%), without findings significant differences between gender. Nevertheless, the results also evidenced that seven of each 10 students considered the tobacco smoke as harmful for their health, seven of each 10 desire to drop the tobacco consumption and in fact seven of each 10 have tried [26]. Not being enough with the exposure to tobacco smoke by direct consumption, it was found that nonsmokers are exposed in a 40% to the tobacco smoke in public places and in a 28% in their homes, fact that urge the need of a legislation that prompts the creation of free smoke places in order to protect those nonsmokers from the exposition equally harmful to the tobacco smoke. In consideration to that, it was found that 63.8% of students (including smokers and nonsmokers) considered that tobacco consumption in public places must be forbidden [26].

Other studies done in Colombia in which the prevalence of tobacco consumption has been determined, have found similar data to CARMELA study. In this way, a paper done in university students in Cartagena de Indias city (a touristic city located in northern Colombia on the Caribbean Coast) and Santiago de Cali (the third city more populated of Colombia, located in the western country) reported prevalence of 23.9% and 23.2%, respectively [27,28]. Another study done in five cities (Bogota, Santiago de Cali, Bucaramanga, Manizales y Valledupar) (Figure 2) reported a prevalence that changes between 7.4% and 34.1% [29]; in this study the onset of tobacco consumption was 11.9 years old. This, added to results that indicate that in Colombia 57.5% of smokers between 11 and 17 years old had acquired cigarette in stores, reflects a poor authority control on the tobacco sale to minors.

As a result of knowledge about the negative impact that tobacco produces on the health of the smoker and nonsmoker population, as well as the failings in relation to the sell control of these products in minors, in Colombia, the authorities tend for optimizing the laws that regulate the policies about tobacco consumption prevention. Thus, on July 21st of 2009, the Colombian Republic Congress issued the law number 1335, law that seeks to regulate the consumption, selling, advertising and promotion of tobacco and its derivatives, as well as the creation and implementation of promotion programs directed to minimize the consumption and promoting the dropping of tobacco [30].

Some measures contained in the 1335 law include the ratification of the ban on the sale of tobacco products to the population under 18 years old, as well as the ban of tobacco products unit sales. It is forbidden that packaging expresses attractive advertising to minor as well as messages suggesting a soft, light or low nicotine product. The law provides that 30% of the packing area must contain clear, explicit and striking messages that warm with images or texts in Spanish about the damage produced by tobacco to the human health. It is forbidden the advertising of tobacco derivatives products on radio, television, film or other media directed to the general public as well as the sponsorship of these products to sporting or cultural events. On the other hand, the law encourages the creation of promotion strategies directed specially to the minor population, where this, may receive quality education about the negative effects of tobacco consumption [30].

Similarly, considering the rights of the nonsmokers are the possibility to breath smoke-free air, the 1335 law forbidden the tobacco consumption in public places like malls, parks, nightclubs, casinos, waiting rooms, among others where nonsmokers people may result affected by the tobacco smoke [30].

Thus, from knowledge about the prevalence of tobacco consumption, the health problems arising from this consumption and the burden of disease generated by this, is duty of the health personnel the promotion of non-consumption of tobacco-based products, in order to reduce the risk that this causes on the Colombians' health.

5. Physical inactivity

Adequate physical activity had been defined as at list 30 minutes of moderate physical activity during five days per week or 20 minutes of vigorous physical activity during three days per week [19]. The physical inactivity is considered as one of the most related factors with inadequate maintenance of the cardiovascular health [3]. It had been calculated that in the world, the physical inactivity produces around 3.2 million of deaths (six per cent of the deaths produced worldwide) and 32.1 million of DALYs (2.1% of the total DALYs in the world) by year, estimating that it causes the 30% of the cases of coronary disease, this fact, added to its association with another chronic diseases like cancer and diabetes mellitus, has placed it as the fourth risk factor of mortality in the world [19].

One of the most relevant aspects about the importance of an adequate physical activity promotion, sedentary is not only an independent risk factor for developing CVD, also is related with the development of another risk factors for CVD as overweight, obesity and high blood levels of glucose and cholesterol.

When evaluating the prevalence of the fulfillment of the recommendations for realization of an adequate physical activity, the National Survey of the Nutritional Situation in Colombia (Encuesta Nacional sobre la Situación Nutricional en Colombia, ENSIN) performed in 2010, reported that when adding the physical activity as a way of transportation and development during the free time [31], the national prevalence was 53.3%, prevalence increased when comparing with the results obtained in the ENSIN done in 2005 with a prevalence of 46.5%; the prevalence of physical inactivity, was found to be associated with female gender, low socioeconomic level and low scholarity [31,32].

Other Colombian studies determined the prevalence of physical inactivity in children, adolescents and adults founding numbers that varies from 26% to 85% [27.33-36]. Nevertheless, such studies can not be compared between them, due that definition of physical activity varies between them. It is noteworthy that as well as reported by the ENSIN, women has the highest prevalence of physical inactivity, in scholars between 7 and 14 years, the same trend is observed with a prevalence in girls of 83.8% and boys of 44.2%.

In Bogota, a study from 2003 evaluated the burden of mortality associated to physical inactivity and found a physical inactivity prevalence of 53.2%, data associated with a population attributable risk of 19.3% for mortality by coronary disease, 24.2% for mortality by stroke and a 13.8% for mortality by arterial hypertension [36]. Additionally, the mortality by NCDs in adults older than 45 years could be reduced between 1.9% and 5.1% if the prevalence of physical inactivity is reduced in a 37.2%. In that way, it must be considered as a priority the implementation of strategies that promote the realization of physical activity in the Colombian population.

In Bogota, during the last years some changes in the policies about transportation and recreation had been implemented, policies that have seek for the generation of spaces for physical activity promotion [36]. As a part of this initiative, the use of the bicycle as an alternative mean of transportation has been promoted with the building of bike paths. Also, some city streets have been intended as bikeways during holidays to promote the recreation and the physical activity as a frequent habit. These and other similar policies, have been extended to another cities of the country with the purpose of improving the population health conditions and reducing the impact of CVD and others non-communicable diseases on Colombians mortality [36]. Nevertheless, studies that allow the evaluation of the effectiveness of these measures must be done, in order to determine if these measures have been enough to reduce in a significant way the prevalence of physical inactivity in Colombian people.

6. Alcohol consumption

Alcohol consumption can be seen as a major public health problem since the consequences of abuse are reflected not only in an increased risk for many types of diseases, but also are related with high violence indexes, sexual abuse, suicide and traffic accidents; events that together affect millions of teenagers and young adults in the world.

It is estimated that during the 2004 the alcohol consumption was responsible of 3.8 %(2.5 million) of the deaths in the world, from which over 50% were due to CVD, liver cirrhosis and cancer [19]. According to the report done by the WHO in the 2009 where, based on the DALYs, the burden of the risk factors over mortality in the world was estimated; the alcohol consumption produced the 4.5% of total DALYs worldwide, being surpassed only by child malnutrition (5.9%) and risk sexual practices, nevertheless, this burden is greater in men, in which the alcohol produces the 6.0% of deaths and the 7.4% of the DALYs, while in women it produces the 1.1% of deaths and the 1.4% of the DALYs, aspects that are related with the study's results in which a higher prevalence of alcohol consumption in men than in women is reported [20].

Multiple diseases have been associated with excessive alcohol consumption, among these are included the CVD like coronary disease, arterial hypertension, cardiac arrhythmias and the cerebrovascular disease, nevertheless, the relation between alcohol consumption and CVD is complex due to there is evidence that supports that a moderate alcohol consumption could reduce the risk of dying by CVD, especially if it is red wine and in quantities not exceeding the 5-30 gr/day. In contrary, high quantities of alcohol consumption have shown a clear association with the risk of developing CVD [19,37].

In Colombia, according to diverse studies done mainly between teenagers and young adults, the lifetime prevalence of alcohol consumption ranges between 63% and 89%, with a past month consumption prevalence that ranges between 33 and 51% [38-42]. In a concerning way, the results of these studies have shown that in most cases, the onset age for alcohol consumption is between 13 and 16 years old [38-42]. Such is the case of a study conducted in Cartagena city, where after studying 1,031 university students, whose ages ranged between 15 and 38 years old, it was found that the 97.6% of those that have consumed alcohol for at least once in their life, have started the consumption before the 19 years old [41], which reflects an exposition to the harmful alcohol effects since very early stages of life and a greater risk for becoming a chronic consumer, since, according to a study done by the Epidemiologic Observatory of Cardiovascular Diseases of the Industrial University of Santander (Bucaramanga, Colombia) (Figure 2), during the years 2005 and 2006 in Bucaramanga city, the probability of being an alcohol consumer increases in a 17% in the individuals whose onset consumption was before the 16 years old and in an 11% in those who get drunk for the first time before this age [43].

Thus, it is clear that in Colombia a greater control on the alcohol drinks consumption in the adolescent population must be applied. Strategies directed to educate this population group about the harmful effects of alcohol consumption have been proposed by the Ministry of Social Protection as part of a policy that aims to reduce the negative impact of the alcoholic beverages consumption on the premature death in the Colombian population [44]. It is expected that these measures are implemented as proposed, and with this, reduce the alcohol beverages consumption in the Colombian territory, as well as the detrimental effects this produces in their inhabitants' health.

7. Unhealthy diet

It is estimated that in the world are produced approximately 16 million DALYs and 1.7 million of deaths related directly with a low fruits and vegetables consumption, which represents 1% of the total DALYs and 2.8% of the total deaths worldwide [19]. The impact of diet over cardiovascular death has been widely studied during the last years, resulting in an important quantity of evidence that shows a relation between the bad dietary habits and an increase of the risk for CVD [19,45,46]. Thus, it has been described that high-calorie diet, rich in trans-fat and with high salt levels is associated with an increase of cardiovascular risk, while a diet rich in vegetables, fruits and unsaturated fatty acids is associated with a decrease of cardiovascular risk.

In the 2010, the results of the ENSIN revealed the dietary habits of the Colombian population evidencing that vegetables and fruits consumption is well below the recommendations that have been considered to prevent the CVD (Figure 3) [31]. Thus, it was found that 66.8% of the population consumes some kind of fruit at least once a day, describing that such consumption has its maximum prevalence during the childhood and decreases steadily as the age advances. Moreover, the daily vegetables consumption was only 25.7%. In contrast, high values for the daily use of sweeteners (94.6%), fried foods (32%), soda drinks (22.1%), packaged food (15.2%) and candies (36.6%) were reported, values that were the highest in the 9 to 18 years old population [31].

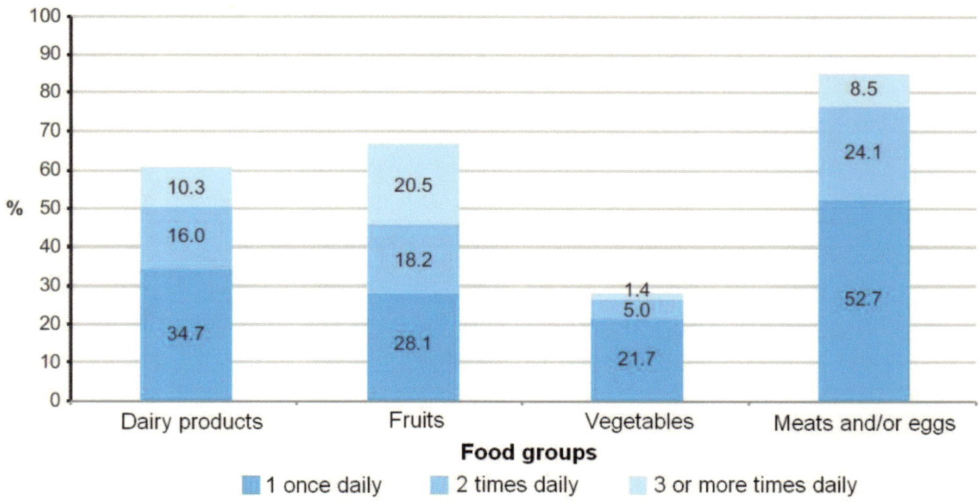

Figure 3. National proportions (5 to 64 years) of the daily frequencies of consumption by food groups in Colombia (Modified from ENSIN 2010) [31].

The previously exposed results, explain why despite existing in Colombia a high malnutrition prevalence, which in the 2010 year was of 13.2% for children between 0 and 4 years old, recently, in a simultaneous way the overweight and obesity are beginning to become a great public health problem because dietary habits as described previously, predispose the population to an alteration in their corporal mass index, with an increase in the cardiovascular risk as a consequence, which will eventually begin to appear in more earlier ages, as it is evidenced by the results in which it is observed that the overweight and obesity prevalence in the children population of 0 to 4 years old, went from 4.9% in the 2005 to 5.2% in the 2010, and is expected to continue rising in the next years as a result of the constant urbanization that exists nationally, and the changes in the lifestyles that this process entails [31].

8. Overweight and obesity

Overweight and obesity represent a great burden concerning the risk of developing CVD because, not only are independent risk factors for the development of these diseases, but also are directly related with an increase of other risk factors as the metabolic syndrome, hyperglycemia, hypertension and hyperlipidemia [22,47]. It is estimated that annually 2.8 million deaths are produced and 35.8 million of DALYs (2.3%) in the world due to overweight and obesity, expecting that this burden keeps increasing through the years as it is estimated that overweight and obesity prevalence will continue rising, affecting people at earlier ages [19,31].

In Colombia, during the last decades a steadily increase in the mass corporal index has been experimented in men as well as in women (Figure 1). The ENSIN, showed the numbers of prevalence of excess weight in the Colombian population, evidencing a continuous increase of such prevalence as the age advances(Table 1), which, associated to the aging population and the increase of others cardiovascular risks factors in the adult population, brings a great burden on the health system [31].

Age (years)	Prevalence %
0 - 4	5.2
5 - 17	17.5
18 - 22	21.4
23 - 27	35.0
28 - 32	48.1
33 - 37	54.9
38 - 42	60.5
43 - 47	63.3
48 - 52	66.4
53 - 57	67.1
58 - 64	65.7

Table 1. Prevalence of excessive weight in Colombian population by age groups [31].

Therefore, strategies through which the population could be educated about the importance of maintaining their weight in normal values must be created, and the consequences that the obesity and overweight bring to their health. Similarly, is the duty of the health personnel to inform the users about the normal values in which their weight should be kept, because, according to the ENSIN, when assessing the self-perception of body weight, the 23.6% of the youths (under 18 years old) and the 32.3% of the adults underestimated their corporal mass index, which may bring as a consequence a lack of motivation for weight losing in those individuals that, even though they have an excess weight, consider this as normal [31].

9. Raised blood pressure

Arterial hypertension is perhaps one of the risk factors for cardiovascular diseases most studied, estimating that it produces 12.8% (7.5 million) of the total deaths in the world and 3.7% (57 million) of the total DALYs [19]. Its prevalence increases with age producing a great impact in the mortality of adult people, estimating that it is present in the 35% of the total cardiovascular events secondary to atherosclerosis and in the 49% of heart failure cases [48].

Multiple studies have assessed the prevalence of arterial hypertension in different Colombian regions. Nationally, the Second National Study of Risk Factors for Chronic Diseases (SNSRFCD II) published in 1999 [49], reported a prevalence of arterial hypertension of 12.3%. Nevertheless, recent publications, evidenced an increase in the prevalence, thus, the report about the Americas Health Situation issued in 2011 by the Pan American Health Organization, showed a prevalence of arterial hypertension in Colombia of 27.8% and 19.1% in men and in women respectively, data that agree with other regional reports like the Study of the Prevalence of Risk Factors for Chronic Diseases done in Santander Department, in which a prevalence of arterial hypertension of 22.9% was reported in men and 17% in women [38]. Besides, is concerning that in this last report, despite the great amount of advances that have been made for the treatment and control of blood pressure, the 58.1% of hypertensive patients was not receiving any kind of antihypertensive treatment and the 18% was receiving a treatment but their blood pressure was not controlled at the time the study was conducted. Thus, the health authorities in Colombia, must implement strategies that seek to ensure that all the hypertensive people receive an adequate antihypertensive treatment, looking forward to reduce the impact that arterial hypertension represents in terms of morbidity and mortality over the Colombian population [38].

10. Raised blood cholesterol

It is estimated that high blood levels of total cholesterol (TC) produce the 4.5% (2.6 million) of the total deaths in the world and the 2 % of the total DALYs (29.7 million) [19]. The high levels of cholesterol represent a factor clearly implicated in the pathophysiology underneath the vascular processes related with the development of cardiovascular diseases like the coronary disease and the cerebrovascular disease. High levels of low density lipoprotein (LDL) (traditionally called 'bad cholesterol') have been related with the CVD due to the atherogenic effect they produce in the blood vessels, while high levels of high density lipoproteins (HDL) (traditionally called 'good cholesterol') represent a protector factor due to their antioxidant, anti-inflammatory, antiproliferative and antithrombotic functions [50].

In Colombia, multiple studies have been conducted with the purpose of assessing the prevalence of cardiovascular risk factors, among which are included the blood measurement of TC, HDL and LDL [38, 51-53]. In studies where those biological indicators have been evaluated, numbers of high TC prevalence have been found in the population over 15 years old, which varies between the 6 and 39%, evidencing an increase of the same with the age [51]. Thus, the study about Prevalence of Risk Factors for Chronic Diseases in Santander showed a prevalence of 14.2%, 36.2% and 32.0% in the age groups of 15 to 24 years old, 25 to 44 years old and 45 to 64 years old respectively [38]. In relation to the high levels of LDL, numbers of prevalence in the population older than 15 years old which varies between the 24% and 39% have been found, showing, as with TC an increase in these values as the age advances. Finally, when assessing the prevalence of low levels of HDL, values between 13% and 22% were found [51,53].

On the other hand, in a concerning way, a study done in children and adolescents between the 6 and 18 years old, found a prevalence of high TC and LDL of 13.5% and 17% respectively, with a prevalence of low HDL levels of 19.1%, evidencing an early presentation of the dyslipidemias as biological factors related to a premature increase of the risk for developing CVD [54].

Considering the facts previously exposed, it is clearly that the alterations in cholesterol blood values represent a risk factor highly prevalent in the Colombian population, which is found even since early ages. It is necessary to intervene early on the factors that may potentially modify these numbers, like consumption of a healthy diet and a regular physical activity, in order to stop the increase that has been showing the prevalence of dyslipidemias in younger population.

11. Raised blood glucose (Diabetes Mellitus)

Diabetes Mellitus is without any doubt one of the main risk factors for CVD. The increase of the cardiovascular risk associated to Diabetes Mellitus is due in part to the coexistence of other risk factors like obesity, hypertension, dyslipidemia and physical inactivity, nevertheless, the increase of blood glucose represents by itself a risk factor for the development of CVD [55], noting for example that glucose blood values at the admission moment of a patient with acute myocardial infarction, behave as an independent predictor of in-hospital mortality [55,56].

It has been estimated that the diabetic population has an increase in the risk for developing a cardiovascular disease that is 2 to 4 times greater, when compared to the rest of the population, because approximately the 80% of the deaths associated to diabetes are related in a direct way to the CVD [19].

In Colombia, the prevalence of Diabetes Mellitus varies between 4.0% and 8.9% in urban areas, and it's around the 1.4% in rural areas, according to the reported by different studies in which the behavior of this risk factor in different cities of the country has been studied [38,51,55]. Such prevalence has shown to vary significantly with age, being higher during the seventh decade of life, where it can reach up to 18.6% [38,51].

The Diabetes Mellitus represents a great economic burden for Colombian society due to the costs generated by the treatment of the disease, as well as by the complications produced, being the CVD the group of complications that more costs generates. Thus, it is estimated that during the 2007, the costs generated by the Colombian population with Diabetes Mellitus reached the 2,708 million dollars, from which, 1,404 million (51.8%) were secondary to coronary disease, cardiac disease and cerebrovascular disease [57]. In turn, the 74.4% (1044 million dollars) of the costs generated by cardiovascular complications previously mentioned, corresponded to direct medical costs (drugs, laboratories, hospitalizations, professional care) while the 25.6% (360 million dollars) were secondary to indirect costs (losses by non-productivity secondary to acquired disability in population under 65 years old and losses by non-productivity secondary to deaths in the population under 65 years old) [57].

Thus, it becomes clearly the need to control the impact that Diabetes Mellitus produces over the Colombian population. It is essential that, the health authorities and also the medical-assistance personnel, consider a priority the early detection of patients with diabetes mellitus through screening strategies, from which an early treatment could be done, looking for to reduce the number of short term, medium term and long term complications, with the purpose of improving life quality in the diabetics and reduce the direct and indirect economic costs secondary to this disease.

12. Conclusion

The NCD and specially the CVD are nowadays the main cause of mortality in Colombia, being these consequence of a high prevalence of the major risk factors that have been related to their development, within the tobacco consumption, alcohol consumption, physical inactivity, unhealthy diet, overweight and obesity, arterial hypertension and high blood cholesterol and glucose levels are the leading ones, which constitute also important risk factors for the development of other NCD.

Thus, as part of a search of cost-effective strategies, that allow to potentially reduce the burden of CVD in Colombia, programs directed specifically to the prevention of each one of the modifiable risk factors identified in the present chapter must be implemented, in order to impact significantly in the reduction of the prevalence of the CVD. Such strategies, must be based in educational programs directed to the general population, making emphasis on children because as seen before, is on this age in which in most cases bad habits that will define the future behavior of this population group are adopted. Besides, is responsibility of authorities to guarantee the fulfillment of the laws by which the alcohol and tobacco products consumption are regulated, looking for to avoid an early onset of tobacco consumption among children and the exposition of non-smokers to the harmful effects of the tobacco smoke, considering the morbidity and mortality associated to these two risk factors.

Finally, is duty of the medical personnel to participate in an active way in the promotion of healthy lifestyles, constantly looking for an excellent adherence of the patients to the indications related to the frequent fruits and vegetables intake and the regular physical activity, educating them about the importance of following these recommendations, in order to guarantee a reduction in their risk profile for the development of NCD and through this reduce the constant increase in the prevalence of this group of diseases in the Colombian population.

Author details

Adrián Bolívar-Mejía[1] and Boris E. Vesga-Angarita[2]

1 Medical School, Faculty of Health, Universidad Industrial de Santander, Bucaramanga, Santander, Colombia

2 Instituto del Corazón de Bucaramanga, Internal Medicine Department, Universidad Industrial de Santander, Bucaramanga, Santander, Colombia

References

[1] World Health Organization. World Health Statistics 2012. http://www.who.int/healthinfo/EN_WHS2012_Full.pdf. (accessed 20 July 2012).

[2] Pan American Health Organization. Regional Consultation: Priorities for Cardiovascular Health in the Americas. Key Messages for Policymakers. http://www.cardiosource.org/acc/international-center/~/media/Files/ACC/International/Priorities.ashx (accessed 20 July 2012).

[3] World Health Organization. State of the Heart: Cardiovascular Disease Report. http://www.world-heart-federation.org/fileadmin/user_upload/documents/WHD2010/FINALStateoftheHeartCVDReport121010.pdf (accessed 20 July 2012).

[4] Pan American Health Organization. Health Situation in the Americas. Basic Indicators 2011. http://ais.paho.org/chi/brochures/2011/BI_2011_ENG.pdf (accessed 20 July 2012).

[5] World Health Organization. Noncommunicable diseases country profiles 2011. http://whqlibdoc.who.int/publications/2011/9789241502283_eng.pdf (accessed 20 July 2012).

[6] Beltrán-Bohórquez JR., García-Ramírez M., Beltrán-Pineda R., Gómez-López E., Bohórquez-Rodríguez R. et al. Guías Colombianas de Cardiología: Síndrome coronario agudo con elevación del ST. Rev Col Cardiol 2010; 17(suppl 3): 121-275

[7] Gómez LA. Las enfermedades cardiovasculares: un problema de salud pública y un reto global. Biomedica 2011;31(4):469-73.

[8] Abegunde DO., Mathers CD., Adam T., Ortegon M., Strong K. The burden and costs of chronic diseases in low-income and middle-income countries. Lancet. 2007; 370(9603):1929-1938.

[9] Dua T., Garrido-Cumbrera M., Mathers C., Saxena S. Global Burden of Neurological Disorders: Estimates and Projections. In Campanini B. (ed.) Neurological Disorders: Public Health Challenges. Geneva: WHO Press; 2006. P27-39.

[10] Uribe CS., Jimenez I., Mora MO., Arana A., Sánchez JL. et al. Epidemiología de las enfermedades cerebrovasculares en Sabaneta, Colombia (1992 1993). Rev Neurol 1997;25(143):1008-1012.

[11] Pradilla G., Vesga BE., Diaz LA., Pinto NX., Sanabria CL. et al. Estudio neuroepidemiológico en comunidad urbana de Piedecuesta Santander. Acta Med Colomb 2002;27(6):407-420.

[12] Pradilla G., Vesga B., Leon FE and GENECO group. ational neuroepidemiological study in Colombia (EPINEURO). Pan Am J Public Health 2003;14(2): 104-111.

[13] Pradilla G., Vesga BE., Leon-Sarmiento FE., Bautista LE., Núñez LC. Neuroepidemiology in the eastern region of Colombia. Rev Neurol 2002;34(11):1035-43.

[14] Silva F., Quintero C., Zarruk JG. Guía Neurológica 8: Enfermedad Cerebrovascular. In Pérez G. (Ed.) Comportamiento Epidemiológico de la Enfermedad Cerebrovascular en la población colombiana. Bogotá: Mavarac LTDA; 2008. p23-29

[15] Ochoa-Vera ME., Otero-Wandarruga JA., Hormiga-Sánchez CM., López-Moreno L. Perfil de morbilidad y mortalidad de Santander. Revista del Observatorio de Salud Pública de Santander 2010;5(2):3-30.

[16] World Bank. Investing in Health. World Development Report, 1993. http://wdronline.worldbank.org/worldbank/a/c.html/world_development_report_1993/back_matter/WB.0-1952-0890-0.back (accessed 20 July 2012).

[17] Acosta-Ramírez N., Peñaloza RE., Rodríguez-García J. Carga de la Enfermedad Colombia 2005: Resultados Alcanzados. http://www.cendex.org.co/GPES/informes/PresentacionCarga_Informe.pdf (accessed 20 July 2012).

[18] World Health Organization. Global status report on noncommunicable diseases 2010. http://www.who.int/nmh/publications/ncd_report_full_en.pdf (accessed 20 July 2012).

[19] World Health Organization. Global Atlas on cardiovascular disease prevention and control. http://www.world-heart-federation.org/fileadmin/user_upload/documents/Publications/Global_CVD_Atlas.pdf (accessed 20 July 2012).

[20] World Health Organization. Global Health Risks Mortality and burden of disease attributable to selected major risks (OMS) http://www.who.int/healthinfo/global_burden_disease/GlobalHealthRisks_report_full.pdf (accessed 20 July 2012).

[21] Unal B., Critchley JA., Capewell S. Explaining the decline in coronary heart disease mortality in England and Wales between 1981 and 2000. Circulation 2004;109(9): 1101-1107.

[22] Yusuf S., Hawken S., Ounpuu S., Dans T., Avezum A. Effect of potentially modifiable risk factors associated with myocardial infarction in 52 countries (the INTERHEART study): case-control study. Lancet 2004;364(9438):937-952.

[23] Doll R., Peto R., Boreham J., Sutherland I. Mortality in relation to smoking: 50 years' observations on male British doctors. BMJ 2004;328(7455): 1519 -1528.

[24] Champagne BM., Sebrié EM., Schargrodsky H., Pramparo P., Boissonnet C. et al. Tobacco smoking in seven Latin American cities: the CARMELA study. Tob Control 2010;19(6):457-462.

[25] World Health Organization. Tobacco Free Initiative (TFI). http://www.who.int/tobacco/surveillance/gyts/en/ (accessed 20 July 2012).

[26] Wiesner C., Peñaranda D. Encuesta mundial de tabaquismo en jóvenes, reporte de Bogotá, Colombia. Rev Col Cancerol 2002;6(4): 5-14.

[27] Hernández-Escolar J., Herazo-Beltrán Y., Valero MV. The frequency of cardiovascular disease-associated risk factors in a university student population. Rev Salud Publica 2010;12(5): 852-864.

[28] Tafur LA., Ordóñez G., Millán JC., Varela JM., Rebellón P. Prevalencia de tabaquismo en estudiantes recién ingresados a la Universidad Santiago de Cali. Colomb Med 2006; 37(2): 126-132.

[29] Pardo C., Piñeros M. Teenage tobacco consumption in five Colombian cities. Biomedica 2010;30(4): 509-518.

[30] Congreso de la República de Colombia. Ley 1335 de 2009. http://www.secretariasenado.gov.co/senado/basedoc/ley/2009/ley_1335_2009.html ((accessed 20 July 2012).

[31] Instituto Colombiano de Bienestar Familiar. Encuesta Nacional de la Situacion Nutricional en Colombia 2010. https://www.icbf.gov.co/icbf/directorio/portel/libreria/pdf/LibroENSIN2010.pdf (accessed 20 July 2012).

[32] Instituto Colombiano de Bienestar Familiar. Encuesta Nacional de la Situacion Nutricional en Colombia 2005. https://www.icbf.gov.co/icbf/directorio/portel/libreria/pdf/1ENSINLIBROCOMPLETO.pdf (accessed 20 July 2012).

[33] Mantilla-Toloza SC., Gómez-Conesa A., Hidalgo-Montesinos. Physical activity and tobacco and alcohol use in a group of university students. Rev Salud Publica 2011;13(5): 748-58.

[34] Alayón AN., Castro-Orozco R., Gaviria-Esquivia L., Fernández-Franco M., Benítez-Peña L. Cardiovascular risk factors among 7-and 14-year old schoolchildren in Cartagena, Colombia, 2009. Rev Salud Publica 2011;13(2): 196-206.

[35] Patiño-Villada FA., Arango-Vélez EF., Quintero-Velásquez MA., Arenas-Sosa MM. Cardiovascular risk factors in an urban Colombia population. Rev Salud Publica 2011;13(3): 433-45.

[36] Lobelo F., Pate R., Parra D., Duperly J., Pratt M. Burden of mortality associated to physical inactivity in Bogota, Colombia. Rev Salud Publica 2006;8(Suppl 2): 28-41.

[37] Böhm M., Rosenkranz S., Laufs U. Alcohol and red wine: impact on cardiovascular risk. Nephrol Dial Transplant 2004;19(1): 11-16.

[38] Hormiga-Sánchez CM., Otero-Wandarraga JA., Rodríguez Villamizar LA., León-Franco MH. Prevalencia de factores de riesgo para enfermedades crónicas en Santander, 2010. Revista del Observatorio de Salud Pública de Santander 2010;5(3): 2-24.

[39] Manrique-Abril FG., Ospina JM., Garcia-Ubaque JC. Children and adolescents' alcohol and tobacco consumption in Tunja, Colombia, 2009. Rev Salud Publica 2011;13(1): 89-101.

[40] López-Maldonado MC., Luis MA., Gherardi-Donato EC. Licit drugs consumption among nursing students at a private university in Bogotá, Colombia. Rev Lat Am Enfermagem 2011;19: 707-13.

[41] Arrieta-Vergara KM. Pathological alcohol consumption amongst students from the University of Cartagena, 2008. Rev Salud Publica 2009;11(6): 878-86.

[42] Observatorio de Drogas de Colombia. Estudio Nacional de Consumo de Sustancias Psicoactivas en Poblacion Escolar Colombia - 2011. http://odc.dne.gov.co/docs/publicaciones_nacionales/Estudio%20Sustancias%20Psicoactivas%20en%20Escolares%202011.pdf (accessed 20 July 2012).

[43] Ardila MF., Herrán OF. Expectancies towards alcohol consumption in Bucaramanga, Colombia. Rev Med Chil 2008;136(1): 73-82.

[44] Ministry of Social Protection. Decreto número 120 de 2010. http://web.presidencia.gov.co/decretoslinea/2010/enero/21/dec12021012010.pdf (accessed 20 July 2012).

[45] Belin RJ., Greenland P., Allison M., Martin L., Shikany JM. et al. Diet quality and the risk of cardiovascular disease: the Women's Health Initiative (WHI). Am J Clin Nutr 2011;94(1): 49-57.

[46] Socarrás-Suárez MM., Bolet-Astoviza M. Healthy feeding and nutrition in cardiovascular diseases. Rev Cubana Invest Bioméd 2010; 29(3): 353-363.

[47] Webber L., Kilpi F., Marsh T., Rtveladze K., Brown M. et al. High Rates of Obesity and Non-Communicable Diseases Predicted across Latin America. PLoS One 2012;7(8): 1-6

[48] Báez L., Blanco MI., Bohórquez R., Botero R., Cuenca G. et al. Guías colombianas para el diagnóstico y tratamiento de la hipertensión arterial. Rev Col Cardiol 2007;13(suppl 1): 187-313

[49] Ministerio de Salud. II Estudio Nacional de Factores de Riesgo de Enfermedades Crónicas - Enfrec II. http://www.col.ops-oms.org/sivigila/IndiceBoletines1999.asp (accessed 20 July 2012).

[50] National Institute of Health. Detection,Evaluation,and Treatmentof High BloodCholesterolin Adults(Adult TreatmentPanel III). http://www.nhlbi.nih.gov/guidelines/cholesterol/atp3full.pdf (accessed 20 July 2012).

[51] Bautista LE., Oróstegui M., Vera LM., Prada GE., Orozco LC. et al. Prevalence and impact of cardiovascular risk factors in Bucaramanga, Colombia: results from the Countrywide Integrated Noncommunicable Disease Intervention Programme (CINDI/CARMEN) baseline survey. Eur J Cardiovasc Prev Rehabil 2006;13(5): 769-75.

[52] Feliciano-Alfonso JE., Mendivil CO., Ariza ID., Pérez CE. Cardiovascular risk factors and metabolic syndrome in a population of young students from the National University of Colombia. Rev Assoc Med Bras 2010;56(3): 293-8.

[53] Alayón AN., Ariza S., Baena K., Lambis L., Martínez L. et al. Active search and assessment of cardiovascular risk factors in young adults, Cartagena de Indias, 2007. Biomedica 2010;30(2): 238-44.

[54] Uscátegui-Peñuela RM., Alvarez-Uribe MC., Laguado-Salinas I., Soler-Terranova W., Martínez-Maluendas L. et al. Cardiovascular risk factors in children and teenagers aged 6-18 years old from Medellin (Colombia). An Pediatr (Barc) 2003;58(5): 411-417.

[55] Aschner P. Epidemiology of diabetes in Colombia. Av Diabetol 2010;26(2): 95-100.

[56] Takada JY., Ramos RB., Avakian SD., dos Santos SM., Ramires JA. et al. BNP and admission glucose as in-hospital mortality predictors in non-ST elevation myocardial infarction. ScientificWorldJournal. 2012;2012: 1-7.

[57] Gozáles JC., Walter JH., Einarson TR. Cost-of-illness study of type 2 diabetes mellitus in Colombia. Rev Panam Salud Publica 2009;26(1): 55-63.

Chapter 20

Topics in Prevention of Diseases in Gastroenterology

Leonardo Sosa Valencia and Erika Rodriguez-Wulff

Additional information is available at the end of the chapter

http://dx.doi.org/10.5772/55138

1. Introduction

Cancer is a disease caused by an uncontrolled division of abnormal cells in a part of the body, in another words, is a malignant growth or tumor resulting from such a division of cells. Is the leading cause of death worldwide. Attributed 7.6 million deaths (approximately 13% of total) occurred worldwide in 2008. The most common types of cancer are shown in Figure 1 [1]

- Gastric (736,000 deaths);
- Liver (695,000 deaths);
- Colorectal (608,000 deaths);
- Pancreas (227,000 deaths).

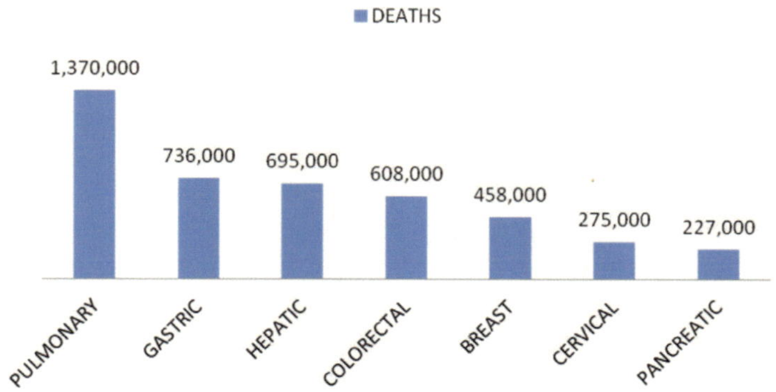

Figure 1. Cancer deaths in 2008

Cancers that cause more deaths per year are lung, stomach, liver, colon and breast.

In this problem, are involving genetic factors and lifestyle of the population, approximately 30% of cancer deaths are due to five behavioral risk factors and diet: high body mass index, reduced intake of fruits and vegetables, sedentary lifestyle, smoking and alcohol use.

More than 50% of cancer could be prevented if people implemented what is already known about cancer prevention, according to researchers at the Union for International Cancer Control (UICC) World Cancer Congress 2012 [2].

In this chapter, we summarize the relationship of some gastrointestinal cancer and factors that can be change in our population to decrease and prevent them in the future.

2. Helicobacter pylori and gastric cancer

Gastric cancer is the second leading cause of cancer death in the world [3,4,5]. A number of environmental factors such as Helicobacter pylori status, smoking, alcohol, decrease vitamin C intake, nitrosamines and nitrates, and salt intake are related to gastric cancer development. Also the presence of a family history of gastric cancer is significantly associated with increased risk of developing the disease [6] Figure 2. Gastric carcinogenesis is a multifactorial process, involving complex interactions between host and environmental factors [7]. It is known that gastric cancer involves the interaction of three major factors: the agent (in the great part of the cases, H. pylori) and its pathogenicity, the characteristics of the host, and the external environment [8].

Among these factors, have been associated with the development of gastric cancer, premalignant conditions within which include chronic atrophic gastritis, intestinal metaplasia, Helicobacter pylori infection and gastric adenoma [3,4,5,8]. Chronic inflammation plays an important role in the development of gastric cancer. Inflammation-induced injury may compromise tissue integrity and drive the multistage process of carcinogenesis by altering targets and pathways crucial to normal tissue homeostasis [7].

Helicobacter pylori (H. pylori), is a spiral, Gram-negative microaerophilic bacterial pathogen that is distributed worldwide and is in particular found in developing countries, infecting the stomach of about 50 % of the world's population [9]. H. pylori infection is closely related to the development of gastric cancer [10]. In 1994 the results of epidemiological studies carried, the World Health Organization's International Agency for Research on Cancer to concluded that H. pylori has a causal link with gastric carcinogenesis and was defined as a type I carcinogen, a definite human carcinogen [10,8]. The evidence in the population of whole world shows that H. pylori infection, has been known to induce chronic gastric inflammation that leads to atrophy, metaplasia, dysplasia, and gastric cancer [3,7]. All patients with H. pylori infection have histological gastritis, which corresponds to classical chronic gastritis and is characterized by the infiltration of neutrophils and other inflammatory cells. However, most patients are asymptomatic for life, while only some will come to develop a digestive disease [8]. The transmission route of H. pylori infection has been the topic of sev-

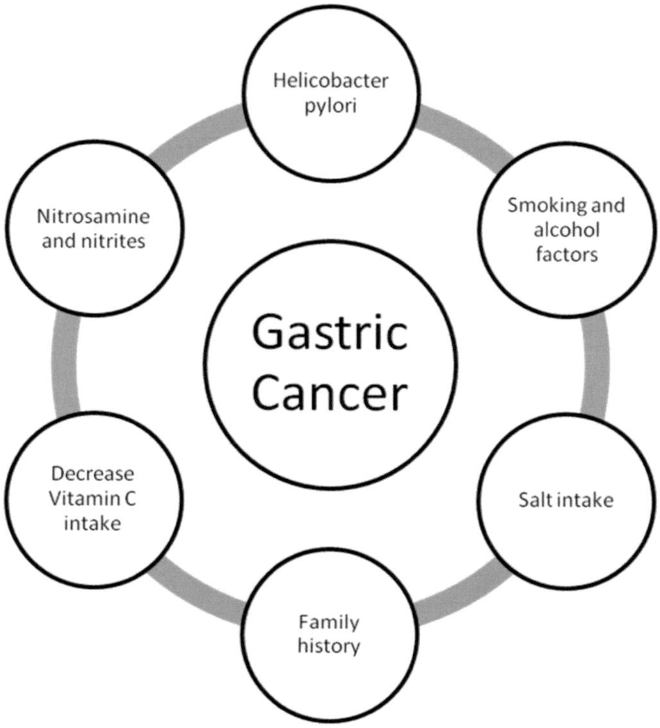

Figure 2. Associated factors in Gastric Cancer

Gastric cancer can develop both in the proximal and the distal region. Dietary factors and H. pylori infection are major risk factors for the development of distal tumors; the major risk factors for proximal cancers are gastroesophageal reflux disease and obesity [5].

The gastric intestinal metaplasia is recognized as a premalignant condition that may be the result of adaptive response to environmental stimuli such as infection by H. pylori, smoking and high concentrations of salt intake. Patients with intestinal metaplasia are up to 10 times greater risk of developing gastric cancer, which may be higher in certain geographical areas and in patients infected with H. pylori [12]. Figure 3.

Despite advances in diagnosis, the disease is usually detected after invasion of the muscular propia, because most patients experience vague and nonspecific symptoms in the early stages and the classic triad of anemia, weight loss, and refusal of meat-based foods is seen only in advanced stages. Furthermore, surgery and chemotherapy have limited value in advanced disease and there is a paucity of molecular markers for targeted therapy. Since cancer of the stomach has a very poor prognosis and the 5-year survival rate is only around 20 per cent, a new look at the results of epidemiological and experimental studies is important to establish strategies for primary prevention [5]. As treatment of gastric cancer at the symptomatic stage represents a significant medical burden, clinicians have been encouraged to focus on designing preventive strategies instead of multimodal therapies [13].

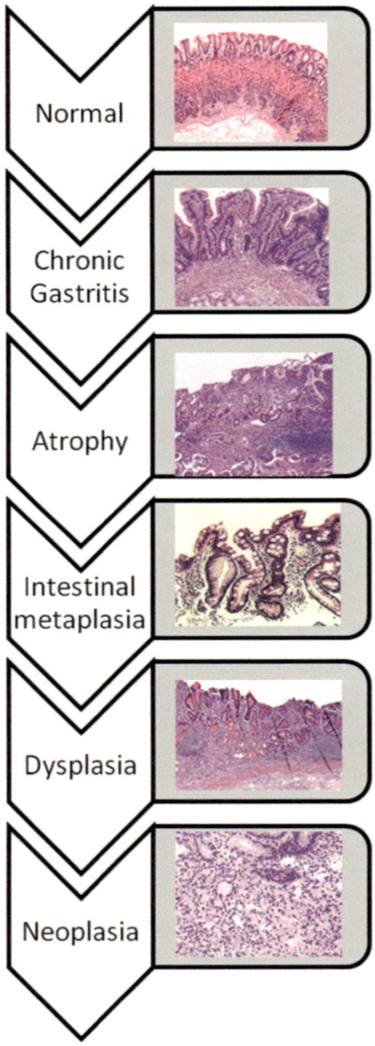

Figure 3. Gastric carcinogenesis: Histologyc changes from normal gastric mucosa to neoplasia.

As a primary prevention, some behavior modifications have been suggested, including reduction of salt intake with the diet, increase of vitamin C consumption, abolition of smoking and H. pylori eradication wich is recommended as it is able to reduce gastric cancer inci-

http://dx.doi.org/10.5772/55138

dence up to 35% [14]. If infection with H. pylori is identified, eradication should be considered the same because it is considered a class I carcinogen [12]. After eradicating H. pylori, precancerous lesions may regress. Testing and treating for the H pylori infection earlier rather than later in life is suggested to be the more beneficial approach [7]. The eradication of H. pylori prophylactically pylori remains controversial in humans, has not shown a significant reduction in the risk of gastric cancer after eradication of H pylori [10], but in a recent population-based study, early H pylori eradication was found to be associated with decreased risk of gastric cancer [7]. There are some studies indicating that the eradication of the microorganisms in the system could reduce the incidence of gastric cancer in patients without precancerous lesions or, when lesions are presents, that the eradication may or may not reduce this incidence. Also, when the eradication is done after endoscopic mucosal resection in patients with early gastric adenocarcinoma, it could decrease the recurrence of metachronous gastric cancer in some patients [8].

3. Hepatitis virus and liver cancer

The hepatocellular carcinoma (HCC), is the most frequent form of primary liver cancer [15], it accounts for up to 90% [16], and is one of the most common malignancies in the world [17], is the third most common cause of cancer-related death worldwide [18,19], results in between 250.000 and one million deaths globally per annum, the increasing incidence rates are in many parts of the world, including the United States and Central Europe. The Incidence of HCC in the United States is expected to continue to rise as a consequence of high hepatitis C infection rates between 1960 and 1990 and the average 20 to 30 year lag time between virus acquisition and the development of cirrhosis and carcinoma.

Cancers caused by viral infections such as infections of hepatitis B virus (HBV), hepatitis C virus (HCV) and human papillomavirus (HPV), are responsible for up to 20% of cancer deaths in middle-income countries low and medium [1]. The major risk factors for the development of HCC include liver cirrhosis of any etiology [16]. Almost 80 percent of cases are due to underlying chronic hepatitis B and C virus infection [19]. Occur with particular frequency in patients with cirrhosis caused by hepatitis virus. HCC can develop in patients with chronic HBV, even in the absence of cirrhosis. However, 70 to 90 percent of patients with HBV who develop HCC will have cirrhosis [18]. The strong association between liver cancer and cirrhosis has been recognized in patients with HCV [17]. Chronic infection of HBV and hepatitis C virus are well-documented major etiologic factors for HCC [20,21].

The majority of HCC occur in patients with chronic liver disease or cirrhosis. Thus, older patients with longstanding liver disease are more likely to develop HCC, it develops commonly, but not exclusively, in a setting of chronic liver cell injury, inflammation which leads to, hepatocyte regeneration, liver matrix remodeling, fibrosis, and ultimately, cirrhosis. The major etiologies of liver cirrhosis are diverse and include chronic HBV and HCV, alcohol consumption, steatosis, diabetes, certain medications or toxic exposures, including dietary aflatoxins and genetic metabolic diseases [22,23]. In addition to cirrhosis, a number of other

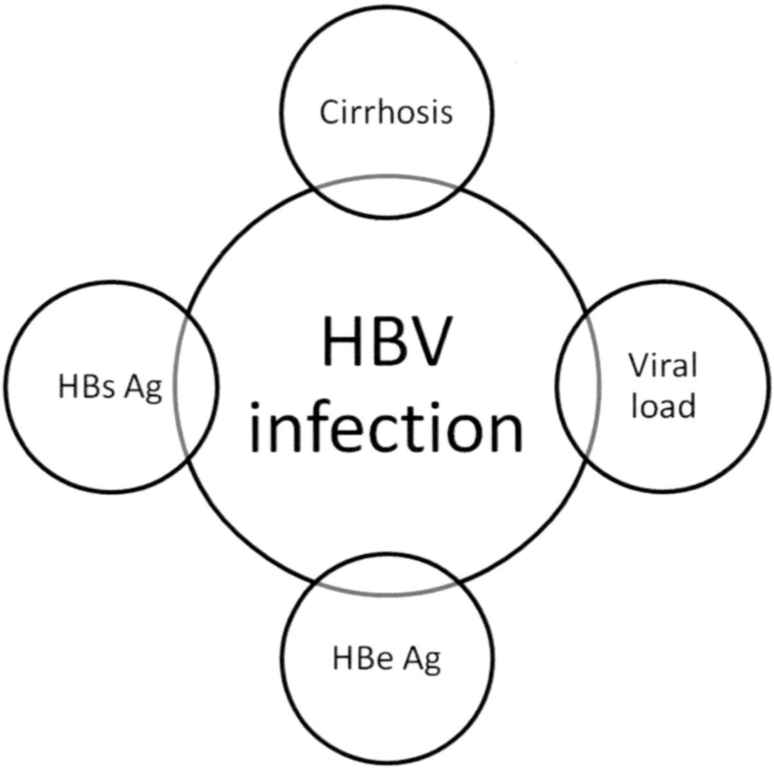

HCC: Hepatocellular Carcinoma. HBV: Virus Hepatitis B. HBs Ag: Hepatitis B surface antigen. HBe Ag: Hepatitis B e antigen

Figure 4. Factors associated with the risk of develop HCC in patients with chronic HBV

The mechanisms by which these varied etiologies lead to cirrhosis and HCC are not yet fully understood [21,22,23]. A common pathway from these varied etiologies to HCC may involve chronic inflammation, which is increasingly recognized as a procarcinogenic condition [21,22]. Both viruses have been classified as human carcinogens by the International Agency for Research on Cancer [20]. Malignant transformation that is induced by chronic HBV infection is a multistage pathogenic process and involves multiple risk predictors [20]. Other many factors determining the risk of developing an HCC are host dependent, some are genetic and not modifiable, other are linked to lifestyle and can be influenced [15]; age, gender, family history of HCC, alcohol consumption habits, serostatus of hepatitis B e anti-

http://dx.doi.org/10.5772/55138

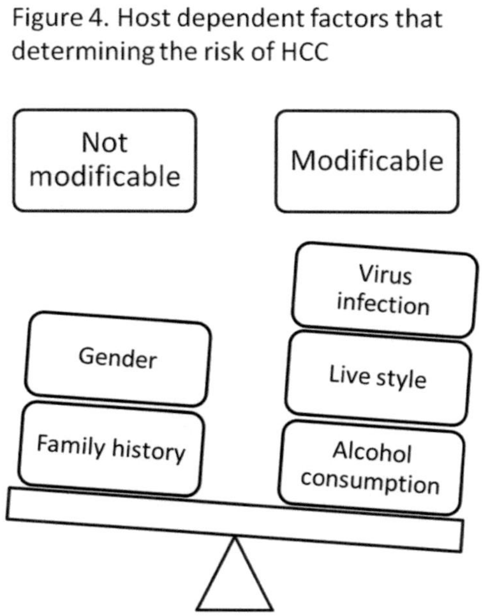

HCC: Hepatocellular Carcinoma. HCC:Hepatocellular Carcinoma.

Figure 5. Host dependant factors that determining risk of HCC

A variety of important risk factors for the development of HCC have been identified. These include viral infections, environmental toxins, comorbid conditions, inherited errors of metabolism, and autoimmune disorders [18]. At one major referral center in the United States, the most commonly seen risk factors for HCC were HCV infection, alcohol use, and nonalcoholic fatty liver disease. In a 5-year cumulative incidence, hepatocellular carcinoma in patients with HCV cirrhosis is about 15%, the risk is increased 2-6 fold in the presence of other risk factors such as alcohol, obesity, diabetes mellitus and HBV [24]. HBeAg positivity, which indicates active viral replication, is also associated with the development of HCC. The risk of HCC is also elevated in patients who are HBsAg positive but HBeAg negative (inactive carriers) compared with the general population.

Because of the association of HBV with HCC, screening for HCC is recommended for many patients with hepatitis B. Currently, it is recommended that patients with high HBV DNA levels and signs of active inflammation (elevated ALT) for several years undergo surveillance for HCC.

Coinfection with HCV has also been associated with an increased risk of HCC. Some studies suggest that patients with dual HBV and HCV infection may have a higher rate of HCC compared with patients infected by either virus alone, particularly those who are anti-HCV and HBeAg positive. Coinfection with hepatitis D virus (HDV) also appears to increase the risk of HCC among patients with HBV. Hepatitis C accounts for at least one-third of the cases of HCC in the United States. An important clinical observation is that HCC in patients with HCV occurs almost exclusively in patients with advanced stages of hepatic fibrosis or cirrhosis.

Symptoms attributable to HCC are usually absent, when symptomatic, is often associated with nonspecific complaints, including right upper abdominal or epigastric pain, early satiety, weight loss, and malaise. Rather, patients typically manifest symptoms related to underlying cirrhosis, a condition present in 80%–90% of patients with HCC. Consequently, the majority of patients are diagnosed with advanced disease, often precluding potentially curative therapies. HCC is associated with a number of paraneoplastic syndromes resulting in hypoglycemia, erythrocytosis, hypercholesterolemia, hypercalcemia, severe watery diarrhea, and cutaneous manifestations. Extrahepatic spread at presentation is relatively uncommon, ranging between 10% and 30% [18].

Eradicating the main viruses associated with cancer worldwide by implementing widespread infant and childhood immunization programs targeting 3 viruses — human papillomavirus and hepatitis B and C — could lead to a 100% reduction in viral-related cancer incidence in 20 to 40 years [2].

4. Colonoscopy and colon cancer

The colonoscopy consists in visualizing the entire large bowel mucosa and the terminal ileum, is widely used for diagnosis and treatment of diseases of the colon; performed properly, is safe, accurate and well tolerated by most patients [25]. Is used for primary colorectal cancer screening, monitoring of patients with colon cancer and for diagnosis in patients with lower gastrointestinal tract symptoms, also used to evaluate patients with screening tests for colorectal cancer such as occult blood positive stool, sigmoidoscopy, fecal DNA, or images studies [26,27,28], having shown in ramdom studies that has been effective in reducing deaths from colorectal cancer [28,29,30].

Colorectal cancer is a leading cause of cancer worldwide [29,31,32,33] increased in both sexes with an increase in incidence and mortality, which is why we have emphasized the need to improve prevention and control in order to modify the course of the disease and improve prognosis [29,31,34]. The rate of colorectal cancer mortality has declined substantially in part by the increase in the performance of studies including screening colonoscopy, which aims to reduce mortality based on a reduction in the incidence of advanced disease [34,35].

There is evidence that most colon cancers develop from adenomatous polyps (adenoma-carcinoma sequence) [36,37] and takes about 10 years when a polyp of 1 cm from becoming invasive colorectal cancer [38], the risk is higher in advanced adenomas, greater than or equal to 1 cm and / or villous component and / or high grade dysplasia [37]. Being a long term process which involves multiple steps, the disease is preventable, on the other hand, if the disease is detected in a first step, the curative is possible [26].

Many colorectal cancer studies focus on symptomatic populations, however, the majority of colorectal adenomas are asymptomatic and are detected by chance during colonoscopy [39].

This finding that adenomatous polyps are precursors to cancer and these are usually asymptomatic, has gained strength in the screening asymptomatic individuals for early cancer detection and prevention [38].

Colonoscopy is considered the preferred tool for colorectal cancer screening [25,29,31,32,33,38,40,41] because it allows us both to make detection and sampling of the lesions and to detect and remove polypoid lesions [25,26,34,35,38,42]. Colonoscopy with removal of adenomas is a useful tool to reduce the incidence and mortality of colorectal cancer, and is recommended as the first choice for screening in patients with intermediate risk of colorectal cancer [36,37,43,44,45].

In individuals with average risk, the U.S. Multi-Society Task Force on Colorectal Cancer and the American Cancer Society recommend screening should begin at age 50 regardless of sex and race [38,46], however, the American College of Gastroenterology suggests to consider these two factors and to be started earlier in blacks because they have a higher incidence and age of onset of colorectal cancer earlier [46]. Other authors suggest could benefit from colorectal cancer screening people with abdominal obesity or metabolic syndrome from 45 years of age reported having these risk factors are independent [45]. In patients at high familial risk, screening is different.

The ASGE publish this guideline for colorectal cancer screening and surveillance [38]:

1. Individuals at Risk for FAP Flexible sigmoidoscopy screening should undergo yearly starting at age 10 to 12 years. The Development of multiple, diffuse adenomas in the colon is an indication for colectomy Total.

2. Individuals at Risk for HNPCC should undergo colonoscopy every 1 to 2 years starting at age 20 to 25 years or 10 years younger than the age of the earliest diagnosis of cancer in the family, whichever is earlier.

3. Individuals with a family history of 1 or more first degree relatives with sporadic CRC regardless of age, should have a colonoscopy beginning at age 40 years or 10 years younger than the affected relative, whichever is earlier. If the index has regular colonoscopy results, repeat colonoscopy should be performed on the basis of the relative age of the affected.

4. Individuals with a first-degree relative age 60 years with adenomatous polyps should undergo colonoscopy at age 40 years or 10 years younger than the affected relative, whichever is earlier. If the index examination is normal, recommend repeat colonoscopy every 5 years.

5. In patients with a first-degree relative more than 60 years old at diagnosis of adenomatous polyps, the timing of screening colonoscopy should be individualized. The timing interval follow-up examinations between should be the same as for average-risk patients.

6. In individuals with UC and Crohn's extensive colitis. Surveillance colonoscopy with multiple biopsy specimens should be performed every 1 to 2 years after beginning 8 to 10 years of disease.

7. A complete colonoscopy should be performed in all patients diagnosed with CRC to rule out synchronous or adenomatous lesions cancers. If a complete examination can not be performed at the time of CRC diagnosis, a colonoscopy should be performed within 6 months after surgical resection.

8. Surveillance colonoscopy after surgical resection of CRC should be performed 1 year after surgery and, if results are normal, every 3 to 5 years thereafter.

Adenomatous polyps are the most frequent neoplasm found during colorectal screening and removal of these lesions have been shown to reduce the risk for future colorectal cancer or advanced adenomas (gastrointestinal). One of the parameters critical to the viability and profitability of colonoscopy for colorectal cancer screening is the time interval for surveillance colonoscopy after resection of an adenoma, surveillance intervals are based primarily on the recurrence of adenoma and not in the incidence of colorectal cancer [43]. In 2006, the U.S. Multi-Society Task Force on Colorectal Cancer joint the American Cancer Society to Provide a broader consensus and thereby increase the use of the recomendations by endoscopists, publishing guidelines for colonoscopy surveillance These after polypectomy:

1. Patients with small rectal polyps should be considered to have normal colonoscopies and therefore, the interval for subsequent colonoscopy should be 10 years. An exception is patients with hyperplastic polyposis syndrome, they are at an increased risk of colorectal adenomas and cancer and need to be identified for more intensive monitoring.

2. Patients with only 1 or 2 small tubular adenomas (less than 1 cm) with only low-grade dysplasia should have their next colonoscopy control in 5 to 10 years, the precise time within this range should be based on other clinical factors such as a result of previous colonoscopy, family history and patient preference and physician's discretion.

3. Patients with 3 or more adenomas, adenomas larger than 1 cm or villous features or adenoma with high grade dysplasia should have their next colonoscopy in control 3 years after complete resection of the adenoma. If the colonoscopy is normal or shows up in 1 or 2 small tubular adenomas or low-grade dysplasia, the interval for further study should be 5 years.

4. Patients who have 10 or more adenomas in an examination, should be reevaluated in a shorter period as 3 years, interval established by clinical judgment, it being necessary to consider an underlying familial syndrome.

5. Patients with sessile adenomas that are removed by picemeal monitoring should be considered for short intervals between 2-6 months to verify complete removal, which, once established, subsequent surveillance should be individualized based on the judgment of the endoscopist, the integrity of elimination by both endoscopy and biopsy evaluations.

6. More intensive monitoring is indicated when the family history may indicate HNPCC.

Subsequent studies suggest that it may be considered to extend surveillance intervals even in people 5 years after detection and elimination of high-risk polyps [43].

It has been reported that colonoscopy could prevent approximately 85% of cases of distal colorectal cancer while the risk reduction for proximal colon is significantly lower ranging from 0-55% [42], but colonoscopy is not perfect have been diagnosed with cancer between the intervals of follow-up examinations, reporting an incidence rate ranging from 1.7 to 2.4 cancers per 1,000 persons / year of observation [44]. The effectiveness of colonoscopy in reducing colon cancer incidence depends on adequate visualization of the mucosa, diligence in examining the mucosa and patient acceptance of the procedure [25]. That is why for the reporting of colonoscopies are suggested previously structured reports that include quality indicators such as colonoscopies specific point as far as progress, quality of bowel preparation, cecal intubation, polyp detection [27], since it has been shown that the quality of colonoscopy is also important in screening, low quality colonoscopies reduce the effectiveness especially in the proximal colon [29]. It has been reported that conventional colonoscopy some lesions may be missed even with adequate colonic preparation, this may be partly because flat lesions which makes them difficult to recognize or be injuries that are located behind the colonic haustral; it is proposes that autofluorescence imaging are better for the detection of colorectal neoplasia than conventional colonoscopy [33]. With the increase of colonoscopy in the general population over 50 years, has contributed to the decreased incidence of colorectal cancer observed since the mid-year 1980 [40].

Should bear in mind the risk cost-benefit of screening colonoscopy for colorectal cancer in elderly patients, remains controversial at this stage because the net benefit of screening reduces the risk of mortality from other diseases, reporting especially in octogenarians, a increased risk of complications during and after colonoscopy [32], the benefits of screening are significantly limited due to their short life expectancy [47].

A recent study showed that after a median follow-up of 11.9 years, there was a 21% relative risk reduction in the incidence of colorectal cancer and a 26% reduction in mortality in adults screened with flexible sigmoidoscopy, with a repeat screening at 3 or 5 years, compared with those treated with the usual care [2].

5. Obesity and pancreatic cancer

Pancreatic cancer is the eighth leading cause of cancer-related death [48], is one of the most lethal malignant diseases due to the high rate of advanced stage disease at diagnosis, and the lack of any affective medical therapy [49]. Currently, there are no methods of screening established for early detection; thus, at present, primary prevention by altering modifiable risk factors will probably be the most effective way of reducing the burden pancreatic cancer [50]. The etiology of pancreatic cancer is complex and poorly understood, therefore the indentification of risk factors, specially those which are modifiable through medication or behavioral change, is important for the development and progression preventing of pancreatic cancer. The risk factors for pancreatic cancer include family history, smoking, obesity, diabetes mellitus and chronic pancreatitis [49,51,52,53] Figure 6.

Figure 5. Risk factors for pancreatic cancer

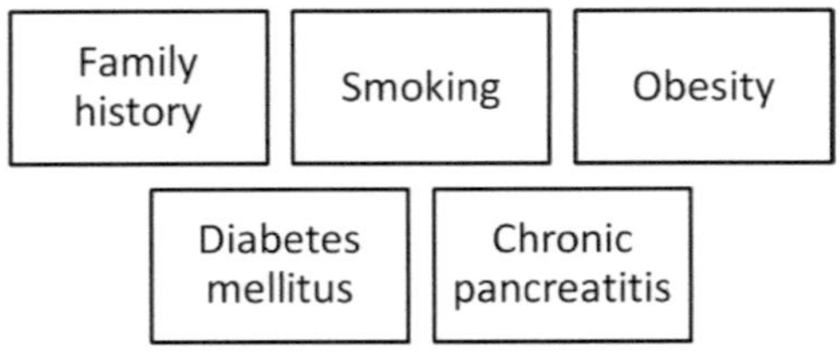

Figure 6. Risk factors for pancreatic cancer

Obesity is defined as abnormal or excessive accumulation of fat that can be harmful to health [48]. A World Health Organization (WHO) report demonstrates that more than 400 million people are obese in the world, with a predicted increase to 700 million by 2015 [52]. Since 1990, the prevalence of obesity has doubled in the United States [12]. Statistics from 2007 to 2008 indicate that 33.8% of american adults are obese [51]. According to WHO/Food and Agriculture Organization (FAO), obesity and overweight conditions can be diagnosed by measuring the body mass index (BMI) of the individual [52]. The BMI is the ratio of calculated with weight in kilograms divided by the square of height in meters kg/m2. The current standard categories of BMI are as follows: underweight <18.5, normal weight 18.5-24.9, overweight 25.0-29.9, obese 30.0-34.9, and severely obese > or = 35.0 [52,54,55].

Many studies based on large population have shown that obesity and insulin resistance are independent risk factors may types of cancer [50,52,55,56], reporting that the strength of the association varies with the organ and histologic type; this evidence supports the notion that controlling obesity can be an important tool for a number of preventing cancers among the populations of modern societies [57].

A number of recent studies indicate that obesity may be an important risk factor for pancreatic diseases including pancreatitis and pancreatic cancer and is associated with a lower age of onset [54,58]. Between the positive association with BMI and high risk of pancreatic cancer has been in at least observed 19 of 29 prospective studies and three meta-analyzes. The magnitude of the association varied from 10 to 45% increased risk for every 5 kg/m2 increase in BMI. It has been reported that people with a BMI greater than 40 kg/m2 in both sexes have higher cancer mortality rate when compared with normal weight [59], associated with a 50-60% death rate from cancer increased of pancreas [49]. Among the many possible mechanisms involved, hyperinsulinemia, diet and nutritional factors, and other hormone abnormalities have been suggested as causal factors [49]. There are sparse data on the association whether between BMI and pancreatic cancer risk is modified by age, sex, smoking, physical activity and history of diabetes [51,60]. Study showed that increased risk of pancreatic cancer was more strongly associated with obesity at younger adulthood (30-40years) than was weight gain at older age (older than 40years) [51].

In the obese patient, becomes important both visceral fat and ectopic fat, as well as waist circumference and the waist-to-hip ratio in relation to pancreatic cancer risk [50]. It has been described that may centralized increased fat distribution pancreatic cancer risk, especially in women [53]. In these patients and have fat deposits in hepatocytes do in pancreatic cells, re-

http://dx.doi.org/10.5772/55138

sulting in an entity called pancreatic steatosis, it has been hypothesized that pancreatic steatosis could promote the development of chronic pancreatitis and pancreatic cancer [61].

Obesity has also been associated with major metabolic abnormalities including insulin resistance and diabetes, and therefore may be associated with the risk of pancreatic cancer.

It has also demonstrated strong association between pancreatic cancer and two medical conditions chronic pancreatitis and diabetes mellitus. Since these conditions are often present many years before the diagnosis of cancer, they should be considered etiologically relevant [58].

Epidemiological studies have demonstrated that diabetes is a risk factor for multiple forms of malignancy including the pancreatic cancer. Previous studies have implicated long-term diabetes as a modifiable risk factor for pancreatic cancer [51]. Roughly half of all the patients with pancreatic cancer are found to have diabetes at the time of diagnosis, and roughly half of the diabetic patients present which is at the time of pancreatic cancer diagnosis is of new onset having developed over the preceding 2-3 years the diagnosis of pancreatic cancer [49]. There has been a long debate about whether diabetes mellitus is a risk factor for, or a consequence of cancer, pancreatic cancer, but there are findings that suggest that diabetic individuals with a history of 5 or more years and have a 2-fold increase risk of pancreatic cancer compared with those with no history of diabetes or with less than 5 years [58], reporting that the long-standing diabetes increases the risk of pancreatic cancer [54]. The association between pancreatic cancer and diabetes has been investigated extensively, but the causal relationships have yet to be fully elucidated [49].

The association between type 2 diabetes and pancreatic cancer risk can be the result of high concentrations of glucose in the after load and gradual alterations glucose tolerance for years. It supports the hypothesis that glucose tolerance and diabetes play a role in carcinogenesis of pancreatic cancer.

Obesity has been associated with a negative prognostic factor, higher BMI is associated with decreased survival and increased mortality in pancreatic cancer [54,62,63]. Furthermore, in pancreatic cancer, increased BMI has been reported to be an adverse prognostic factor for survival after surgery in two surgical series [63].

A majority of prospective epidemiological studies have found that a high body mass index and/or a lack of physical activity are associated with an increased risk of pancreatic cancer incidence or mortality, independently of prior history of diabetes [53]. Physical activity and reduced caloric intake have to been shown to reduce the risk of pancreatic cancer especially in those who are overweight [49,54]. The successful treatment of obesity and diabetes has been shown to reduce the risk of pancreatic cancer, but the treatment with insulin, insulin analogs, and insulin secretagogues maintains or increases the risk. Metformin as well as livestyle alterations has been shown to reduce the risk of pancreatic cancer [49].

It is estimated that being overweight or obese causes approximately 20% of cancer today. If people could maintain a healthy body mass index (BMI), the incidence of cancer could be reduced by approximately 50% in 2 to 20 years [2].

6. Conclusion

Having the knowledge of the cancer associated factors, interventions could be implemented to prevent and treat it, in order to reduce and control the disease. We should apply science-based strategies for the prevention of disease as well as early detection and treatment of these patients.

A percentage of all cancer deaths could be prevented by modifying or avoiding key risk factors, such as: smoke, overweight or obese, unhealthy diets with a low consumption of fruit and vegetables, physical inactivity, consumption of alcoholic beverages, HPV infection and HBV, air pollution in cities.

It is critical the knowledge of the risk factors to apply prevention strategies in the future to modify the morbidity of this disease.

Author details

Leonardo Sosa Valencia and Erika Rodriguez-Wulff

CITE (National Center of Ecoendoscopia), Caracas, Venezuela

References

[1] Organización Mundial de La SaludNota descriptiva N°297, Febrero de (2012).

[2] Pam HarrisonLifestyle Changes Could Prevent 50% of Common Cancers . Medscape Medical News, September 5, 2012. Union for International Cancer Control (UICC) World Cancer Congress 2012 August (2012). Montreal, Canada, 27-30.

[3] Kenichi SaitoMD, PhD, Kazuko Arai, MD, Masatomo Mori, MD, PhD, Ryouta Kobayashi, MD, Ichiro Ohki, MD, PhD. Effect of Helicobacter pylori eradication on malignant transformation of gastric adenoma. *Gastrointestinal Endoscopy*; (2000).

[4] Anna, D. Wagner, Wilfried Grothe, Johannes Haerting, et al. Chemotherapy in Advanced Gastric Cancer: A Systematic Review and Meta-Analysis Based on Aggregate Data. *Journal Of Clinical Oncology*. 24 (18): 2903-2909, (2006).

[5] Siddavaram NaginiCarcinoma of the stomach: A review of epidemiology, pathogenesis, molecular genetics and chemoprevention. World J Gastrointest Oncol. 4(7): 156-169, (2012).

[6] Mi Ah HanMyueng Guen Oh, Il Ju Choi, et al. Association of Family History With Cancer Recurrence and Survival in Patients With Gastric Cancer. *Journal Of Clinical Oncology*. 30 (7): 701-708, (2012).

[7] Chun-Ying WuMing-Shiang Wu, Ken N. Kuo, et al. Effective Reduction of Gastric Cancer Risk With Regular Use of Nonsteroidal Anti-Inflammatory Drugs in Helicobacter Pylori-Infected Patients. *Journal Of Clinical Oncology.* , 28(18), 2952-2957.

[8] BrunaMaria RoeslerSandra Cecilia Botelho Costa and Jose Murilo Robilotta Zeitune. Eradication Treatment of Helicobacter pylori Infection: Its Importance and Possible Relationship in Preventing the Development of Gastric Cancer. ISRN Gastroenterol. (2012).

[9] Aneta TargoszTomasz Brzozowski, Piotr Pierzchalski et al. Helicobacter pylori promotes apoptosis, activates cyclooxygenase (COX)-2 and inhibits heat shock protein HSP70 in gastric cancer epithelial cells. Inflamm. Res. 61:955-966, (2012).

[10] Yuji MaehataShotaro Nakamura, Kiyoshi Fujisawa, Motohiro Esaki, Tomohiko Moriyama, Kouichi Asano, Yuta Fuyuno et al. Long-term effect of Helicobacter pylori eradication on the development of metachronous gastric cancer after endoscopic resection of early gastric cancer. *Gastrointestinal Endoscopy*; (2012).

[11] Hassan MomtazNegar Souod, Hossein Dabiri et al. Study of Helicobacter pylori genotype status in saliva, dental plaques, stool and gastric biopsy samples. World J Gastroenterol. 18(17): 2105-2111, (2012).

[12] ASGE guideline: the role of endoscopy in the surveillance of premalignant conditions of the upper GI tract*Gastrointestinal Endoscopy*; (2006).

[13] Yi-Chia LeeTony Hsiu-Hsi Chen, Han-Mo Chiu, Chia-Tung Shun, et al. The benefit of mass eradication of Helicobacter pylori infection: a community-based study of gastric cancer prevention. Gut doi:10.1136/gutjnl-, 2012-302240.

[14] Angelo ZulloCesare Hassan, Adriana Romiti et al. Follow-up of intestinal metaplasia in the stomach: When, how and why. World J Gastrointest Oncol. 4(3): 30-36, (2012).

[15] Lorenz KuskeArmand Mensen, Beat Müllhaupt et al. Characteristics of patients with chronic hepatitis C who develop hepatocellular carcinoma. Swiss Med Wkly. 142: 1-9, (2012).

[16] Chung-Hwa ParkSeung-Hee Jeong, Hyeon-Woo Yim et al. Family history influences the early onset of hepatocellular carcinoma. World J Gastroenterol. 18 (21): 2661-2667, (2012).

[17] Katsuya ShirakiAtsuya Shimizu, Koujiro Takase, Atsushi Suzuki, Yukihiko Tameda, Takeshi Nakano. Prospective study of laparoscopic findings with regard to the development of hepatocellular carcinoma in patients with hepatitis C virus-associated cirrhosis. *Gastrointestinal Endoscopy*; (2001).

[18] Christopher L Tinkle and Daphne Haas-KoganHepatocellular carcinoma: natural history, current management, and emerging tools. Biologics: Targets and Therapy. 6: 207-219, (2012).

[19] So Young BaeMoon Seok Choi, Geum-Youn Gwak et al. Comparison of usefulness of clinical diagnostic criteria for hepatocellular carcinoma in a hepatitis B endemic area. Clinical and Molecular Hepatology. 18: 185-194, (2012).

[20] Chien-Jen Chen and Mei-Hsuan LeeEarly Diagnosis of Hepatocellular Carcinoma by Multiple microRNAs: Validity, Efficacy, and Cost-Effectiveness. J Clin Oncol. 29 (36): 4745-4747, (2011).

[21] Hany ElewaManal Abd-Elmeneem, Ahmed Murad Hashem et al. Study of interleukin 8 (IL8) serum level in patients with chronic liver disease due to hepatitis C virus (HCV) with and without hepatocellular carcinoma (HCC). International Journal of Hepatology.

[22] Melanie, B. Thomas and James L. Abbruzzese. Opportunities for Targeted Therapies in Hepatocellular Carcinoma. Journal of Clinical Oncology. 23 (31): 8093-8108, (2005).

[23] Jing GaoLi Xie, Wan-Shui Yang et al. Risk Factors of Hepatocellular Carcinoma- Current Status and Perspectives. Asian Pacific J Cancer Prev. 13: 743-752, (2012).

[24] Thuluvath Paul JEUS-guided FNA could be another important tool for the early diagnosis of hepatocellular carcinoma. *Gastrointestinal Endoscopy* ; (2007).

[25] Douglas, K. Rex, John L. Petrini, Todd H. Baron et al. Quality indicators for colonoscopy. Gastrointest Endosc. 63 (4): SS28, (2006)., 16.

[26] Christian StockUlrike Haug and Hermann Brenner. Population-based prevalence estimates of history of colonoscopy or sigmoidoscopy: review and analysis of recent trends. Gastrointest Endosc. 71 (2): 366-381, (2010).

[27] David, A. Lieberman, Douglas O. Faigel, Judith R. Logan et al. Assessment of the quality of colonoscopy reports: results from a multicenter consortium. Gastrointest Endosc. 69 (3): 645-653, (2009).

[28] Andrew, N. Freedman, Martha L. Slattery, Rachel Ballard-Barbash et al. Colorectal Cancer Risk Prediction Tool for White Men and Women Without Known Susceptibility. Journal of Clinical Oncology. 27 (5): 686-693, (2009).

[29] Nancy, N. Baxter, Joan L. Warren, Michael J. Barrett et al. Association Between Colonoscopy and Colorectal Cancer Mortality in a US Cohort According to Site of Cancer and Colonoscopist Specialty. Journal of Clinical Oncology. 30 (21): 2664-2669, (2012).

[30] Hye Won ParkSeungbong Han, Jong-Soo Lee et al. Risk stratification for advanced proximal colon neoplasm and individualized endoscopic screening for colorectal cancer by a risk-scoring model. Gastrointest Endosc (2012). in press

[31] Wei-Chih LiaoHan-Mo Chiu, Chien-Chuan Chen et al. A prospective evaluation of the feasibility of primary screening with unsedated colonoscopy. Gastrointest Endosc. 70 (4):724-731, (2009).

[32] Lukejohn, W. Day, Annette Kwon, John M. Inadomi et al. Adverse events in older patients undergoing colonoscopy: a systematic review and meta-analysis. Gastrointest Endosc. 74 (4): 885-896, (2011).

[33] Yoji TakeuchiTakuya Inoue, Noboru Hanaoka et al. Autofluorescence imaging with a transparent hood for detection of colorectal neoplasms: a prospective, randomized trial. Gastrointest Endosc 72 (5): 1006-1013, (2010).

[34] Binu, J. Jacob, Rahim Moineddin, Rinku Sutradhar et al. Effect of colonoscopy on colorectal cancer incidence and mortality: an instrumental variable analysis. Gastrointest Endosc. 76 (2): 355-364, (2012).

[35] Christian StockAmy B. Knudsen, Iris Lansdorp-Vogelaar et al. Colorectal cancer mortality prevented by use and attributable to nonuse of colonoscopy. Gastrointest Endosc. 73 (3): 435-443, (2011).

[36] Christine, N. Manser, Lucas M. Bachmann, Jakob Brunner et al. Colonoscopy screening markedly reduces the occurrence of colon carcinomas and carcinoma-related death: a closed cohort study. Gastrointest Endosc. 76 (1): 110-117, (2012).

[37] Franco ArmelaoCorrado Paternolli, Gaia Franceschini et al. Colonoscopic findings in first-degree relatives of patients with colorectal cancer: a population-based screening program. Gastrointest Endosc. 73 (3): 527-34, (2011).

[38] ASGE guideline: colorectal cancer screening and surveillance*Gastrointestinal Endoscopy*; (2006).

[39] Wai, K. Leung, Khek Yu Ho, Won-ho Kim et al. Colorectal neoplasia in Asia: a multicenter colonoscopy survey in symptomatic patients. Gastrointest Endosc. 64 (5): 751-759, (2006).

[40] Christian StockDianne Pulte, Ulrike Haug et al. Subsite-specific colorectal cancer risk in the colorectal endoscopy era. Gastrointest Endosc. (2012)., 75(3), 621-630.

[41] Hermann BrennerJenny Chang-Claude, Christoph M. Seiler et al. Long-Term Risk of Colorectal Cancer After Negative Colonoscopy. Journal of Clinical Oncology. 29 (28): 3761-3767, (2011).

[42] Eveline, J. A. Rondagh, Mariëlle W.E. Bouwens, Robert G. Riedl et al. Endoscopic appearance of proximal colorectal neoplasms and potential implications for colonoscopy in cancer prevention. Gastrointest Endosc. 75 (6): 1218-1225, (2012).

[43] Hermann BrennerJenny Chang-Claude, Alexander Rickert et al. Risk of Colorectal Cancer After Detection and Removal of Adenomas at Colonoscopy: Population-Based Case-Control Study. Journal of Clinical Oncology. 30 (24): 2969- 2976, (2012).

[44] Keith LeungPaul Pinsky, Adeyinka O. Laiyemo et al. Ongoing colorectal cancer risk despite surveillance colonoscopy: the Polyp Prevention Trial Continued Follow-up Study. Gastrointest Endosc. 71 (1): 111-117, (2010).

[45] Sung Noh HongJeong Hwan Kim, Won Hyeok Choe et al. Prevalence and risk of colorectal neoplasms in asymptomatic, average-risk screenees 40 to 49 years of age. Gastrointest Endosc. 72 (3): 480-489, (2010).

[46] Iris Lansdorp-VogelaarMarjolein van Ballegooijen, Ann G. Zauber et al. Individualizing colonoscopy screening by sex and race. Gastrointest Endosc. 70 (1): 96-108, (2009).

[47] Charles, J. Kahi, Faouzi Azzouz, Beth E. Juliar et al. Survival of elderly persons undergoing colonoscopy: implications for colorectal cancer screening and surveillance. Gastrointest Endosc. 66 (3): 544-550, (2007).

[48] Organización Mundial de La SaludNota descriptiva N°311, Mayo de (2012).

[49] YunFeng Cui and Dana KAndersen. Diabetes and Pancreatic Cancer. Endocr Relat Cancer. (2012). doi:ERC-, 12-0105.

[50] Aune, D, Greenwood, D. C, & Chan, D. S. M. et al. Body mass index, abdominal fatness and pancreatic cancer risk: a systematic review and non-linear dose-response meta-analysis of prospective studies. Annals of Oncology. 23: 843-852, (2012).

[51] Hongwei TangXiaoqun Dong, Manal Hassan et al. Body Mass Index and Obesity- and Diabetes-Associated Genotypes and Risk for Pancreatic Cancer. Cancer Epidemiol Biomarkers Prev. 20(5):779-792, (2011).

[52] Bin BaoZhiwei Wang, Yiwei Li et al. The complexities of obesity, diabetes, and the development and progression of pancreatic cancer. Biochim Biophys Acta. 1815(2): 135-146, (2011).

[53] Alan, A. Arslan, Kathy J. Helzlsouer, Charles Kooperberg et al. Anthropometric Measures, Body Mass Index and Pancreatic Cancer: a Pooled Analysis from the Pancreatic Cancer Cohort Consortium (PanScan). Arch Intern Med. 170(9): 791-802, (2010).

[54] Ho Gak Kim and Jimin HanObesity and Pancreatic Diseases. Korean J Gastroenterol. 59 (1): 35-39, (2012).

[55] Carolyn, C. Gotay. Behavior and Cancer Prevention. *Journal Of Clinical Oncology*. 23 (2): 301-310, (2005).

[56] Sang Min ParkMin Kyung Lim, Kyu Won Jung et al. Prediagnosis Smoking, Obesity, Insulin Resistance, and Second Primary Cancer Risk in Male Cancer Survivors: National Health Insurance Corporation Study. *Journal Of Clinical Oncology*. 25 (30): 4835-4843, (2007).

[57] Sang Woo OhYeong Sook Yoon, and Soon-Ae Shin. Effects of Excess Weight on Cancer Incidences Depending on Cancer Sites and Histologic Findings Among Men: Korea National Health Insurance Corporation Study. *Journal Of Clinical Oncology*. 23 (21): 4742-4754, (2005).

[58] Michaud Dominique SThe epidemiology of pancreatic, gallbladder, and other biliary tract cancers. *Gastrointestinal Endoscopy*; (2002). S6)

[59] Lauren, B. Gerson. Impact of obesity on endoscopy. *Gastrointestinal Endoscopy*; (2009).

[60] Body mass indexeffect modifiers, and risk of pancreatic cancer: a pooled study of seven prospective cohorts. Li Jiao, Amy Berrington de Gonzalez, Patricia Hartge et al. Cancer Causes Control. 21(8): 1305-1314, (2010).

[61] Paul, S. Sepe, Ashray Ohri, Sirish Sanaka, Tyler M. Berzin, Sandeep Sekhon, Gayle Bennett, et al. A prospective evaluation of fatty pancreas by using *Eus. Gastrointestinal Endoscopy*; (2011).

[62] Wen-Ko ChiouJawl-Shan Hwang, Kuang-Hung Hsu et al. DiabetesMellitus IncreasedMortality RatesMore in Gender-Specific than in Nongender-Specific Cancer Patients: A Retrospective Study of 149,491 Patients. Exp Diabetes Res. (2012). doi:

[63] Robert, R. McWilliams, Martha E. Matsumoto, Patrick A. Burch et al. Obesity Adversely Affects Survival in Pancreatic Cancer Patients. Cancer. 116 (21): 5054-5062, (2010).

Section 6

Environmental Public Health

Pathogen Management in Surface Waters: Practical Considerations for Reducing Public Health Risk

Matthew R. Hipsey and Justin D. Brookes

Additional information is available at the end of the chapter

http://dx.doi.org/10.5772/55367

1. Introduction

Pathogen contamination of water systems is a major public health challenge in both developing and developed countries across the globe [1-9]. The pathogens of concern to human health vary between aquatic systems depending on the nature of the pathogen source and the intended use of the water. Due to their persistence in the environment and resistance to conventional treatment technologies, the (oo)cysts of the protozoan organisms *Cryptosporidium* spp. and *Giardia* spp. are a typical concern in water bodies used for drinking water [10-11]. In poorly treated drinking water storages and recreational waters (both fresh and marine), other problem organisms include bacteria such as *Salmonella* spp., *Shigella* spp., *Vibrio* spp. *Clostridium* spp. and *Staphylococcus aureus,* and numerous human enteric viruses such as those from the genera *Enterovirus, Hepatovirus, Rotavirus* and *Norovirus* [12-13]. Accordingly, the nature of disease caused by these organisms is also widely variable (Table 1).

Most concern is given to allochthonous enteric microorganisms, those that enter surface waters via external loading. However, depending on the environmental context, some autochthonous pathogens, those that develop internally, may also be important (*e.g. Vibrio cholerae*). The allochthonous sources typically occur when heavy rains wash infected material from surrounding agricultural and/or urban catchments into the runoff waters that ultimately supply the waterbody, or when effluent is discharged directly into watercourses (Figure 1). Inputs to lakes and rivers from recreational users can also lead to a significant increase in pathogen concentrations [14]. These major pathogen sources present a risk to humans through three main routes of exposure: direct consumption of microorganisms within drinking water, recreational contact, and consumption of microorganisms that have bio-accumulated within the tissues of consumable shellfish (Figure 2).

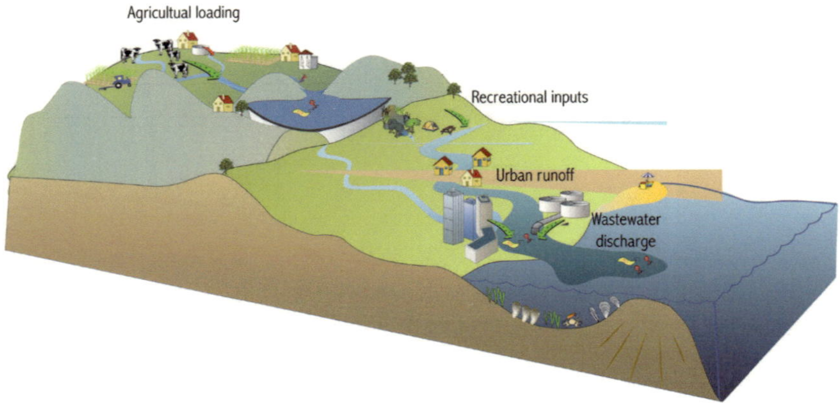

Figure 1. Schematic overview of allochthonous microbial sources and receiving aquatic environments from the catchment to the ocean.

Disease	Agent	Symptoms
Amebiasis	Protozoan (*Entamoeba histolytic*)	Abdominal pain, fatigue, weight loss, diarrhoea
Campylobacteriosis	Bacterium (*Campylobacter jejuni*)	Fever, Abdominal pain, fatigue, diarrhoea
Cholera	Bacterium (*Vibrio cholerae*)	Fever, Abdominal pain, vomiting, diarrhoea
Cryptosporidiosis	Protozoan (*Cryptosporidium parvum*)	Abdominal pain, vomiting, diarrhoea
Diarrhoeagenic *Escherichia coli*	Bacterium (*Escherichia coli* O157:H7)	Acute bloody diarrhoea, abdominal cramps
Giardiasis	Protozoan (*Giardia lamblia*)	Abdominal pain, vomiting, diarrhoea
Hepatitis	Virus (Hepatitis A)	Fever, chills, abdominal pain, jaundice
Salmonellosis	Bacterium (*Salmonella* sp.)	Fever, abdominal cramps, bloody diarrhoea
Shigellosis	Bacterium (*Shigella* sp.	Fever, diarrhoea, bloody stools
Viral Gastroenteritis	Virus (rotavirus etc.)	Vomiting, diarrhoea, headache, fever

Table 1. Summary of common water-borne diseases.

Pathogen distribution and transport in surface waters is a function of the pathogen load in the source water (*e.g.* agricultural runoff or direct wastewater discharge), the settling or entrainment characteristics of the particles that they may attach to, and resuspension from sediment-associated organisms by turbulence at the benthic boundary layer. The distribution of organisms will also be impacted by predation [15] and degradation due to sunlight exposure, or mortality due to undesirable physico-chemical conditions [16]. For some organisms, in situ growth may also need to be considered.

Contamination of rivers, lakes and reservoirs that are primarily used for drinking water is a particular challenge for environmental scientists and water managers charged with supplying water that minimises the risk of infection to downstream consumers. The nature of the contamination and the mechanisms that control contaminant dynamics may vary considerably due to either site-specific or contaminant-specific properties and hence there is a need to better understand how to assess and mitigate the risks.

As indicated above, microbial contaminants such as the (oo)cysts of the pathogens *Crytposporidium* or *Giardia*, are mainly derived from allochthonous (external) sources, whereas others may be generated autochthonously (internally) within the water storage. It is therefore not surprising that a fundamental principle of drinking water supply is to use high quality, protected source waters as a means of reducing the potential load of drinking water contaminants and thus reducing treatment costs and subsequent health risks to consumers. In reference [17], it was reported that the mean concentration of *Cryptosporidium* oocysts in protected reservoirs (0.52/100L) and pristine lakes (0.3 – 9.3/100L) was considerably lower compared to polluted rivers (43 – 60/100L) and polluted lakes (58/100L), which demonstrates the merit of this strategy. However, with increasing pressures on catchments, aquatic systems are not always sufficiently protected and pathogen risks must therefore be appropriately managed. In developing countries this is further confounded since both drinking and recreational waters may be subject to substantial direct and unregulated effluent discharges that are difficult to control at the source.

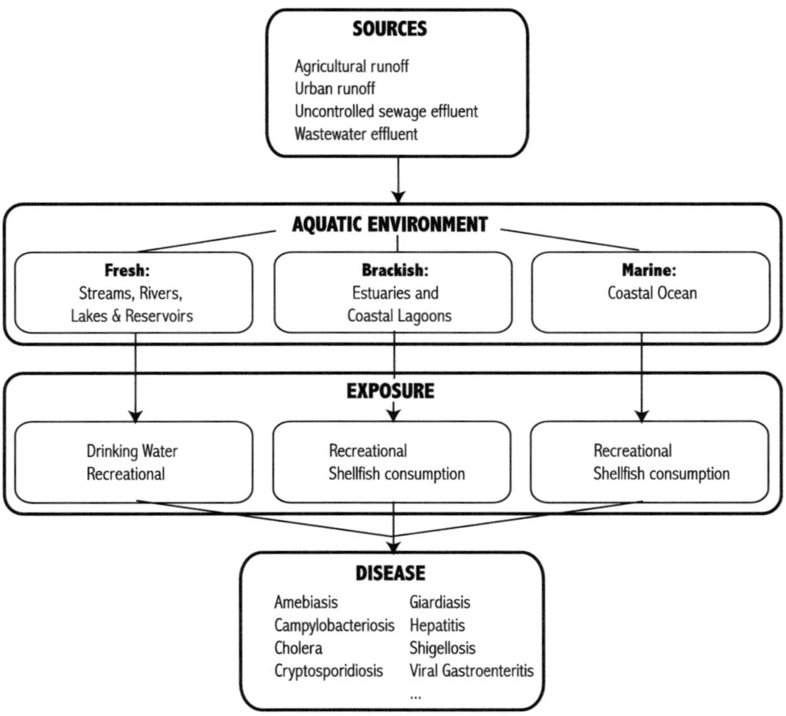

Figure 2. Conceptual breakdown of routes of exposure of microbial pollutants.

When planning management measures or policies it is important to consider that the presence or absence of pathogens within the aquatic environment does not always translate directly to a high risk to human health. For example, *Cryptosporidium* and *Giardia* (oo)cysts have been identified at hazardous levels in Lake Kinneret, which has historically supplied around half of Israel's water, however no major outbreaks were reported in Israel during an equivalent period [5]. Conversely, outbreaks of cryptosporidiosis have been documented where the water met guidelines based on standard bacterial indicator concentrations [3-4]. It must therefore be recognized that contaminant data and risk assessment procedures need to consider the wider management framework that encompasses the entire system, from source to exposure. To obtain a more realistic assessment of the overall contaminant risk it is necessary to understand the critical variables controlling contaminant fate and distribution once they enter the aquatic environment.

Allen *et al.* [18] went further, and described pathogen monitoring alone as being of little value and highlighted several cases where monitoring had misled regulatory authorities as to the actual risk, including both false positives and false negatives. They highlight several technical and administrative barriers why this is the case, and instead suggest that the human and financial resources would be better invested in enhancing treatment processes and gaining a better understanding of the system (such as the major pathogen sources and sinks, and inactivation processes). Within a drinking water system this is fairly clear since there are many points at which the quality of the source water can be controlled before the public is ultimately exposed, but for other environmental waters there is only limited ability for intervention. However, aquatic systems have an inherent natural assimilative capacity and, there are a number of beneficial water quality changes that can occur when water is stored in reservoirs, which may ultimately attenuate pathogen concentrations [16,19]. Reduced water movement increases the rate of sedimentation of particulate material. This reduces turbidity and may also result in the sequestering of the microbes associated with the particles. Many of the pathogens of concern are attenuated by environmental conditions with mortality linked to temperature, grazing by protozoa, and incident ultra violet radiation being the most critical factors. Of particular importance is having a good knowledge of the hydrodynamic processes that control water transport in the aquatic environment as this will ultimately determine the length of time the water is retained and the environmental conditions that it will be subjected to. In reservoirs, issues such as the thermal stratification and the short-circuiting of inflows have been identified as being significantly important [20].

The question then becomes whether or not it is possible to optimise the performance of aquatic systems as barriers to pathogen transmission by manipulating river or reservoir conditions. The climatic and hydrological conditions that lead to the development of a specific contamination threat are highly diverse and it is necessary to have a clear understanding of the origin and dynamics of the potential contaminants in relation to environmental conditions in order to understand the most appropriate control methodologies to implement of the range that are available. Further, it is often the case where multiple contaminants occur within a single storage or system, and the optimum solution for minimising risk is a compromise between minimising exposure to individual contaminants and may involve implementation of several management options. As a result it is necessary to manage the associated risks through development of a suitable risk management framework. To address the complexities and variability inherent in pathogen transmission requires a detailed quantitative understanding of contaminant fate and distribution through surface water systems, yet this is rarely achieved in practice and there is a need for improved assessment and mitigation of pathogen threats.

The aim of this chapter is to describe how to best gather specific information to support structured risk assessment programs for dealing with pathogen distribution in surface water systems. With this knowledge we summarise several control measures and discuss how they may be implemented within a structured framework to minimise the risk of contamination to humans. It is important to understand the key dynamics of contaminants, as described next, to provide the necessary context for the risk management framework and control measures.

2. Controls on fate and transport of microbial contaminants

Hydrodynamic controls on pathogen distribution: Hydrodynamics are a key driver in shaping distribution of pathogens in aquatic systems [21] and determine the horizontal transport, rates of dispersion and dilution, and their vertical distribution. In lakes and reservoirs horizontal transport is predominantly driven by basin-scale circulation patterns including wind-driven currents, inflows and basin-scale internal waves [22]. Although wind-driven currents only influence the surface layer, inflows can occur at any depth in a stratified water column [23], and internal waves can generate significant internal currents that may act in different directions at different depths. In stratified lakes and reservoirs, internal waves have been shown to be responsible for the vertical advection of pathogens past offtake structures resulting in periodic variations in water quality [24].

Dispersion describes both the turbulent dispersion (for example in the surface mixed layer) and shear dispersion due to the presence of a horizontal or vertical velocity shear, (*e.g.* rivers or in tidally forced systems). In river-floodplain systems sharp velocity gradients between the floodplain and main river cause substantial horizontal dispersion and mixing.

Since the source of most pathogens to reservoirs is via catchment inflows or engineered outfalls, the behaviour of inflowing water as they enter the water column is of particular importance. Inflow dynamics are controlled by their density and momentum relative to that of the ambient water. For example, warm inflows will flow over the surface as a buoyant surface flow, and cold dense inflows will sink beneath the ambient water where they will flow along the bottom towards the deepest point. In either case, as it propagates the gravity current will entrain ambient water, increasing its volume, changing its density and diluting the concentration of pathogens and other properties. A further complication is introduced where the density difference is derived from particulate matter (turbidity current), in which case the settling of these particles will influence the density and propagation of the inflow [25]. The speed at which the inflowing water travels, its entrainment of ambient water and resulting dilution of its properties, and its insertion depth are all of critical importance in determining the hydrodynamic distribution of pathogens. Prediction therefore requires a detailed numerical solution, often in three dimensions, which can resolve processes controlling momentum, mixing, and thermodynamics.

Kinetics: As particles are advected and mixed throughout a waterbody they are also subject to 'non-conservative' behaviour, *i.e.* growth or decay. Organisms become inactivated as they are exposed to the range of biotic and abiotic pressures that face them within the aquatic environment. In particular, organisms are known to be sensitive to temperature, salinity, pH, oxygen, turbidity, sunlight, and they are also subject to predation by larger autochthonous microorganisms [15]. Some bacteria may also be able to support growth through assimilation of nutrients from the water [26-30].

Sedimentation & association with particles: The settling rate of free-floating organisms is relatively small [31]. Association with inorganic and organic aquatic particles however can considerably increase the losses due to sedimentation, with particle settling being affected by their size and density according to Stoke's law [32-33]. Pathogens may be associated with particles via adsorption at the surface, or they may be physically enmeshed within the organic matrix of faecal material. Differences in dynamic aggregation rates between different organism classes (*i.e.* protozoan, bacterial, viral) are thought to be an important determinant when deciding the applicability of surrogates [21].

Resuspension: Since pathogens may remain viable for significant periods in aquatic sediments [34-36], the resuspension and subsequent re-distribution of pathogens and indicator organisms can potentially be an important process. Sediment resuspension occurs when the shear stress due to currents and turbulent velocity fluctuations reaches a critical level. In rivers and estuaries, large currents are capable of generating significant critical bed-shear that exceeds the critical level regularly. In lakes and stratified environments such high velocities are reached less frequently, but can be caused by large underflow events and by basin-scale internal waves motions, for example after a period of significant wind forcing. Turbulent motions within the benthic boundary layer driven by currents and internal wave breaking [37] result in the resuspension of particulate material [38]. In environments with an active surface wave field such as the coastal ocean and estuarine environments, then oscillatory currents due to wind-wave action will also be important in periodically redistributing pathogen-laden sediments near coastal cities [39-40].

3. Hazard analysis and risk assessment framework

In drinking supply reservoirs the major contaminant risks not only originate from the introduction of pathogens, but also from the release of dissolved iron and manganese from sediment, growth of cyanobacteria and subsequent release of associated toxins, and from natural organic matter (NOM) reaction with the chlorine used for treatment. Risk management of pathogens therefore cannot be considered in isolation. The timescale over which these hazards generate varies from days to weeks, or even months. Problems associated with iron, manganese and cyanobacteria typically develop with the evolution of thermal stratification. It may take a number of days or weeks for cyanobacteria to grow to concentrations that may cause a taste and odour or toxin problem. Problematic concentrations of iron and manganese develop under anoxic conditions from long periods of stratification typically ranging from weeks to months. On the other hand, the greatest risk of transport of pathogens from catchment to the treatment plant is after significant inflow events, which may present a water quality issue within the timescale of hours to days depending upon the reservoir size and flow magnitude. Similarly the highest loading of NOM and turbidity occurs during inflow events.

In addition to the variable time scales that must be considered when deciding control measures and developing a risk management framework, the potential for large spatial heterogeneity must also be considered. In long, drowned-valley reservoirs, the concentration of a contaminant introduced from upstream may pass through a long reach of standing water and be progressively attenuated prior to reaching the offtake location(s), depending on the hydrodynamics and stratification at the time of the event. If the shape of the supply is more circular then circulation patterns may be more complex and considerable variability and patchiness may develop and influence the observed trends. For cyanobacteria and metal contaminants, the dynamics are strongly governed by vertical gradients in temperature and other physicochemical properties that will vary based on meteorological conditions.

In many cases there maybe coinciding water quality issues that pose different risks and require the implementation of control measures that minimize exposure to one threat but which may actually increase exposure to another. For example, in a single reservoir, cyanobacterial toxins may exist in the surface, pathogens within an inflow intrusion at mid-depth, and anoxia and soluble metals in the deepest regions. In such instances care must be taken to ensure the management strategies that are implemented are well founded and the individual risks are well quantified. In these more complicated situations cost-benefit analyses may help guide the most appropriate action and help assess the relative benefits for public health, also set within context of reducing treatment costs at the downstream treatment facility.

Informed management not only requires knowledge on the spatial distribution, but also the temporal variability of threats. As the threat changes, so may the most suitable control measure, and it is therefore logical that any management framework that is implemented is adaptable and able to respond to changes in risk. To be effective in this regard, monitoring must also be flexible and reflect the nature of the risk at any given time [41].

Catchment-reservoir systems are complex and it is important to note that given the high variability in these systems one can never reduce all risk(s) to zero, however by strategic identification of potential problems, one can mitigate risk with knowledge of some basic hydrodynamics, the evolution of hazards, and careful monitoring. In drinking water supplies that are deemed critical and face multiple pressures, more sophisticated options such as real-time management systems are emerging to assist with the assessment of risks and the ongoing monitoring of the implemented control measures.

Successful risk management of water supply reservoirs and recreational waters requires a systematic approach to contaminant monitoring and prediction in order to reduce the risk of exposure to the public. This is best achieved through a quantitative understanding of the critical processes involved in contaminant distribution and transport, such as dilution rates and time scales for inactivation or contaminant decay. Such information would enable water managers to quantify the risk to water quality associated with a contaminant threat in source water, revise monitoring protocols to detect the organisms or chemicals of concern, and to manage water treatment or recreational closures proactively based upon detected or, ideally, modelled (anticipated) risk. Due to their flexibility, such 'adaptive' management strategies are more effective than their rigid counterparts [42], yet they are rarely adopted due to numerous uncertainties in our understanding and due to poor numerical model predictions.

The critical fist step in developing an adaptive management strategy for water supply is identifying the hazards of concern, articulating the hydrodynamic and biogeochemical conditions that lead to the development of the hazard and understand how these are influenced by the prevailing meteorology and hydrology (Figure 3). Within a drinking water supply reservoir the important processes can be summarised as loads entering the reservoir; transport, growth or attenuation with the reservoir and the distribution of the hazard relative to the offtake (Figure 3). Each of the parameters contributing to risk can be monitored and the processes measured and modelled.

4. Management framework

Routine monitoring and targeted measurement of the major processes systematically builds up a bank of knowledge to support reservoir management and detect and mitigate risks in a timely fashion. The aim is to measure the processes and hazards identified in Figure 3 which contributes to knowledge of the system (Figure 4).

System knowledge can be used to inform on catchment hydrology and contaminant loads, reservoir behaviour and can help focus the monitoring effort on the key variables. Monitoring for those variables will vary depending upon the timescales for which different hazards present, the cost associated with monitoring and the ease at which the parameter can be monitored. Typically these fall with three classes; routine monitoring for analytes that are sampled and then measured within a laboratory, online monitoring where sensors are deployed in the reservoir and log key parameters at relatively short time intervals (typically 10 min) and ad hoc monitoring in response to an event, such as a rain event inflow.

This monitoring serves two purposes; it allows for detection of the hazard so the appropriate risk assessment can be undertaken, and it also allows the managers to draw correlations between when the hazard is present and the reservoir and catchment conditions at the time. Upon detection of the hazard the situation needs to be assessed with respect to what risk it poses to water quality. This stage of the management framework can draw upon expert knowledge, specific process understanding derived from online monitoring and simulation of the event with hydrodynamic models. Armed with this knowledge and a prediction about the severity of the event, decisions on the operational response can be made. Points of control include attenuation of inflows in engineered wetlands and biofilters, alteration of the inflow dynamics, in reservoir treatment or manipulation of the offtake depth to select the best quality water to send to the treatment plant.

http://dx.doi.org/10.5772/55367

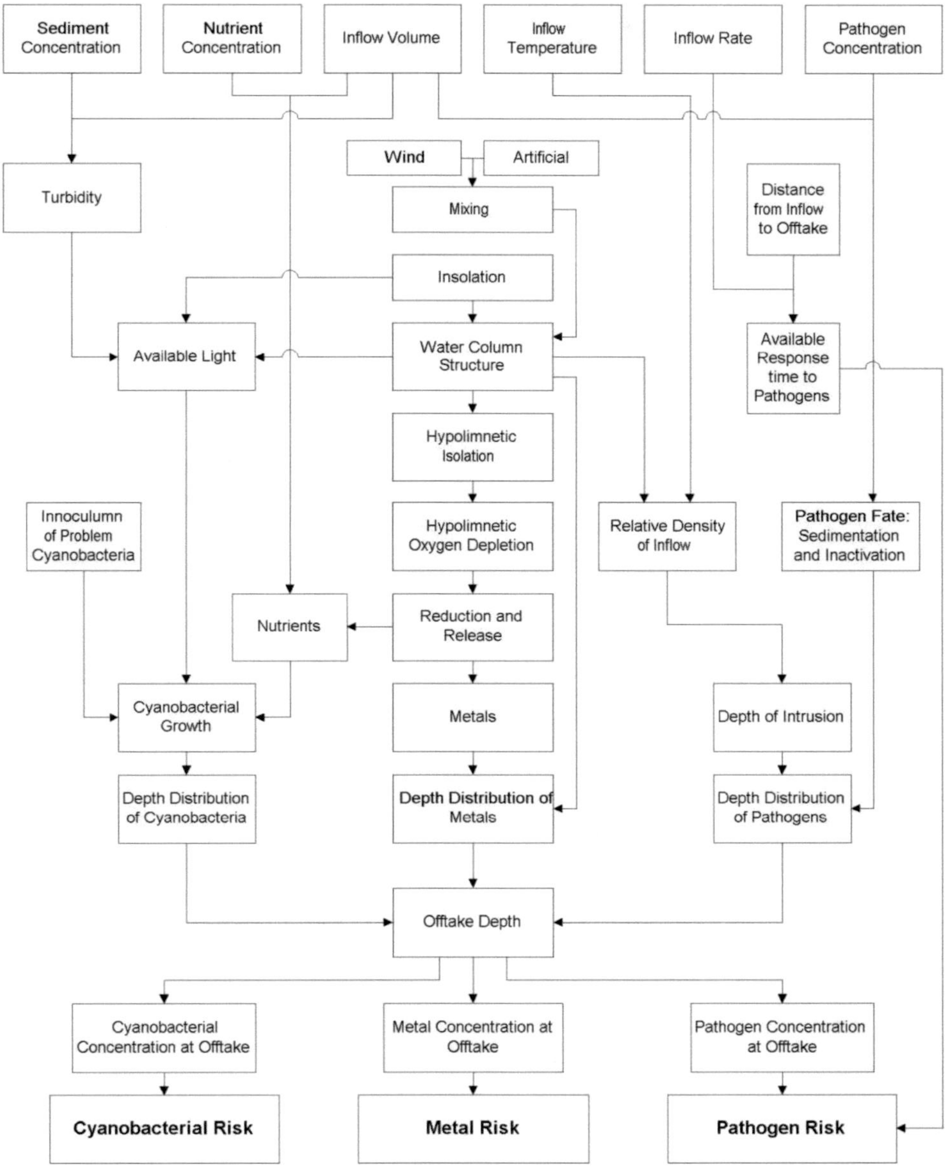

Figure 3. Conceptual model of the major hazards challenging drinking water supplies and their links to meteorology, hydrodynamics and biogeochemistry.

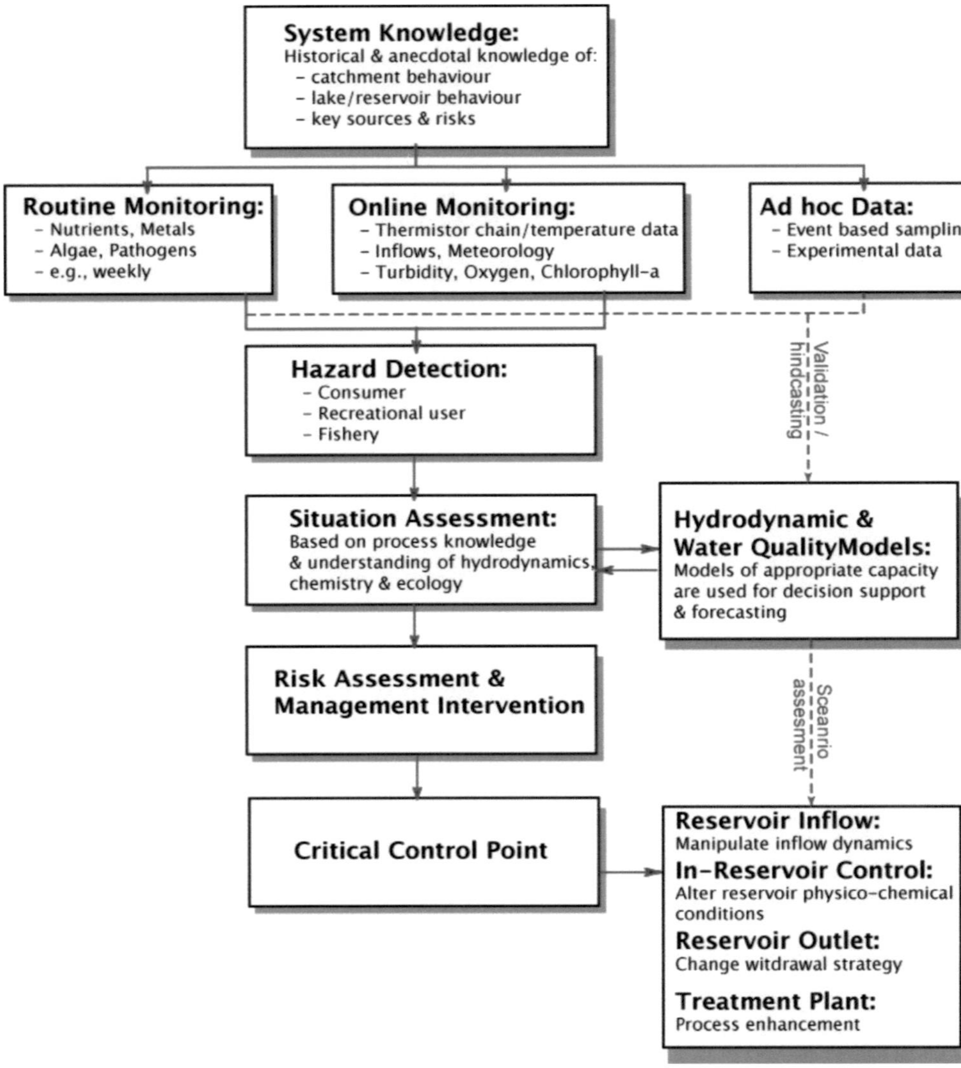

Figure 4. Management framework for assessing and responding to health threats to drinking water sources (modified from [20]).

5. Gathering information for risk assessment

The above risk assessment framework is built around suitable streams of information that are used to inform decision making and guide mitigative measures. There are numerous types of information that contribute to the understanding of an aquatic system, ranging from static information that characterises the domain, to routinely collected water quality samples and real-time sensors, through to strategically collected data related to a particular threat. In addition to general environmental or direct microbial data measurements, microbial surrogates (or bio-indicators) also have an important place in risk assessments. The application of hydrodynamic and water quality models have also significantly increased in recent years to supplement direct measurements. The hydrodynamic models are now well developed and tested and there are now numerous published models of pathogen dynamics in aquatic systems. These various information sources are discussed in this section.

5.1. System characterisation and baseline monitoring

Catchment: In most cases, the quality of water and public health risks that may exist within a lake, river or reservoir used for drinking water will reflect land-use practices and their distribution within the surrounding catchment. Any risk determination or control measure assessment must therefore give careful consideration to the nature of the activities within the catchment and identify key sources of contaminants or contaminant precursors and whether they are point-source or diffuse in nature. This analysis need not be complex and may simply involve plotting topography, land-use type, vegetation and soil type within a Geographical Information System (GIS), and assessing them within the context of the stream and drainage network and proximity to the water supply. The distribution of land-use activities that provide large quantities of contaminants will vary widely depending on the site-specific catchment properties and it is therefore not possible to generalise risk profiles with certain land-use activities. Using the case of *Cryptosporidium* within areas used for dairying as an example, animal husbandry practices vary from farm to farm, and how these activities are managed relative to the stream will largely determine the downstream pathogen numbers. Nonetheless it is useful information to have to help identify potential contaminant 'hot-spots'. Areas of urbanisation are generally major sources of diffuse inputs and easily identifiable.

Other attributes that should not be overlooked included catchment vegetation distribution, since this influences contaminant attenuation, runoff quality and concentrations of natural organic matter and suspended material. More specific indicators such as riparian integrity can also be considered as it is well documented that this correlates with turbidity [43] and pathogen attenuation [44-45]. When considering catchment properties that may contribute to downstream contaminant loading, it is important to not only look for potential sources of contaminants, but also to search for opportunities to implement management measures. Preventing contaminant loading by reducing the source may in fact be the most cost-effective and sustainable solution rather than purely relying on engineering interventions or avoidance procedures in downstream locations [42].

Rivers & Reservoirs: For most situations it is critical to understand the nature of inflows entering a river reach, lake or reservoir. They are of direct relevance from a health point of view as they are the mechanism for seeding downstream water bodies with pathogens washed from the catchment. The relationship between flow and pathogens is well established and different phases of the hydrograph may be identified from a risk perspective [46]. For example, the first-flush concept highlights that risk is concentrated around times of large rainfall events and is therefore linked with the stochastic nature of climatic drivers for the location of interest. As pathogen concentrations vary with flow stage, so to do factors such as suspended particles, dissolved organic carbon and other variables such as predatory microorganisms. Highly turbid water is effective at attaching bacteria and viruses [33], but may be ineffective at removing protozoan (oo)cysts. Dissolved organic carbon is also critical in attenuating UV light, which is an important mechanism for inducing mortality in a range of microbial organisms.

In addition to the river flow rate measurement (or stage-height should a suitable height-flow rating relationship exist), it is essential to regularly measure the temperature and salinity (or electrical conductivity) of the inflow for characterisation of its density for later comparison with the stratification profile present at downstream stations. Depending on the nature of the site, the characteristic concentration of suspended particles in the inflow water may also be insightful since highly turbid waters not only influence sedimentation, but also can impact the density and ultimate fate of the inflow water [25]. This may be easily measured using an optical turbidity probe, or ideally an *in situ* particle analysis instrument (e.g., [47]). Developing a relationship between the particle size distribution and the optical turbidity signal is also able to provide further information about the dynamics of suspended sediment [25].

In stratified water bodies such as estuaries and deep lakes or reservoirs, the fate of inflowing water is largely determined by the stratification profile and the domain morphology. The vertical structure of density, and how it varies seasonally, will ultimately determine whether the inflow water will flow along the surface, along the bottom thalweg of the site, or at some level in between (Figure 5). It will also control the travel time, and level of entrainment that the inflow water experiences within the ambient water profile. The environmental conditions the pathogens experience will also vary accordingly and this may impact on the ability of the site to attenuate pathogens successfully or otherwise [23]. To best understand the vertical structure it is essential to have vertically resolved information of temperature (and salinity where relevant), and ideally a thermistor chain with a surface meteorological station to understand the dynamics of wind mixing and surface heat fluxes.

The information detailed above permits the development a clear picture of how the system is interfacing with the surrounding catchment and the key controls on transport processes. This can be improved by collection of water quality samples that provide specific information on microbiological concentrations in the water. They should generally be collected upstream and at various locations along the waterbody. Given that they are more resource intensive (both cost and time) than typical environmental measurements, it is essential they are targeted to specific points of concern and the monitoring program should be designed within the context of the transport dynamics.

http://dx.doi.org/10.5772/55367

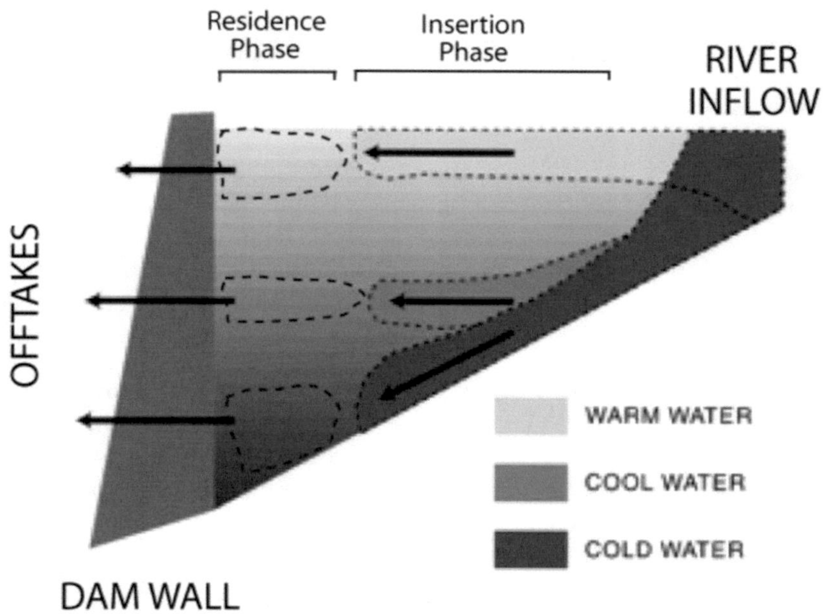

Figure 5. Schematic of inflow scenarios that may be observed entering a lake or reservoir, illustrating the surface overflow, interflow and underflow.

5.2. Real-time sensors

Often *ad hoc* monitoring, such as that described above, will miss 'events' that occur at a frequency below the monitoring interval unless they are specifically programmed to coincide with the event. Generally, the timescales of horizontal transport in rivers and lakes during flood events are significantly less than the routinely implemented monitoring frequencies. Remotely deployable sensors are therefore attractive to supplement other sources of information. Logistical challenges may also make deployable sensors better value as they save travel and manpower expenses, although maintenance and regular calibration is essential for these to be reliable and useful.

Instrumentation used to collect *in situ* data are available from numerous sources. Real-time sensors for meteorology, temperature, conductivity, turbidity and chlorophyll-a are commercially available from numerous vendors to provide high temporal resolution data, which in many cases, may be transmitted automatically to managers via telemetry. Such instrumentation is already being used widely across the globe to support decision-making activities. Advances in sensor technology continue and sensors are now available for examining *in situ* concentrations for nutrients, metals and other contaminants although they are yet to be widely adopted. As these become more widely available, practitioners will be able to take advantage of high-resolution time-series of many physical and chemical constituents. Even without the implementation of more advanced sensors, real-time information of core environmental properties (temperature, salinity, oxygen and turbidity) can provide considerable insight into the dynamics that will ultimately control pathogen fate and transport.

5.3. Strategic data collection

Strategic sampling may be undertaken to improve process understanding about the dynamics of the system. For example, routine sampling may not be able to provide sufficient information on hydrodynamic or biogeochemical processes at a scale required to truly assess the risk of a threat developing. Commonly, site-specific experimental data is collected to supplement other information on items such as the particle size distribution of suspended sediment, fine to medium scale horizontal and vertical mixing processes, and important ecological processes.

It is often the case that routine monitoring programs do not accurately portray the actual risk and strategic data can help to build knowledge about a system and improve the management practices. As an example, the reservoir shown in Figure 5 would typically be monitored by the managing water utility by collecting microbial samples at the inflow and at the surface near the centre of the basin. Although noticeable inflow concentrations would be recorded, surface grab samples from the main body of lake would be near the minimum level of detection, and it would therefore be assumed the reservoir had sufficiently attenuated the inflowing load. Experimentation of pathogen transport by [21] has showed that in fact in the case the reservoir may have attenuated little of the incoming load, and that significant concentrations existed below the surface layer [48]. Furthermore, most microbial monitoring programs are based on regular, often weekly, sampling. Although this is a good idea, and is acceptable for the case where there is a constant pollution source, for lakes and reservoirs fed by rivers, the highest risk is from large runoff events. It is therefore also recommended that event based monitoring be implemented. Even for large reservoirs that have considerable residence times, it can take just a few days for contaminated inflow water to reach the extraction point (e.g., [20,23,49]).

Often models (discussed below) can be used to assist in the design of an effective and targeted monitoring programme that reflects the dynamics of the system and can more accurately portray the risk. Sophisticated monitoring programmes also include capacity to logically adapt the monitoring regime as a particular threat is observed to develop. This approach acknowledges that we are more interested in the spatial and temporal variability in the contaminant of concern as the probability of exposure increases, and accordingly the monitoring effort intensifies to ensure the actual risk is being portrayed accurately.

5.4. Surrogate measurements for indicating threats to health

Often it is not possible or practical to directly detect the presence of a certain contaminant within a water body and so surrogates or other indirect indicators of the dynamics may be defined. In particular, the complexity, cost and time constraints associated with the direct enumeration of pathogens to identify their distribution in large water bodies, frequently limits the ability of water managers to detect the intrusion of poorer quality water inflows into the aquatic environment. As a result, there is considerable discussion in regulatory organizations and water utilities as to the value of using surrogates, such as microbial indicator organisms

http://dx.doi.org/10.5772/55367

or even physical properties such as turbidity, as a way of detecting the presence of microbial contamination and hence the threat of actual pathogenic organisms. Microbial indicators have the advantage of being low-risk, present in high concentrations relative to other organisms of concern and simple and cheap to enumerate.

The most widely used indicator organisms of microbial pollution are the enteric coliform bacteria, which are gram-negative bacilli that belong to the family *Enterobacteriaceae* (*e.g. Klebsiella* spp., *Enterobacter* spp. *Citrobacter* spp., *Escherichia coli*). Specific coliform measurements include total coliforms, faecal coliforms, and in particular the specific organism *E. coli* [50]. The latter two are the most common since they are abundant in the faeces of humans and other warm blooded animals, and are hence thought to be a reliable indicator of faecal pollution. Total coliforms are used less frequently since they include organisms from soil and cold-blooded animals. Except for certain strains of pathogenic *E. coli* (*e.g.* O157), coliform bacteria are not a threat to human health, but their high abundance means that they are easy to detect, thereby alerting regulatory authorities to pollution events that may contain other organisms of concern. Other routinely used indicator bacteria include the gram-positive cocci, including Enterococci and faecal streptococci. However, it is now apparent that these bacterial indicators are not suitable for assessing the risk posed by protozoan pathogens and some enteric viruses [21,51-52].

Various bacteriophages are used as index organisms for enteric viruses [53-56]. The single-stranded F-specific RNA (F^+ RNA) bacteriophages (*e.g.* strains *MS-2*, *F2* and *Q beta*) and the double-stranded somatic coliphages (*e.g.* strains T_2, T_7 and $\phi X174$) are routinely measured in fresh and coastal waters. However, faecal bacteriophages are not always suitable index organisms since they are present in a range of animal as well as human faeces, whereas human enteric viruses only originate from human faeces. There have also been reports of human enteric viruses being detected in waters in the absence of bacteriophages [57]. The rationale for their use as model organisms is based on their similar size and morphology, along with the low cost, ease and speed of detection compared to human enteric virus assays. The ideal host bacteria would be of human faecal origin only, consistently present in sewage in sufficient numbers for detection, and only lysed by phages that do not replicate in another host or the environment. While bacteriophages to *Bacteroides fragilis* strain HSB40 appear to be human specific and do not replicate in the environment [58], their phage numbers are too low for general use. Due to their high abundance, studies have focused on the coliphage systems, including the double and single-stranded DNA and RNA-containing phages listed above, and for a range of bacterial hosts. The F^+ RNA coliphages attach to the sides of the bacterial pili that only occur on exponentially growing specific (F^+) strains of *E. coli* or an engineered *Salmonella typhimurium* (strain WG49), and are therefore the current models of choice [53,57].

The use of spores of the gram-positive bacilli *Clostridium perfringens* has been suggested as a good indicator of human faecal contamination and may correlate with human parasitic protozoa and enteric viruses [21,58-59]. However, two confounding factors must be considered; first, *C. perfringens* spores are very persistent [35] and second, they may be excreted by various animals [60]. Hence, they may show little relationship with parasitic protozoa in animal-impacted raw waters, and could be misleading about the likely presence of infective human viruses.

Particle counting and turbidity levels have also been identified as potential surrogates of microbial pollution and weak epidemiological evidence exists that suggests waterborne illness from drinking water may be associated with the raw water turbidity [61]. The use of turbidity alone to predict pathogen presence is difficult because turbidity is dependent on a range of processes that are independent of pathogen presence. For example, it is well established that many young calves are infected with *Cryptosporidium* [62], however, calving is timed to coincide with the period when feed is abundant and cows are on a rising plane of nutrition. Consequently, calving and high oocyst numbers occur when catchments are well vegetated, yet this is typically when turbidity is low. Additionally, surrogates such as turbidity are influenced by catchment specific factors such as soil-type distribution and non-grazing land-use such as horticulture that do not correlate with pathogen input. In shallow systems, turbidity may be caused through resuspension of sediment during high wind events or strong currents, and therefore may exist unrelated to any catchment or wastewater discharges. Nonetheless, turbidity is a readily measurable parameter that warrants investigation as a potential early warning mechanism of increased risk.

While no single water quality indicator can reliably assess the bacterial, protozoan and viral contamination of aquatic environments in all circumstances, it is feasible that a suite of surrogates may be identified that will estimate levels of microbial contamination within defined circumstances, such as within a storage reservoir with well characterized inputs [21]. To understand how they relate to each other, it is necessary to develop a process-based understanding of surrogate organisms in order to develop a model of their behaviour and assess their dynamics relative to their pathogenic counterparts [16].

5.5. Role of numerical models

Although the processes influencing enteric organism fate and distribution are fairly well established, much uncertainty remains as to the relative importance of each process on a system-wide scale, and the spatial and temporal variability that is present. Furthermore, a detailed understanding of how pathogen dynamics vary between systems, which may differ in their loading, salinity, temperature and trophic status, remains elusive. As a result, *ad hoc* monitoring routines are often employed that rarely give an indication of the true risk. Numerical models are attractive since they offer to integrate the myriad of interacting and non-linear processes and place them within a system-wide context.

The use of numerical models to augment existing monitoring and risk-management activities is becoming increasingly widespread since they are able to highlight dominant processes controlling organism dynamics, and can be used to fill knowledge gaps and test catchment management scenarios or examine engineering interventions. There have been several models used to simulate different components of microbial pollution reported in the literature that range in sophistication and that are relevant for different surface water environments, including freshwater lakes and reservoirs [16,63-64], streams and rivers [65], and estuaries and coastal lagoons [66-68].

http://dx.doi.org/10.5772/55367

Models are used by a range of organizations for a variety of applications:

- *as a scientific tool to explore the dominant processes within a given system* – for managers interested in understanding the spatial and temporal variability in the dynamics that control enteric organism behaviour, and conducting pathogen budgets and exploring sensitivities;
- *to guide the design targeted monitoring programs* – the model can be run to provide information about expected transport and kinetic controls to ensure that the sampling locations and frequency is focused on the areas that present the largest risk;
- *to quantify differences between species* – the model can be used to 'correct' the observed microbial indicator organism data so that the true risk by actual pathogenic organisms can be quantified;
- *to quantify the impact of proposed management scenarios* – scenarios such as catchment remediation, climate change and engineering interventions can be compared to the base case system as part of a cost-benefit analysis prior to any remedial action;
- *to support real-time decision-making* – the model can be used to provide now- and fore-casts of conditions within an aquatic system to enable managers to alter pumping regimes or issue recreational closures.

Models for assisting with the understanding of contaminant dynamics within a system range from simple web-based tools to full three-dimensional (3D) hydrodynamic-water quality models. To demonstrate their ability to describe pathogen transport dynamics, here we focus on a case-study of a medium sized Australian reservoir, Myponga Reservoir in South Australia, where pathogen transport dynamics have been measured and modelled using various approaches. The model developed to simulate pathogen kinetics is shown in Figure 6.

INFLOW: This is a simple web-based tool written in JavaScript (http://www.cwr.uwa.edu.au/) developed by [23], that estimates the entrainment experienced by a riverine intrusion as it enters and progresses through a standing body of water (*e.g.* lake or reservoir) and the final insertion depth and inflow thickness. The model simply requires the inflow parameters including temperature, salinity and channel parameters (*e.g.* bed slope, roughness), and reservoir information such as the vertical temperature and salinity profiles. This information is used to estimate whether the inflow will act as an overflow, interflow or underflow (Figure 5), the approximate entrainment rate (and hence the dilution), and the timescale for transport and insertion. In addition, since the model is able to estimate the time-scale of transport, a simplified loss-model (simplified version of Figure 6) is included that estimates the loss due to settling and inactivation. Therefore, with relatively simple input information, the user is able to assess reservoir risk reduction of pathogen concentrations by dilution, settling and inactivation. This tool is only applicable where the lake is weakly forced at the surface, and doesn't tell you what happens to the contaminated inflow water once it has inserted. However, the simplicity of knowing if the water will travel at the surface, mid-regions or at depth and an approximate dilution factor is a surprisingly powerful management tool.

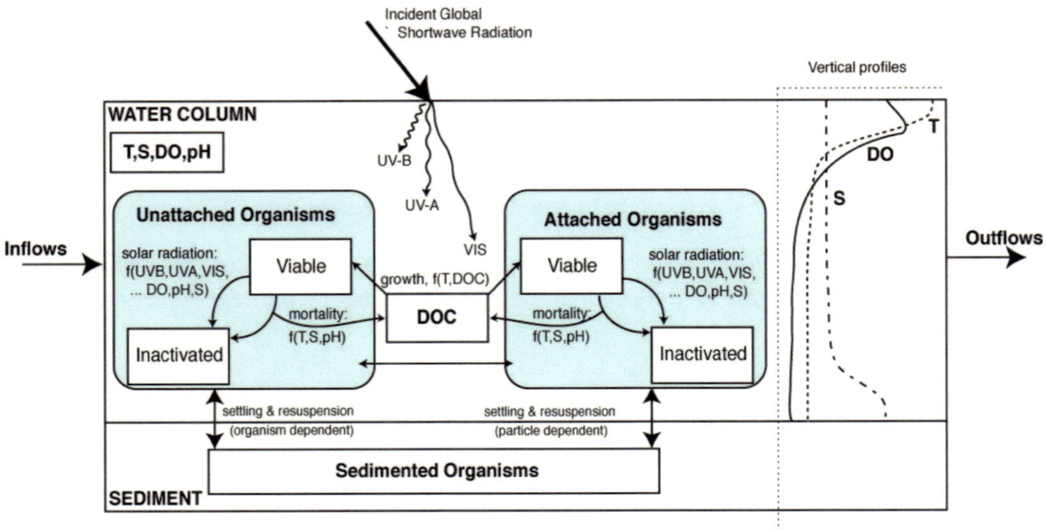

Figure 6. Schematic indicating organism dynamics showing the major pools and kinetic processes that occur in response to sunlight (UV-B, UV-A and VIS), temperature (T), salinity (S), dissolved oxygen (DO), pH and available carbon (DOC) (modified from [16]).

CAEDYM: The Computational Aquatic Ecosystem Dynamics Model (CAEDYM) is a comprehensive water quality model available from the Centre for Water Research at The University of Western Australia [69], able to couple with a 1D lake stratification model (DYRESM) and a 3D hydrodynamic model (ELCOM). ELCOM is specifically designed for modelling circulation patterns in stratified lakes and reservoirs and can be easily run on a desktop computer. The pathogen sub-model includes inactivation due to different solar radiation bandwidths (including UV), natural mortality, sedimentation and aggregation onto suspended particles, and resuspension as described in [16]). ELCOM-CAEDYM is well suited to applications where topographic effects may be important or where lake circulation is a dominant process over inflow forcing. For example, if the source is a recreational area or a lakeside canal estate, then three-dimensional effects may be important in determining the mixing of the contaminated water around the lake. Similarly, if the source is a discrete effluent discharge, then the prevailing hydrodynamics will need to be well understood in order to accurately characterize the risk of the contaminated water reaching an off-take or recreational area. As an example, the application to Myponga Reservoir (Figure 7) describes a contaminated inflow entering from a side tributary before it begins to interact with a large peninsula and migrate into the main basin. Output from the model highlights the strong vertical gradients that result. Hipsey et al [16] use this platform to further investigate the controls on *E. coli* dynamics over a range of time-scales for different sized reservoirs and showed that a different combination of transport and kinetic processes could ultimately shape the response of the microbial concentrations observed at the offtake.

http://dx.doi.org/10.5772/55367

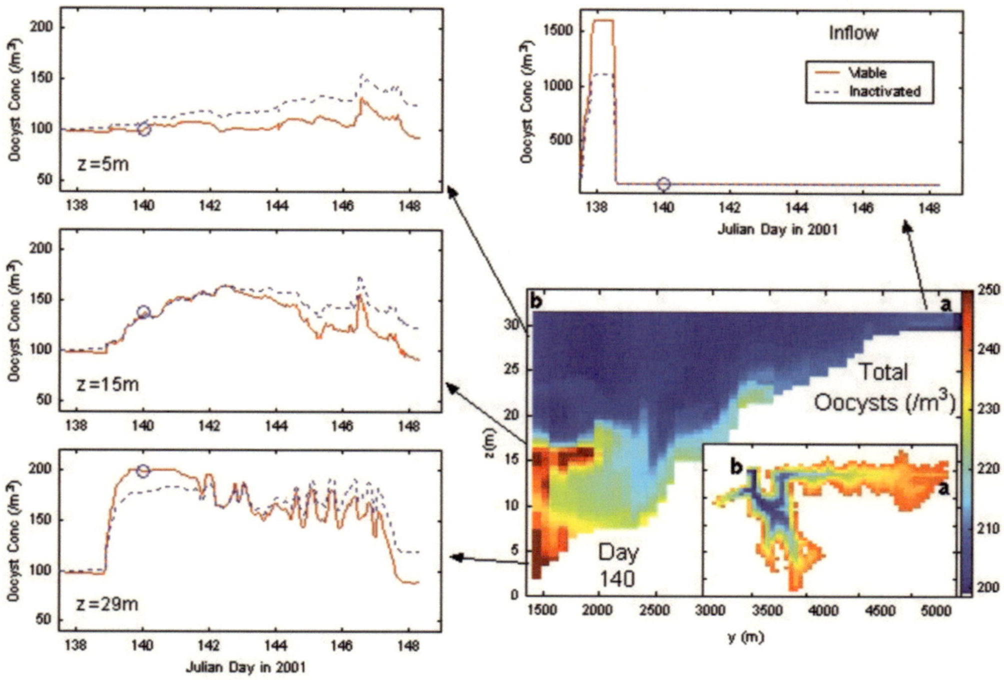

Figure 7. ELCOM-CAEDYM *Cryptosporidium* concentrations (oocysts/10L) presented as a slice through Myponga Reservoir (bottom-right, colour scale reflects oocyst concentration), South Australia (see inset), following a large runoff event, and highlighting *Cryptosporidium* oocyst concentrations as a function of time for three depths near the offtake (left).

DYRESM, is a 1D hydrodynamic model that has been shown to accurately capture the temperature and salinity dynamics of large and small lakes and reservoirs [70]. It accommodates horizontal motions caused by inflows and outflows, in addition to a Lagrangian vertical mixing model and a surface thermodynamics module. CAEDYM couples with DYRESM and includes the same detailed microbial sub-model as outlined in Figure 6. The horizontal averaging used in DYRESM-CAEDYM significantly improves computational efficiency and means that seasonal or even multi-decadal simulations can be performed with reasonable run-times. This model is therefore well suited to applications that look at the long-term impact of different watershed management or climate change scenarios for example, and its ease of use makes it particularly useful to reservoir and lake managers.

GLM-FABM: The General Lake Model (GLM) is coupled with the open-source ecological model FABM as described in [71]. The model GLM is similar to DYRESM but based on [72], and a simplified version of the pathogen kinetic model [16] is implemented within FABM. Output from the model as applied to Myponga Reservoir for the year of 2003 (Figure 8) demonstrates how the incoming oocyst load manifests in the water column concentrations and highlights the temporal and vertical variability that may be expected. The figure indicates the variability seen in the off-take *Cryptosporidium* concentrations at three different depths, and demonstrates the potential benefits of selective withdrawal and adaptive reservoir management to minimize the potential risks.

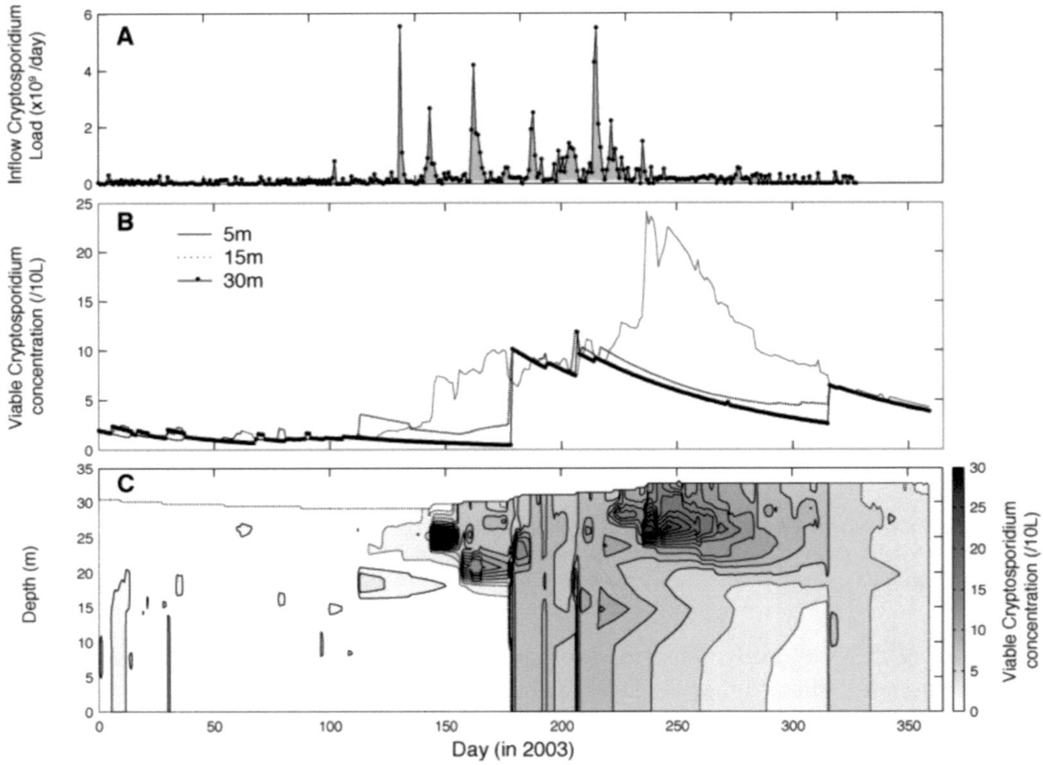

Figure 8. Time-series of A) viable inflow oocyst load as estimated from data; B) simulated concentrations of viable oocysts at the dam wall for three different depths, and C) the viable oocyst concentrations (oocysts/10L) throughout the water column as simulated by GLM-FABM.

6. Control measures and considerations to minimise exposure

There are a range of control measures that can be implemented to mitigate the risk of contaminants passing through to delivery systems. Here we provide a broad overview of the different

http://dx.doi.org/10.5772/55367

approaches and their relevance to different contamination issues. The different control methods can be characterised based on the nature of the intervention:

- reducing the delivery of contamination to the exposure point (water storage);
- improved attenuation of the contaminant within the storage;
- and optimal extraction of water to reduce exposure.

The methods around these are discussed next, including a discussion on operational monitoring and the potential for real-time management of water bodies for risk minimization.

6.1. Catchment management

Most contamination within drinking water storages is linked to the surrounding catchment land-use. The contamination can either originate from the catchment and enter the tributaries to the storage, or a precursor of the contamination may originate within the catchment that is later transformed to the end product that constitutes a health risk. There is therefore much scope to reduce contamination within drinking waters through strategic assessment and management of catchment land-use and the condition of tributary streams.

For *Cryptosporidium* and other pathogens the biggest threat is when heavy rains wash viable cells from agricultural catchments within the surrounding river basin into the floodwaters that feed the reservoirs [73-74], or in some cases when effluent from wastewater treatment plants is discharged directly into upstream watercourses (75-76). For many reservoirs, prevention of the contaminant source from entering the hydrological network is the ultimate method for reducing downstream health risks. In particular this involves improving agricultural practices and the best example is related to improvement of the methods used in animal husbandry. Farm-scale alleviation techniques such as improved drainage and runoff recharge may prevent or delay contaminated runoff from entering the stream network. At the sub-catchment scale, policies for suitable riparian management are also recommended since it has been shown that suitable riparian buffers can act to filter contaminated farm water from entering streams [46].

In urban environments, principles of Water Sensitive Urban Design (WSUD) are increasingly being adopted with numerous innovations in the design of stormwater management features including biofilters and constructed wetlands at critical catchment points [77].

6.2. Inflow manipulation

A significant critical control point for managing contaminant transfer into the main reservoir body is through strategic engineering based interventions where catchment tributaries meet a standing water body. Several flow management options exist here that can reduce the delivery of contaminants, including:

- *flow diversions* – as seen in pathogen concentrations over the course of an inflow event, higher values occur at the leading edge of the peak in the hydrograph, and so there is potential for 'first-flush' flows to be diverted away from the water body under consideration. After the initial peak in cell numbers are reduced, then the flow diversion can be removed. The disadvantage of this approach is the potential loss of valuable water, however it could be considered as an environmental flow.

- *sedimentation basins, or 'pre-reservoirs'* –can be used to slow incoming water down and encourage sedimentation of particulates. The water that overflows the basin is usually of a higher quality and passes into the main water body with a lower concentration. There are potential complications with this approach, particularly considering that oocysts have a long life in the sediment and a very high may mobilise previously sedimented organisms in a single event.
- *constructed wetlands* – like pre-reservoirs are useful at slowing the inflowing water and enhancing attenuation (e.g., [78]), also mentioned above.

To assess the efficiency of any of these controls and the loading reduction, it is a simple case of measuring water at the outlet relative to the influent water.

6.3. In-lake controls

Aside from manipulating the inflow concentrations (above) or offtake strategy (below), there is some potential to manipulate concentrations by using in-lake interventions. However, there are no standard methods for controlling the concentration of pathogens within standing waters and these are more commonly applied for management of nuisance cyanobacteria, for example, but also offer potential to support management of high pathogen loads. The most common method for managing stratified waters is destratification, generally achieved through the introduction of compressed air on the lake bottom. The air-water mixture with lowered specific weight causes a rising water curtain, destroying stratification. Similarly, impellers have also be suggested as a method to disperse contaminated water that is concentrated within highly important areas to regions where they are less of a concern. They operate by enhancing the water exchange rate (potentially the littoral water exchange rate, depending upon the flushing technique and the location of the devices), which, if important enough, can prevent the formation of high concentration patches. Some flushing devices also increase also vertical mixing and this may impact on incident light received by organisms.

Where hypolimnetic contaminants become unmanageable, for example following a large, dense flood intrusion, then historically there has been examples of hypolimnetic release or purging to remove these from the system. It can be done in natural lakes by pipes called Olszewski-tubes [79], and by selecting an appropriate height of the discharge on the dam for reservoirs. However, this potentially involves losing valuable water resources and may also lead to enhanced downstream contamination.

Morillo *et al* [80] numerically demonstrated the use of a suspended geo-textile curtain to manipulate the flow path of contaminated inflow water, thereby increasing time taken for natural attenuation processes to occur. These curtains change the internal flow-paths by compartmentalisation, and either slow down or redirect highly contaminated inflow pulses. They may also contribute to address other contamination concerns, since they can have an impact on the nutrient distribution and the residence time of the lake [80-81]. In addition to

http://dx.doi.org/10.5772/55367

controlling the path of inflowing water, they constitute a barrier to internal waves, and thus can prevent enhanced mixing due to seiching and subsequent sediment resuspension.

However, such measures are logistically difficult and may incur considerable cost, and for pathogens in particular, management of the offtake location usually remains a more practical and effective means to reduce risk.

6.4. Adapting the location of drinking-water offtakes and bathing sites

The vertical variability in reservoir water quality can be exploited to select an offtake depth with the lowest contaminant concentrations. Selective withdrawal is a widely used method for controlling transmission of contaminants downstream of surface storages. This is mostly applicable for reservoirs with sufficient depth and the capability in the dam offtake structure for multiple offtake depths.

The simple INFLOW model described above enables prediction of the depth at which the riverine inflow will occur and the anticipated dilution as it travels through the reservoir. Consideration should be given to the time of transport. Appropriate monitoring is necessary to ensure stratification and intrusion type is known to the operator. The speed at which an inflow travels through a lake, the degree of entrainment of ambient lake water, the dilution, and the insertion depth are all important in determining the distribution of pathogens in lakes and reservoirs. Consequently it is important to know the depth of the riverine intrusion so water can be harvested outside of this intrusion.

Similarly, where bathing sites are situated around the system of interest, the best solution is temporary closure upon detection of high concentrations with the monitoring data, or from the model predictions.

6.5. Real-time management systems

Given the complexity of managing environmental waters it is not surprising that there has been a considerable proliferation of decision support systems (DSS) in the water resources sector over the past several decades. In general DSSs integrate databases, models, and data visualization tools through a user-friendly interface. The complexity of the models and the databases ranges greatly depending on the intended use. A distinction exists between 'real-time' DSSs that provide advanced warning of deleterious impacts and 'non-real-time' DSSs that serve as planning and operational development tools. Real-time flood prediction DSSs have emerged as commonplace technology, which provide advance warning to save life and property. However, the development of real-time systems for water quality concerns has been less common, but is increasing as data acquisition systems and the associated cyber-infrastructure associated with such developments improves.

The purpose of the DSS is to accurately predict the fate and transport of floods and contaminant dynamics. Because these types of incidents have high spatial and temporal variability in inland standing waters, complex three-dimensional simulations are often also implemented. In this case the DSS performs all of the tasks to maintain simulations of the current conditions in an automated manner so that when incidents occur, the system provides useful predictions to aid in mitigation measures (Figure 9).

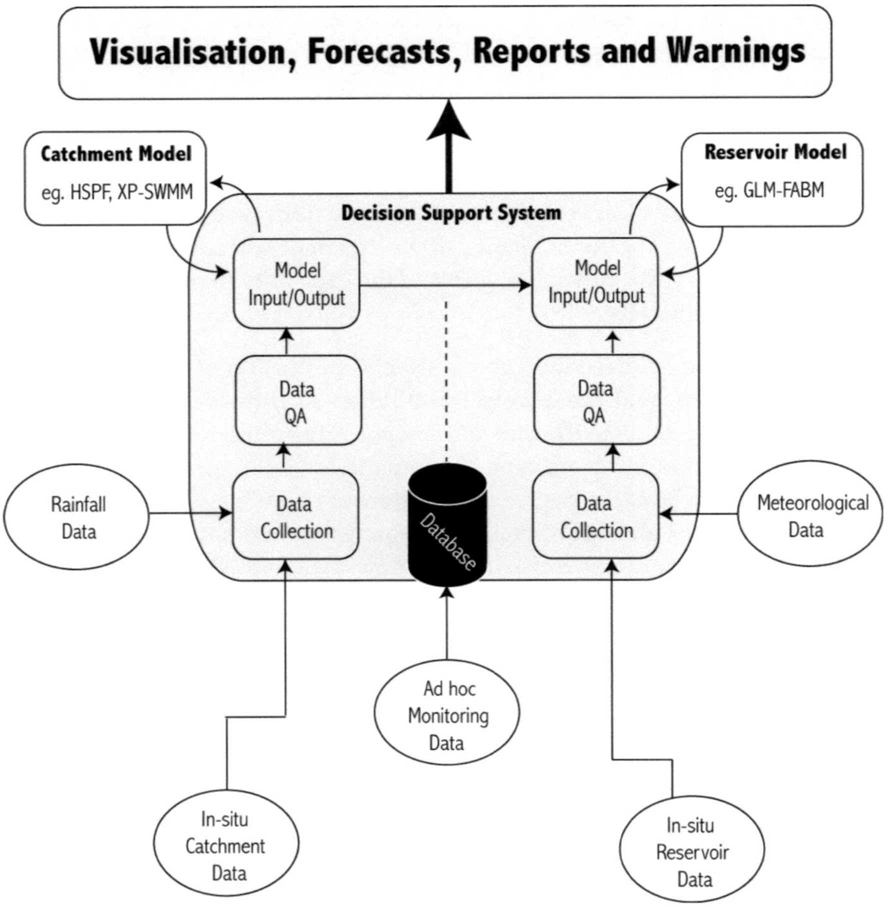

Figure 9. Framework for a Decision Support System (DSS) that has inputs from a range of monitoring programs which inform and input to hydrodynamic and management models to visually represent predictions of risk, and report exceedance of contaminant thresholds and send warnings to managers.

7. Conclusions

It is apparent that contaminant risk to drinking water supply needs to consider a broad management framework that encompasses the entire system, from source to exposure. Reducing the corporate and human health risk associated with these contaminants requires a realistic assessment of the overall contaminant risk which can only be achieved with an understanding of the critical variables controlling contaminant fate and distribution once they

http://dx.doi.org/10.5772/55367

enter the aquatic environment. Whilst it is near impossible to reduce the pathogen risk to zero, it is possible to manage the load of pathogens entering the water body, understanding and predicting where they go within a drinking water supply reservoir and managing the withdrawal of water to ensure the best quality of water is treated and distributed for potable supply. Sanitation and water treatment have dramatically reduced the burden of water borne disease on the human population. However, the water industry cannot afford to be complacent or not implement risk management strategies for contaminants in drinking water supply catchments and reservoirs. Failure to do so has significant cost, can lead to outbreaks and at worst cost human lives [82]. Tragically water borne disease still takes an enormous toll in developing countries but with implementation of some of the simple technologies and approaches presented here, an integrated risk management framework, and in combination with treatment and disinfection, this toll can be reduced.

Author details

Matthew R. Hipsey[1] and Justin D. Brookes[2]

1 School of Earth and Environment, The University of Western Australia, Nedlands, Australia

2 School of Earth and Environmental Science, The University of Adelaide, Adelaide, Australia

References

[1] Herwaldt, B. L, Craun, G. F, Stokes, S. L, & Juranek, D. D. (1992). Outbreaks of waterborne disease in the United States: 1989-90, *J. Amer. Water Works Assoc.* , 64(4), 129-135.

[2] Moore, A. C, Herwaldt, B. L, Craun, G. F, Calderon, R. L, Highsmith, A. K, & Juranek, D. D. (1994). Waterborne disease in the United States, 1991-1992, *J. Amer. Water Works Assoc.* , 86(2), 87-99.

[3] MacKenzieW. R., Hoxie, N. J., Procter, M. E., Gradus, M. S., Blair, K. A., and Peterson, D. E., (1994). A massive outbreak of Milwaukee *Cryptosporidium* infection transmitted through the public water supply, *N. Engl. J. Med.* , 331(3), 161-167.

[4] Lisle, J. T, & Rose, J. B. (1995). *Crytposporidium* contamination of water in the USA and UK- a mini review, *Aqua* , 44(3), 103-117.

[5] Zuckerman, U, Gold, D, Shelef, G, & Armon, R. (1997). The presence of *Giardia* and *Cryptosporidium* in surface waters and effluents in Israel, *Water Sci. Technol.* 25(11-12): 381-384.

[6] Gibson, C. J, Haas, C. N, & Rose, J. B. (1998). Risk assessment of waterborne protozoa: current status and future trends, *Parasitol.* , 117, 205-212.

[7] Hsu, B. M, Huang, C, Hsu, Y. F, & Hsu, C. L. L. (2000). Examination of *Giardia* and *Cryptosporidium* in water samples and faecal specimens in Taiwan, *Water Sci. Technol.* , 41(7), 87-92.

[8] Howe, A. D, Forster, S, Morton, S, Marshall, R, Osborn, K. S, & Wright, P. (2002). *Cryptosporidium* oocysts in a water supply associated with cryptosporidiosis outbreak, *Emerg. Infect. Dis.* , 8(6), 619-624.

[9] Belkin, S, & Colwell, R. R. eds., (2005). *Oceans and health: pathogens in the marine environment*, Springer, New York, 464p.

[10] Robertson, L. J, Campbell, A. T, & Smith, H. V. (1992). Survival of *Cryptosporidium parvum* oocysts under various environmental pressures, *Appl. Environ. Microbiol.* , 58(11), 3494-3500.

[11] Castro-hermida, J. A, Garci, a-P. r. e. s. e. d. o, Almeida, I, & Gonzalez-warleta, A. M., Correia Da Costa, J. M., Mezo, M., (2008). Contribution of treated wastewater to the contamination of recreational river areas with *Cryptosporidium* spp. and *Giardia duodenalis*. *Water Res.* , 42, 3528-3538.

[12] Soller, J. A, Schoen, M. E, Bartrand, T, Ravenscroft, J. E, & Ashbolt, N. J. (2010). Estimated human health risks from exposure to recreational waters impacted by human and non-human sources of faecal contamination. *Water Res.* , 44(16), 4674-4691.

[13] Fong, T, & Lipp, E. K. (2006). Enteric viruses of humans and animals in aquatic environments: health risks, detection, and potential water quality assessment tools, *Microbiol. Mol. Biol. Rev.* , 69(2), 357-371.

[14] Sunderland, D, Graczyk, T. K, Tamang, L, & Breysse, P. N. (2007). Impact of bathers on levels of *Cryptosporidium parvum* oocysts and *Giardia lamblia* cysts in recreational beach waters. *Water Res.* , 41(15), 3483-3489.

[15] Bichai, F, Payment, P, & Barbeau, B. (2008). Protection of waterborne pathogens by higher organisms in drinking water: a review. *Can. J. Microbiol.* 2008, 54(7): 509-524.

[16] Hipsey, M. R, Antenucci, J. P, & Brookes, J. D. process-based model of microbial pollution in aquatic systems, Water Resour. Res. 44: W07408.

[17] Edzwald, J. K, & Kelley, M. B. (1998). Control of *Cryptosporidium*- from reservoirs to clarifiers to filters, *Water Sci. Technol.* , 37(2), 1-8.

[18] Allen, M. J, Clancy, J. L, & Rice, E. W. (2000). The plain, hard truth about pathogen monitoring, *J. Amer. Water Works Assoc. 92*(9), 64-76.

[19] Kay, D, & Mcdonald, A. (1980). Reduction of coliform bacteria in two upland reservoirs: the significance of distance decay relationships, *Water Res.* , 14, 305-318.

[20] Brookes, J. D, Antenucci, J. P, Hipsey, M. R, Burch, M. D, Ashbolt, N, & Ferguson, C. M. (2004). Fate and transport of pathogens in lakes and reservoirs, *Environ. Intl.* , 30, 741-759.

[21] Brookes, J. D, Hipsey, M. R, Burch, M. D, Regel, R. H, Linden, L, Ferguson, C. M, & Antenucci, J. P. (2005). Relative value of surrogate indicators for detecting pathogens in lakes and reservoirs, *Environ. Sci. Technol.* , 39(22), 8614-8621.

[22] Wuest, A, & Lorke, A. (2003). Small-scale hydrodynamics in lakes. *Ann. Rev. Fluid Mech.* , 35, 373-412.

[23] Antenucci, J, Brookes, J. D, & Hipsey, M. (2005). A simple model for quantifying *Cryptosporidium* transport, dilution, and potential risk in reservoirs. *Journal of the American Water Works Association* , 97(1), 86-93.

[24] Deen, A, Craig, R, & Antenucci, J. P. (2000). The Sydney Water contamination incident of monitoring and modelling. *In "Hydro 2000: 3rd International Hydrology and Water Resources Symposium"*. Institution of Engineers Australia, Perth, Australia., 1998.

[25] Chung, S. W, Hipsey, M. R, & Imberger, J. (2009). Modelling the propagation of turbid density inflows into a stratifuied lake: Daecheong Reservoir, Korea. Environ. Model. Softw. , 24, 1467-1482.

[26] Evison, L. M. (1988). Comparative studies on the survival of indicator organisms and pathogens in fresh and sea water, *Water Sci. Technol.* 20(11-12): 309-315.

[27] Lopez-torres, A. J, Prieto, L, & Hazen, T. C. (1988). Comparison of the in situ survival and activity of *Klebsiella pneumoniae* and *Escherichia coli* in tropical marine environments, *Microb. Ecol.* , 15, 41-57.

[28] Camper, A. K, Mcfeters, G. A, Characklis, W. G, & Jones, W. L. (1991). Growth kinetics of coliform bacteria under conditions relevant to drinking water distribution systems, *Appl. Environ. Microbiol.* , 57(8), 2233-2239.

[29] Ashbolt, N, Dorsch, M. R, Cox, P. T, & Banens, B. Blooming *E coli*, what do they mean?' *In Coliforms and E. coli: problem or solution?* (D. Kay and C. Fricker, eds.), The Royal Society of Chemistry, Cambridge, UK., 78-85.

[30] Solo-gabriele, H. M, Wolfert, M. A, Desmarais, T. R, & Palmer, C. J. (2000). Sources of *Escherichia coli* in a coastal subtropical environment, *Appl. Environ. Microbiol.* , 66(1), 230-237.

[31] Brookes, J. D, Davies, C, Antenucci, J, & Hipsey, M. (2006). Association of *Cryptosporidium* with bovine faecal particles and implications for risk reduction by settling within water supply reserviors. *Water and Health* , 4, 87-98.

[32] Reynolds, C. S. (1984). *The ecology of freshwater phytoplankton*, Cambridge Univ. Press, Cambridge, 390p.

[33] Hipsey, M. R, Brookes, J. D, Regel, R. H, Antenucci, J. P, & Burch, M. D. (2006). In situ evidence for the association of total coliforms and *Escherichia coli* with suspended inorganic particles in an Australian reservoir, *Water Air Soil Pollut.* 170(1-4): 191-209.

[34] Gerba, C. P, & Mcleod, J. S. (1976). Effect of sediments on the survival of *Escherichia coli* in marine waters, *Appl. Environ. Microbiol.* , 32(1), 114-120.

[35] Davies, C. M, Long, J. A. H, Donald, M, & Ashbolt, N. J. (1995). Survival of fecal microorganisms in marine and freshwater sediments, *Appl. Environ. Microbiol.* , 61(5), 1888-1896.

[36] Howell, J. M, Coyne, M. S, & Cornelius, P. L. (1996). Effect of sediment particle size and temperature on fecal bacteria mortality rates and the fecal coliform/fecal streptococci ratio, *J. Environ. Qual.* , 25, 1216-1220.

[37] Lemckert, C. J, & Imberger, J. (1998). Turbulent benthic boundary layer mixing events in fresh water lakes', *In Physical Processes in Lakes and Oceans* (J. Imberger, ed.), American Geophysical Union, Washington., 54, 503-516.

[38] Michallet, H, & Ivey, G. N. (1999). Experiments on mixing due to internal solitary waves breaking on uniform slopes, *J. Geophys. Res.* 104(C6): 13467-13478.

[39] Beach, R. A, & Sternberg, R. W. (1992). Suspended sediment transport in the surf zone: response to incident wave and longshore current interaction, *Mar. Geol.* , 108, 275-294.

[40] Grant, S. B, Litton, R. M, & Ahn, J. H. (2011). Measuring and modeling the flux of fecal bacteria across the sediment-water interface in a turbulent stream. *Water Resour. Res.* 47: W05517.

[41] Hobson, P, Fabris, R, Develter, E, Linden, L. G, Burch, M. D, & Brookes, J. D. (2010). Reservoir inflow monitoring for improved management of treated water quality-A South Australian experience. *Water Resour. Manag.* , 24(14), 4161-4174.

[42] Bryan, B. A, Kandulu, J, Deere, D. A, White, M, Frizenschaf, J, & Crossman, N. D. (2009). Adaptive management for mitigating Cryptosporidium risk in source water: a case study in an agricultural catchment in South Australia. *J Environ. Manage.* , 90(10), 3122-3134.

[43] Pusey, B. J, & Arthington, A. J. (2003). Importance of the riparian zone to the conservation and management of freshwater fish: a review. *Mar. Freshwater Res.* , 54(1), 1-16.

[44] Ferguson, C. M, Davies, C. M, Kaucner, C, Krogh, M, Rodehutskors, J, Deere, D. A, & Ashbolt, N. (2007). Field scale quantification of microbial transport from bovine faeces under simulated rainfall events. *J. Water Health* , 5, 83-95.

[45] Winkworth, C. L, Matthaei, C. D, & Townsend, C. R. (2008). Recently planted vegetation strips reduce giardia runoff reaching waterways. *J. Environ.* Qual. , 37(6), 2256-2263.

[46] Bach, P. M, Mccarthy, D. T, & Deletic, A. (2010). Redefining the stormwater first flush phenomenon. *Water Res.* , 44(8), 2487-2498.

[47] Agrawal, Y. C, & Pottsmith, H. C. (2000). Instruments for particle size and settling velocity observations in sediment transport. *Mar. Geol.* , 168, 89-114.

[48] Hipsey, M. R, Brookes, J. D, Antenucci, J. P, Burch, M. D, & Regel, R. model of Cryptosporidium dynamics in lakes and reservoirs: a new model for risk management. *Intl. J. River Basin Manage.* , 2(3), 181-197.

[49] Romero, J. R, Antenucci, J. P, & Imberger, J. (2004). One- and three- dimensional biogeochemical simulations of two differing reservoirs, *Ecol. Model.* , 174(1), 143-160.

[50] Baudisova, D. (1997). Evaluation of *Escherichia coli* as the main indicator of faecal pollution, *Water Sci. Technol.* 35(11-12): 323-336.

[51] Helmi, K, Skraber, S, Burnet, J, Leblanc, L, Hoffmann, L, & Cauchie, H. (2011). Two-year monitoring of *Cryptosporidium parvum* and *Giardia lamblia* occurrence in a recreational and drinking water reservoir using standard microscopic and molecular biology techniques. *Environ. Monit. Assess.* , 179, 163-175.

[52] Ashbolt, N. J, Grabow, W. O. K, & Snozzi, M. (2001). Indicators of microbial water quality', *In WHO | Water Quality: Guidelines, Standards and Health. Risk assessment and management for water-related infectious disease* (L. Fewtrell and J. Bartram, eds.). IWA Publishing, London.

[53] Havelaar, A. H, Van Olphen, M, & Drost, Y. C. (1993). F-specific RNA bacteriophages are adequate model organisms for enteric viruses in fresh water, *Appl. Environ. Microbiol.* , 59(9), 2956-2962.

[54] Armon, R, & Kott, Y. (1995). Distribution comparison between coliphages and phages of anaerobic bacteria (*Bacteroides fragilis*) in water sources, and their reliability as faecal pollution indicators in drinking water, *Water Sci. Technol.* 31(5-6): 215-222.

[55] Tartera, C, Lucena, F, & Jofre, J. (1989). Human origin of *Bacteroides fragilis* bacteriophage present in the environment, *Appl. Environ. Microbiol.* , 55, 2696-2701.

[56] Cornax, R, & Morinigo, M. A. (1991). Significance of several bacteriophage groups as indicator of sewage pollution in marine waters, *Water Res.* , 25(6), 673-678.

[57] Grabow, W. O. K, Taylor, M. B, & De Villiers, J. C. (2001). New methods for the detection of viruses: call for review of drinking water quality guidelines, *Water Sci. Technol.* , 46(12), 1-8.

[58] Payment, P, & Franco, E. (1993). *Clostridium perfringens* and somatic coliphages as indicators of the efficiency of drinking water treatment for viruses and protozon cysts, *Appl. Environ. Microbiol.* , 59(8), 2418-2424.

[59] Ferguson, C. M, Coote, B. G, Ashbolt, N. J, & Stevenson, I. M. (1996). Relationships between indicators, pathogens and water quality in an estuarine system, *Water Res.* , 30(9), 2045-2054.

[60] Leeming, R, Nichols, P. D, & Ashbolt, N. J. (1998). Distinguishing sources of faecal pollution in Australian inland and coastal waters using sterol biomarkers and microbial faecal indicators'. Water Services Association of Australia, Melbourne.

[61] Juranek, D. D, & Mackenzie, W. R. (1998). Drinking water turbidity and gastrointestinal illness, *Epidemiol.* , 9(3), 228-231.

[62] Ongerth, J. E, & Stibbs, H. (1989). Prevalence of *Cryptosporidium* infection in dairy calves in western Washington, *Am. J. Vet. Res. 50*, 1069-1070.

[63] Auer, M. T, & Niehaus, S. L. (1993). Modeling fecal coliform bacteria- I. Field and laboratory determination of loss kinetics, *Water Res.* , 27(4), 693-701.

[64] Jin, G, Englande, A. J, & Liu, A. (2003). A preliminary study on coastal water quality monitoring and modeling, *J. Environ. Sci. Health* A, 38(3), 493-509.

[65] Wilkinson, J, Jenkins, A, Wyer, M, & Kay, D. (1995). Modelling faecal coliform dynamics in streams and rivers, *Water Res.* , 29(3), 847-855.

[66] Salomon, J. C, & Pommepuy, M. (1990). Mathematical model of bacterial contamination of the Morlaix Estuary (France), *Water Res.* , 24(8), 983-994.

[67] Steets, B. M, & Holden, P. A. (2003). A mechanistic model of runoff-associated fecal coliform fate and transport through a coastal lagoon, *Water Res.* , 37, 589-608.

[68] Mccorquodale, J. A, Georgiou, I, Carnelos, S, & Englande, A. J. (2004). Modeling coliforms in storm water plumes, *J. Environ. Eng. Sci.* , 3, 419-431.

[69] Hipsey, M. R, & Hamilton, D. P. (2008). Computational Aquatic Ecosystem Dynamic Model: CAEDYM Science Manual v3.3. Centre for Water Research Report, Perth, Australia, 140pp.

[70] Gal, G, Imberger, J, Zohary, T, Antenucci, J. P, Anis, A, & Rosenberg, T. (2003). Simulating the thermal dynamics of Lake Kinneret. Ecol. Model. , 162, 69-86.

[71] Hipsey M. R, Bruce L. C, Boon C, Bruggeman J, Bolding K, & Hamilton D. P. (2012). GLM-FABM - Model Overview and User Documentation. The University of Western Australia Technical Manual, Perth, Australia. 44pp.

[72] Hamilton, D. P, & Schladow, S. G. (1997). Water quality in lakes and reservoirs. Part I Model description. *Ecol. Model.* , 96, 91-110.

[73] Atherholt, T. B. LeChevalier, M. W., Norton, W. D., and Rosen, J. S., (1998). Effect of rainfall on Giardia and Crypto, *J. Amer. Water Works Assoc.* , 90(9), 66-80.

[74] Walker, M. J, Montemagno, C. D, & Jenkins, M. B. (1998). Source water assessment and non-point source of acutely toxic contaminants: A review of research related to survival and transport of *Cryptosporidium parvum*, *Water Resour. Res.* , 34(12), 3383-3392.

[75] Rajala, R. L, & Heinonen-tanski, H. (1998). Survival and transfer of faecal indicator organisms of wastewater effluents in receiving lake waters, *Water Sci. Technol.* , 38(12), 191-194.

[76] Medema, G. J, & Schijven, J. F. (2001). Modelling the sewage discharge and dispersion of *Cryptosporidium* and *Giardia* in surface water, *Water Res.* , 35(18), 4307-4316.

[77] Li, Y. L, Deletic, A, Alcazar, L, Bratieres, K, Fletcher, T. D, & Mccarthy, D. T. (2012). Removal of *Clostridium perfringens, Escherichia coli* and *F-RNA coliphages* by stormwater biofilters. *Ecol. Engng.* , 49, 137-145.

[78] Wu, C. Y, Liu, J. K, Cheng, S. H, Surampalli, D. E, Chen, C. W, & Kao, C. M. (2010). Constructed wetland for water quality improvement: a case study from Taiwan. *Water Sci Technol.* , 62(10), 2408-18.

[79] Olszewski, P, & Sikorowa, A. (1973). Drawing off of hypolimnion waters as a method for improving the quality of lake waters. In: International Symposium on Eutrophication and Water Pollution Control, October 16-20, 1973, Castle Reinhardsbrudnn: , 136-141.

[80] Morillo, S, Imberger, J, & Antenucci, J. P. (2006). Modifying the residence time and dilution capacity of a reservoir by altering internal flow-paths. *Intl. J. River Basin Manage.* , 4(4), 255-271.

[81] Asaeda, T, Pham, H. S, Priyanthac, D. G. N, Manatunge, J, & Hocking, G. C. (2001). Control of algal blooms in reservoirs with a curtain: a numerical analysis. *Ecol. Engng.* , 16(3), 395-404.

[82] Hrudey, S, & Hrudey, E. J. (2004). Safe drinking water: lessons from recent outbreaks in affluent nations. IWA publishing 1-84339-042-6, 486.

Chapter 22

Biological Responses of in vivo Studies to Contaminants: A Contribution to Improve Public Health Knowledge

Maria de Lourdes Pereira,
Irvathur Krishnananda Pai and
Fernando Garcia e Costa

Additional information is available at the end of the chapter

http://dx.doi.org/10.5772/53446

1. Introduction

Global climate changes and ecosystems deterioration due to several human activities involving environmental hazards have a great impact on human welfare [1]. These factors added to many other stressors are responsible for emerging diseases worldwide, which represent an important endeavour. For this reason the risk of contaminants on human health is an expanding area of environmental epidemiology. This sub-field of epidemiology addresses, not only the environmental factors affecting the health and illness of populations but also offers public education on environmental issues. Matters such as sources of environmental contaminants, assessment of how exposure to a hazardous chemical may occur, measurement of health effects, and applying appropriate controls are relevant issues of this branh [2]. Surveillance platforms for hazardous environmental factors involving data collection and analyses, and public health promotion through evidence-based approaches are also within the scope of this growing field. Nowadays, attention to chemical and physical factors have gained special care within the scope of environmental epidemiology due to the myriad of pollutants persisting in water bodies, air, crop lands, and other environmental settings.

The example of the adverse effects on humans and other species induced by heavy metals, and metalloids spread within environment [3-12] illustrates the intersection between the environmental and human health issues. Another example, based on epidemiological studies has revealed that pesticides may cause birth deficiencies, and cancer [13].

Latest advances in scientific research and new developments on important environmental and human health topics such as the potential risk to humans from toxic chemicals in the environment were recently communicated [14]. In this matter, research elucidating the cellular and molecular mechanisms by which these environmental agents induce toxicity, mutagenesis, and carcinogenesis, among others were underlined.

Human exposure to environmental contaminants and their potentially harmful impacts on public health was more recently discussed by a panel of international experts on the conference "Human Biomonitoring: Political benefits – scientific challenges", held in Berlin 2010 [15]. In fact, health measures surveys have been implemented worldwide, and the role of human biomonitoring data has been underlined due to important risk assessment, and risk management procedures. Quantitative measure of exposure to environmental chemicals by measuring them or their metabolites in tissues (eg. hair, nails), fluids (e.g., saliva, breast milk, blood, and urine) or exhaled air are indicators of the degree of human exposure to potentially hazardous chemicals. Some widespread health impacts like diabetes, obesity, attention deficit, or hyperactivity are related to chemical exposure, as evidenced by linking human biomonitoring and epidemiological data to health effects [16].

Additionally to this topic, the importance of sentinel animal species for evaluating the potential human health impacts of chemical stressors was previously debated and the possible use of animal data into the human risk assessment process was emphasized [17]. In fact, the scientific literature evidences reports on a wide range of animal sentinels and their relevance as models for epidemiologic studies of human diseases and environmental exposures. For example, domestic and wild animals may be sensitive indicators of environmental hazards and provide an early warning system for public health, corroborating or informing epidemiologic studies in humans [18]. For example, the suitability of pet dogs was focussed since they share the same environment as humans. Additionally, large mammals were pointed in these studies due to the role as top predator species.

Advances in the development of environmental epidemiology are then illustrated by the interrelationships between humans and other forms of life sharing the same environment. In this context, several effects occurring in organisms (eg. mortality, reproductive dysfunction) in a particular ecological niche may alert to potential harmful effects on human health.

Comparison between human and wildlife exposure models revealed similarities in exposure endpoints, chemical stressors (i.e., pesticides and metals), and extent of model validation (for review see) [19].

More recently the topic "Contaminant and Pollutant effects" was discussed in a workshop organised by the Society of Environmental Toxicology and Chemistry (SETAC e Italian Branch), and newly reported [20]. Under this concern, this working group underlined that almost all the contaminants thought to be of concern in large marine vertebrates (eg. pelagic fish, whales) is of great relevance to contaminant-related human diseases. In addition, concerns over newly emerging threats such as perfluorinated compounds and nanomaterials

http://dx.doi.org/10.5772/53446

were debated. Workshop participants also highlighted the role of biomarkers to accomplish this study. To reinforce this idea the relevance of biological responses of some species was mentioned to clarify questions concerning the behaviour of persistent organic pollutants, and emerging contaminants and their impact on humans and the environment [21].This report focussed on the importance of archiving biological and environmental samples (eg. plankton, fish, marine mammals, water, sediment) for monitoring anthropogenic contaminants and a global coordination need in environmental research.

The measurement of the health consequences due to contaminants exposure is a very hard task, since different actors play in this scenario. Factors such as complexes mixtures within the environment (including chemical and biological agents), added to physical parameters (eg. see level rise, heat), and individual factors (eg. species, gender, age, nutritional, and immunological status) take an important part in this evaluation.

Apart from field studies, the use of laboratory animals in biomedical research for the benefit of human health conducted in accordance with ethical procedures, and based on the 3Rs (replacement, reduction, and refinement) remain vital. These reports emphasize the crucial value of research findings on animal species for understanding the extent and burden of health-related problems induced by xenobiotics. In fact, decisions in public health based on these findings contribute for a better formulation of health policy planning and intervention.

Although substantial progress has been devoted to the production, management, and disposal of chemicals, added to the Directives and other regulations aiming to minimise threats, past and present experiences revealed that, it is still a very multifaceted process due to several interacting factors among genetic features and environmental exposures, which deserve much attention.

This chapter is a contribution for the *in vivo* data knowledge on the relevance of both experimental laboratory mice and field studies including wildlife species in which concern to contaminants. Although some exposure models for either wildlife or humans are available following regulatory guidelines focussing on relevant endpoints, some examples, offered as a case study, include, among others, those based on our experiments. For example, the disease potential of some copepods due to their role as vectors of waterborne pathogens of humans is focussed; some fish species used as pollutants indicators are mentioned; finally, some experimental studies conducted on laboratory mice exposed to some contaminants are analysed. Those reports based on interdisciplinary techniques including histopathological, ultrastructural, biochemical, molecular and/or analytical approaches aims to characterize the biological responses to several contaminants within target organs. The last goal intends to integrate these experimental findings for environmental monitoring, and is a contribution for the understanding of human health impacts.

Finally, some issues for a more robust public health-based interdisciplinary research are recommended.

2. Relevance of animal studies for human health

A growing body of research focuses on the impact of chemical contamination on a wide range of animal species among different phyla and habitats. Adverse effects have been described alerting for the risk to humans. In this part, some representative examples are given with special emphasis for zooplankton, and fish. In addition, studies on the toxicity of contaminants on laboratory mice are presented.

Birds have been used to evaluate the presence of heavy metals in some habitats [22]. Some marine gastropod molluscs such as *Nucella lapillus* (L.) are used as bioindicators of tributyltin pollution in the North Atlantic coastlines through an important imposex assessment index [23]. Amphibians can serve as crucial and valuable research models for understanding the ecological effects of persistent contaminants such as mercury amplifying the risk of transfer of accumulated contaminants to higher trophic levels [24]. Amphibians living near uranium mines were used to assess the impacts of the locally produced acidic and metal-rich materials [25]. Copepods have broad geographic ranges, and sustain the world fisheries that nourish and support human populations [26]. They are key sensitive indicators of local and global climate change, and potential vectors of waterborne diseases. Mussels such as *Mytilus galloprovincialis,* and *Mytilus edulis* are key bivalves widely used as sentinel species [27, 28]. Mussels are suitable test species for monitoring persistent pollutants because they are sessile, filter feeders with low rates of metabolic transformation [29].

The biological signals of exposure in the above mentioned species include suitable biomarkers (eg. subcellular, cellular, functional levels) added to pollutant analysis in species. Of course, parameters such as biological cycles must be regarded as for a proper interpretation of data. Another factor to consider when dealing with wild animals is the availability of food once it may have a great influence on the immune system condition of animals [25].

2.1. Role of zooplankton with special reference to copepods in human health

The name plankton is derived from the Greek adjective - *planktos*, meaning "errant", and by extension "wanderer" or "drifter". This is in contrast to nekton organisms that can swim against the ambient flow and control their position (e.g. squid, fish, and marine mammals). Though many planktic or planktonic species are microscopic in size, plankton includes organisms covering a wide range of sizes, including large organisms such as jellyfish.

Plankton are any drifting organisms (animals, plants, or bacteria) that, inhabit the pelagic zone of oceans, seas, or bodies of freshwater. That is, plankton are defined by their ecological niche rather than phylogenetic or taxonomic classification. They provide a crucial source of food to larger, more familiar aquatic organisms such as fish and whales. Freshly hatched fish larvae are also plankton for a few days as long as they cannot swim against currents. Their density and distribution pattern varies horizontally, vertically and seasonally. This variability is mainly due to the availability of light, availability of nutrient. Besides from representing the bottom few levels of a food chain that supports commercially important fisheries, plankton ecosystems play a role in the biogeochemical cycles of many important chemical elements, including the ocean's carbon cycle. In addition, plankton species play important role in the disposal of sewage and in the natural purification of polluted water. But, some of them like dinoflagellates, their harmful bloom causes high mortality in the aquatic environment. They also act as indicator of petroleum too [30]. They are responsible for causing various diseases to animals and human beings.

Plankton are primarily divided into broad functional (or trophic level) groups: Phytoplankton (from Greek *phyton*, or plant), autotrophic, prokaryotic or eukaryotic algae that live near the water surface, where there is sufficient light to support photosynthesis. E.g. diatoms, cyanobacteria, dinoflagellates and coccolithophores; Zooplankton (from Greek *zoon*, or animal), small protozoans or metazoans (e.g. crustaceans and other animals) that feed on other plankton; Bacterioplankton, bacteria and archaea, which play an important role in remineralising organic material down the water column.

Plankton are further classified into holoplankton, which spend their entire life cycle as plankton (e.g. most algae, copepods, salps, and some jellyfish) and meroplankton, which lead a planktonic life only for a part of their lives (usually the larval stage), and then develop in to a nektic or sea floor living benthic form (eg: larvae of sea urchins, starfish, crustaceans, marine worms, and most fish.

Plankton are also classified into the following groups, based on the size of these organisms (Table 1).

Plankton inhabits in ponds, lakes, seas and oceans too and their density and distribution pattern varies horizontally, vertically and seasonally. This variability is mainly due to the availability of light, availability of nutrient.

Zooplankton can also act as a disease reservoir. They have been found to house the bacterium *Vibrio cholerae,* which causes cholera, by allowing the cholera vibrio to attach to their chitinous exoskeletons. This symbiotic relationship enhances the bacterium's ability to survive in an aquatic environment, as the exoskeleton provides the bacterium with carbon and nitrogen.

Copepods are known for extensive and varied type of parasitism. In this process they show all degrees of modifications right from slight reduction to complete disappearance. Several marine animals such as anemones, annelids, crustaceans mollusks, tunicates, fishes and even whales and sharks too are being parasitized by the copepods. They can be ectoparasites or endoparasites. Members Lernaeopodidae and Lernaeidae family (Or: Copepoda) are well known ectoparasites. Copepods of Family Caligidae are ectoparasites found on the gills, buccal cavity, and opercular cavity [31].

Copepods are multicellular animals, more abundant than any other groups including insects and nematodes [32]. Though they are mostly inhabit in natural and man-made aquatic systems, they can also inhabit nutrient-rich black oozes of abyssal ocean depths to the nutrient-poor waters of the highest mountain tarns. Some of them are found on canopies of some rain forests, hot springs, leaf-litter, in caves, between sand grains (Figure 1).

They also exhibit symbiotic associations with other animal and plant species. Their density can be as high as 92,000 individuals/L [33].

Copepods form a subclass belonging to the subphylum Crustacea (crustaceans). Copepods are divided into ten orders. Some 13,000 species of copepods are known, and 2,800 of them live in freshwaters [34].

Group	Size Range	Example
Megaplankton	(>20 mm)	Metazoans; e.g. Jellyfish; Ctenophores; Salps (e.g. Cyclosalps, Members of genus Thalia) Pelagic Tunicates (e.g. Sea Tulip, Sea Squirts or Sea Pork); Cephalopodes (e.g. Octopus, squid, Cuttle fish)
Macroplankton	(2–20 mm)	Metazoans; Chaetognaths (eg: Sagitta); Euphausids (e.g.: Antarctic krill), Medusae (e.g. Coelenterates); ctenophores; salps, doliolids (e.g. Doliolum) Tunicata Cephalopoda
Mesoplankton	(0.2 -2 mm)	Metazoans; e.g. copepods; Medusae; Cladocera; Ostracoda; Chaetognaths; Pteropods; Tunicata; Heteropoda
Microplankton	(20–200)	Large eukaryotic protists; most phytoplankton; Protozoa (Foraminifera); ciliates; Rotifera; juvenile metazoans - Crustacea (copepod nauplii)
Nanoplankton	(2–20 μm)	Small eukaryotic protists; Small Diatoms; Small Flagellates; Pyrrophyta; Chrysophyta; Chlorophyta; Xanthophyta
	(0.2–2 μm)	Small eukaryotic protists; bacteria; Chrysophyta

Table 1. Classification of plankton based on the size of organisms [30].

(a)

(b)

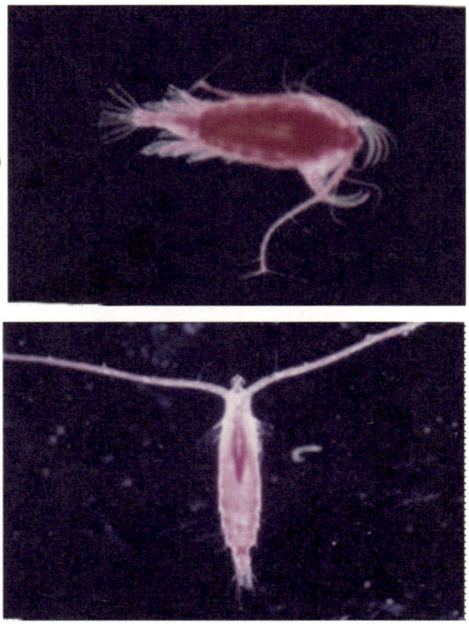

Figure 1. (a) and (b). Representative specimens of copepods: *Euchaeta marina* (a), and *Rhinocalanus cronutus* (b).

Copepods are known to carry pathogenic strains of *Vibrio* and have the potential to play important roles in cholera transmission [35]. This acute bacterial infection of the intestine caused by a few strains of bacterium *Vibrio cholerae* is transmitted through consumption of contaminated water. The bacteria needs chitinous surface of copepods to replicate. In Asia and Africa due to seasonal blooms of phytoplankton, which happen to be the food of the main food source of copepods, increases the amount of cholera-causing bacteria in waterways. When people consume bacteria infected copepod colonized water, they get cholera. The bacteria cause severe watery diarrhea, known as "rice water" diarrhea, and vomiting. Fluid loss can lead to severe dehydration and death within 24 hours of the onset of symptoms if dehydration is not treated. Poor sanitation, mixing up of sewage containing feces from cholera infected patients further contaminates water sources, allowing cholera to continue to propagate.

Apart from this aspect they are vectors of relevant human diseases. Fasciolasis also known as Distomatosis and Liver rot is an important disease caused by trematode helminthes viz., *Fasciola hepatica* (the common liver fluke or sheep live fluke) and *Fasciola gigantica*. This disease belongs to the plant-borne trematode zoonoses. In Europe, the Americas and Oceania only *F. hepatica* is common while in Asia and Africa both species have found in common. Estimated loss by this disease is pegged around US$3.2 billion per annum. As around 2.4 million people are infected ad over 180 million people are at risk, WHO has considered this disease as an emerging human disease. *Fasciola hepatica* is a parasitic flatworm (Cl: Trematoda, Ph.: Platyhelminths), that infects the liver of various mammals, including humans. *F. hepatica* is distributed worldwide, and has been known as an important parasite of sheep and cattle for hundreds of years, causing great economic losses in sheep and cattle. Thus has been the subject of many scientific investigations and may be the best known of any trematode species. They have a wide range of definitive host, which includes many herbivorous mammals, including humans. They have freshwater snails such as *Galba truncatula*, (in which the parasite can reproduce asexually) as an intermediate host for completion of their life cycle. For completion of liver fluke they pass through cercaria and miracidium larval stages, which are also considered as planktonic stages. Though a freshwater snail is required as a intermediate host, for the *F. hepatica* to complete its life cycle, Species in the family Lymnaeidae include: *Austropeplea tomentosa, Austropeplea ollula, Austropeplea viridis, Radix peregra, Radix lagotis, Radix auriculari, Radix natalensis, Radix rubiginosa, Omphiscola glabra, Lymnaea stagnalis, Stagnicola fuscus, Stagnicola palustris, Stagnicola turricul, Pseudosuccinea columella, Lymnaea viatrix, Lymnaea neotropica, Fossaria bulimoides, Lymnaea cubensis, Galba truncatula, Lymnaea cousini, Lymnaea humilis· Lymnaea diaphana, Stagnicola caperata* and *Lymnaea occulta* that serve as naturally or experimentally intermediate hosts of *Fasciola hepatica*.

Adult specimens live in bile passages of the liver of many kinds of mammals in general and ruminants in particular. Humans are also occasionally infected. In fact, fascioliasis is one of the major causes of hypereosinophilia in France. The flukes feed on the lining of biliary ducts. Their eggs are passed out of the liver with bile and into the intestine to be voided with feces. If they fall into water where the eggs complete their development and turn into miracidia, which hatch in 9 to 10 days during warm weather. During cold season it takes longer period. On hatching, miracidia have 24 hours in which find a suitable snail host. Mother sporocysts produce first generation rediae, which in turn produce daughter rediae that develop in snail's digestive gland. From the snail, minute cercariae emerge, which swim through pools of water to pasture and encyst as metacercariae on near-by vegetation. When ruminants feed on this vegetation or when human eat uncooked/semi cooked food prepared out of these plants from the pasture, the metacercariae find their way into ruminants or in human beings. In the liver, due to low pH, these encysted metacercaria start excystement. Later, these parasites break free of the metacercariae and burrows through the duodenum and intestinal lining into the peritoneal cavity. Though the newly excysted juvenile does not feed at this stage. After some days, once they find the liver parenchyma, they start feeding. This immature stage in the liver tissue is the pathogenic stage, causing anaemia and clinical signs sometimes observed in infected animals. The parasite feeds on liver tissue for a period of about six weeks, and later moves into bile duct, where it matures into an adult and begins to produce eggs. Under mild infection, these organisms can produce up to 25,000 eggs per day per fluke and can produce and deposit up to 500,000 eggs onto a pasture by a single sheep.

Trypanosomiasis also called as Chagas disease is caused in several vertebrates like horses, buffalo, dogs, cats and also human beings by parasitic protozoan trypanosomes of the genus *Trypanosoma*. It is reported that around 500,000 men, women, and children in 36 countries of sub-Saharan Africa suffer from human African trypanosomiasis and around 21,000 die due to this disease. The main casual agents are T*rypanosoma brucei gambiense* and *Trypanosoma brucei rhodesiense*.

Basically there are two types of trypanosome species viz. salivarian species and the stercorarian species trypanosoma exists. Stercorarian trypanosomes infect the insects like triatomid kissing bug, develop in its posterior gut and infective organisms are released into the faeces and deposited on the skin of the host. The organism then penetrates and can disseminate throughout the body. Insects become infected when taking a blood meal. While the second type, namely Salivarian trypanosomes develop in the anterior gut of insects, most importantly the Tsetse fly and infective organisms are inoculated into the host by the insect bite before it feeds.

As trypanosomes progress through their life cycle they undergo a series of morphological changes as is typical of trypanosomatids. The life cycle often consists of the trypomastigote form in the vertebrate host and the trypomastigote or promastigote form in the gut of the invertebrate host. Intracellular lifecycle stages are normally found in the amastigote form. The trypomastigote morphology is unique to species in the genus *Trypanosoma*.

The role of copepods as intermediate hosts of the fish parasite *Diphyllobothrium latum* is well known [36]. The life cycle of this tapeworm include copepod, and fish as first and second hosts, respectively. Human consumers of raw or lightly processed fish are final hosts. The debilitating disease, dracunculosis is vectored by freshwater copepods such as *Mesocyclops kieferi*, *M. aspericornis*, *Thermocyclops incisus*, *T. inopinus* and *T. oblongatus* of the Guinea worm, *Dracunculus mediensis* [35]. Though stomach digestive juices destroy the copepods, the larvae of the Guinea worm survive and penetrate the stomach or small intestinal wall, migrating to the subcutaneous tissue of the abdomen and thorax.

Other adverse impacts on human health of copepods include their potential as important allergens [37].

2.2. Relevance of edible fish

This section deals, mainly, with the relevance on contaminants on fish, due to the relationship between the environment and human populations through diet.

Contaminants are among the anthropogenic stresses with negative impact on water quality, thus contributing for general decline on several fish species which economical value is well recognised [38]. Moreover, hazardous chemicals alter the chemical composition of water, thus may render them susceptible to infectious diseases, being a source for several zoonotic diseases agents.

Fish is considered as one of the best indicators of heavy metal contamination in coastal milieu [39]. A number of fish species has been used as relevant bio-indicators in monitoring programs around the world. For example, skipjack tuna (*Katsuwonus pelamis*) has been used for global monitoring of wide range pollutants (eg. PCBs and organochlorine pesticides, polybrominated diphenyl ethers, polychlorinated dibenzo-p-dioxins, furans, and coplanar polychlorinated biphenyls [40-43]. Red mullets (*Mullus barbatus*) were used as sentinel organisms from anthropogenic impacted areas at Mediterranean Sea [44]. The Atlantic cod, *Gadus morhua* has been used in the Barents Sea sub-Arctic location for PAHs and metals monitoring [28]. *Anguilla anguilla, Platichthys flesus* and *Dicentrarchus labrax* are other bioindicadors of contaminants in different geographical areas [45-48].

Bottom feeders such as mullets, and flounders concentrate contaminants to a higher degree than other species.

To evaluate the biological responses of contaminants on fish a wide range of techniques have been used namely histopathology, and biochemistry of enzymes. Biomarkers such as DNA integrity and detoxification enzyme status in fish tissues have also frequently been used. Other biomarkers of aquatic pollution including fish phagocytes-induced ROS, peroxidative damage, and oxidative stress were reported on the European eel *Anguilla anguilla* [49, 50]. A battery of biomarkers together with gonad histology was used to characterize the responses of red mullets (*Mullus barbatus*) to anthropogenic pollutants [44].

The effects of some stressors were evaluated on *Platichthys flesus,* using several biomarkers [46]. Different patterns of response, namely enzymatic, genotoxic, and cytotoxic were observed on fish from impacted areas, underlying the role of reliable biomarkers for future biomonitoring studies. Other studies reported on biological responses of this flatfish to chemical stress including gene expression, genotoxicity, cholinesterase, and growth rate [51].

Novel biomarkers at molecular level, such as alterations in the expression of *xpf* gene and some of the genes found by SSH, such as HGFA were described in *Dicentrarchus labrax* and *Liza aurata* exposed to environmental contaminants [52].

Adverse changes on liver of *Poecilia vivipara* assessed semi-quantitatively using the (Histopathological Alterations Index – HAI) were described and the possibility of relationship to pesticides, heavy metals, sewage and others factors were postulated [53]. Other potential markers on environmental pollution were illustrated by analyse of matrix metalloproteinases on fish bile from *Mugil liza* and *Tilapia rendalli* [54].

High concentration values of heavy metals exceeding the permissive levels and the allowable maximum concentrations of these pollutants on organs of edible fish were reported in different species worldwide, suggesting that fishes could cause serious problems to human health, due to bioaccumulation over time; for example high levels of the most hazardous metals on muscular tissue of *Oreochromis niloticus* were reported (1.315 Cd 2.053 Pb 1.159 Hg mg/kg) representing an hazard at human health point of view [55]. Among nine commercially important species, the concentration of Mn, Fe, and Pb in a few species exceeded the WHO guideline values for safe human consumption [39]. For example muscle samples of *Lepturacanthus savala* displayed maximum levels of Pb (2.29 μg g−1). Similarly, chemical analyzes on four species (*Sarda sarda, Mulus barbatus ponticus, Trachurus trachurus* and *Merlangius merlangus* using flame and graphite furnace atomic absorption spectrometry revealed acceptable values of trace element levels. However, lead and cadmium (e.g. 0.28 ± 0.03 μg/g Pb and 0.35 ± 0.04 μg/g Cd/ *Sarda sarda*) in fish samples were higher than the recommended legal limits [56].

High mercury levels in organs of *Liza aurata* inhabiting a contaminated estuary were reported, and human risk associated to the ingestion of fish was not excluded [57].

Other reports mention lower concentration of some pollutants on fish tissues, namely muscle, being suitable for human diet. However, the influence of chemical interactions must be considered. For example heavy metal concentrations in different tissues of *Labeo rohita* and *Ctenopharyngodon idella* of Upper Lake of Bhopal were within the recommended limit values for fish consumption [58]. Although the results of this study confirm the safety for human health, these authors alert for the need of further preventive measures, since it is quite evident that there was accumulation of heavy metals in fish tissues.

Studies on heavy metals and metalloid (mercury, cadmium, lead, and arsenic) levels in the muscles of three relevant economically pelagic species (*Sardine pilchardus, Scomber japonicus* and *Trachurus trachurus*) from the Northeast and Eastern Central Atlantic Ocean revealed different patterns of contamination according to feeding behaviour [59]. Values of As>Pb>Hg>Cd for sardine, and As>Hg>Pb>Cd for chub mackerel and horse mackerel were reported. This elegant survey also estimated the potential public health risks via consumption of the mentioned species. From those studies it was concluded the safety for human consumption in terms of the amounts of cadmium and lead although moderate intake was recommended due to possible health risks derived from arsenic and mercury.

Another survey, aiming to evaluate potential risk–benefit of fish consumption was conducted using 24 common fish species collected from Chinese markets on 2007 [60]. Nutritional value and contaminants levels (DDT, PCB_7, arsenic and cadmium) were evaluated. Although mercury concentration in common carp exceeded the upper limit of the Chinese national standard these studies indicated that fish, particularly marine oily fish can be regularly consumed to achieve optimal nutritional benefits, without causing significant contaminant related health risks. Nevertheless, potential health warning was referred for people consuming large amounts of fish, namely wild fish.

Some physiological alterations such as, breathing, gastrointestinal, and skin disorders were reported as associated to individuals consuming As-contaminated fish daily and the potential risk of arsenicosis among poor people was underlined [61].

Some of the examples above mentioned illustrate the significance of pollutants release into the environment on edible fish species which may represent a warning for public health. Therefore, these findings may lead to public health interventions and policy initiatives for safeguarding human health.

2.3. Experimental studies with laboratory mice

The following section presents some examples of our experimental studies conducted with laboratory mice, aiming to illustrate the effects of some hazardous compounds at different levels of biological response (cellular, tissue, and/or physiological). Efforts aiming a cross-disciplinary interaction were done and several techniques were used, such as histology, transmission electron microscopy, and flow cytometry. These approaches complemented with chemical analysis of the toxicants or its metabolits on tissues exemplify the relationship between contamination, and injury.

Apart from our experience using this model the scientific evidence of adverse health effects from ubiquitous anthropogenic pollutants (eg. metals, metaloids, and pesticides) on both animal species and humans has been largely documented, thus, contributing to identify potential harmful chemicals for human health.

Some environmental toxicants have been shown to exhibit deleterious effects on testis, namely spermatogenesis, and fertility.

There is growing evidence that lead ($PbCl_2$) and cadmium compounds ($CdCl_2$) adversely affects spermatogenesis and fertility parameters of mice indicated by severe degenerative changes on seminiferous tubules, and poor quality of semen [62, 63]. Histopathological studies were also conducted in order to explore the extension of damage. In addition, flow cytometry (FCM) studies were performed using buffered formalin fixed and paraffin embedded paraffin samples of testicular tissue from mice exposed to cadmium and lead chloride per se, in order to establish the ploidy level of germ cells. Significant alterations in germ cell percentages in mice exposed to cadmium were detected by FCM, supporting the histopathological data [62]. However, no alterations in the percentages of testicular germ cells detected by FCM were evident in animals exposed to lead chloride, excepting of an increase in the percentage of cells in S phase.

Further reports, by using several biomarkers at subcellular level of sperm physiology such as DNA fragmentation, and chromatin integrity, assessed by the terminal deoxylnucleotidyl transferase-mediated deoxyuridine triphosphate (dUTP) nick-end labelling (TUNEL), and sperm chromatin structure assays (SCSA), respectively, coupled to other techniques for evaluation of sperm function authors demonstrated that lead chloride affects physiological parameters such as motility, morphology, and acrosome status, although no significant genotoxic effects were noted [63]. In fact, sperm DNA is in general resistant due to its highly compacted nature. Those reports also evidenced the role of flow cytometry as a powerful tool for quantitative analyses of different cell types and an insight on cell cycle status, added to the measurement of DNA content of cell subpopulations in the testis.

More recently the genotoxic effects induced by cadmium were reported using a panel of suitable microsatellites as markers of genetic instability [64].

The effects on testis after co-exposure to lead and cadmium were also described on mice through a histological approach [65]: seminiferous epithelium degeneration, exfoliation of germ cells into the lumen, distorted morphology of tubules was accompanied by atrophy. Work in progress in our laboratory demonstrated adverse effects of this mixture on other target organs such as kidney, spleen, and liver, comparing with respective controls (Figures 2 and 3). Degenerative aspects were noted on renal cortical area; splenic sections denoted cell loosening and numerous macrophages; hepatic parenchyma displays several haemorrhagic foci. Overall, the histopathological study revealed several adverse changes pointing obviously for dysfunctions.

Another illustration of a toxicant targeting the male reproductive function of mice was the research conducted with sodium arsenite [66]. Awareness was directed to spermatogenesis, a multipart process involving delicate cells such as germ cells, often targets of a wide range of contaminants. Impairment of spermatogenesis was found on testis sections, complemented with biochemical parameters. Those issues have been established as suitable in the evaluation of physiological disorders in mice.

Further studies aiming to explore and characterize possible recovery of sperm morphology and functional parameters after withdrawal of the toxicant revealed several changes at ultrastructural level, namely irregular pattern of chromatin, and altered acrosome [67]. In addition, a molecular approach demonstrated high DNA fragmentation index revealing abnormal chromatin structure. In this work, as in present studies on this topic, transmission electron microscopy studies were pertinent to identify fine changes on cell organelles (Figure 4).

Work in progress also demonstrated the effects of sodium arsenite on splenic structure of dosed animals (Figure 5). The degree of lesions was irregular: some areas of the spleen evidenced reduced cellular concentration (Figure 5a) and disruption (Figure 5b), respectively, within white pulp comparing with controls (data not shown). In addition, an increase of megakaryocytes was observed, probably due to the required phagocytic activity.

Histopathology coupled with ultrastructural studies were sensitive tools for the detection of adverse effects of sodium arsenite on target organs (eg. testis) allowing information on the nature of the lesions, and its eventual recovery.

http://dx.doi.org/10.5772/53446

(a)
(b)
(c)

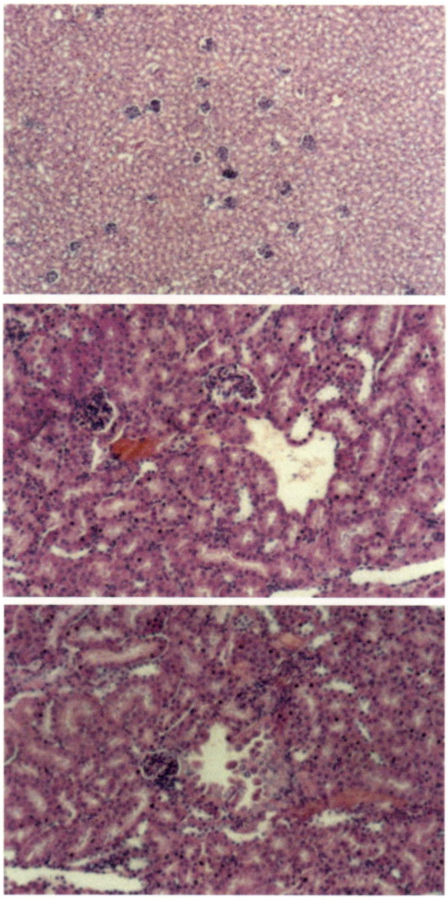

Figure 2. Representative histological section from kidneys of controls where regular pattern of organization is observed (a), and lead and cadmium co-exposure on mice ((b), and (c)). Figures (b), and figure (c) display haemorrhagic focus, and strong dilation of intertubular spaces. Cell detachment is evident. Haematoxylin & eosin staining (HE). Original magnification: Figure (b) – 40x; Figure (c), and 5 – 100x.

The relevance of toxicity of some chromium compounds, namely hexavalent chromium generated by production industries such as leather tanning, and chrome plating, were investigated on mice [68-70]. In these studies Cr(VI), a proved strong carcinogenic, was investigated in vivo in order to evaluate Cr(VI), and Cr(V) reduction effects on the target organs such as testis, liver, and kidneys. For example it was demonstrated that Cr(V), in the form of $[CrV\text{-}BT]^{2-}$ is a male reprotoxicant, causing several histological and ultrastructural changes in mice spermatogenesis [68]. One of the most representative lesions was the loss of acrosome sperm integrity, as demonstrated by electron microscopy studies. Adverse effects were also observed on cauda epididymis, namely epithelial vacuolation. Altogether, these lesions confirm the potent toxicity of this compound.

(a) (b) (c) (d)

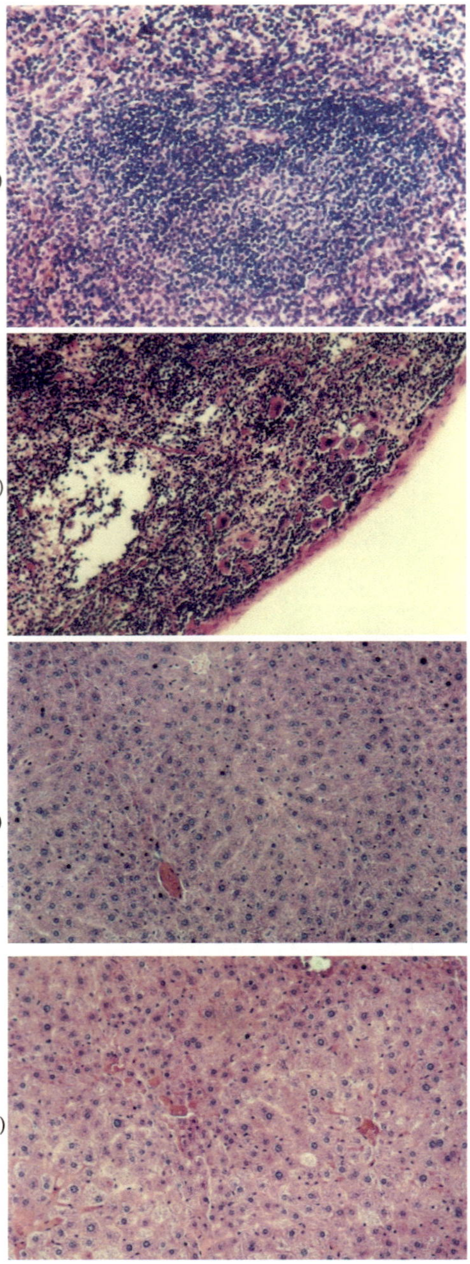

Figure 3. Representative histological sections from spleen, and liver from controls (Figures a,c), and cadmium-lead exposed mice (Figures b,d). A great number of megakaryocytes are evident in spleen (Figure b); WP – White pulp. Several hemorrhagic areas are seen in hepatic parenchyma (Figure d). Original magnification: Figures a-d – 100x; haematoxylin & eosin staining.

http://dx.doi.org/10.5772/53446

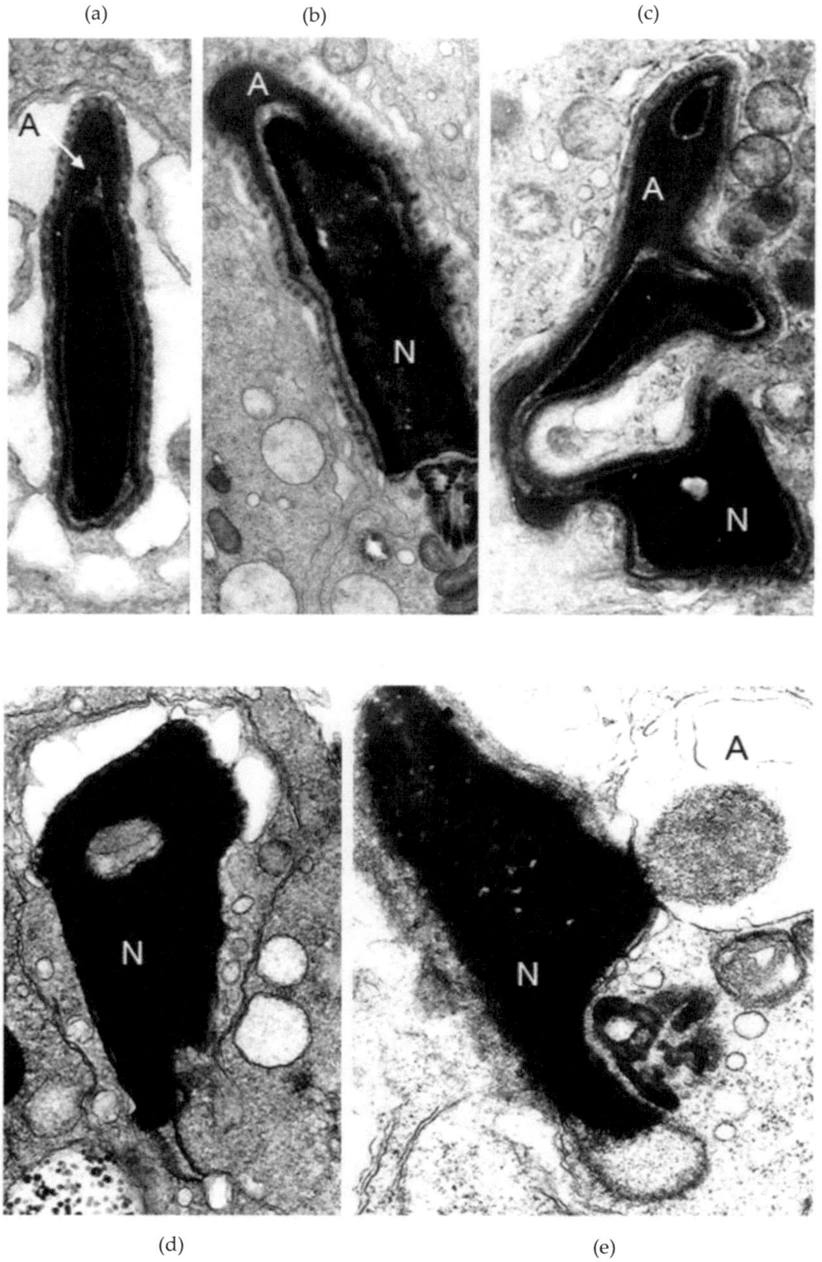

Figure 4. Transmission electron micrographs from spermatozoa and late spermatids in control (a) and sodium arsenite exposed animals during seven days where some morphological irregularities are seen (b-e). N – nucleus; A – acrosome; double staining with uranyl acetate and lead citrate. Original magnification : Figures a -c – x6,700; Figure d – x10,000 ; Figure e – x14,000.

(a)

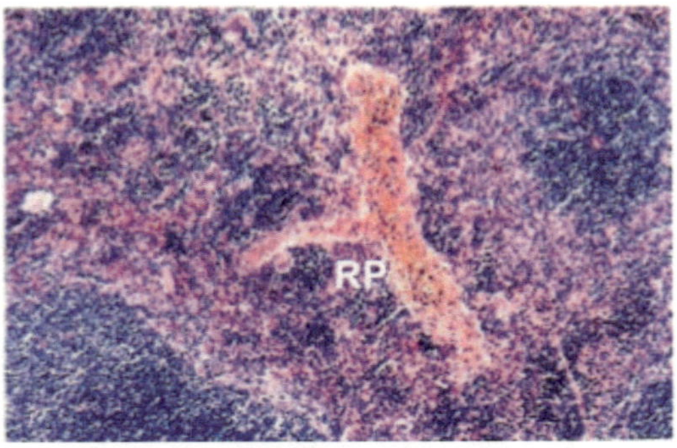

(b)

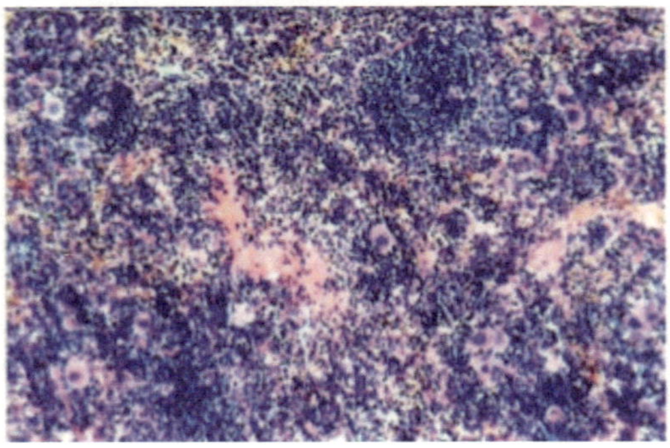

Figure 5. Representative sections of spleen from sodium arsenite dosed group, displaying injury of red pulp (RP) (a), and altered morphology pattern of white pulp (b). Original magnification Figure 5 –x100; haematoxylin & eosin staining.

In a subsequent study the reproductive toxicity on testis and sperm cell's function was evaluated on mice exposed to potassium chromate through a wide range of approaches for a more comprehensive analysis of its effects [70]. Chromium contents on mice testes were determined by inductively coupled plasma mass spectrometry (ICP-MS), and higher levels of chromium were found on K_2CrO_4 exposed group. Histology data of testis were supported by the analysis of testicular cellular subpopulations by flow cytometry. Multiple abnormalities were noted on sperm cells after one cycle of spermatogenic process, such as decreased motility, and percentage of cells with intact acrosome, revealing a premature acrosome reaction. Although no DNA damage on sperm cells assayed by SCSA was observed, altogether those results underlined the reprotoxic effects of hexavalent chromium compounds. Although no histopathological changes on testis or epididymis were noted, a reduction in seminiferous tubules diameter occurred on exposed animals, as determined by software based on deformable models (Snakes) as previously reported [71]. These authors have demonstrated the suitability of this method for evaluation of seminiferous tubules diameter in mice exposed to chromium compounds, one of the relevant parameters for testis damage. Also, the functional properties of Sertoli cells from mice exposed to Cr(V) were investigated using ultrastructural tracer techniques [72]. Horseradish peroxidase added in vitro to the medium was used to follow the route of macromolecules. Seminiferous tubules were then placed into this medium, and the marker penetrated freely on the blood-testis barrier compared to controls, evidencing the toxicity induced by the reduction of Cr(VI) compounds.

Other organs such as kidneys were also affected by hexavalent chromium [69].

Similar approaches were conducted to clarify the nephrotoxicity of chromium copper arsenate (CCA), and its constituents *per se* using mice as models [73-75]. Although this mixture (CCA type C - 34.0% As_2O_5, 47.5% CrO_3 and 18.5% CuO, w/w) was broadly used in the past, as a wood preservative, elevate levels of residues as arsenic still remain in the environment posing a great hazard for public health. For example, CCA, arsenic pentoxide, and chromium trioxide were studied per se on kidneys, based on histopathology, and histochemistry. Correlating histology, and histochemistry with the chromium and arsenic analyses (ICP-MS and GFAAS) on kidney, the synergetic effect of the components (pentavalent arsenic and hexavalent chromium) within the mixture conducted to acute tubular necrosis. The histochemistry assay confirmed the presence of carbohydrate, and proteins filling the tubular lumen; the degeneration of epithelial cells (both in cortex and medulla) was also noted. In addition, higher values of arsenic in CCA-exposed group when noted to those submitted to As_2O_5 one of the components of CCA.

Some of the abovementioned studies based case-by-case underline the contribution of animal research for the understanding of the adverse effects of harmful chemicals on human health.

3. Conclusion and future perspectives

Globally, the field of environmental epidemiology has gained substantial attention in current days due to the adverse effects on human health induced by the myriad of pollutants persisting in air, oceans and freshwater, and agriculture soils. In addition, natural resources which safeguard and support human life are also affected by contaminants. A growing body of research focuses on how the environment can damage human life, through the understanding of toxicity signs in other animal species among different taxa. In this concern, a wide range of biological responses were described (eg. reduction of the population, changes in reproductive pattern, and loss of some species). Surveillance programs have been conducted around the world using key species for contaminants monitoring. These studies showed that accumulation and biomagnification of current hazardous chemicals occurs in many species.

Zooplankton can very well act as bio indicators for probable and possible spread of diseases. Breaking the link between such kind of zooplankton and the hosts will result in non-completion of the life cycle of several such disease causing agents which are threatening the human kind. This will also help in having a healthy world.

Other relevant aspect to report is the overall benefits on human health populations due to regular fish consumption. Trials conducted worldwide based on the nutrients value suggests that fish intake based on policy recommendation lowers the risk of some diseases. Several international regulatory agencies such as the Codex Alimentarius Commission, and European Commission, Council and Parliament and Food and Agriculture Organization/ World Health Organization conventioned maximum limits for numerous contaminants on edible fish.

On the other hand, the accumulation of harmful residues in fish fillets, even below the maximum limit, may alert for future surveillance. A comprehensive risk–benefit evaluation of fish intake is essential and consumption advisories for specific populations such as pregnant women, and children are required.

The last part of this chapter outlines the contribution of laboratory studies using mice for the knowledge of biological mechanisms and toxicity of several hazardous chemicals. The use of laboratory rodents in biomedical research still remains useful to identify potential responses of harmful chemicals under controlled conditions. However, ethics in animal care and procedures must be considered.

The examples mentioned in this chapter highlight that changes occurring in lower levels of biological organization such as copepods, fish, and mammals, added to the environment surrounding affecting humans, may predict, or may alert to potential harmful effects on human health highlighting the role of environmental epidemiology as an emergent discipline. In fact, monitoring health problems within fauna, and health hazards may contribute for searching new solutions, thus improving the quality of live. An integrated monitoring of species from different taxa with trophic relevance permit a more comprehensive outlook of environmental health problems, and is an important step forward to protect wildlife and human health. However, these approaches comparing effects among different species that might occurs in humans as well, needs a special attention in extrapolating result in animals to humans.

In conclusion, this chapter clearly shows that, the contribution of the need for further local, and global multi-and inter-disciplinary research involving critical representative trophic chain species within impacted areas, since they offer important data. The valuable information of human biomonitoring combined with watchfulness on different species and humans sharing the same environment is needed. A continued focus to promote coordination of biobanks, and data harmonisation is encouraged aiming to formulate public health strategies in the future. In addition, new technologies including analytical methods for detection of contaminants, and multiplicity of biomarkers at different biological levels of organization represent decisive advances in this field.

Acknowledgements

This work was funded by the Research Centre on Ceramic and Composite Materials (CICECO) from Aveiro University (Portugal). Pest-C/CTM/LA0011/2011- FCT is acknowledged. Thanks to Mr. Aldiro Pereira for preparing photographs. Thanks to Mr. Aldiro Pereira for preparing photographs.

Author details

Maria de Lourdes Pereira[1], Irvathur Krishnananda Pai[2] and Fernando Garcia e Costa[3]

*Address all correspondence to: mlourdespereira@ua.pt

1 Departament of Biology & CICECO, Aveiro University, Aveiro, Portugal

2 Department of Zoology, Goa University, Goa, India

3 Departament of Morphology & Function, CIISA, Faculty of Veterinary Medicine, Technical University of Lisbon, Portugal

References

[1] Smol J.P. A planet in flux. Nature 2012; 483, S12-S15.

[2] Merrill R.M. Introduction to Environmental Epidemiology. In: Environmental Epidemiology: Principles and Methods, Jones & Bartlett Learning; 2008. p3-25.

[3] Kah M, Levy L & Brown C. Potential for effects of land contamination on human health. 1. The case of cadmium. Journal of Toxicology & Environmental Health B Critical Reviews 2012; 15(5), 348-363.

[4] Eisler R. Mercury hazards to living organisms. CRC Press, Boca Raton; 2006.

[5] Mudgal V., Madaan N., Mudgal A., Singh R.B. & Mishra S. Effect of Toxic Metals on Human Health. The Open Nutraceuticals Journal 2010; 3, 94-99.

[6] Jomova K. & Valko M. Advances in metal-induced oxidative stress and human disease. Toxicology 2011; 283, 65–87.

[7] Harmanescu M., Alda L.M., Bordean D.M., Gogoasa I., & Gergen I. Heavy metals health risk assessment for population via consumption of vegetables grown in old mining area; a case study: Banat Country, Romania. Chemistry Central Journal 2011; 5: 64-74.

[8] Huss J. Health hazards of heavy metals and other metals. Council of Europe. Doc. 12613, 12 May 2011. http://assembly.coe.int/Documents/WorkingDocs/Doc11/EDOC12613.pdf (accessed 6 September 2012).

[9] Cooksey C. Health concerns of heavy metals and metalloids. Science Progress 2012; 95(1), 1–16.

[10] Argos M., Ahsan H., Graziano J.H. Arsenic and human health: epidemiologic progress and public health implications. Reviews on Environmental Health 2012. http://www.ncbi.nlm.nih.gov/pubmed/22962196 (accessed 7 September 2012).

[11] Morais S., Costa F.G. & Pereira M.L. Heavy Metals & Human Health. In: Jacques O. (ed.) Environmental Health - Emerging Issues and Practice, 1st Ed.; InTech; 2012a. p227-246.

[12] Morais S., Costa F.G. & Pereira M.L. Thoughts on Evaluation of Heavy Metals Toxicity. In: James C. (ed.) Advances in Chemistry Research 14, Taylor; Nova Science Publishers; Inc. 2012b. https://www.novapublishers.com/catalog/product_info.php?products_id=30588&osCsid= (accessed 2 September 2012).

[13] Environmental Protection Agency. Pesticides and Food: Health Problems Pesticides May Pose. http://www.epa.gov/pesticides/food/risks.htm (accessed 7 September 2012).

[14] Tchounwou P.B. Editorial. International Journal of Environmental Research & Public Health 2010; 7, 2131-2135.

[15] Schulz C., Calafat A.M., Haines D., Becker K.B. & Kolossa-Gehring M. Editorial. International Conference on Human Biomonitoring, Berlin 2010. International Journal of Hygiene & Environmental Health 215; 91– 92.

[16] Meeting report. Human biomonitoring: Political benefits—Scientific challenges. September 26–28, 2010. International Journal of Hygiene & Environmental Health 2012; 215: 247– 252.

[17] van der Schalie W.H., Gardner Jr. H.S., Bantle J.A., De Rosa C.T., Finch R.A., Reif J.S., Reuter R.H., Backer L.C., Burger J., Folmar L.C. & Stokes W.S. Animals as Sentinels of Human Health Hazards of Environmental Chemicals. Environmental Health Perspectives 1999; 107: 309-315.

[18] Reif J.S. Animal sentinels for environmental and public health. Public Health Reports 2011; Supplement 1, 126, 50-57.

[19] Loos M., Schipper A.M., Schlink U., Strebel K. & Ragas Ad.M.J. Receptor-oriented approaches in wildlife and human exposure modelling: a comparative study. Environmental Modelling & Software 2010; 25: 369–382.

[20] Fossi M.C., Casini S., Caliani I., Panti C., Marsili L., Viarengo A., Giangreco R., di Sciara G.N., Serena F., Ouerghi A. & Depledge M.H. The role of large marine vertebrates in the assessment of the quality of pelagic marine ecosystems. Marine Environmental Research 2012; 77, 156-158.

[21] Tanabe S. & Ramu K. Monitoring temporal and spatial trends of legacy and emerging contaminants in marine environment: Results from the environmental specimen bank (es-BANK) of Ehime University, Japan. Marine Pollution Bulletin 2012; 64, 1459–1474.

[22] Costa R.A., Petronilho J. M. S., Soares A. M. V. M. & Vingada J. V. The use of passerine feathers to evaluate heavy metal pollution in Central Portugal. Bulletim of Environmental Contamination & Toxicology 2011; 86, 352–356.

[23] Galante-Oliveira S., Oliveira I., Santos J.A., Pereira M.L., Pacheco M. & Barroso C. Factors affecting RPSI in imposex monitoring studies using Nucella lapillus (L.) as bioindicator. Journal of Environment Monitoring 2010; 12, 1055-1063.

[24] Todd B.D., Bergeron C. M. & Hopkins W.H. Use of toe clips as a nonlethal index of mercury accumulation and maternal transfer in amphibians. Ecotoxicology 2012; 21, 882–887.

[25] Marques S.M., Antunes S.C., Pissarra H., Pereira M.L., Gonçalves F. & Pereira R. Histopathological changes and erythrocytic nuclear abnormalities in Iberian green frogs (Rana perezi Seoane) from a uranium mine pond. Aquatic Toxicology 2009, 91, 187-195.

[26] Bron J.E., Frisch D., Goetze E., Johnson S.C., Lee C.M. & Wyngaard G. A. Observing copepods through a genomic lens. Frontiers in Zoology, 2011; 8:22, 1-15.

[27] Zorita I., Apraiz I., Ortiz-Zarragoitia M., Orbea A., Cancio I., Soto M., Marigómez I. & Cajaraville M.P. Assessment of biological effects of environmental pollution along the NW Mediterranean Sea using mussels as sentinel organisms. Environmental Pollution 2007; 148, 236-250.

[28] Nahrganga J., Brooks S.J., Evenseta A., Camusa L., Jonssona M., Smitha T.J., Lukinaa J., Frantzena M., Giarratano E. & Renauda P.E. Seasonal variation in biomarkers in blue mussel (Mytilus edulis), Icelandic scallop (Chlamys islandica) and Atlantic cod (Gadus morhua)—Implications for environmental monitoring in the Barents Sea. Aquatic Toxicology 2012. http://www.sciencedirect.com/science/article/pii/S0166445X12000227# (accessed 2 September 2012).

[29] Galloway, T.S. Biomarkers in environmental and human health risk assessment. Marine Pollution Bulletin (2006); 53, 606–613.

[30] Battish S.K. Freshwater zooplankton of India. New Delhi, India, Oxford and IBH publishing Co; 1992.

[31] Nair N.B. & Thumpy D.M., A textbook of Marine Ecology, New Delhi, India. The MacMillan Company: 1990.

[32] Humes A. How many copepods? In: F.D. Ferrari & B.P. Bradley (eds.). Ecology and morphology of copepods: proceedings of Fith International Conference on Copepoda, 292/293, London: Springer: 1-7, 1994.

[33] Buskey E.J., Peterson, J.O. & Ambler J.W. The swarming behavior of the copepod Dioithona oculata: In situ and laboratory studies. Limnology and Oceanography 1996; 41: 513-521.

[34] Boxhall, G.A. & Defaye D. Global diversity of copepods (Crustacea: Copepoda) in freshwater. Hydrobiologia 2008; 595 (1): 195–207.

[35] Bron J., Boore J., Boxshall G., Bricknell I., Frisch D., Goetze E., Hansen B., Johnson S., Lee C.E., Lee J., Lenz P., Skern R., Willet C. & Wyngaard G. Copepod Genome Initia-

tive. White Paper for the Development of Large-Scale Genomics Resources for Copepods. World Association of Copepodologists, 2009; July 2nd.1-53.

[36] Piasecki, W.,Goodwin A.E., Eiras J.C. & Nowak B.F. Importance of Copepoda in Freshwater Aquaculture. Zoological Studies 2004; 43(2): 193-205.

[37] Muthiah, R., Kagen S., Burton, R. S. Copepods: Worldwide Sources of Allergens - Partial Sequences of Three Unique Proteins. Journal of Allergy & Clinical Immunology 2005; 115(2): PS91.

[38] ICES, 2010. Report of the ICES Advisory Committee, ICES Advice 2010; Book 9, pp. 115–123.

[39] Biswas S., Prabhu R.K., Hussain K.J., Selvanayagam M., & Satpathy K.K. Heavy metals concentration in edible fishes from coastal region of Kalpakkam, southeastern part of India. Environmental Monitoring Assessment 2012; 184, 5097–5104.

[40] Ueno D., Takahashi S., Tanaka H., Subramanian A., Fillman G., Nakat H., Lam P.K.S., Zheng J., Muchtar M., Prudente M., Chung K.H. & Tanabe S. Global pollution monitoring of PCBs and organochlorine pesticides using skipjack tuna as a bioindicator. Archives of Environmental Contamination and Toxicology 2003; 45: 378–389.

[41] Ueno D., Kajiwara N., Tanaka H., Subramanian A., Fillmann G., Lam P.K.S., Zheng G.J., Muchtar M., Razak H., Prudente M., Chung K.H. & Tanabe S. Global pollution monitoring of polybrominated diphenyl ethers using skipjack tuna as a bioindicator. Environmental Science & Technology 2004; 38: 2312–2316.

[42] Ueno D., Watanabe M., Subramanian A., Tanaka H., Fillmann G., Lam P.K., Zheng G.J., Muchtar M., Razak H., Prudente M., Chung, K.H. & Tanabe S. Global pollution monitoring of polychlorinated dibenzo-p-dioxins (PCDDs), furans (PCDFs) and coplanar polychlorinated biphenyls (coplanar PCBs) using skipjack tuna as bioindicator. Environmental Pollution 2005; 136: 303–313.

[43] Ueno D., Alaee M., Marvin C., Muir D.C., Macinnis G., Reiner E., Crozier P., Furdui V.I., Subramanian A., Fillmann G., Lam P.K., Zheng G.J., Muchtar M., Razak H., Prudente M., Chung K.H. & Tanabe S. Distribution and transportability of hexabromocyclododecane (HBCD) in the Asia-Pacific region using skipjack tuna as a bioindicator. Environmental Pollution 2006; 144: 238–247.

[44] Zorita I., Ortiz-Zarragoitia M., Apraiz I., Cancio I., Orbea A., Soto M., Marigómez I. & Cajaraville M.P. Assessment of biological effects of environmental pollution along the NW Mediterranean Sea using red mullets as sentinel organisms. Environmental Pollution 2008; 153 157-168.

[45] Pacheco M., Santos M.A., van Der Gaag M.A., The ecotoxicological relevance of Anguilla anguilla L. as a proposed model for brackish-water genetic toxicological studies. Science of Total Environment 1993; (Suppl.) Part 1: 817–822.

[46] Napierska D., Janina Barsiene J., Mulkiewicz E., Podolska P. & Rybakovas A. Biomarker responses in flounder Platichthys flesus from the Polish coastal area of the Baltic Sea and applications in biomonitoring. Ecotoxicology 2009; 18, 846–859.

[47] Dabrowska H., Ostaszewska T., Kamaszewski M., Antoniak A., Napora-Rutkowski L., Kopko O., Lang T., Fricke N.F., Lehtonen K.K. Histopathological, histomorphometrical, and immunohistochemical biomarkers in flounder (Platichthys flesus) from the southern Baltic Sea. Ecotoxicology and Environmental Safety 2012; 78, 14–21.

[48] Abreu S.N., Pereira E., Vale C. & Duarte A.C. Accumulation of Mercury in Sea Bass from a Contaminated Lagoon (Ria de Aveiro, Portugal). Marine Pollution Bulletin 2000; 40(4), 293-297.

[49] Ahmad I., Pacheco M. & Santos M.A. Anguilla anguilla L. oxidative stress biomarkers: An in situ study of freshwater wetland ecosystem (Pateira de Fermentelos, Portugal). Chemosphere 2006; 65: 952–962.

[50] Santos M.A., Pacheco M. & Ahmad I. Responses of European eel (Anguilla anguilla L.) circulating phagocytes to an in situ closed pulp mill effluent exposure and its association with organ-specific peroxidative damage. Chemosphere 2006; 63, 794–801.

[51] Evrard E., Devaux A., Bony S., Burgeot T., Riso R., Budzinski H., Du M.L., Quiniou L. & Laroche J. Responses of the European "flounder Platichthys flesus to the chemical stress in estuaries: load of contaminants, gene expression, cellular impact and growth rate. Biomarkers, 2010; 15(2): 111–127.

[52] Nogueira P., Pacheco M., Pereira M.L., Mendo S. & Rotchell J.M. Novel potential molecular biomarkers of aquatic contamination in Dicentrarchus labrax and Liza aurata. In: Hamamura N., Suzuki S., Mendo S., Barroso C.M., Iwata H. and Tanabe S. (eds.) Interdisciplinary Studies on Environmental Chemistry — Biological Responses to Contaminants. Terrapub; 2010. p127–138.

[53] Paulo D.V., Fontes F.M. & Flores-Lopes F. Histopathological alterations observed in the liver of Poecilia vivipara (Cyprinodontiformes: Poeciliidae) as a tool for the environmental quality assessment of the Cachoeira River, BA. Brazilian Journal of Biology 2012; 72, 131-140.

[54] Hauser-Davisa R.A., Lima A.A., Ziolli R.L. & Campos R.C. First-time report of metalloproteinases in fish bile and their potential as bioindicators regarding environmental contamination. Aquatic Toxicology 2012; 110-111: 99-106.

[55] Authman M.M.N., Wafa T. Abbas, W.T. & Gaafar A.Y. Metals concentrations in Nile tilapia Oreochromisniloticus (Linnaeus, 1758) from illegal fish farm in Al-Minufiya Province, Egypt, and their effects on some tissues structures. Ecotoxicology & Environmental Safety 2012; 84: 163–172.

[56] Mendil D., Demirci Z., Tuzen M. & Soylak M. Seasonal investigation of trace element contents in commercially valuable fish species from the Black sea, Turkey. Food and Chemical Toxicology 2010; 48: 865–870.

[57] Mieiro C.L., Pacheco M., Pereira M.E. & Duarte A.C. Mercury distribution in key tissues of fish (Liza aurata) inhabiting a contaminated estuary-mplications for human and ecosystem health risk assessment. Journal of Environmental Monitoring 2009; 11: 1004–1012.

[58] Malik N., Biswas A.K., Qureshi T.A., Borana K. & Virha R. Bioaccumulation of heavy metals in fish tissues of a freshwater lake of Bhopal. Environmental Monitoring Assessment 2010; 160, 267–276.

[59] Vieira C., Morais S., Ramos S., Delerue-Matos C. & Oliveira M.B.P.P. Mercury, cadmium, lead and arsenic levels in three pelagic fish species from the Atlantic Ocean: intra- and inter-specific variability and human health risks for consumption. Food & Chemical Toxicology 2011; 49, 923-932.

[60] Du Z.Y., Zhang J., Wang C., Li L., Man Q., Lundebye A.K. & Frøyland L. Risk–benefit evaluation of fish from chinese markets: nutrients and contaminants in 24 fish species from five big cities and related assessment for human health. Science of the Total Environment 2012; 416, 187–199.

[61] Shah A.Q., Kazi T.G., Baig J.A. & Afridi H.I. Correlation between arsenic concentration in fish and human scalp hair of people living in arsenic-contaminated and non-contaminated areas of pakistan. Biology of Trace Elements Research 2011; 144(1-3): 197-204.

[62] Oliveira H., Loureiro J., Filipe L., Santos C., Ramalho-Santos J., Sousa M. & Pereira M.L. Flow cytometry evaluation of lead and cadmium effects on mouse spermatogenesis. Reproductive Toxicology 2006a; 22, 529–535.

[63] Oliveira H., Spanò M., Santos C. & Pereira M.L. Lead affects mice sperm motility and acrosome reaction. Cell Biology & Toxicology 2009; 25, 341–353.

[64] Oliveira H., Lopes T., Almeida T., Pereira M.L. & Santos C. Microsatellite instability in mice exposed to cadmium. Human & Experimental Toxicology 2012. doi: 10.1177/0960327112445937.

[65] Pereira M.L., Rodrigues N.V. & Garcia e Costa F. Histomorphological evaluation of mice testis after co-exposure to lead and cadmium. Asian Pacific Journal of Reproduction 2012; 1: 35-38.

[66] Ferreira M., Matos R.C., Oliveira H., Nunes B., & Pereira M.L. Impairment of mice spermatogenesis by sodium arsenite. Human and Experimental Toxicology 2012; 31, 290-302.

[67] Pereira M.L. & Garcia e Costa F. Cytotoxic effects of sodium arsenite on mice sperm cells: conference proceedings. 10th International Congress on Cell Biology, July 25-28, 2012, Rio Convention & Exhibition Centre, Brazil; 2012.

[68] Pereira M.L., das Neves R.P., Oliveira H., Santos T.M. & de Jesus J.P. Effect of Cr(V) on reproductive organ morphology and sperm parameters: an experimental study in mice. Environmental Health 2005; 27, 4-9.

[69] Oliveira H., Santos T.M., Ramalho-Santos J. & Pereira M.L. Histopathological effects of hexavalent chromium in mice kidney. Bulletin of Environmental Contamination and Toxicology 2006b; 76, 977–983.

[70] Oliveira H., Spano M., Guevara M.A., Santos T.M., Santos C. & Pereira M.L. Evaluation of in vivo reproductive toxicity of potassium chromate in male mice. Experimental & Toxicologic Pathology 2010; 62: 391-404.

[71] Guevara M.A., Silva A., Oliveira H., Pereira M.L. & Morgado F. Segmentation and morphometry of histological sections using deformable models: a new tool for evaluating testicular histopathology. In: Sanfeliu A, Shulcloper JR, editors. Progress in pattern recognition, speech and image analysis: Ciarp 2003. Lecture Notes in Computer Science 2003; 2905, 282–290.

[72] Pereira M.L., Santos T.M., Garcia e Costa F. & Pedrosa de Jesus J. Functional Changes of mice Sertoli cells induced by Cr(V). Cell Biology & Toxicology 2004; 20: 285-291.

[73] Matos R.C., Vieira C., Morais S., Pereira M.L. & Pedrosa de Jesus J.P. Nephrotoxicity of CCA-treated wood: a comparative study with As_2O_5 and CrO_3 on mice. Environmental Toxicology & Pharmacology 2009a; 27, 259–263.

[74] Matos R.C., Vieira C., Morais S., Pereira M.L. & Pedrosa de Jesus J.P. Nephrotoxicity effects of the wood preservative chromium copper arsenate on mice: histopathological and quantitative approaches. Journal of Trace Elements in Medicine & Biology 2009b; 23, 224-230.

[75] Matos R.C., Vieira C., Morais S., Pereira M.L. & Pedrosa de Jesus J.P. Toxicity of chromated copper arsenate: A study in mice. Environmental Research 2010; 110, 424-427.

Chapter 23

Atmospheric Nanoparticles and Their Impacts on Public Health

Klara Slezakova, Simone Morais and
Maria do Carmo Pereira

Additional information is available at the end of the chapter

http://dx.doi.org/10.5772/54775

1. Introduction

The World Health Organization (WHO) estimates that every year around two million people die annually due to the effects of atmospheric pollution (Tranfield & Walker, 2012). These estimates are based on epidemiological studies that showed associations between air pollution exposure and respiratory and cardiovascular illnesses and deaths. Special efforts thus have been made in order to reduce air pollution on a global level (Slezakova et al., 2012) and, more importantly, aiming to reduce the adverse impacts of atmospheric pollutants. Although these efforts have been leading to a reduction of risks and effects, air pollution is still a matter of great concern, mainly to relative impacts on human health.

Air pollution is a mixture of various gases such as ozone, carbon monoxide, sulphur dioxide, and nitrogen dioxide combined with airborne particles in sizes range of few nanometers to hundreds of micrometers. According to the WHO, these particles are one of the most important pollutants of present times and their presence in the atmosphere has harmful effects both on human health and environment. Nanosized particles (i.e. smaller than 100 nm) are a subgroup of atmospheric particles. Though humans have been exposed to nanosized particles throughout their evolutionary stages, the respective exposure has dramatically increased over the last century due to contribution from various anthropogenic sources. In addition, the rapidly developing field of nanotechnology is likely to become another source of these particles through increased use of engineered nanomaterials. Thus information about safety and potential hazards is urgently needed. Apart from their role for possible adverse health effects (Hoek et al., 2010; Knol et al., 2009), nanoparticles are important precursors for the formation of coarser particles that are known to strongly influence global climate (Intergovernmental Panel on Climate Change [IPCC], 2007; Strawa et al., 2010) and urban visibility (Horvath, 1994). They may also influence the atmospheric chemistry in general as their chemical composition and reactivity are different from coarser particles, thus opening novel chemical transformation pathways in the atmosphere (Anastasio & Martin, 2001).

This chapter focuses specifically on airborne nanosized particles and their importance to public health. Various aspects are discussed in the following sections including sources, levels, chemical compositions, regulations, and health and environmental impacts.

2. Characteristics of atmospheric particles

2.1. Particle sizes

The size of particles in the atmosphere ranges from few nanometers up to hundred micrometers. There is no doubt that the particle size is an important parameter. It controls much of the dynamic behavior of particles as well as their chemical and physical impacts upon the environment. It is also certainly an important parameter for the health consequences of the respective human exposure as particle size determines: (i) the deposition of particles within human respiratory system; (ii) the amount of surface area that can contact tissues; and (iii) the rate of particle clearance from lungs (Oberdörster et al., 2005). Particles have many irregular shapes so their aerodynamic behavior is expressed in terms of the diameter of an idealized sphere (i.e. aerodynamic diameter), which is usually simply referred to as "particle size". Up to this date various terminologies in relation to particle size are used to describe atmospheric particles. Medical sciences use terms such as inhalable or respirable particles that derived from particles classification according to the entrance into various compartments of the respiratory system (WHO, 2000). Toxicologists typically describe particles as ultrafine, fine and coarse whereas regulatory agencies, namely WHO, US Environmental Protection Agency (USEPA) and European Union (EU) use terms such as PM_X where PM stands for particulate matter and the subscripts identifies the upper 50% cutpoint. The aerosol science uses classification of particles into the modes based on the particles diameter. Each mode has distinctive size range, formation mechanisms, sources, chemical composition and deposition pathways (Hinds, 1999).

Typically, the mass-based size distribution of atmospheric particles is bimodal, with a minimum point that generally occurs in the size range of 1000–3000 nm (i.e. 1–3 μm; Sioutas et al., 2005), which distinguishes the coarse and fine modes (Fig. 1). By convention, the coarse mode consists of particles larger than 2500 nm in aerodynamic diameter. Based on their size, the coarse mode particles can be further subdivided into supercoarse and coarse particles. The coarse particles have diameter between 2500 nm and 10000 nm (Fig. 1). These particles are usually produced by mechanical processes such wind erosion. Particles from sea salt sprays, pollen and spores also belong to this mode as do coarse particles from plant fibers and leaves. As coarse particles are large, they settle out of the atmosphere typically within few hours of formation. Coarse particles deposit in the upper airways of the human respiratory system and they are cleared from human body through nose or by coughing or swallowing. The supercoarse particles are those with aerodynamic diameter bigger than 10000 nm (i.e. 10 μm; USEPA, 2012a). As these particles are too large to enter human respiratory system they are not considered as relevant from the health point of view. However, due to their possible environmental impacts, supercoarse particles are partly assessed when evaluating total suspended particulate matter (TSP) which includes particles of size range up to 30000 nm (i.e. 30 μm).

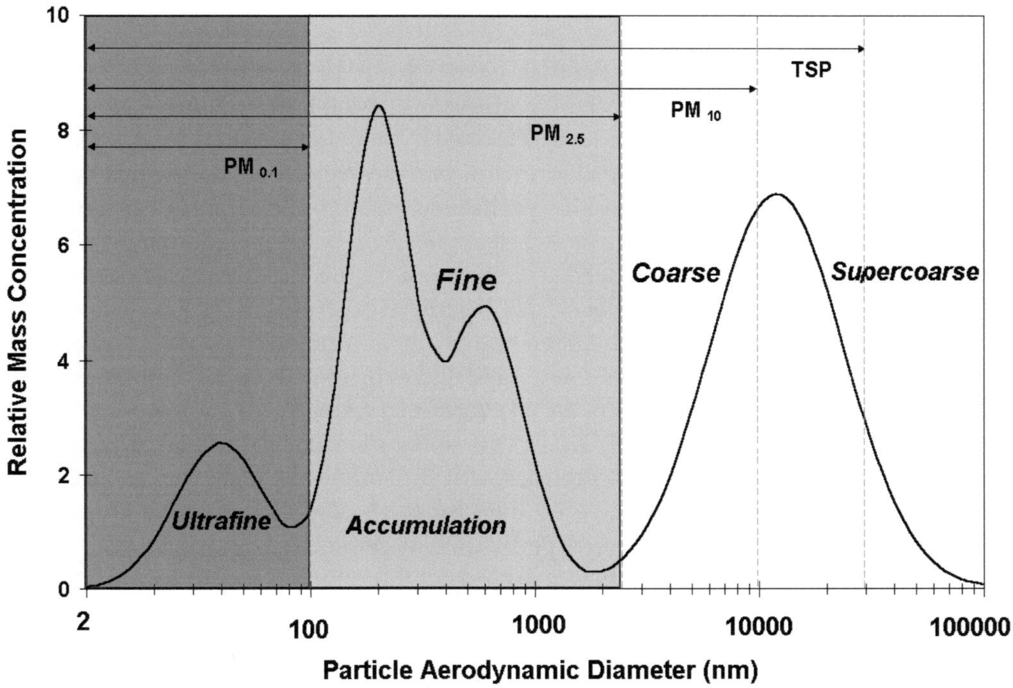

Figure 1. Schematic representation of the size distribution of atmospheric particles.

Fine mode is composed of particles with aerodynamic diameter smaller than 2500 nm (Fig. 1). Typically, these particles are generated by anthropogenic sources. The small sizes of the particles make them less susceptible to the gravitational settling resulting in atmospheric lifetimes in range of days up to weeks and the ability to travel over very long distances in the atmosphere (Anastasio & Martin, 2001). When inhaled fine particles deposit in the conducting airways of the lungs but some of them can penetrate beyond conducting airways into the alveolar region. Based on the formation mechanisms fine mode particles are further subdivide into accumulation and nuclei modes. Accumulation mode consists of particles with aerodynamic diameter between 100-1000 nm. They result from anthropogenic sources (combustions of engine fuel and lubricant oil by diesel-fuelled or direct injection petrol-fuelled vehicles; Kumar et al., 2010, 2011) but can be formed by natural formations, i.e. by coagulation of nuclei-mode particles or by condensation of gas or vapor molecules on the surface of existing particles.

Coagulation is most efficient for large numbers of particles, and condensation is most efficient for large surface areas. Thus the efficiency of both coagulation and condensation decreases as the particle size increases which produces an upper limit of approximately 1000 nm beyond which particles do not grow by these processes. Particles in the range of 100-1000 nm are important because they can represent a significant fraction of the particulate emissions from some types of industrial processes. In addition, sizes of particles in accumulation mode are comparable with the wavelengths of visible light, and hence they account for much of the anthropogenic visibility impairment problem in many urban areas (Seinfeld & Pandis, 2006).

Nuclei mode consist of particles smaller than 100 nm that are also called as ultrafine particles or nanoparticles. In the atmosphere these particles are formed through nucleation, i.e. condensation of low-vapor-pressure substances formed by high temperature vaporization or by chemical reactions in the atmosphere to form new particles (nuclei). These particles are traditionally considered as fresh emissions that yet have to undergo chemical reactions or modification processes. They are mostly composed of nitrates, sulphates, ammonium, organic compounds as well as trace metals when formed from combustion processes (Sioutas et al., 2005; Seinfeld & Pandis, 2006). Nucleation mode particles accounts for the greatest number of atmospheric particles and are found in high number concentrations near their sources. Their concentration in air is most commonly measured and expressed in terms of number concentrations of particles per unit volume of air (in contrast larger particles are measured in terms of mass concentration) (Kumar et al., 2011). Due to their small sizes and large surface area, they are highly chemically reactive. Collisions with each other and with particles in the accumulation mode are largely responsible for their relatively short atmospheric life time (few minutes up to hours). When inhaled these particles are deposited on the alveolar surface (Naga et al., 2005; West, 2008), thereafter, they can transport through the bloodstream or lymphatic system to vital organs (Oberdörster et al., 2004). In addition to their great efficiency to penetrate deep into the lungs, the large surface area may also account for their negative impacts on human health; the scientific evidence indicates that the larger the superficial area the greater the health impacts of particles (Tranfield & Walker, 2012).

The first research studies used the term *ultrafine particles* (Granqvist et al., 1976, 1977). Nowadays this term is still being predominantly used in aerosol and environmental sciences. However, in 1990's the term *nanoparticles* became vastly popular as substitution of ultrafine particles and quickly became adopted in many fields, such as in medicine, material sciences and engineering. Both terms constitute a somewhat arbitrary classification of particles in terms of their size, indicating the significant role of this physical characteristic on particle fate in the air. Theoretically, nanoparticle is any particle with size range in nanometer scale (i.e. bellow 1000 nm; Anastasio & Martin, 2001; Kumar et al., 2010). British Standards Institution (BSI, 2005) defined nanoparticles as those that have one or more dimensions in the order of 100 nm or less. However in current scientific works, the size range definitions for nanoparticles differ significantly. The term nanoparticles was used for atmospheric particles in size ranges such as below 100 nm, 50 nm, 10 nm or occasionally even for particles smaller than 1 μm (Anastasio & Martin, 2001; British Standards Institution, 2005; Morawska et al., 2008). It is worth mentioning that Kumar et al. (2010) recently defined atmospheric nanoparticles as those bellow

http://dx.doi.org/10.5772/54775

300 nm (Fig. 2). Though this size range represents an overlap between particles from nuclei and accumulation mode, authors rationalized that the respective range includes more than 99% of the total number concentration of particles in the ambient atmospheric environments (Kumar et al., 2008a, 2008b, 2009, 2011), being potentially relevant for future regulations.

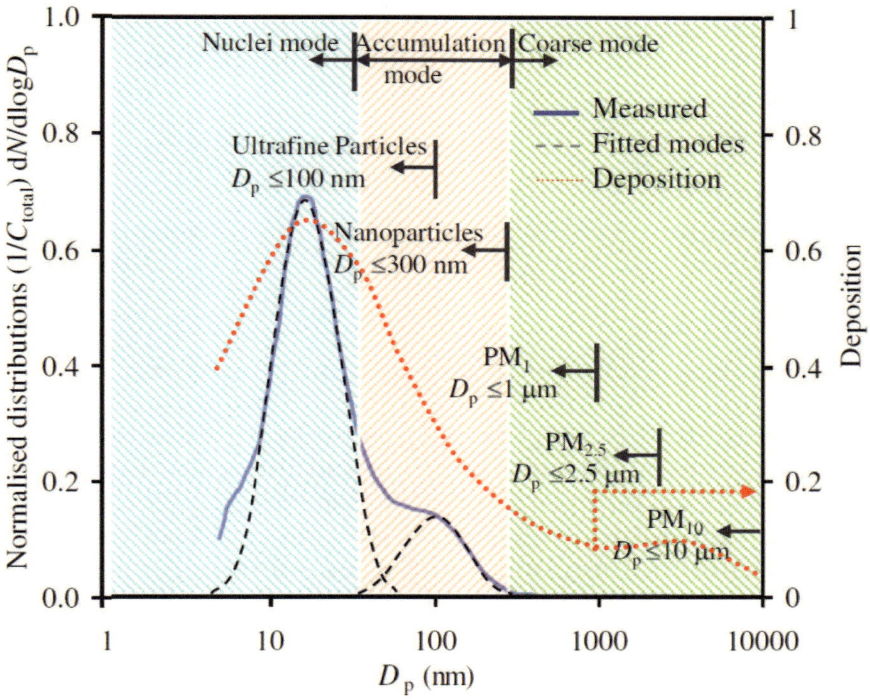

Figure 2. Distribution of atmospheric particles in street canyon in Cambridge, UK (Kumar et al., 2008); Dp, is particle diameter. Definitions of atmospheric particles and their size dependent deposition in alveolar and trancheo-bronchial regions are also shown. Adapted from Kumar et al. (2010).

Therefore, when using the term nanoparticles it is necessary to define the size range of the particles in question. For the purposes of this chapter the term nanoparticles includes ambient nanosized particles < 100 nm (Oberdörster et al., 2005).

2.2. Sources and levels of nanoparticles

The major natural sources of atmospheric nanoparticles (Table 1) are atmospheric formations, vegetation and sea sprays. Volcanic eruptions or forest fires also produce, though sporadically, a large number of atmospheric nanoparticles (Kumar et al., 2011; Oberdörster et al., 2005).

The atmospheric formations of the particles include condensation of semi-volatile organic aerosols, photochemically induced nucleation, and/or nucleation through gas-to particle conversion (Holmes, 2007). Concerning the latter, different nucleation mechanisms have been assumed for the formation of atmospheric nanoparticles (Kumala et al., 2004): (i) binary nucleation of sulphuric acid and water; or (ii) ternary nucleation involving a third molecule, most likely is ammonia that is abundant in the troposphere and has been shown to enhance nucleation rates of sulphuric acid.

Natural sources	Anthropogenic sources	
Atmospheric formations Sea spray Vegetation Forest fires Volcanoes (hot lava) Viruses	Engine combustions	Vehicles (petrol-, diesel-, alternative fuels) Trains, ships, airplanes
	Industrial emissions	Power plants Incinerators Various processes (smelting, heating, welding)
	Commercial productions	

Table 1. Sources of nanoparticles (Buseck & Adachi, 2008; Kumar et al., 2011; Oberdörster et al., 2005)

In remote sites, the formation of new particles is preceded by an increase in the atmospheric concentration of sulphuric acid (Holmes, 2007). Various studies reported an increase in particles number occurring about 1–2 h after an increase in sulphuric acid (Weber et al., 1996), being followed by a relatively small particle growth rate (between 1 and 2 nm h^{-1}; Birmili & Wiedensohler, 2000a; Weber et al., 1996, 1997). These findings point towards a linear relationship between the number of newly formed particles and the production rate of sulphuric acid. It is still not clear though whether at these environments the binary nucleation (i.e. water–sulphuric acid nucleation) is solely responsible for the formation of new particles or if a third specie, such as ammonia or an organic compound, is involved (i.e. ternary nucleation). In forests the mechanisms responsible for the formation and growth of atmospheric nanoparticles are not completely understood. Although sulphuric acid is one of the most likely candidates that might be responsible for the formation of the initial nanometre-sized particles (Riipinen et al., 2007), sulphur chemistry does not sustain enough sulphuric acid in the atmosphere to explain more than a small fraction of the observed particle size growth rate (Morawska et al., 2008). Several forest studies have concluded that particle formation can commonly occur from biogenic precursors (O'Dowd et al., 2002), some of them suggesting a direct relation between emissions of monoterpenes and gas-to-particle formation in regions substantially lacking in anthropogenic aerosol sources (Tunved et al., 2006). In addition the authors also estimated that forests provide an aerosol population of $1–2\times10^3$ cm^{-3} of climatically active particles (during the period of late spring to early autumn) thus representing a considerable source of global importance. In the marine environments the possible particle formation mechanisms are (Morawska et al., 2008): seawater bubble-burst process (Clarke et al., 2006; O'Dowd et al., 2004), ternary nucleation producing a reservoir of undetectable particles upon which vapours can condense (Kulmala et al., 2000, 2004), free tropospheric production with mixing down to the boundary layer (Raes, 1995), and generation of coastal iodine particles from macroalgal iodocarbon emissions (Kulmala et al., 2000; O'Dowd et al., 2004; O'Dowd & Hoffmann, 2005). Whereas the iodine-containing particles are not likely to play an important role globally, wind produced bubble-burst particles containing salt are ubiquitous in the marine environments. Clarke et al. (2006) have shown that sea salt aerosols produced by breaking waves are a significant constituent of particles with sizes as small as 10 nm, with 60% of the particles smaller than 100 nm in diameter. The authors estimated that in marine regions between 5% and 90% of the nuclei particles originate from the sea salt flux.

The implication of the above referred text is that nanoparticles are formed in the environments due to natural processes. Therefore, they are always present at some concentration levels even in the atmosphere of environments free from the immediate influence of anthropogenic activities. These concentrations should be considered as "natural background". In addition, because the rates of formation and growth of nanoparticles differ significantly between various natural environments, there are significant variations in number concentrations of atmospheric particles. Whereas in marine environments particle number concentrations typically range between 10^2 and 10^3 particles cm^{-3} (O'Dowd et al., 2004; Seinfeld & Pandis, 2006), the usual ranges in forests and rural continental regions are 10^3-10^4 (Birmili & Wiedensohler, 2000b; O'Dowd et al., 2002; Riipinen et al., 2007), though occurrence of forest fires may temporally increased these levels. Meteorological parameters, such as wind speed, precipitation, relative humidity and temperature also influence particle concentrations. Therefore, when evaluating particle concentrations in urban environments it is important to assess the respective background levels and to compare them with concentrations in urban environments in order to correctly estimate the magnitude of the anthropogenic impacts.

The number concentrations of nanoparticles in the atmosphere can vary by up to five or more orders of magnitude (from 10^2 to 10^7 particles cm^{-3}) depending on environmental conditions and source strengths (Kumar et al., 2010) but typically, in natural environments the particle number concentrations are approximately to 1-2 orders of magnitude smaller than those in urban areas (Kumar et al., 2010). Morawska et al. (2008) analysed concentration levels of 71 studies performed on nanoparticles in various environments, including those from clean background and rural background sites (Table 2). The authors found (Morawska et al., 2008), respectively, the mean concentrations of 2.6×10^3 and 4.8×10^3 particles cm^{-3} for clean background and rural background sites compared to 42.1×10^3 and 48.2×10^3 particles cm^{-3} for urban and street canyons; in urban areas anthropogenic sources, such as vehicular emissions are strong contributors of nanoparticles, thus much higher particle concentration levels were observed (Table 2). Road tunnels (167.7×10^3 particles cm^{-3}) account for the highest concentrations. They can act as a trap for pollutants from vehicular emissions that is enhanced by the surrounding built-up environment that limits the dispersion of exhaust emissions (Van Dingenen et al., 2004).

There is no doubt that anthropogenic emissions constitute the major source of atmospheric nanoparticles in urban environments (Table 2). With respect to urban sites various studies have concluded that vehicle exhaust emissions represent a primary source of nanoparticle pollution in urban environments (Harrison et al., 1999; Shi & Harrison, 1999; Shi et al., 2001; Wåhlin et al., 2001) that might be responsible up to 86% of total particle number concentrations (Pey et al., 2009). The vehicle emissions depend on many factors such as type of engines, fuels, lubricating oil, after-treatment or driving conditions. Typically particles emitted from diesel engines are in the size range 20–130 nm (Kittelson, 1998; Harris & Maricq, 2001). Diesel-fuelled vehicles make by far the greatest contributions to total number concentrations (Kumar et al., 2010) although in most of European countries their proportion is lower. In 2009 passenger diesel-fuelled cars in Europe accounted for to 9-10% (Sweden and Cyprus) to 62% (Luxemburg) but in 16 out of 21 European countries (where data is available) their proportion was less than 50% (EU, 2011). Large part of nanoparticles is also produce by heavy duty diesel vehicles (trucks, buses) that exhibit particle number emission factors one to two orders of magnitude larger than a typical petrol car (Ristovski et al., 2005, 2006). In comparison, particles from petrol-fuelled vehicles are in the size range 20–60 nm (Harris & Maricq, 2001; Ristovski et al., 2006), and their emissions vary significantly depending on the engine operating conditions; Graskow et al. (1998) reported that when driven at higher speed (~120 km h^{-1}) or during acceleration, the particle number emissions from petrol vehicles were similar to those observed from diesel vehicles.

Site	Number of analyzed studies	Estimated concentration × 10^3 (particles cm^{-3})	
		Mean	Median
Clean background	5	2.6	3.2
Rural background	8	4.8	2.9
Urban background	4	7.3	8.1
Urban	24	10.8	8.8
Street canyon	7	42.1	39.3
Roadside	18	48.2	34.6
On-road	2	71.5	47.0
Tunnel	3	167.7	99.1

Table 2. Particle number concentrations in different environments (Morawska et al., 2008)

In general particles from vehicle exhaust may be divided into two main categories. Primary particles are directly emitted from the engines. These particles are mostly submicrometer agglomerates (30-500 nm) of solid phase carbonaceous material containing metallic ash (from lubricating oil additives and engine wear) and adsorbed or condensed hydrocarbons and sulphur compounds (Morawska et al., 2008). Secondary particles are formed in the atmosphere when hot exhaust gases are expelled from vehicle tailpipe; as they cool and condensate they form nuclei mode particles (typically smaller than 30 nm) that consists mainly of hydrocarbons and hydrated sulphuric acid (Morawska et al., 2008). On-roads studies (e.g. when a vehicle is being followed by a mobile laboratory; Kittelson et al., 2004, 2006; Casati et al., 2007) and those performed near busy roads (Harrison et al., 1999; Ntziachristos et al., 2007; Rosenbohm et al., 2005; Westerdahl et al., 2005) reported large number of these particles.

The interactions between vehicle tyres and road can also generate particles of submicron sizes, although it was generally believed that tyre wear on the road contributes mainly to larger size (> 2.5 μm). Some more recent studies report (Gustafsson et al., 2008; Dahl et al., 2006) that considerable emissions of nanoparticles might be generated from road and tyre interactions, depending on surface, vehicle and driving conditions. As this source could be a significant contributor to particle number emissions, more research on this topic is needed.

The industrial sources of atmospheric nanoparticles include power plants, incinerators, or various industrial processes such as smelting or welding, heating operations (Oberdörster et al., 2005). Compared to vehicle exhaust emissions, their contribution to atmospheric nanoparticles is though much lower. In a study performed in Barcelona, Spain, Pey et al. (2009) investigated source apportionment of atmospheric particles in size range 13-800 nm (i.e. nuclei and accumulation mode) at an urban background site. The authors identified vehicular exhaust emissions (65%) and regional/urban background (24%) as the largest contributors to total particle number concentrations (mean of 17×10^3 particles cm^{-3}); industrial emissions accounted only for 2% of the total particle number. The levels of this contribution were similar in the study (Pey et al. (2009) to: photochemically induced nucleation (3%), sea spray (2%), and mineral dust (1%); unidentified sources accounted for 3%.

In the last decade nanoscience has been a dynamically developing field of scientific interest in the entire world (Aguar-Fernandez & Hullmann, 2007). Small size and relatively large reactive surface area of nanoparticles led to their increased use in a variety of fields such as in medicine, material sciences, electronics or energy storage (Helland et al., 2007). Thus engineered (i.e. manufactured) nanoparticles have become (apart from vehicle exhaust and industrial emissions) another important anthropogenic source of atmospheric nanoparticles. These nanoparticles are not intentionally released into the environment, though some release may occur during production, use and disposal phases of nanomaterial-integrated products (Bystrzejewska-Piotrowska et al., 2009). Their characteristics (sources, composition, homogeneity or heterogeneity, oxidant potential, exposure and emissions) differ from other atmospheric nanoparticles (Oberdörster et al., 2005). The engineered nanoparticles are nowadays incorporated into many products of daily use (pharmaceuticals, lubricants, cosmetics, pharmaceuticals, fillers, catalysts, electronic devices or other domestic appliances; Nel et al., 2006). The widespread use of manufactured nanoparticles in consumer products may dramatically increase potential environmental, occupational, and public exposures to these particles that may result in adverse health effects if they are not appropriately controlled. In addition, as nanotechnology has being nowadays used in various industries, it becomes responsible for the production of waste containing residue of nanomaterials; considering the unprecedented application of nanoparticles in various products, significant amounts of new-generation-waste will be certainly created in the near future (Bystrzejewska-Piotrowska et al., 2009).

In view of the comprehensive utilizations of nanotechnological applications, concerns regarding the potential health effects of engineered nanoparticles have been raised (Helland et al.,

2005). The available toxicological studies indicate (Nel et al., 2006; Oberdörster et al., 2005) that toxicity of engineered nanoparticles depends on specific physiochemical and environmental factors, implying that toxic potential of each type of nanoparticle has to be evaluated individually (Helland et al., 2007). Due to the great variability in used materials (e.g. titanium dioxide, silver, carbon, gold, cadmium and heavy metals; Kumar et al., 2010) it is thus not possible to generalize the toxicological impacts of the engineered nanoparticles. In addition size, shape, surface characteristics, inner structure and chemical composition may also play an important role in determining toxicity and reactivity (Maynard & Aitken, 2007; Nel et al., 2006).

2.3. Chemical composition of nanoparticles

The composition of atmospheric nanoparticles is highly variable. The source and formations influence their chemical composition and nanoparticles include components such as inorganic compounds (sulphates, nitrates, ammonium, chloride, trace metals), elemental and organic carbon, crystal materials, biological components (viruses), and volatile and semivolatile organic compounds (Oberdörster et al., 2005). They can carry toxic compounds such as heavy metals, dioxins, hydrocarbons and other organic chemicals (some of which are potentially carcinogenic) adhered to their surfaces which then increase their toxicity (Terzano et al., 2010). Apart the source-specificity, composition of nanoparticles also depends on geographical and meteorological parameters which in general lead to great differences in physicochemical properties among nanoparticles.

Several studies including a number of recent ones (Chen et al., 2010; Kim et al., 2011; Klems et al., 2011; Kudo et al., 2011) have evaluated the composition of atmospheric nanoparticles. However, at present, the knowledge on nanoparticles composition is far from comprehensive. The existent scientific studies are conducted at different ways, sample particles in a different size range, use different samplers, and focus on different aspects of particle chemical composition. Thus the reported data are not completely comparable across the studies. In their attempt to improve the current knowledge, Chow & Watson (2007) review and summarized the results of the existent studies. The authors analyzed 25 studies performed at various environments (rural, urban, industrial, coastal, roadside, traffic, city-centre, urban background, and etc.) and in various regions: two studies were conducted in Europe (Finland), four in Japan, three in Asia (one in China, two in Taiwan) and sixteen in USA; eleven US studies were performed in California, eight of them were from different locations within the Los Angeles metropolitan area. Concerning the chemical composition the authors concluded that organic material including polycyclic aromatic hydrocarbons was the most abundant portion of atmospheric nanoparticles in most, but not all environments. High elemental concentrations were found in nanoparticles from industrial sites with potassium, calcium and iron as important elements. Potassium originates from biomass burning, and calcium is used as an oil additive; condensed iron vapors are often found in industrial processes. Much of the nanoparticles appeared to be semi-volatile, consistent with being comprised of organic materials such as hopanes from engine oils or condensed secondary organic aerosol such as organic acids. However, authors emphasize the necessity to conduct more studies on particle chemical

http://dx.doi.org/10.5772/54775

composition in to order to provide a more complete understanding on the chemistry of atmospheric nanoparticles and local variations.

3. Regulatory aspects

During last two decades the exponentially growing interdisciplinary research on air quality and health has clearly demonstrated increased incidence and the prevalence of respiratory diseases along with increased air pollution. Particles have emerged as the most dangerous pollutants due their adverse health effects going far beyond the simple toxicity to the lung. The results of the conducted epidemiology studies were so relevant that USEPA and EU have implemented strategies to protect public health which resulted in establishment of regulatory limits of atmospheric particles (PM_{10}). As the ongoing research emphasized the importance of smaller (i.e. fine) particles the new $PM_{2.5}$ standards were proposed and implemented in most of developed countries (Table 3). However, the reduction of atmospheric particulate emissions is nowadays required especially in rapidly developing countries, such as Brazil, China or India but they are only slowly moving towards implementation of these standards (Slezakova et al., 2012); there are still a number of countries, such as Pakistan where any regulatory limits for atmospheric particles have not been proposed yet.

Country	Pollutant	Targeted limit	Note	Reference
European Union	PM_{10}	24h mean: 40 μg/m^3	Not to be exceeded more than 35 times per calendar year	Directive 2008/50/EC
		Annual mean: 50 μg/m^3		
	$PM_{2.5}$	Annual mean: 25 μg/m^3	(in force from 2015)	
USA	PM_{10}	24h mean: 150 μg/m^3		USEPA, 2006
	$PM_{2.5}$	24h mean: 35 μg/m^3		
		Annual mean : 15 μg/m^3		
Canada	$PM_{2.5}$	24h mean : 30 μg/m^3		Canadian Council of Ministries of Environment, 2003
Australia	PM_{10}	24h mean: 50 μg/m^3		Australian Government, 2012
	$PM_{2.5}$	24h mean: 25 μg/m^3		
		Annual mean: 8 μg/m^3		
Japan	PM_{10}	24 h mean: 100 μg/m^3		Government of Japan, 2012
	$PM_{2.5}$	24h mean: 35 μg/m^3		
		Annual mean: 15 μg/m^3		

Table 3. Air quality standards for atmospheric particles in selected countries

Unlike fine or coarse particles, the regulatory aspect of nanoparticles has not been addressed yet. The difficulty lies as to which metric of nanoparticles would be the most adequate. Several generic and specific characteristics of particles such as chemical composition, size, geometry or surface area have been discussed (Kumar et al., 2010, 2011) but no conclusion has been reached yet. The mass-based paradigm of PM_{10} and $PM_{2.5}$ regulator limits is not applicable to nanoparticles as their distribution is not dominated by mass but particle number. Some studies have suggested that the particle number concentrations of ultrafine particles (i.e. smaller than 100 nm) are an important parameter as size range comprises the major proportion (about 80%) of the total number concentration of ambient nanoparticles, but negligible mass concentration. Reliable characterization of nanoparticles in the air is thus vital for developing a regulatory framework. At national levels air quality agencies should be encouraged to integrate nanoparticle measurements in their monitoring networks (number and size distributions measurements). Such initiatives might provide comprehensive data and information necessary to correctly address regulatory aspects of atmospheric nanoparticles in order to prevent the public exposures.

4. Health impacts

Due to intensive research, there is an emerging evidence that exposure to nanoparticles may adversely affect human health (Stölzel et al., 2007). The nanoparticles enter human body through the skin, lung and gastrointestinal tract (Nel et al., 2006). When they are inhaled, their behavior differs from coarse particles. Their small size allows them to be breathed deeply into the lungs where they are able to penetrate alveolar epithelium and enter the pulmonary interstitium and vascular space to be absorbed directly into the blood stream (Terzano et al., 2010). They may also translocate within the body to the central nerve system, the brain, into the systemic circulation and to organs like the liver (Helland et al., 2007; Figure 3). They are more reactive and toxic due to the larger surface areas, leading to detrimental health effects such as oxidation stress, pulmonary inflammation and cardiovascular events (Buseck & Adachi, 2008; Nel et al., 2006).

Though the toxicological studies have provided evidence of the toxicity of nanoparticles, epidemiological evidence of the health effects is limited. Currently, there is also no quantitative summary of concentration-response functions for these particles that could be used in health impact assessment (Hoek et al., 2010). Unlike for coarse and fine particles there are relatively few epidemiological studies on the health effects of atmospheric nanoparticles. The first conducted studies on atmospheric nanoparticles have been panel studies, which generally showed associations between short-term exposure to nanosized particles and occurrence of acute respiratory symptoms and lung function (Ibald-Mulli et al., 2002; Peters et al., 1997; Penttinen et al., 2001a, 2001b). Some of these studies have suggested that nanoparticles might be even more strongly associated with adverse respiratory outcomes than fine particles (Peters et al., 1997; Penttinen et al., 2001a) whereas other studies found similar associations in health outcomes of nano and fine particles (von Klot et al., 2002; Pekkannen et al., 1997, Penttinen et al., 2001b).

Up to this date, only few epidemiological studies have assessed more severe end points such as daily, and cause specific mortality and hospital admissions (Stölzel, et al., 2007; Wichman et al., 2000); there are no epidemiological studies on long-term exposure to atmospheric nanoparticles.

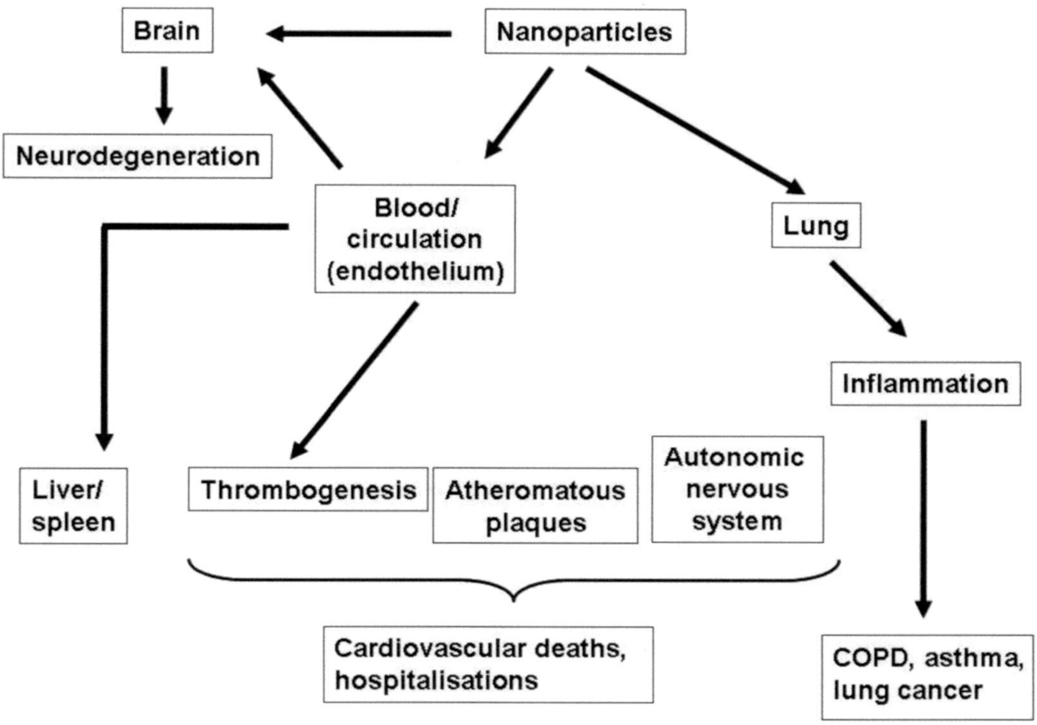

Figure 3. Systemic health effects of atmospheric nanoparticles. Adapted from Terzano et al. (2010).

Although lungs are the primary target of nanoparicles, cardiovascular detrimental consequences due exposure to nanoparticles have been also observed in some epidemiological studies (Kettunen, et al., 2007; Rückerl et al., 2007). Specifically, the "Exposure and Risk Assessment for Fine and Ultrafine Particles in Ambient Air" (i.e. ULTRA) study investigated the health effects of nanoparticles in three European cities (Amsterdam, Erfurt, Helsinki), where daily number concentrations levels of nanoparticles in air were similar (Ruuskanen et al., 2001). The authors followed a cohort of 131 patients aged 40-84 with established coronary heart disease with biweekly submaximal exercise tests over a 6-months period. It was observed that the risk of developing ischemia during exercise was significantly elevated at 2 days after exposure to increased environmental levels of nanoparticles (Pekkanen et al., 2002). The importance of this observation is that it highlights myocardial ischemia as a significant potential mechanism responsible for the adverse cardiac outcomes associated with poor air quality (Terzano et al., 2010). In addition particulate pollution including nanoparticles was associated with decrease in blood pressure (Ibald-Mulli et al., 2004). The study thus started to provide an understanding of how nanoparticles may affect cardiovascular health.

5. Environmental impacts

5.1. Visibility impairment

Impairment of the visibility involves degrading of the ability to perceive the environment. Atmospheric suspended particles are the most important factor in the visibility reduction (Boubel et al., 1994). The reduction of visibility is caused by build-up of the atmospheric particles that absorb or scatter light from the sun (Horvath, 2008); though light scattering by particles is the most important phenomenon responsible for impairment of visibility. The size of particles plays a crucial role for the interaction with light, but so far the existent links between visibility impairment and mass concentrations have been established for larger particles (Boubel et al., 1994; Strawa et al., 2010). Shape and composition of particles are also relevant for visibility reduction; carbon particles may contribute 5–40% of overall visibility reduction through light absorption in polluted areas, whereas particles containing sulphate, organic carbon and nitrate species may cause 60-95% of visibility reduction (Kumar at al., 2010). Finally, visibility impairment is affected by meteorological parameters; it increases with relative humidity and atmospheric pressure and decreases with temperature and wind speed (Kim et al., 2002; Tsai, 2005). In general the role of nanoparticles in visibility impairment is still unclear. However, diesel vehicles emit large number of sulphate and carbonaceous nanoparticles. Particles of these compositions reduce visibility which suggests that nanoparticles might be relevant for visibility impairment. Therefore, deeper understanding of nanoparticles role in visibility impairment is necessary.

5.2. Climate change

Climate system, atmospheric chemistry and even life on the Earth are dependent on solar radiation (Boubel et al., 1994). Approximately 30% of the incoming solar energy is reflected back to space. The remaining 70% is absorbed by the surface–atmosphere system of the Earth. This energy heats the planet and the atmosphere. As the surface and the atmosphere become warm, they release the energy in form of infrared radiation. This process continues until the incoming solar energy and the outgoing heat radiation are in balance. This radiation energy balance provides a powerful constraint for the global average temperature of the planet (Ramanathan & Feng, 2009). Atmospheric greenhouse gases (such as like carbon dioxide and methane) and particles affect the climate by altering the incoming solar and outgoing thermal radiations. In other words changing the atmospheric abundance or properties of these gases and particles can lead to a warming or cooling of the climate system. The influence of a factor (pollutant) that cause change of climate system are typically evaluated in terms of its radiative forcing, which is an estimate of how the energy balance of the Earth-atmosphere system is influenced when the factor in question is altered (IPCC, 2007).

Atmospheric nanosized particles are the main precursors of larger particles. They promote their growth and modify the optical properties thus affecting the radiative properties of the atmosphere. It was generally believed that particles reflect sunlight back to space before it reaches the surface, and thus contribute to a cooling of the surface (i.e. negative radiative forcing; Monks et al., 2009). During time as the concentrations of particles increased (along with greenhouse gases) their cooling effect has masked some of the greenhouse warming (Ramanathan & Feng, 2009). This masking effect could be relative large considering that estimated negative radiative forcing of particles is –1.2 W m^{-2} compared with +2.63 W m^{-2} for greenhouse gases (+1.66 W m^{-2} for carbon dioxide, +0.48 W m for methane and +0.16 W m^{-2} for nitrous oxide, +0.34 W m^{-2} for halocarbons; IPCC, 2007). However, in the last years the view of particle role in climate change has deepened. It was found that atmospheric particles may also enhance scattering and absorption of solar radiation thus causing direct warm-up (i.e. positive radiation; IPPC, 2007). Especially, carbonaceous particles are considered as one of the major contributors to global warming (i.e. +0.34 W m^{-2}); if they are coated with sulphate or organic compounds their radiative forcing can increase up to about +0.6 W m^{-2} (Kumar et al., 2010).

Indirectly nanoparticles can also cause a negative radiative forcing through changes in cloud formations and properties (IPCC, 2007). They can act as cloud condensation nuclei and modify size and number concentrations of cloud droplets. In clean air, clouds are composed of a relatively small number of large droplets. As a consequence, the clouds are somewhat dark and translucent. In polluted air with high concentrations of particles (such as urban areas) water can easily condense on the particles, creating a large number of small droplets. These clouds are dense, very reflective, and bright white. Due to the decrease of the size of water droplets these clouds are less efficient at releasing precipitation. They cause large reductions in the amount of solar radiation reaching Earth's surface, a corresponding increase in atmospheric solar heating, changes in atmospheric thermal structure, surface cooling, disruption of regional circulation systems such as the monsoons, suppression of rainfall, and less efficient removal of pollutants (Ramanathan & Feng, 2009). In general the indirect effects of particles are only partially understood. The interactions between aerosol particles (natural and anthropogenic in origin) and clouds are complex and most instruments cannot measure aerosols within the clouds. Climatologists thus consider the role of clouds to be the largest single uncertainty in climate prediction.

The close relation between climate and air quality also reflects on the impacts of climate change on air pollution levels. For example particle pollution levels are strongly influenced by shifts in the weather (e.g., heat waves or droughts; EEA, 2012a). While closely related, climate change and air pollution have mostly been treated as separate problems. At the international level, various efforts have helped to reduce air pollution levels. The largest reductions have been achieved for emissions of sulphur dioxide which decreased in Europe by 82% between 1990 and 2010 (EEA, 2012b). The implementation of EU regulation limits setting levels of sulphur dioxide in urban areas and various political actions to control urban atmospheric emissions (i.e. sulfur abatement technologies in industrial facilities, EEA, 2011; introduction of fuels with reduced levels of sulfur, Directive 98/70/EC; EN 590/2004) have contributed to these reductions. In addition, significant reductions were also obtained for emissions of air pollutants that are primarily responsible for formation of harmful ground-level ozone: non-methane volatile organic compounds (56% reduction) and nitrogen oxides (47% reduction; EEA, 2012b). However, based on the future climate scenarios (and in the absence of additional emissions reductions) the IPCC still projected declining air quality in cities into the future as a result of climate change (USEPA, 2012b). In agreement, USEPA has concluded that climate change could have various negative impacts on national air quality levels that included both increases and decreases in particle pollution (USEPA, 2009). Thus in order to protect human health and environment, joined efforts to control air pollution and mitigate climate change have to be done in future: air pollution abatement measures may help protect the regional and global climate whilst taking certain climate change measures may yield additional benefits through improved local and regional air quality.

6. Conclusion

Atmospheric nanoparticles represent an area of growing health concern. Although our understanding of the ambient nanoparticles and their behavior has increased considerably in recent years, the magnitude of the impacts of nanoparticles on human health and the environment has still not been fully understood. Lack of answers from epidemiological studies in relation to atmospheric nanoparticles and the absence of the exposure-response relationships also mean that currently it is not possible to develop health guidelines, a basis for national regulations. Thus, a multidisciplinary approach including atmospheric scientists, nanomaterial engineers, epidemiologists, clinicians and toxicologists is necessary to further investigate sources, generation, physicochemical characteristics and potential harmful effects of nanoparticles. This knowledge would allow better understanding of the potential impacts of the particles on the environment and health and would provide scientific foundation for development of strategies to protect public health.

The knowledge on the characteristics of engineered nanoparticles is in general very limited. Though these nanoparticles appear in smaller concentrations than other atmospheric nanoparticles they may pose much larger health risks (Oberdörster et al., 2005). Therefore, the future studies need to consider the specificity of these nanoparticles and the new kinds of environmental and health impacts resulting from the release of these nanoparticles.

Acknowledgements

The authors would like to thank to Fundação para Ciência e Tecnologia for the financial support through grants number PEst-C/EQB/LA0006/2011 and PEst-C/EQB/UI0511/2011, and fellowship SFRH/BPD/65722/2009.

Author details

Klara Slezakova[1,2], Simone Morais[2] and Maria do Carmo Pereira[1]

1 LEPAE, Departamento de Engenharia Química, Faculdade de Engenharia, Universidade do Porto, Portugal

2 REQUIMTE, Instituto Superior de Engenharia do Porto, Instituto Politécnico do Porto, Portugal

References

[1] Aguar-Fernandez, M.A. & Hullmann, A. (2007). A boost for safer nanotechnology. *Nano Today*, Vol. 2, No. 1, (February 2007), pp. 56, ISSN 1748-0132

[2] Anastasio, C. & Martin, S.T. (2001). Atmospheric nanoparticles, In: *Nanoparticles and the Environment*, J.F. Banfield, A. Navrotsky (Eds.), pp. 293–349, Mineralogical Society of America, ISBN 0-939950-56-1, Washington, DC.

[3] Australian Government, National Environment Protection Council. (2012). *Ambient Air Quality Standards*, August 2012, available from <http://www.environment.gov.au/atmosphere/airquality/standards.html>

[4] Birmili, W. & Wiedensohler, A. (2000a). Evolution of newly formed aerosol particles in the continental boundary layer: a case study including OH and H2SO4 measurements. *Geophysical Research Letters*, Vol. 27, No. 15, (August 2000), pp. 2205–2208, ISSN 0094-8276

[5] Birmili, W. & Wiedensohler, A. (2000b). New particle formation in the continental boundary layer: meteorological and gas phase parameter influence. *Geophysical Research Letter*, Vol. 27, No. 20, (October 2000), pp. 3325-3328, ISSN 0094-8276

[6] Boubel, R.W., Fox, D.L., Turner, D.B. & Stern, A.C. (1994). *Fundamentals of Air Pollution* (3rd edition), Academic Press, ISBN 0-12-118930-0, London, United Kingdom

[7] British Standards Institution. (2005). *Vocabulary — Nanoparticles*. British Standards Institution, ISBN 0 580 45925 X, London, United Kingdom

[8] Buseck, P.R. & Adachi, K. (2008). Nanogeoscience: nanoparticles in the atmosphere. *Elements*, Vol. 4, No. 6, (December 2008), pp. 389-394, ISSN 1811-5209

[9] Bystrzejewska-Piotrowska, G., Golimowski, J. & Urban, P.L. (2009). Nanoparticles: their potential toxicity, waste and environmental management. *Waste Management*, Vol. 29, No. 9, (September 2009), pp. 2587–2595, ISSN 0956053X

[10] Canadian Council of Ministries of Environment. (2000). *Canada-wide Standards for Particulate Matter (PM) and Ozone.* CCME Council of Ministers, Quebec City, August 2012, available from < http://www.ccme.ca/assets/pdf/pmozone_standard_e.pdf>

[11] Casati, R., Scheer, V., Vogt, R. & Benter, T. (2007). Measurement of nucleation and soot mode particle emission from a diesel passenger car in real world and laboratory in situ dilution. *Atmospheric Environment,* Vol. 41, No. 10, (March 2007), pp. 2125–2135, ISSN 1352-2310

[12] Chen, S.-C., Tsai, C.-J., Chou, C.C.-K., Roam, G.-D., Cheng, S.-S. & Wang, Y.-N. (2010). Ultrafine particles at three different sampling locations in Taiwan. *Atmospheric Environment,* Vol. 44, No. 4, (February 2010), pp. 533-540, ISSN 1352-2310

[13] Chow, J.C. & Watson, J.G. (2007). Review of measurement methods and Compositions for ultrafine particles. *Aerosol and Air Quality Research,* Vol. 7, No. 2, (June 2007), pp. 121-173, ISSN 2071-1409

[14] Clarke, A.D., Owens, S.R. & Zhou, J. (2006). An ultrafine sea-salt flux from breaking waves: implications for cloud condensation nuclei in the remote marine atmosphere. *Journal of Geophysical Research D: Atmospheres,* Vol. 111, No. D6, (March 2006), pp. 1–2, ISSN 0148-0227

[15] Dahl, A., Gharibi, A., Swietlicki, E., Gudmundsson, A., Bohgard, M., Ljungman, A., Blomqvist, G. & Gustafsson, M. (2006). Traffic-generated emissions of ultrafine particles from pavement-tire interface. *Atmospheric Environment,* Vol. 40, No. 7, (March 2006), pp. 1314-1323, ISSN 1352-2310

[16] Directive 2008/50/EC. (2008). Directive of the European Parliament and of the Council on Ambient Air Quality and Cleaner Air for Europe. *Official Journal of the European Union,* L152, (June 2006), pp. 1-44

[17] Directive 98/70/EC. (1998). Directive of the European Parliament and of the Council Relating to the Quality of Petrol and Diesel Fuels. *Official Journal of the European Communities,* L350, (December 1998), pp. 58–68

[18] EN Standard 590/2004. (2004). *Automotive Fuels. Diesel. Requirements and Test methods,* European Committee for Standardization, ISBN 05-8044-119-9, Brussels, Belgium

[19] Environmental European Agency (EEA). (2011). *European Union Emission Inventory Report 1990–2009 under the UNECE Convention on Long-range Transboundary Air Pollution (LRTAP).* EEA Technical report No. 9/2011, Office for Official Publications of the European Union, ISBN 978-92-9213-216-3, Luxemburg

[20] Environmental European Agency (EEA). (2012a). *Evaluation of progress under the EU National Emission Ceilings Directive.* EEA Technical report No. 14/2012, Publication Office of the European Union, ISBN 978-92-9213-336-8, Luxemburg

[21] Environmental European Agency (EEA). (2012b). *Urban adaptation to climate change in Europe.* EEA Report No. 2/2012, Office for Official Publications of the European Union, ISBN 978-92-9213-308-5, Luxemburg

[22] European Union (EU). (2011). *Energy, Transport, and Environmental Indicators* (2011 ed.), European Union, ISBN 978-92-79-21384-7, Luxemburg

[23] Government of Japan, Ministry of Environment. (2012). *Environmental Quality Standards in Japan - Air quality,* August 2012, available from <http://www.env.go.jp/en/air/aq/aq.html>

[24] Granqvist, C.G., Buhrman, R.A., Wyns, J. & Sievers, A.J. (1976). Far-infrared absorption in ultrafine Al particles. *Physical Review Letters,* Vol. 37, No. 10, (September 1976), pp. 625–629, ISSN 0031-9007

[25] Granqvist, C.G., Buhrman, R.A., Wyns, J. & Sievers, A.J. (1977). Far-infrared absorption in ultrafine Al particles: Drude model versus Gor'kov-Eliashberg theory. *Journal de Physique Colloque,* Vol.38, pp. C2 93–96, DOI: 10.1051/jphyscol:1977219

[26] Graskow, B.R., Kittelson, D.B., Abdul-Khaleek, I.S., Ahmadi, M.R. & Morris, J.E. (1998). Characterization of exhaust particulate emissions from a spark ignition engine. *SAE Special Publications,* Vol. 1326, (February 1998), pp. 155-165

[27] Gustafsson, M., Blomqvist, G., Gudmundsson, A., Dahl, A., Swietlicki, E., Bohgard, M., Lindbom, J. & Ljungman, A. (2008). Properties and toxicological effects of particles from the interaction between tyres, road pavement and winter traction material. *Science of The Total Environmen*t, Vol. 393, No. 2-3, (April 2008), pp. 226-240, ISSN 0048-9697

[28] Harris, S.J. & Maricq, M.M. (2001). Signature size distributions for diesel and gasoline engine exhaust particulate matter. *Journal of Aerosol Science,* Vol. 32, No. 6, (June 2001), pp. 749–764, ISSN 0021-8502

[29] Harrison, R., Jones, M. & Collins, G. (1999). Measurements of the physical properties of particles in the urban atmosphere. *Atmospheric Environment,* Vol. 33, No. 2, (January 1999), pp. 309–321, ISSN 1352-2310

[30] Helland, A., Kastenholz, H., Thidell, A., Arnfalk, P. & Deppert, K. (2006). Nanoparticulate materials and regulatory policy in Europe: an analysis of stakeholder perspectives. *Journal of Nanoparticle Research,* Vol. 8, No. 5, (October 2006), pp. 709–719, ISSN 1388-0764

[31] Helland, A., Wick, P., Koehler, A., Schmid, K. & Som, C. (2007). Reviewing the environmental and human health knowledge base of carbon nanotubes. *Environmental Health Perspectives,* Vol. 115, No. 8, (August 2007), pp. 1125-1131, ISSN 0091-6765

[32] Hinds, W.C. (1999). *Aerosol Technology: Properties, Behaviour and Measurement of Airborne Particles,* John Wiley & Sons, ISBN 978-0-471-19410-1, Hoboken, USA

[33] Hoek, G., Boogaard, H., Knol, A., de Hartog, J., Slottje, P., Ayres, J.G., Borm, P., Brunekreef, B., Donaldson, K., Forastiere, F., Holgate, S., Kreyling, W.G., Nemery, B., Pekkanen, J., Stone, V., Wichmann, H.E. & van der Sluijs, J. (2010). Concentration response functions for ultrafine particles and all-cause mortality and hospital admissions: results of a European expert panel elicitation. *Environmental Science and Technology*, Vol. 44, No. 1, (January 2010), pp. 476-482, ISSN 0013-936X

[34] Holmes, N.S. (2007). A review of particle formation events and growth in the atmosphere in the various environments and discussion of mechanistic implications. *Atmospheric Environment*, Vol. 41, No. 10, (March 2007), pp. 2183-2201, ISSN 1352-2310

[35] Horvath, H. (1994). Atmospheric aerosols, atmospheric optics visibility. *Journal of Aerosol Science*, Vol. 25, Suppl. 1, (May 1994), pp. 23-24, ISSN 0021-8502

[36] Horvath, H. (2008). Conference on visibility, aerosols, and atmospheric optics, Vienna, September 3–6, 2006. *Atmospheric Environment*, Vol. 42, No. 11, (April 2008), pp. 2569-2570, ISSN 1352-2310

[37] Ibald-Mulli, A., Timonen, K.L., Peters, A., Heinrich, J., Wölke, G., Lanki, T., Buzorius, G., Kreyling, W.G., de Hartog, J., Hoek, G., ten Brink, H.M. & Pekkanen, J. (2004). Effects of particulate air pollution on blood pressure and heart rate in subjects with cardiovascular disease: A multicenter approach. *Environmental Health Perspectives*, Vol. 112, No. 3, (March 2004), pp. 369-37, ISSN 0091-6765

[38] Ibald-Mulli, A., Wichmann, H.E., Kreyling, W. & Peters, A. (2002). Epidemiological evidence on health effects of ultrafine particles. *Journal of Aerosol Medicine: Deposition, Clearance, and Effects in the Lung*, Vol. 15, No. 2, (June 2002), pp. 189–201, ISSN 0894-2684

[39] Intergovernmental Panel on Climate Change (IPCC). 2007. *Climate Change 2007: The Physical Science Basis. Contribution of Working Group I to the Fourth Assessment Report of the Intergovernmental Panel on Climate Change*, Cambridge University Press, ISBN 978-0-521-88009-1, Cambridge, United Kingdom

[40] Kettunen, J., Lanki, T., Tiittanen, P., Aalto, P.P., Koskentalo, T., Kulmala, M., Salomaa, V. & Pekkanen, J. (2007). Associations of fine and ultrafine particulate air pollution with stroke mortality in an area of low air pollution levels. *Stroke*, Vol. 38, No. 3, (March 2007), pp. 918-922, ISSN 0039-2499

[41] Kim, K.H., Sekiguchi, K., Furuuchi, M. & Sakamoto, K. (2011). Seasonal variation of carbonaceous and ionic components in ultrafine and fine particles in an urban area of Japan. *Atmospheric Environment*, Vol. 45, No. 8, (March 2011), pp. 1581-1590, ISSN 1352-2310

[42] Kim, Y.J., Kim, K.W. & Oh, S.J. (2001). Seasonal characteristics of haze observed by continuous visibility monitoring in the urban atmosphere of Kwangju, Korea. *Environmental Monitoring and Assessment*, Vol. 70, No. 1-2, (July 2001), pp. 35-46, ISSN 0167-6369

[43] Kittelson, B.D. (1998). Engines and nanoparticles: a review. *Journal of Aerosol Science*, Vol. 29, No. 5-6, (June 1998), pp. 575–588, ISSN 0021-8502

[44] Kittelson, D., Watts, W. & Johnson, J. (2006). On-road and laboratory evaluation of combustion aerosols – Part1: summary of diesel engine results. *Journal of Aerosol Science*, Vol. 37, No. 8, (August 2006), pp. 913–930, ISSN 0021-8502

[45] Kittelson, D.B., Watts, W.F. & Johnson, J.P. (2004). Nanoparticle emissions on Minnesota highways. *Atmospheric Environment*, Vol. 38, No. 1, (January 2004), pp. 9–19, ISSN 1352-2310

[46] Klems, J.P., Pennington, M.R., Zordan, C.A., McFadden, L. & Johnston, M.V. (2011). Apportionment of motor vehicle emissions from fast changes in number concentration and chemical composition of ultrafine particles near a roadway intersection. *Environmental Science and Technology*, Vol. 45, No. 13, (July 2011), pp. 5637-5643, ISSN 0013-936X

[47] Knol, A., de Hartog, J., Boogaard, H., Slottje, P., van der Sluijs, J., Lebret, E., Cassee, F., Wardekker, J.A., Ayres, J., Borm, P., Brunekreef, B., Donaldson, K., Forastiere, F., Holgate, S., Kreyling, W., Nemery, B., Pekkanen, J., Stone, V., Wichmann, H.E., Hoek, G., 2009. Expert elicitation on ultrafine particles: likelihood of health effects and causal pathways. *Particle and Fibre Toxicology*, Vol. 6, No. 19, (July 2009), 16 pp., ISSN 1743-8977

[48] Kudo, S., Sekiguchi, K., Kim, K.H. & Sakamoto, K. (2011). Spatial distributions of ultrafine particles and their behavior and chemical composition in relation to roadside sources. *Atmospheric Environment*, Vol. 45, No. 35, (November 2011), pp. 6403-6413, ISSN 1352-2310

[49] Kulmala, M., Pirjola, L., Makela & J. (2000). Stable sulphate clusters as a source of new atmospheric particles. *Nature*, Vol. 404, No. 6773, (March 2000), pp. 66–69, ISSN 0028-0836

[50] Kulmala, M., Vehkamäki, H., Petäjä, T., Dal Maso, M., Lauri, A., Kerminen, V.-M., Birmili, W. & McMurry, P.H. (2004). Formation and growth rates of ultrafine atmospheric particles: a review of observations. *Journal of Aerosol Science*, Vol. 35, No. 2, (March 2004), pp. 143-176, ISSN 0021-8502

[51] Kumar, P., Fennell, P. & Britter, R. (2008a). Effect of wind direction and speed on the dispersion of nucleation and accumulation mode particles in an urban street canyon. *The Science of The Total Environment*, Vol. 402, No. 1, (August 2008), pp. 82–94, ISSN 0048-9697

[52] Kumar, P., Fennell, P. & Britter, R. (2008b). Measurements of particles in the 5–1000 nm range close to road level in an urban street canyon. *Science of The Total Environment*, Vol. 390, No. 2-3, (February 2008), pp. 437-447, ISSN 0048-9697

[53] Kumar, P., Fennell, P., Hayhurst, A.N. & Britter, R.E. (2009). Street versus rooftop level concentrations of fine particles in a Cambridge street canyon. *Boundary-Layer Meteorology,* Vol. 131, No. 1, (April 2009), pp. 3-18, ISSN 0006-8314

[54] Kumar, P., Robins, A., Vardoulakis, S. & Britter, R. (2010). A review of the characteristics of nanoparticles in the urban atmosphere and the prospects for developing regulatory controls mode particles in an urban street canyon. *Atmospheric Environment,* Vol. 44, No. 1, (August 2008), pp. 5035-5052, ISSN 1352-2310

[55] Kumara, P., Robins, A., Vardoulakis, A., Paul Quincey, P. (2011). Technical challenges in tackling regulatory concerns for urban atmospheric nanoparticles. *Particuology,* Vol. 9, No. 6, (December 2011), pp. 566– 571, ISSN 1674-2001

[56] Maynard, A.D. & Aitken, R.J. (2007). Assessing exposure to airborne nanomaterials: current abilities and future requirements. *Nanotoxicology,* Vol. 1, No. 1, (March 2007), pp. 26-41, ISSN 1743-5390

[57] Monks, P.S., Granier, C., Fuzzi, S., Stohl, A., Williams, M.L, Akimoto, H., Amanni, M., Baklanov, A. & et al. (2009. Atmospheric composition change – global and regional air quality. *Atmospheric Environment,* Vol. 43, No. 33, (October 2009), pp. 5268–5350, ISSN 1352-2310

[58] Morawska, L., Ristovski, Z., Jayaratne, E.R., Keogh, D.U. & Ling, X. (2008). Ambient nano and ultrafine particles from motor vehicle emissions: characteristics, ambient processing and implications on human exposure. *Atmospheric Environment,* Vol. 42, No. 35, (November 2008), pp. 8113–8138, ISSN 1352-2310

[59] Naga, S., Guptaa, K. & Mukhopadhyay, U.K. (2005). Size distribution of atmospheric aerosols in Kolkata, India and the assessment of pulmonary deposition of particle mass. *Indoor and Built Environment,* Vol. 14, No. 5, (October 2005), pp. 381-389, ISSN 1420-326X

[60] Nel, A., Xia, T., Madler, L. & Li, N. (2006). Toxic potential of materials at the nanolevel. *Science,* Vol. 311, No. 5761, (February 2006), pp. 622–627, ISSN 0036-8075

[61] Ntziachristos, L., Ning, Z., Geller, M.D. & Sioutas, C. (2007). Particle concentration and characteristics near a major freeway with heavy duty diesel traffic. *Environmental Science and Technology,* Vol. 41, No. 7, (April 2007), pp. 2223–2230, ISSN 0013-936X

[62] O'Dowd, C. & Hoffmann, T. (2005). Coastal new particle formation: a review of the current state-of-the-art. *Environmental Chemistry,* Vol. 2, No. 4, pp. 245–255, ISSN 1448-2517

[63] O'Dowd, C., Aalto, P., Hameri, K., Kulmala, M. & Hoffmann, T. (2002). Aerosol formation: atmospheric particles from organic vapours. *Nature,* Vol. 416, No. 6880, (April 2002), pp. 497-498, ISSN 0028-0836

[64] O'Dowd, C., Facchini, M.C., Cavalli, F., Ceburnis, D., Mircea, M., Decesari, S., Fuzzi, S., Yoon, Y.J. & Putaud, J.-P. (2004). Biogenically driven organic contribution to marine aerosol. *Nature*, Vol. 431, No. 7009, (October 2004), pp. 676–680, ISSN 0028-0836

[65] Oberdörster, G., Oberdörster, E. & Oberdörster, J. (2005). Nanotoxicology: an emerging discipline evolving from studies of ultrafine particles. *Environmental Health Perspectives*, Vol. 113, No. 7, (July 2005), pp. 823–839, ISSN 0091-6765

[66] Oberdörster, G., Sharp, Z., Atudorei, V., Elder, A., Gelein, R., Kreyling, W. & Cox, C. (2004). Translocation of inhaled ultrafine particles to the brain. *Inhalation Toxicology*, Vol. 16, No. 6-7, (June 2004), pp. 437-445, ISSN 0895-8378

[67] Pekkanen, J., Peters, A., Hoek, G., Tiittanen, P., Brunekreef, B., De Hartog, J., Heinrich, J., Ibald-Mulli, A., Kreyling, W.G., Lanki, T., Timonen, K.L. & Vanninen, E. (2002). Particulate air pollution and risk of ST-segment depression during repeated submaximal exercise tests among subjects with coronary heart disease: The exposure and risk assessment for fine and ultrafine particles in ambient air (ULTRA) study. *Circulation*, Vol. 106, No. 8, (August 2002), pp. 933-938, ISSN 00097322

[68] Pekkanen, J., Timonen, K.L., Ruuskanen, J., Reponen, A. & Mirme, A. (1997). Effects of ultrafine and fine particles in urban air on peak expiratory flow among children with asthmatic symptoms. *Environmental Research*, Vol. 74, No. 1, pp. 24-33, ISSN 0013-9351

[69] Penttinen, P., Timonen, K.L., Tiittanen, P., Mirme, A., Ruuskanen, J. & Pekkanen, J. (2001a). Ultrafine particles in urban air and respiratory health among adult asthmatics. *European Respiratory Journal*, Vol. 17, No. 3, (March 2001), pp. 428-435, ISSN 0903-1936

[70] Penttinen, P., Timonen, K.L., Tiittanen, P., Mirme, A., Ruuskanen, J. & Pekkanen, J. (2001b). Number concentration and size of particles in urban air: Effects on spirometric lung function in adult asthmatic subjects. *Environmental Health Perspectives*, Vol. 109, No. 4, (April 2001), pp. 319-323, ISSN 0091-6765

[71] Peters, A., Wichmann, H.E., Tuch, T., Heinrich, J. & Heyder, J. (1997). Respiratory effects are associated with the number of ultrafine particles. *American Journal of Respiratory and Critical Care Medicine*, Vol. 155, No.4, (April 1997), pp. 1376-83, ISSN 1073-449X

[72] Pey, J., Querol, X., Alastuey, A., Rodríguez, S., Putaud, J.P. & Van Dingenen, R. (2009). Source apportionment of urban fine and ultra fine particle number concentration in a Western Mediterranean City. *Atmospheric Environment*, Vol. 43, No. 29, (September 2009), pp. 4407–4415, ISSN 1352-2310

[73] Raes, F. (1995). Entrainment of free tropospheric aerosols as a regulating mechanism for cloud condensation nuclei in the remote marine boundary layer. *Journal of Geophysical Research*, Vol. 100, No. D2, (February 1995), pp. 2893–2904, ISSN 0148-0227

[74] Ramanathan, V. & Feng, Y. (2009). Air pollution, greenhouse gases and climate change: Global and regional perspectives. *Atmospheric Environment*, Vol. 43, No. 1, (January 2009), pp. 37–50, ISSN 1352-2310

[75] Riipinen, S., Kulmala, M., Arnold, F., Dal Maso, M., Birmili, W., Saarnio, K., Teinilä, K., Kerminen, V., Laaksonen, A. & Lehtinen, K. (2007). Connections between atmospheric sulphuric acid and new particle formation during QUEST III-IV campaigns in Heidelberg and Hyytiälä. *Atmospheric Chemistry and Physics*, Vol. 7, No. 8, (April 2007) pp. 1899–1914, ISSN 1680-7316

[76] Ristovski, Z.D., Jayaratne, E.R., Lim, M., Ayoko, G.A. & Morawska, L. (2006.) Influence of diesel fuel sulphur on the nanoparticle emissions from city buses. *Environmental Science and Technology*, Vol. 40, No. 4, (February 2006), pp. 1314–1320, ISSN 0013-936X

[77] Ristovski, Z.D., Jayaratne, E.R., Morawska, L., Ayoko, G.A., Lim, M. (2005). Particle and carbon dioxide emissions from passenger vehicles operating on unleaded petrol and LPG fuel. *Science of The Total Environment*, Vol. 345, No. 1-3, (June 2005), pp.93–98, ISSN 0048-9697

[78] Rosenbohm, E., Vogt, R., Scheer, V., Nielsen, O., Drieseidler, A., Baumbach, G., Imhof, D., Baltensperger, U., Fuchs, J. & Jaeschke, W. (2005). Particulate size distributions and mass measured at a motorway during the BAB II campaign. *Atmospheric Environment*, Vol. 39, No. 31, (October 2005), pp. 5696–5709, ISSN 1352-2310

[79] Rückerl, R., Phipps, R.P., Schneider, A., Frampton, M., Cyrys, J., Oberdörster, G., Wichmann, H.E. & Peters, A. (2007). Ultrafine particles and platelet activation in patients with coronary heart disease--results from a prospective panel study. *Particle and Fibre Toxicology*, Volume 4, (January 2007), pp. 1, ISSN 17438-977

[80] Ruuskanen, J., Tuch, Th., Ten Brink, H., Peters, A., Khlystov, A., Mirme, A., Kos, G.P.A., Brunekreef, B., Wichmann, H.E., Buzorius, G., Vallius, M., Kreyling, W.G. & Pekkanen, J. Concentrations of ultrafine, fine and PM2.5 particles in three European cities. *Atmospheric Environment*, Vol. 35, No. 21, (July 2001), pp. 3729-3738, ISSN 1352-2310

[81] Seinfeld, J.H. & Pandis, S.N. (2006). *Atmospheric Chemistry and Physics: From Air Pollution to Climate Change* (2nd edition), John Wiley & Sons, ISBN 978-0-471-72018-8, Hoboken, New Jersey

[82] Shi, J. & Harrison, R.M. (1999). Investigation of ultrafine particle formation during diesel exhaust dilution. *Environmental Science and Technology*, Vol. 33, No. 21, (September 1999), pp. 3730–3736, ISSN 0013-936X

[83] Shi, J., Evans, D., Khan, A., Harrison, R., 2001. Sources and concentration of nanoparticles (<10 nm diameter) in the urban atmosphere. *Atmospheric Environment*, Vol. 35, No. 7, (July 2001), pp. 1193–1202, ISSN 1352-2310

[84] Sioutas, C., Delfino, R. J. & Singh, M. (2005). Exposure assessment for atmospheric ultrafine particles (UFPs) and implications in epidemiologic research. *Environmental Health Perspective*, Vol. 113, No. 8, (August 2005), pp. 947-955, ISSN 0091-6765

[85] Slezakova, K., Morais S. & Pereira M.C. (2012). Traffic–related air pollution: legislation versus health and environmental effects, In: *Environmental Health – Emerging Issues and Practice*, J. Oosthuizen (Ed.), pp. 103–124, Intech, ISBN 978-953-307-854-4, Rijeka, Croatia

[86] Slezakova, K., Morais S. & Pereira M.C. (2012). Air pollution: particulate matter, In: *Encyclopedia of Environmental Management*, S.E. Jorgensen (Ed.), in press, CRC Press, ISBN 9781-439-829-271, Boca Raton, Florida

[87] Stölzel, M., Breitner, S., Cyrys, J., Pitz, M., Wölke, G., Kreyling, W., Heinrich, J., Wichmann, H.E. & Peters, A. (2007). Daily mortality and particulate matter in different size classes in Erfurt, Germany. *Journal of Exposure Science and Environmental Epidemiology*, Vol. 17, No. 5, (August 2007), pp. 458-467, ISSN 1559-0631

[88] Strawa, A.W., Kirchstetter, T.W., Hallar, A.G., Ban-Weiss, G.A., McLaughlin, J.P., Harley, R.A. & Lunden, M.M. (2010). Optical and physical properties of primary on-road vehicle particle emissions and their implications for climate change. *Journal of Aerosol Science* Vol. 41, No. 1, (January 2010), pp. 36-50, ISSN 0021-8502

[89] Terzano, C., Di Stefano, F., Conti, V., Graziani, E. & Petroianni, A. (2010). Air pollution ultrafine particles: Toxicity beyond the lung. *European Review for Medical and Pharmacological Sciences*, Vol. 14, No. 10, (October 2010), pp. 809-821, ISSN 1128-3602

[90] Tranfield, E.M. & Walker D.C. (2012). Understanding of Human Illness and Death Following Exposure to Particulate Matter Air Pollution, In: *Environmental Health – Emerging Issues and Practice*, J. Oosthuizen (Ed.), pp. 81-102, Intech, ISBN 978-953-307-854-4, Rijeka, Croatia

[91] Tsai, Y.I. (2005). Atmospheric visibility trends in an urban area in Taiwan 1961-2003. *Atmospheric Environment*, Vol. 39, No. 30, (September 2005), pp. 5555-5567, ISSN 1352-2310

[92] Tunved, P., Hansson, H., Kerminen, V., Strom, J., Dal Maso, M., Lihavainen, H., Viisanen, Y., Aalto, P., Komppula, M. & Kulmala, M. (2006). High natural aerosol loading over boreal forests. *Science*, Vol. 312, No. 5771, (April 2006), pp. 261–263, ISSN 0036-8075

[93] United States Environmental Protection Agency (USEPA). (2006). *National Ambient Air Quality Standards for Particulate Matter; Final Rule*, Federal Register, Vol. 71, No. 200 (October 2006), pp. 61144, August, 2012, available from <http://www.gpo.gov/fdsys/pkg/FR-2006-10-17/html/06-8477.htm>

[94] United States Environmental Protection Agency (USEPA). (2009). *Assessment of the Impacts of Global Change on Regional U.S. Air Quality: A Synthesis of Climate Change Impacts on Ground-Level Ozone*, EPA 600-R-07-094F, Office of Research and Develop-

ment, National Centre for Environmental Assessment, Research Triangle Park, North Carolina

[95] United States Environmental Protection Agency (USEPA). (2012a). *Characteristics of Particles - Particle Size Categories*, June 2012, Available from: <http://www.epa.gov/apti/bces/module3/category/category.htm>

[96] United States Environmental Protection Agency (USEPA). (2012b). *Our Nation's Air: Status and Trends through 2010*, EPA-454/R-12-001, Office of Air Quality Planning and Standards, Research Triangle Park, North Carolina

[97] Van Dingenen, R., Raes, F., Putaud, J.-P., Baltensperger, U., Charron, A., Facchini, M.-C., Decesari, S., Fuzzi, S., Gehrig, R., Hansson, H.-C. & et al. (2004). A European aerosol phenomenology - 1: physical characteristics of particulate matter at kerbside, urban, rural and background sites in Europe. *Atmospheric Environment*, Vol. 38, No. 16, (May 2004), pp. 2561–2577, ISSN 1352-2310

[98] von Klot, S., Wölke, G., Tuch, T., Heinrich, J., Dockery, D.W., Schwartz, J., Kreyling, W.G., Wichmann, H.E. & Peters, A. (2002). Increased asthma medication use in association with ambient fine and ultrafine particles. *European Respiratory Journal*, Vol. 20, No. 3, (September 2002), pp. 691-702, ISSN 0903-1936

[99] Wåhlin, P., Palmgren, F., Dingenen, R., & Raes, F. (2001). Pronounced decrease of ambient particle number emissions from diesel traffic in Denmark after reduction of the sulphur content in diesel fuel. *Atmospheric Environment*, Vol. 35, No. 21, (July 2001), pp. 3549–3552, ISSN 1352-2310

[100] Weber, R., Marti, J.J., McMurray, P., Eisele, F.L., Tanner, D.J. & Jefferson, A. (1996). Measured atmospheric new particle formation rates: implications for nucleation mechanisms. *Chemical Engineering Communications*, Vol. 151, No. 1, (January 1996), pp. 53–64, ISSN 0098-6445

[101] Weber, R., Marti, J.J., McMurray, P., Eisele, F.L., Tanner, D.J. & Jefferson, A. (1997). Measurement of new particle formation and ultrafine particle growth rates at a clean continental site. *Journal of Geophysical Research D: Atmospheres*, Vol. 102, No. 4, (February 1997), pp. 4375–4386, ISSN 0148-0227

[102] West, J.B. (2008). *Pulmonary Pathophysiology: the Essentials*, (7th edition), Lippincott Williams & Wilkins, ISBN 978-0-7817-6414-8, Baltimore, Philadelphia

[103] Westerdahl, D., Fruin, S., Sax, T., Fine, P. & Sioutas, C. (2005). Mobile platform measurements of ultrafine particles and associated pollutant concentrations on freeways and residential streets in Los Angeles. *Atmospheric Environment*, Vol. 39, No. 20, (June 2005), pp. 3597–3610, ISSN 1352-2310

[104] Wichmann and Peters, H.E., Spix, C., Tuch, T., Wolke, G., Peters, A., Heinrich, J., Kreyling, W.G & Heyder, J. (2000). Daily mortality and fine and ultrafine particles in Erfurt, Germany part I: role of particle number and particle mass. *Research report*

(Health Effects Institute), No. 98, (November 2000), pp.5-86; discussion 87, ISSN 1041-5505

[105] World Health Organization (WHO). 2000. *Particulate Matter, Chapter 7.3*; WHO Regional Publications, European Series: Copenhagen, Denmark; pp. 1–40, August 2012, <http://www.euro.who.int/__data/assets/pdf_file/0019/123085/AQG2ndEd_7_3Particulate-matter.pdf>

Chapter 24

Cyanobacterial Toxins in Food-Webs: Implications for Human and Environmental Health

John Berry

Additional information is available at the end of the chapter

http://dx.doi.org/10.5772/55111

1. Introduction

Cyanobacteria (or "blue-green algae") are among the oldest known groups of organism on Earth, with fossil records spanning approximately 3.5 billion years, and inhabit nearly every ecological niche on the planet. In addition to their conspicuous occurrence as aquatic "blooms" (e.g. visible scums on ponds and lakes; Fig. 1), as well as various colonial or macrophytic forms, in marine and freshwater habitats, these photosynthetic prokaryotes are widely found in terrestrial soils, and as part of numerous symbiotic relationships with a range of organisms including animals, plants and fungi. To illustrate the extent of their global abundance and importance, approximately 50% of all primary productivity, and related oxygen production, occurs in the ocean, and the majority of this is derived from two genera of cyanobacteria, *Synechococcus* and the picophytoplankton, *Prochlorococcus* (Ting et al., 2002). Likewise, nitrogen-fixing cyanobacteria, and particularly the genus, *Trichodesmium*, are the largest source of nitrogen in ocean systems (Carpenter and Romans, 1991). Moreover, several lines of evidence (see, for example, Paerl and Huisman, 2009) point to an increase in the abundance, distribution and persistence of cyanobacterial blooms in marine and freshwater system, specifically driven by regional and global changes in climate (e.g. elevated water temperature, stratification of the water column, changes in interseasonal weather patterns). The latter, in particular, underscores the potential of cyanobacteria – and specifically toxin-producing cyanobacterial blooms (discussed below) – as a rapidly emerging concern for public health.

Alongside their global biological importance, the cyanobacteria are widely recognized as producers of a chemically diverse array of biologically active secondary metabolites (see, for example, reviews by Gerwick et al., 2001; Tan, 2007; Tan, 2010). Considerable work over the past four decades (see Tan, 2007) has, in particular, focused on exploring this chemical diversity as a source of bioactive compounds with possible relevance to biomedicine, and specifically development of potential chemotherapeutics. Furthermore, a rather convincing body of evidence (Proksh et al., 2002; Simmons et al., 2008) also suggests that many of the pharmacologically active marine natural products, originally isolated from various marine animal sources – and including several currently either in clinical trials, or being commercially developed as drugs - may, in fact, originate from cyanobacterial (or other microbial) sources as a result of trophic transfer (e.g. herbivory, filter-feeding), and symbiotic or commensal relationships.

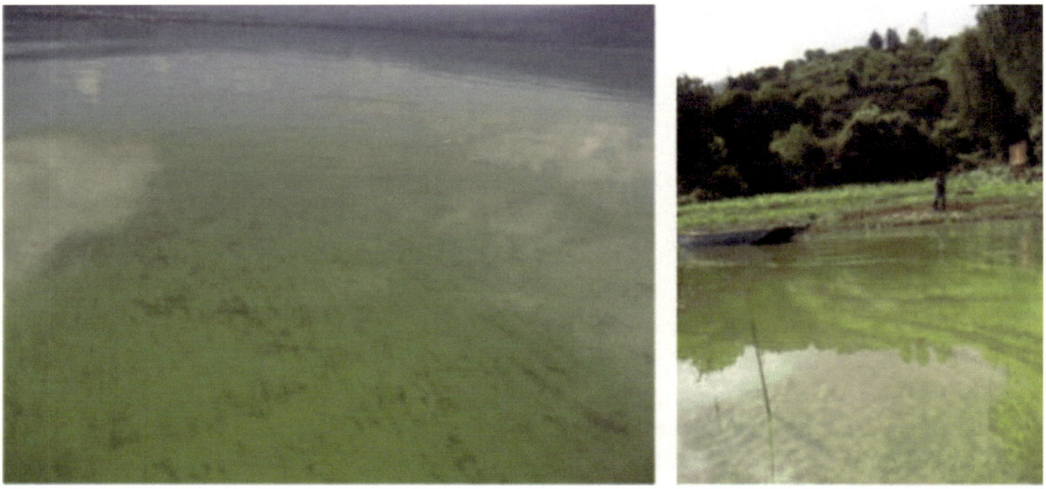

Figure 1. Bloom of toxin-producing cyanobacteria on Lake Patzcuaro (Michoacan, Mexico), and subsistence fishing occurring within the bloom. Photo courtesy of Alan Wilson (Auburn University).

In addition to their potential in biomedicine, however, a number of these bioactive metabolites have been identified as naturally occurring toxins, and have been associated – as so-called "cyanotoxins" - with various human and environmental health concerns. Perhaps most notably, in freshwater systems, cyanobacterial populations can proliferate to the extent that they form large "blooms," typically manifesting as "films" or "scums" on lakes, ponds and other freshwater systems (see Fig. 1). When comprised of toxin-producing representatives, their occurrence is generally categorized as "harmful algal blooms" (HABs), or frequently as "cyanoHABs" (to distinguish from similar blooms of several, unrelated, but likewise toxigenic, marine microalgae). In particular, toxins from cyanoHABs - or even simply high abundance of cyanobacterial cells – can contaminate water, and exposure to toxins via drinking water, recreational exposure and related routes has been linked to various cases of human and animal intoxication, as well as possible sub-acute and/or chronic health effects (e.g. increased rates of certain cancers, effects on fetal development). As these direct routes of exposure are beyond the scope of this chapter, and have been thoroughly covered by many previous authors, the reader is direct to several good reviews on the topic (e.g. Rao et al., 2002; Stewart et al., 2006; Funari and Testai, 2008).

Although the vast majority of studies related to the health impacts of cyanobacteria have focused on direct exposure to cyanotoxins via drinking water and related routes, there is a growing body of evidence to suggest that toxic cyanobacterial metabolites can bioaccumulate in aquatic food-webs, and may consequently pose additional health concerns as food-borne contaminants. The relatively limited number of studies on food-borne cyanobacterial contaminants may be attributed, in part, to the perceived lack of a mechanism for their bioaccumulation. Unlike more lipophilic contaminants, many of the recognized, water-soluble cyanotoxins would, as such, not be expected to biomagnify by otherwise well-documented mechanisms (i.e. storage, and subsequent transfer, in fatty tissues of animals) to higher trophic levels most frequently consumed by humans. However, despite the lack of a clear means transfer of these hydrophilic toxins in food webs, numerous studies have, indeed, demonstrated presence and apparent bioaccumulation in a range of trophic levels. Also likely limiting the attention paid to cyanobacterial toxins in food-webs is the fact that best documented cases of intoxication have been generally limited to direct exposure to these toxins, and specifically acute human or animal poisonings with clear links to consumption of contaminated water, or various related route, whereas there are - at present - few, if any, clear cases of recognized human intoxication by food-borne cyanotoxin. That said, growing recognition that cyanobacterial toxins may contribute to a sub-acute and/or chronic health effects – ranging from increased rates of cancers, neurodegeneration and development toxicity - which are considerably more difficult to identify, would suggest that, despite the lack of currently documented toxicoses, health threats posed by diet-derived toxins remains a very real concern.

The following chapter will present the current state of knowledge regarding the bioaccumulation of cyanobacterial toxins in the food web, and the possible role of these food-borne toxins as it relates to human and environmental health. To begin, the chapter will present a brief summary of the recognized cyanobacterial toxins, and their known toxicology and health effects. Subsequently, the current evidence related to the bioaccumulation, trophic transfer and bioavailability of these cyanobacterial toxins in food webs will be reviewed, along with related methodologies (including methodological limitations and innovations) for investigating these aspects. In addition to the widely recognized water-soluble cyanotoxins, cyanobacteria produce a host of bioactive metabolites, including a number of lipophilic representatives. Accordingly, the discussion will include a consideration of the less characterized bioactive metabolites that, despite relatively unknown health effects, may represent – due to their potential for biomagnification –relevant food-web contaminants. Finally, the chapter will summarize the current state of knowledge regarding the impacts of cyanobacterial toxins as it relates to human and environmental (i.e. ecosystem, animal) health.

2. Recognized cyanobacterial toxins: Chemistry and toxicology

2.1. Hepatotoxins

Detoxification of a wide range of toxic metabolites occurs - via multiphasic enzymes, and associated processes (e.g cellular transporter and "pumps") - in the liver or equivalent organ systems in animals. Accordingly, many toxic metabolites are actively transported (for subsequent detoxification) to, and thus accumulate primarily in, hepatocytes. Not surprising, therefore, two of the most commonly recognized cyanobacterial toxins are, in fact, associated with hepatotoxicity. However, aside from active transport of these toxins to – and consequent toxicity in - hepatocytes, it is becoming increasingly clear that the same metabolites may accumulate in a range of tissues (even if not associated with acute toxicity in these cells), and may – along with their generally uncharacterized toxicology in these tissues - be thusly transferred to higher trophic levels.

2.1.1. Microcystins (MCs) and nodularin (NOD)

Perhaps the most widespread, and consequently well studied, of the cyanobacterial toxins, microcystins (MCs) and nodularin (NOD) are, respectively, hepatotoxic hepta- and pentapeptide toxins. Both share structural similarity (Fig. 2), specifically characterized by a peptide macrocyle incorporating common and unusual amino acids. However, the former (i.e. MCs) represents a chemically diverse group of toxins, comprised of more than ninety variants (Welker and Van Dohran, 2006). Although structural variation throughout the macrocycle of the MCs has been reported, the primary differences occur in "X" and "Y" positions (Fig. 2), as per the accepted nomenclature for the group. As an example, the most common, and generally considered the most toxic, of these variants is MC-LR in which the X and Y positions, respectively, are occupied by leucine (L) and arginine (R) residues. Although chemical variations exist, both NOD and most MC variants are characterized by a relatively well-conserved unusual β-amino acid, 3-amino-9-methoxy-2,6,8-trimethyl-10-phenyldeca-4,6-dienoic acid (Adda), which is involved (see below) in the toxicology of these metabolites (Gulledge et al., 2003). Finally, whereas NOD is generally limited to a single late summer blooming species, *Nodularia spumigens*, the MCs are produced by a taxonomically wide array of cyanobacterial species including, most notably, the widespread species, *Microcystis aeruginosa*, but also a growing list of other diverse taxa (e.g. *Aphanizomenon, Oscillatoria, Planktothrix, Anabaena, Nostoc*).

Toxiologically, both NOD and the MCs are inhibitors of Ser/Thr type 1 and 2A protein phosphatases (PPases). Data generally suggest that Adda of NOD and MCs are involved in the binding of the metabolite to the active site of PPases (Nishiwaki-Matsumishi et al., 1991; Gulledge et al., 2003). To demonstrate this, several analogues of the MCs, specifically comprised of only a single amino acid (i.e. Gly, or L- or D-Ala) coupled via peptidyl linkage to the carboxylic acid of the *N*-acetylated Adda, were synthesized (Gulledge et al. 2003) and evaluated for toxicity. Although orders of magnitude lower than intact MC-LR, these analogs retained substantial PPase inhibitory activity, suggesting that Adda significantly contributes to the toxicophore of the MCs and NOD. On the other hand, the unusual amino acid, N-methyldehydroalanine (Mdha), found in many MC variants has been shown to covalently bind via a Michael addition to Cys_{273} of type 1/2A Ser/Thr PPases (MacKintosh et al., 1995). Accordingly, it has been suggested that this distal (to Adda) amino acids is, therefore, also involved in irreversible binding of the toxin to the PPase targets, as well as considerable

http://dx.doi.org/10.5772/55111

underestimation of bioaccumulation (as a non-extractable "bound" form) in organisms exposed to the toxin (see 4.2 *Methodologies for evaluating cyanobacterial toxins in food-webs*, below).

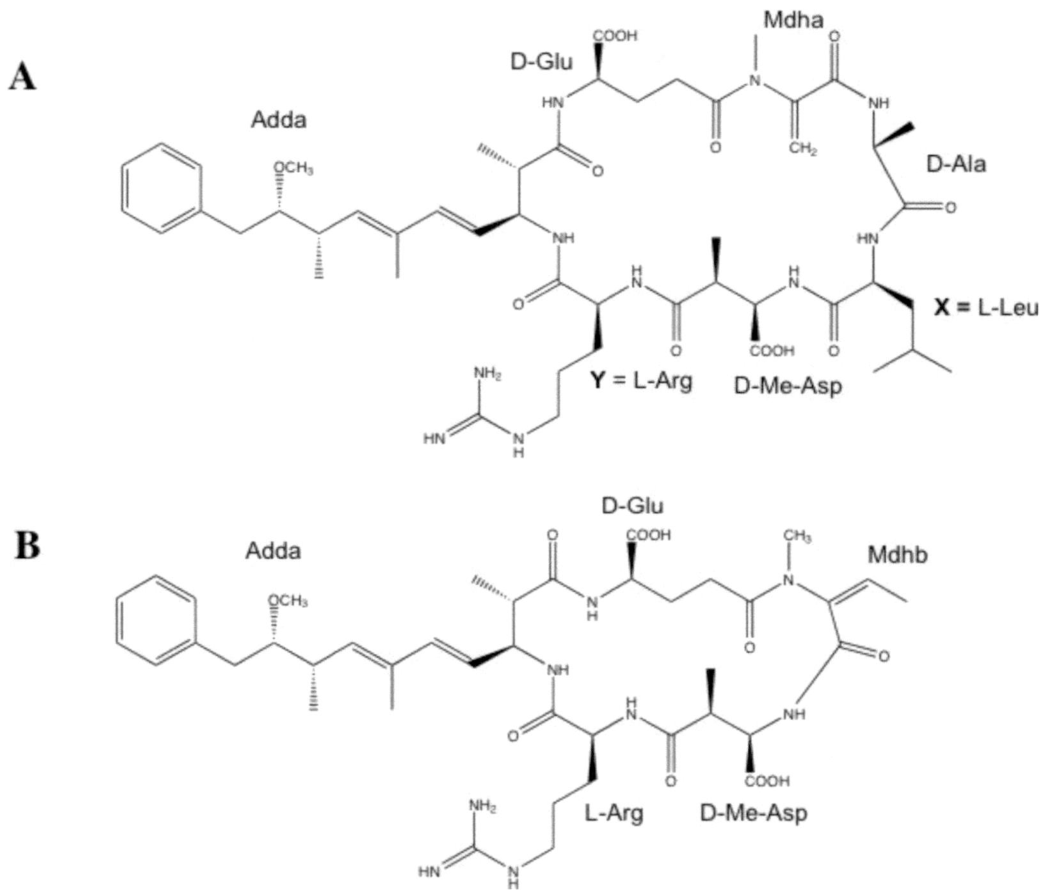

Figure 2. Chemical structures of hepatotoxic microcystins (A) and nodularin (B). In the former, structural variability is primarily based on variation in the "X" and "Y" amino acid positions indicated; for reference, the common variant, MC-LR, in which X and Y positions are leucine (L) and arginine (R) is shown.

Given the importance of PPases in a wide range of cellular functions, inhibition of these enzymes, following exposure to NOD/MCs, can result in a range of acute toxicoses. Accumulating primarily in hepatocytes (i.e. liver) and associated organ systems, inhibition of PPase by MCs and NOD most typically manifests as acute failure and hemorrhaging in these systems. However, recent studies, specifically pointing to the presence of similar active transporters in mammalian (e.g. rat) brains, have proposed a possible connection between MC uptake and apparent inhibitory effects on short- and long-term memory (Maidana et al., 2006). Moreover, emerging evidence supports an additional role of MCs in various chronic health effects, and particularly, as recognized tumor promoters, increased rates of certain cancers. Most notably, studies in China (Yu, 1995; Ueno et al., 1996; Yu et al., 2001) have linked chronic exposure to MC through ingestion of contaminated surface (i.e. ditch) waters to endemically high rates of primary liver cancers. These studies suggest, in particular, that health concerns associated with exposure to even quite low (e.g. sub-picogram per day) doses of cyanobacterial toxins, such as MC/NOD, may promote negative health effects that might not clearly manifest as acute intoxication. This may be particularly germane to discussion of the bioaccumulation of these toxins since there have been to-date no known cases of overt intoxication from food-borne MCs or NOD, whereas the possible long-term effects associated with chronic exposure to these toxins (and others, e.g. BMAA) in the diet continues to present a possible concern.

2.1.2. Cylindrospermopsin (CYN)

Cylindrospermopsin (CYN) is a zwitterionic tricyclic alkaloid, specifically containing a unique hydroxyuracil (Fig. 3). It was first identified following a relatively large intoxication event (the so-called "Palm Island Mystery") in Queensland, Australia. In this original case, children from more than one hundred families on Palm Island, and nearby mainland community of Townsville, were stricken with severe gastroenteritis. Subsequent studies (Bourke et al., 1983; Hawkins et al., 1985) linked the illness to the Solomon Dam – the primary water reservoir for the community – and identified several bloom-forming species of cyanobacteria. Among these, a toxic (in mouse bioassay) strain of the species, *Cylindrospermospsis raciborskii,* was identified (Hawkins et al., 1985). More than ten years after the incident, CYN was identified as the toxic principle of the *C. raciborksii* blooms in the reservoir (Ohtani et al., 1992), and following subsequent stereoselective synthesis (Heintzelman et al., 2001), assigned the structure shown in Figure 3. Originally thought to be a strictly tropical species, *C. raciborskii,* has been subsequently shown to occur worldwide in both tropical and temperate freshwater systems, possibly the result of recent expansion in its geographic distribution (Gugger et al., 2005). Moreover, since its initial identification from *C. raciborskii,* CYN has been subsequently found to be produced by several other members of the Nostocales, including the closely related *Aphanizomenon* and *Anabaena* (Banker et al., 1997; Spoof et al., 2006; Preußel et al., 2006), as well as at least one member of the Stigonometales (i.e. *Umezakia*; Harada et al., 1994), suggesting relatively widespread production of the toxin.

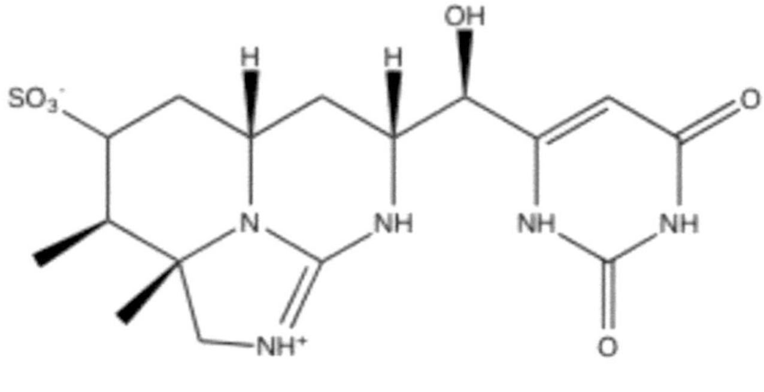

Figure 3. Chemical structure of the hepatotoxin, cylindrospermopsin (CYN).

Toxicological studies primarily suggest that CYN is an inhibitor of protein synthesis (Terao et al., 1994; Froscio et al., 2001). Specifically, Terao et al. (1994) demonstrated ribosomal detachment (from endoplasmic reticula) in hepatocytes treated with CYN, and *in vitro* studies using the rabbit reticulocyte translation system showed that CYN inhibits protein synthesis at nanomolar concentrations (e.g. IC_{50} = 120 nM; Froscio et al., 2001). However, a range of possible mechanisms of toxicity, and associated biomarkers of the toxin, have been additionally identified and/or proposed. In accordance with inhibition of protein synthesis, Runnegar et al. (1994, 1995) showed a reduction of the tripeptide, glutathione (GSH), in rat hepatocytes exposed to CYN, particularly via apparent inhibition of GSH synthesis, leading to a presumptive reduction in the detoxifying capacity of cells. Studies (e.g. Shaw et al., 2000; Humpage et al., 2005) have similarly pointed to possible interaction of CYN with cytochrome P450, and suggested a role of this detoxifying enzyme system. Based on structural similarity to nucleotides, specifically as guanidine alkaloid, and more specifically the hydroxyuracil moiety contained in the tricyclic structure (Fig. 3), it has been suggested that CYN may additionally exert toxicity by means of interaction with DNA and/or RNA. Indeed, CYN has been found to form covalent linkages with DNA, leading to consequent chromosomal strand breakage (Shaw et al., 2000; Shen et al., 2002), as well as other apparent genotoxic effects (Bazin et al., 2010). This is notable as the uracil moiety of CYN has been shown as required for toxicity (Banker et al., 2001). Finally, *in vivo* studies, particularly in the mouse model, point to a range of histopathological effects, particularly in cells of the liver, but additionally in several organ systems (e.g. kidney, adrenal glands, lungs, intestines), following exposure via intraperitoneal or oral exposure (Hawkins et al., 1985; Shaw et al, 2000; Humpage and Falconer, 2003). Moreover, recent studies (in mice) show that long-term oral exposure to low-doses of CYN leads to measurable effects (e.g. reduced hematocrit levels; Sukenik et al., 2006), and, likewise, exposure to CYN during gestation induces fetal toxicity (Rogers et al., 2007), indicating that (similar to MCs) sub-acute effects may occur with relatively low doses, but may be missed by simple assessment of intoxication.

2.2. Neurotoxins

Several of the prominent cyanobacterial toxins are known to presumably cross the blood-brain barrier, and have been consequently associated with neurotoxicity. Neurotoxic cyanotoxins have been particularly identified based on observation of acute toxicity following exposure to these toxins (see below). However, in at least one case (i.e. BMAA; see below), toxicity has been associated with possible chronic neurodegeneration.

2.2.1. Anatoxin-a (ATX-a) and anatoxin-a(s)

Although chemically unrelated, two of the most active neurotoxins produced by cyanobacteria are related both in name and mode of action. First identified from species of *Anabaena*, anatoxin-a (ATX-a) is a tropane alkaloid (Fig. 4) with structural, but not pharmacological, similarity to cocaine. In contrast, the relatively less common anatoxin-a(s), so-named due to hyper-*salivation* associated with its neurotoxicity, is a phosphate ester of N-hydroxyguanine (Fig. 4), likewise, isolated primarily from *Anabaena* spp. Although structurally very different, the two metabolites (along with a few chemically related variants, e.g. homoanatoxin-a) share related toxicological mechanisms of action. Known as the "very fast death factor," ATX-a and its analogues are potent inhibitors of nicotinic acetylcholine receptors (nAChRs), specifically mimicking the endogenous neurotransmitter, acetylcholine, whereas anatoxin-a(s) inhibits related acetylcholinesterases (Aráoz et al., 2010). Interestingly, ATX-a is not degraded by acetylcholinesterases, and thus irreversibly inhibits nAChRs (Aráoz et al., 2010). With regards to food-webs, it should be noted that – compared to other cyanobacterial toxins – the "anatoxins" are relatively unstable chemically, as well as being generally limited in their distribution and occurrence, and thus rather few studies have reported their bioaccumulation (e.g. Mejean et al., 2010; Osswald et al., 2011). That said at least one case of apparent bioaccumulation of ANTX-a and its analogue (i.e. homoANTX-a) is, in fact, among the very few cases of acute intoxications being possibly linked to food-borne cyanotoxins (see *3. Evidence for bioaccumulation of cyanobacterial toxins in aquatic food-webs,* below).

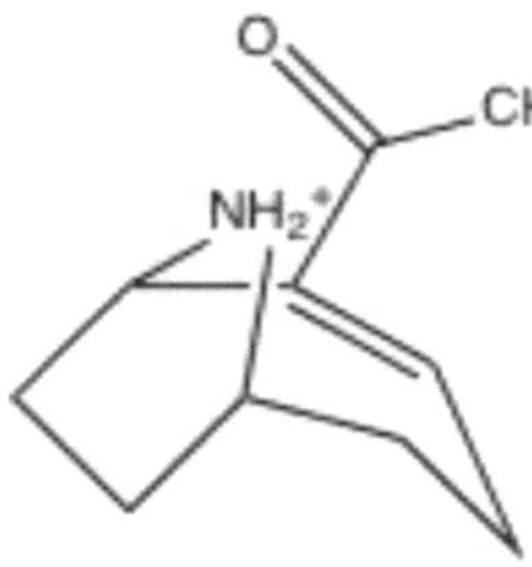

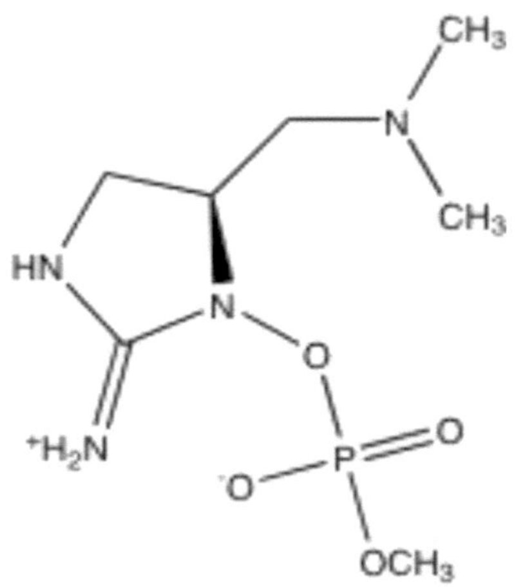

Figure 4. Chemical structure of the neurotoxins, anatoxin-a (ATX-a, left) and anatoxin-a(s) (right).

2.2.2. Saxitoxin (STX) and "Paralytic Shellfish Toxins" (PSTs)

Potent inhibitors of voltage-gated sodium channels, saxitoxin (STX) and several chemically related metabolites have been frequently associated with contamination of shellfish, and consequent toxicity (i.e. "paralytic shellfish poisoning" [PSP]), as the so-called "paralytic shellfish toxins" (PSTs). Specifically, in marine systems, the origins of STX/PSTs have been identified as *Alexandrium* and several related species of dinoflagellates. However, in the late 1960s, apparent STX was identified (Jackim and Gentile, 1968) in the cyanobacterial species, *Aphanizomenon flos-aquae*. Over the subsequent four decades, STX and related PSTs have been identified from a wide range of cyanobacterial genera (e.g. Mahmood and Carmichael, 1986; Humpage et al., 1994; Negri et al., 1995; Carmichael et al., 1997; Lagos et al., 1999; Beltran and

Neilan, 2000; Pomati et al., 2000; Smith et al., 2011) including members of the Nostocales (e.g. *Anabaena, Scytonema, Cylindrospermopsin*) and Oscillatoriales (e.g. *Lyngbya, Planktothrix*).

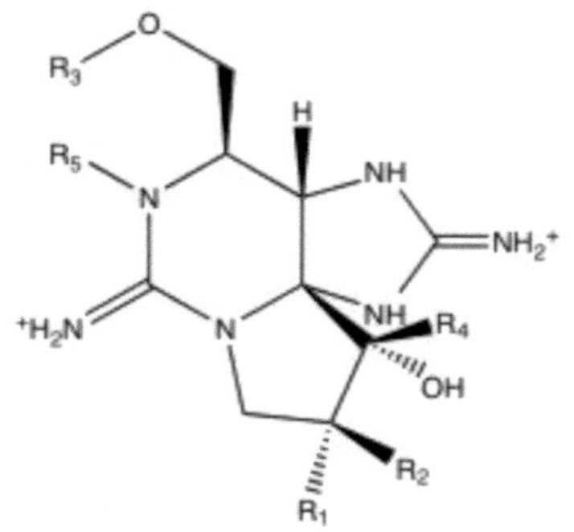

PST Variant	R1	R2	R3	R4	R5
STX	H	H	$CONH_2$	OH	H
neoSTX	H	H	$CONH_2$	OH	OH
Gonyautoxin 1 (GTX1)	H	OSO_3^-	$CONH_2$	OH	OH
GTX2	H	OSO_3^-	$CONH_2$	OH	H
GTX3	OSO_3^-	H	$CONH_2$	OH	H
GTX4	OSO_3^-	H	$CONH_2$	OH	OH
B1	H	H	$CONHSO_3^-$	OH	H
B2	H	H	$CONHSO_3^-$	OH	OH
C1	H	OSO_3^-	$CONHSO_3^-$	OH	H
C2	OSO_3^-	H	$CONHSO_3^-$	OH	H
C3	H	OSO_3^-	$CONHSO_3^-$	OH	OH
C4	OSO_3^-	H	$CONHSO_3^-$	OH	OH
dcSTX	H	H	H	OH	H

Figure 5. Chemical structure of saxitoxin (STX) and selected variants of the related "paralytic shellfish toxins" (PSTs).

STX/PSTs are potent inhibitors of voltage-gated sodium channels in neuronal cells, specifically acting on (via binding to, and consequent blockage of) sodium passage through channel pores (Aráoz et al., 2010). Inhibition of sodium channels, by blocking sodium influx involved in the propogation of action potentials in neurons, leads to the aforementioned PSP syndrome which manifests in a range of neurotoxic symptoms including numbness, tingling, weakness and difficulty breathing as a result of the neuromuscular paralysis (Etheridge, 2010). Interestingly, STX/PST binds to the nearly identical location as the equally potent neurotoxin, tetrodotoxin (TTX), associated with poisoning by consumption of several species of pufferfish (Stevens et al., 2011), and STX has, in fact, been identified alongside TTX in pufferfish (Nakamura et al., 1984; discussed below). Notably, despite the identification of STX/PSTs from numerous cyanobacteria species found in freshwater sytems, as well as apparent bioaccumulation of presumptively cyanobacteria-derived toxin in fish and shellfish consumed by humans, reported poisoning by the PSTs has been generally limited to ingestion of shellfish contaminated by apparent marine dinoflagellate sources.

2.2.3. *β-Methylamino-L-alanine (BMAA)*

As perhaps the best studied case of apparent long-term toxicity resulting from a cyanobacterial toxin bioaccumulated within food webs, the non-essential, non-protein amino acid, β-methylamino-L-alanine (BMAA; Fig. 6) has been linked to high rates of the otherwise rare amyotrophic lateral sclerosis (ALS), and possibly other related neurodegenerative diseases (e.g. Parkinson's Disease, Alzheimer's Disease). Indeed, the first reports of BMAA as a neurotoxic cyanobacterial metabolite specifically stemmed from studies of extraordinarily high rates of ALS amont the indigenous Chamorro populations on the island of Guam. BMAA was originally identified as a plant-derived natural product, and specifically found in non-flowering plants of the genus, *Cycas* (Vega & Bell, 1967). However, the origin of the metabolite was ultimately traced to an endosymbiotic species of the cyanobacterial genus, *Nostoc*, found within roots these cycads. The occurrence of BMAA in this cycad species (Spencer et al., 1987), and its apparent biomagnification by fruit bats (or "Flying Foxes") which consume the fruits of the cycad, which are, in-turn, consumed as a delicacy by the Chamorro of Guam (Cox et al., 2003; discussed below), has been suggested to provide a route of exposure to the neurotoxin, and was consequently linked to ALS among the Chamorro. Indeed, subsequent studies have accordingly identified both apparent biomagnification of the metabolite in this rather short "food chain" (i.e. an approximately 10^4-fold increase from cyanobacteria to cycad to fruit bat), as well as measurable levels of BMAA in the brains of Chamorro patients that died from ALS and related syndromes (Cox et al., 2003).

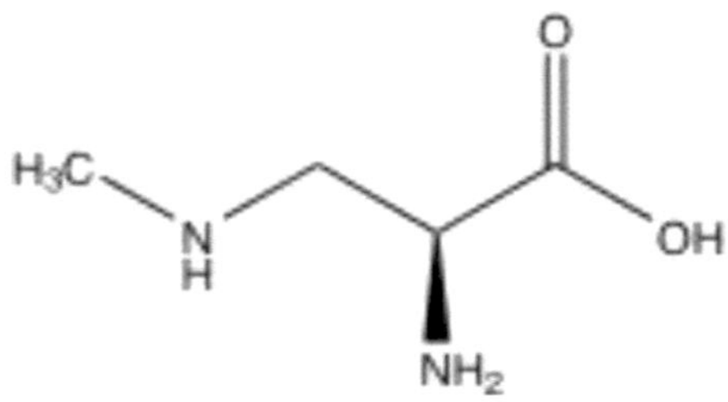

Figure 6. Chemical structure of β-Methylamino-L-Alanine (BMAA).

Toxicologically, BMAA is a recognized agonist of glutamate receptors. Staton and Bristow (1997) found that BMAA excited glutamate receptors, leading to apoptotic and necrotic cell death, in cerebellar granule cells. Subsequent studies (e.g. Rao et al., 2006; Lobner et al., 2007; Cucchiaroni et al., 2010) have confirmed a similar effect in a range of relevant neurons (e.g. spinal motor neurons, cortical neurons, dopaminergic substantia nigra pars compacta cells). More recently, however, it has been proposed that BMAA – as an amino acid – may become erroneously incorporated via translation into proteins. One of the hallmarks of several related neurodegenerative diseases (including ALS, Alzheimer's Disease, Parkinson Disease/Dementia) is the formation of misfolded protein aggregates, and it has consequently been proposed that the possible mis-incorporation of BMAA may represent an alternative mechanism of action for this putative toxin.

Although first identified in the Chamorro/ALS case, potential health concerns associated with BMAA have continued to grow with recent reports of a widespread occurrence of the metabolite among cyanobacteria, and its bioaccumulation in a wide range of systems, as well as additional epidemiological findings that link the compound to a complex of related neurodegenerative diseases. In a study by Cox et al. (2005) chemical analysis of a wide range of cyanobacteria, including marine, freshwater and terrestrial representatives, indicated that as many as 95% of the genera produce BMAA, and pointed to a potentially widespread occurrence of the metabolite. Since this study, the analytical techniques used with respect to BMAA have rapidly evolved (see *5. Methodologies for analyis of cyanobacterial toxins in food-webs*, below). Accordingly, several investigators (e.g. Li et al., 2012) have, in fact, argued - specifically based on re-evaluation of the analytical methods previously used - that these prior estimates regarding occurrence among cyanobacteria are perhaps exaggerated. However, despite this standing controversy, a growing number of studies have concurrently pointed to the apparent bioaccumulation of the metabolite in food webs and relevant human foods (discussed below) which, along with increasing experimental evidence to support toxicological effects related to neuronal and memory function (e.g. Karlsson et al., 2009 and 2009b; Liu et al., 2009; Purdie et al., 2009 and 2009b; Karlsson et al., 2011), and links to additional clusters of these disease, have continued to fuel emerging hypotheses regarding BMAA and neurodegeneration. With regards to the latter, *post mortem* studies have identified BMAA in the brain tissues of patients who had died from ALS and Alzheimer's Diesease (AD), but not from either strictly hereditary neurodegenerative disease (e.g. Huntington's Disease) or unrelated causes (Pablo et al., 2009). Several studies have, likewise, suggested links between BMAA and so-called "sporadic" occurrence of these diseases ranging from Canadian AD patients (Murch et al., 2004) to clusters of ALS associated with exposure to water blooms in New England (Caller et al., 2009) to sporadic occurrence among Gulf War veterans purportedly exposed to BMAA through cyanobacteria in desert dust (Cox et al., 2009). As these questions regarding occurrence of BMAA among cyanobacteria, as well as its toxicological relevance, continue to be answered, it is becoming clear that understanding the potential role of food-web bioaccumulation, as a route of exposure to this metabolite, will be particularly critical.

3. Evidence for bioaccumulation of cyanobacterial toxins in aquatic food-webs

Toxins from a number of marine HAB species – particularly including diverse eukaryotic taxa within the dinoflagellates and diatoms (Bacilliariophyta) – bioaccumulate and/or biomagnify in marine food-webs, and have been clearly linked to contamination of fish and seafood, and consequent intoxication of humans and wildlife (Van Dolah, 2000). Notably, marine algal toxins are (1) frequently associated with commercially important seafood species, including filter-feeding/grazing shellfish (e.g. clams, mussels) and several plantivorous fish species, and/or (2) alternatively characterized by relatively high lipophilicity enabling uptake and storage in fat tissues as a means of biomagnifications to higher trophic levels, including marine fish species eaten by humans (Van Dolah, 2000). Relevant examples of the former include dinophysotoxins and various other metabolites associated with "diarrhetic shellfish poisoning" (DSP), domoic acid associated with "amnesic shellfish poisoning" (ASP) and contamination of shellfish by so-called PSP toxins (i.e. STX and other PSTs, see above) derived from dinoflagellates (e.g. *Alexandrium* spp.). Examples of the latter, on the other hand, include biomagnification of ciguatoxin, and several chemically related lipophilic metabolites (e.g. maitotoxin), by various top-level predator species of fish in relation to the well documented "ciguatera poisoning."

Compared to marine HAB toxins, bioaccumulation of cyanobacterial toxins in food webs, and its consequent relevance to human and environmental health, has been relatively much less studied. There are likely several reasons for this. The most obvious is that, in contrast to the well-documented contamination of fish and other seafood by marine algal toxins, there are very few recognized cases of acute human or animal intoxication via consumption of bioaccumulated cyanobacterial toxins. It is further proposed that this may be due, in part, to less commercial fishing in freshwater water habitats - and thus consumption of freshwater fish and shellfish - compared to marine fisheries. Indeed, a recent report by the United Nations' Food and Agriculture Organization (FAO) estimated the 2008 global fisheries catch as approximately 90 million tonnes, but it was comprised of only a "record 10 million tonnes from inland waters," compared to more than 80 million tonnes from marine sources (FAO, 2010).

Regardless of the relatively limited focus on cyanobacterial toxins in freshwater fish and shellfish, a growing body of knowledge – summarized in Table 1 – does, in fact, support the occurrence of cyanobacterial toxins in a range of trophic levels, including species with direct potential for human exposure, as well as possible implications for ecosystem health (see *7. Implications for Ecosystem Health*, below). Indeed, a number of thorough reviews on the topic have recently appeared (e.g. Ibelings and Chorus, 2007; Ferrao-Filho et al., 2011; Kozlowsky-Suzuki et al., 2012). Owing to the relatively polar (i.e. water-soluble) nature of the recognized cyanobacterial toxins, it has been generally suggested that bioaccumulation in the food-web will be limited to relatively "low" trophic positions. Indeed, in freshwater food webs, this has included particularly high rates of bioaccumulation of toxins in planktivorous fish, and filter-feeding or other grazing invertebrates (Table 1). Reported concentrations of accumulated cyanobacterial toxins are, at first glance, typically quite low (Table 1). However, levels are obviously expected to vary - as shown in experimental studies (e.g. Osswald et al., 2011) - with concentrations of toxins and/or algal cell density to which animals are exposed. Moreover, it is suggested by various studies that levels may be sufficient for long-term (and consequently difficult to study) health effects, and that these reported data (as discussed further below) may underestimate - due to limitations of typical analytical methodologies, food preparation techniques used and other variables - the possible contribution of these food-borne toxins.

From inspection of the available data on the accumulation of cyanobacterial toxins in fish and shellfish (Table 1), it is clear that MCs are, by far, the most commonly reported. Indeed, MCs are generally considered the most widespread of the freshwater cyanobacterial toxins. Frequently, these data are reported in terms of "MC-LR equivalents," as typical quantitative analyses (e.g. ELISA, LC-MS) use this common variant as a reference standard, despite the fact that as many as ninety variants have been reported (see Welker and von Döhren, 2006). In addition to being among the most commonly detected of the microcystins, MC-LR is also one of the most toxic variants (Zurawell et al., 2005). That said, studies suggest variability in the uptake and detoxification of the variants. Xie et al. (2004), for example, studied MC-LR and MC-RR distribution and depuration in phytoplanktivorous carp, and proposed, based on these findings, a possible preferential uptake of MC-RR, or inhibited uptake of and/or active mechanism to "degrade" MC-LR.

Fish	Toxin(s)[a]	Tissue(s)	Toxin Conc. (μg g^{-1})[b]	Reference(s)
Silverside (*Odontesthes bonariensis*)	MC-RR	Muscle	0.05 (mean) 0.34 (max)	Cazenave et al., 2005
Silver Carp (*Hypophthalmichthys molitrix*)	MC-LR/RR MC-LR (eq)	Muscle Muscle	0.00025-0.097 0.0016	Chen et al., 2005 Shen et al., 2005
Carp (*Cyprinus carpio*)	MC-LR (eq) MC-LR (eq) ATX-a	Muscle Muscle Whole (juvenile)	0.038 0.005 0.005	Li et al., 2004 Berry et al., 2011a Osswald et al., 2007 (experimental studies)
Goodea spp.	MC-LR (eq)	Muscle Viscera[c]	0.157 0.867	Berry et al., 2011a
"Charales" (*Chirostoma* sp.)	MC-LR (eq)	Whole[c]	0.0185	Berry et al., 2011a
Redbreast Tilapia (*Tilapia rendalli*)	MC-LR (eq)	Muscle	0.002-0.337	Magalhaes et al., 2001
Nile Tilapia (*Oreochromis niloticus*)	MC-LR (eq)	Muscle	0.102	Mohammed et al., 2003
Blue Tilapia (*Oreochromis aureus*)	CYN STX/PSTs	Muscle Muscle	0.00009 0.00003	Berry et al., 2011b
Topote (*Dorosoma mexicana*)	CYN STX/PSTs	Muscle	0.0008 0.0003	Berry et al., 2011b
Flounder (*Platichthys flesus*)	NOD	Muscle	0.0005-0.1	Sipia et al., 2006
Roach (*Rutilus rutilus*)	NOD	Muscle	0.0004-0.2	Sipia et al., 2006
Trout (*Oncorhynchus mykiss*)	MC-LR (eq) ATX-a	Muscle Whole (juveniles)	0.035 3.9-23.6	Wood et al., 2006 Osswald et al., 2011 (experimental studies)
Yellow Perch (*Perca flavescens*)	MC-LR (eq)	Muscle	0.0008 (max)[d]	Wilson et al., 2008
Unidentified species	MC-LR (eq)	Muscle	0.04	Magalhaes et al., 2003
	NOD	Muscle	0.0007-0.025	Van Buynder et al, 2001
Shellfish				
Bivalves: Mussels				
Anodonta woodiania	MC-LR (eq)	Muscle/foot Whole[c]	0.009 (mean) 0.026 (max) 0.064	Chen & Xie, 2005a
Anodonta cygnea	STX/PSTs	Whole[c]	2.6	Pereira et al., 2004 (experimental study)
Alathyria condola	STX/PSTs	Whole[c]	57	Negri & Jones, 1995 (experimental study)
Hyriopsis cumingii	MC-LR (eq)	Muscle/foot Whole[c]	0.022 (mean) 0.039 (max) 0.188	Chen & Xie, 2005a
Cristaria plicata	MC-LR (eq)	Muscle/foot Whole[c]	(mean) 0.023 (max) 0.096	Chen & Xie, 2005a

Fish	Toxin(s)[a]	Tissue(s)	Toxin Conc. (μg g-1)[b]	Reference(s)
Lamprotula leai	MC-LR (eq)	Muscle/foot Whole[c]	0.021 (mean) 0.058 (max) 0.131	Chen & Xie, 2005a
Mytilus galloprovincialis	MC-LR ATX-a	Whole Soft tissue[c]	1.8 (max)e 0.006 (max)	Vasconcelos, 1995 (experimental study) Osswald et al., 2008 (experimental study)
Unidentified mussel species	CYN	Whole[c]	0.247	Saker et al., 2004
Unidentified mussel species	NOD	Whole[c]	2.5	Van Buynder et al., 2001
Gastropods: Snails				
Apple Snails (*Pomacea patula catemacensis*)	CYN STX/PSTs	Wholec Wholec	0.003 0.001	Berry and Lind, 2010
Crustaceans: Shrimp, Crab and Crayfish				
Crayfish *(Procambarus clarkia*)	MC-LR (eq)	Muscle	0.005 (mean) 0.010 (max)	Chen & Xie, 2005b
Red Claw Crayfish (*Cherax quadricarinatus*)	CYN	Muscle Hepato-pancreas	0.18[f] (mean) 0.86[f] (mean)	Saker & Eaglesham, 1999
Freshwater Shrimp (*Palaemon modestus*)	MC-LR (eq)	Muscle Whole	0.006 (mean) 0.026 (max) 0.0114	Chen & Xie, 2005b
Freshwater Shrimp (*Macrobrachium nipponensis*)	MC-LR (eq)	Muscle Whole	0.004 (mean) 0.012 (max) 0.051	Chen & Xie, 2005b
Unidentified crab species	MC-LR (eq)	Muscle	0.103	Magalhaes et al., 2003
Unidentified prawn species	CYN NOD	Muscle Muscle	0.205 0.005-0.022	Saker et al., 2004 Van Buynder et al., 2001

[a] Total MC content frequently reported as MC-LR equivalents ("MC-LR(eq)" in the table).

[b] Toxin concentrations given as either range, or maximum ("max") or mean (if not otherwise indicated).

[c] Fish or shellfish eaten whole including muscle and viscera. In the case of shellfish, shell or exoskeleton/carapace is typically removed, and the inner flesh consumed.

[d] Converted from dry weight to wet weight using conversion factor of 5 as per U.S. EPA recommendation, assuming ~80% water content of fish (Holcomb et al., 1976).

[e] Conversion from dry weight to wet weight using conversion factor of 5.8 as per Ricciardi and Bourget (1998).

[f] Conversion from dry weight to wet weight using conversion factor of approximately 5 as per Headon and Hall (xxx)

Table 1. Measured concentrations of cyanobacterial toxins in freshwater fish and aquatic invertebrates eaten by humans. Adapted, in part, from Ibelings and Chorus (2007).

As shown in Table 1, concentrations of MC in these tissues are generally quite low, and might imply a consequently low concern with respect to human exposure. However, there is evidence – as discussed above - to suggest that chronic expoure to low levels of these toxins may pose concern for long-term health (e.g. increased rates of cancer). Moreover, not shown in this table is the generally higher accumulation of MCs by liver and associated organ systems due to active transport of these toxins to hepatocytes and related cells (as discussed above). Although, in the case of fish, in particular, muscle tissues (i.e. "flesh," e.g. filets, etc.) are most typically eaten, there are exceptions. Berry et al. (2011a), for example, evaluated the MC content (see Table 1) of fish caught from a persistent cyanobacterial bloom in Lake Patzcuaro (Mexico), and specifically reported considerable levels for those fish (i.e. "charales" and *Goodea* spp.) that are locally eaten in their entirety, including muscle and associated viscera. Accordingly, these results suggest that preparation technique can have a key role in assessing the potential for human exposure.

Bioaccumulation, however, is not limited to the MCs, and a growing number of studies (see recent review by Kinnear, 2010) have, for example, also reported variable levels of the hepatotoxic CYN in relevant fish and shellfish species (Table 1). In fact, soon after the identification of CYN as the toxin responsible for the Palm Island Mystery (Ohtani et al., 1992), Saker and Eaglesham (1999) reported quite high levels of the toxin in both fish ("Rainbow Fish," *Melanotaenia eachemensis*) and invertebrate (i.e. "Red Claw Crayfish," *Cherax quadricarinatus*) species. Although, the former is not generally considered edible, the latter is, in fact, extensively aquacultured as freshwater "seafood" commercially. Since that time, the potential for bioaccumulation CYN has been reported in several field and laboratory studies (Norris et al., 2001; Nogueira et al., 2004; White et al., 2006; White et al., 2007), although most have focused on species not – or rarely (e.g. Swan Mussel, *Anodonta cygnea;* Saker et al., 2004) – eaten by humans, and therefore, not generally relevant to human diet and health. As a notable exception, Seifert et al. (2007) reported CYN from Eel-Tailed Catfish (*Tandanus tandanus*), an omnivorous species of game fish; the toxin, however, was not detected in several other less planktivorous species of fish (e.g. perch, bass). More recently, evaluation of CYN in the endorheic lake system of Lake Catemaco (Mexico) identified the toxin in species of both finfish (Berry et al., 2012) and relevant species of invertebrates (i.e. freshwater snails; Berry and Lind, 2010) consumed in this region.

Although not as well recognized (nor investigated), emerging evidence suggests that cyanobacterial neurotoxins may also accumulate in relevant freshwater species (Table 1). With regards to human health, STX and related "paralytic shellfish toxins" (PSTs) are – based on their well-described association to intoxication via seafood – perhaps of most obvious concern. STX/PSTs have widely documented as contaminants of marine shellfish, and particularly bivalves, representing a recognized concern for public health (Van Dolah, 2000). More recently, there have been increasing reports of STX/PSTs in fish, and particularly species of "pufferfish" (Family Tetraodontidae), alongside the toxicologically related (i.e. voltage-gated sodium channel blocking) tetrodotoxins that have been well described from these species. Similar to contamination of shellfish, however, it has been recently shown (Landsberg et al., 2006) that marine dinoflagellates (e.g. *Pyrodinium* spp.) are likely the source of STX/PSTs in the case of these typically estuarine fish. That said, studies (Negri and Jones, 1995; Pereira et al., 2004) have shown that – like marine bivalves – freshwater mussels can also accumulate cyanobacterially derived STX/PSTs. Although the mussel species (*Alathyria condola*) examined in these studies (e.g. Negri and Jones, 1995) are not one typically eaten by humans (although frequently by other animal species), more recent studies (Pereira et al., 2004) have measured considerable levels of PSTs (fed via PST-producing *Aphanizomenon issatschenkoi*) in the Swan Mussel (*Anodonta cygnea*) that, as previously mentioned, is occasionally consumed within certain human populations in Europe and elsewhere. Even more recently, while evaluating the apparent bioaccumulation of CYN associated with a bloom of *C. raciborskii* in Lake Catemaco (Mexico), it was found that both edible "tegogolo" snails (Berry and Lind, 2010), and locally consumed species of freshwater finfish (Berry et al., 2012), were found to accumulate STX/PSTs. These studies, furthermore, point to a shared source of CYN and STX/PSTs, and specifically *C. raciborskii* that is abundant in this lake system (Berry et al., 2012).

In addition to STX/PSTs, cyanobacteria are known to produce several other neurotoxic metabolites, including (as discussed above) the toxicologically related ATX-a and anatoxin-a(s). Compared to other cyanotoxins, the neurotoxic ATX-a is generally considered chemically quite labile, and it is generally anticipated that the potential for bioaccumulation of this unstable toxin would be, accordingly, rather low. That said, in experimental studies, it has been shown that both fish – including trout (*Oncorhynchus mykiss*; Osswald et al., 2011) and juvenile carp (*Cyprinus carpio*; Osswald et al, 2007) - and shellfish (e.g. mussel, *Mytilus galloprovincialis;* Osswald et al., 2008) can, in fact, accumulate the toxin presented in either dissolved (added to tank water) or cell-bound form. Moreover, in a recent study (Mejean et al., 2010), bioaccumulation of this toxin in the giant clam (*Tridacna maxima*), frequently consumed in the South Pacific, was evaluated in relation to several "ciguatera-like" intoxication cases reported in the region, and found to contain the potently toxic analog, homoanatoxin-a, as well as possible traces of ATX-a. Though confirmation of these toxins, as the causative agent of these reported poisoning, remains to be made, this study represents of the very few examples of possible acute intoxication by a food-borne cyanobacterial toxin.

Similarly, despite the emerging picture of its biomagnification in terrestrial species (e.g. fruit bats feeding on cycads; see above) over the past several decades, as well as the particularly conspicuous abundance of cyanobacteria in aquatic systems, relatively limited attention has been paid to the possible bioaccumulation of neurotoxic BMAA in aquatic food-webs. Several recent studies (Jonasson et al., 2010; Brand et al., 2010; Mondo et al., 2012), however, have suggested both accumulation, and possible biomagnifications of BMAA in marine systems, including those species (i.e. fish, seafood) directly related to human health. In one very recent case, the fins of several species of sharks, as "apex" marine predators, were examined, and found to be laden with BMAA (Mondo et al, 2012), and consequently proposed to present – via widespread consumption in the form of "sharkfin soup" – a potentially important route of exposure to this toxin, and thus a public health concern, in Asian countries where shark fins are considered a delicacy. Likewise, one of these studies, specifically evaluating BMAA in South Florida waters, and more specifically including Caloosahatchee River, did, in fact, detect this putatively toxic amino acid in both invertebrate (i.e. mussel) and fish species, including those consumed – at least occasionally - by humans (e.g. bass, bowfin, alligator gar) in this freshwater system. Most interestingly perhaps, it was found in this, as well as concurrent studies of marine food-webs, that measured BMAA levels were, in fact, higher in higher trophic levels suggesting the possibility of biomagnifications of this metabolite. As a highly water-soluble amino acid - with a low octanol/water-partitioning coefficient - it is not expected that BMAA would biomagnify by conventional means (i.e. via deposition in fat bodies, etc.); however, alternative mechanisms to this end are proposed (discussed below).

Finally, it bears mention that a growing number of studies have documented apparent uptake of cyanobacterial toxins by various plant species via toxin-contaminated irrigation water. Uptake of cyanobacterial toxins by plants was first suggested in a study by Pflugmacher et al. (2001) that reported both uptake - and associated metabolism - of MC-LR by the water reed (*Phragmites australis*). Subsequently, uptake and metabolism was similarly found to occur in several agriculturally important species including various legumes, maize, wheat and alfalfa (Peuthert et al., 2007). Similarly, it was recently reported that various cruciferous vegetables (e.g. *Brassica* spp., *Sinapsis alba*) are capable of accumulating 10-21% of CYN provided to roots, reaching as high as 49 μg/g (fresh weight) in the leafy components (Kittler et al., 2012). Although not bioaccumulation *per se* (i.e. via trophic transfer), the rather high levels of these compounds found in exposed plants, and specifically several agriculturally important crop plant species, suggest that exposure to cyanotoxins through plant crops may pose a very real public health concern.

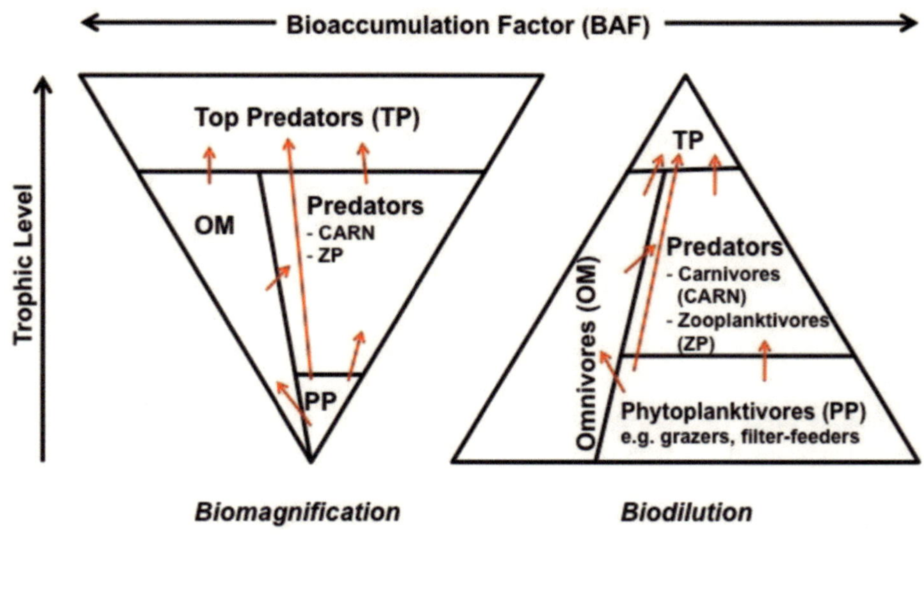

Figure 7. Depiction of biomagnification (left) and biodilution (right) of toxins in food-webs.

4. Trophic transfer and bioavailability of cyanobacterial toxins

Despite emerging evidence to suggest the bioaccumulation of cyanobacterial toxins within food webs (as summarized above; Table 1), relatively little is known regarding the process of trophic transfer, and the subsequent bioavailability of "food-derived" cyanotoxins. For lipophilic contaminants, including recognized anthropogenic pollutants (e.g. PCBs, DDT) and even some HAB toxins (e.g. ciguatoxins), uptake and storage in fat tissues have been largely implicated as a means of trophic transfer. However, there is no clear mechanism for bioaccumulation and/or biomagnification of the most widely recognized and, moreover, typically water-soluble cyanobacterial toxins. Likewise, although growing evidence suggests that cyanobacterial toxins are, in fact, present in relevant components of freshwater food webs (see section 3. *Evidence for bioaccumulation of cyanobacterial toxins in food-webs,* above), a very limited number of studies have investigated whether toxins contained within ingested tissues are, in fact, released, available and/or taken up in the digestive process. The following sections will summarize the current state of knowledge regarding both of these aspects.

4.1. Trophic transfer

As discussed in the previous section, a growing number of studies do, indeed, suggest that cyanobacterial toxins are transferred via dietary/trophic transfer within aquatic food-webs. It has been shown, in particular, that a range of phytoplanktivorous species, including zooplankton, fish, benthic grazers and filter-feeders consume toxin-laden algal cells, and directly accumulate these toxins. Alternatively, it has been shown (Karjalainen et al., 2003) that certain species, specifically including zooplankton, can accumulate, i.e. *bioconcentrate,* dissolved toxins directly from water as might be found, in particular, during algal bloom senescence. However, given the generally water-soluble (i.e. non-lipophilic) nature of the best known cyanobacterial toxins (see 2. *Recognized cyanobacterial toxins: chemistry and toxicology,* above), as well as currently available data on the apparent accumulation of these toxins within food webs (see 3. *Evidence for accumulation of cyanobacterial toxins aquatic food-webs,* above), it has been largely argued that transfer of these toxins follows a trophic pattern of *biodilution* rather than biomagnification (e.g. Ibelings et al., 2005; Ibelings and Chorus, 2007; Kozlowsky-Suzuki et al., 2012; Fig. 7). In a very recent, and particularly thorough, meta-analysis of existing data by Kozlowsky-Suzuki et al. (2012), it was shown that biodilution generally prevails. However, the authors of this study do highlight several exceptions and related caveats with relevant implications for potential exposure to toxins via food webs. Likewise, although concerns regarding human exposure to aquatic toxins – particularly in freshwater systems – are most frequently focused on higher trophic levels (i.e. sport and commercially caught fish species) as sources of toxins, a growing number of studies (Ibelings and Chorus, 2007; Berry and Lind, 2009; Berry et al., 2011; Berry et al., 2012) have documented accumulation of cyanobacterial toxins by species from lower trophic levels (i.e. freshwater shellfish, phytoplanktivorous fish) that are, indeed, consumed by humans, such that lack of biomagnification would not preclude possible human dietary exposure.

The potential for trophic transfer of cyanobacterial toxins is, generally speaking, controlled by three interrelated factors: *selection, chemical availability, toxin uptake* and *detoxification/elimination* (Fig. 8). Chemical availability will be discussed in the next section (*4.2. Bioavailability*). With regard to the former (i.e. selection), this factor would be most likely expected to be limited to initial consumption of toxin-producing algal cells by planktivores (that can subsequently serve as vectors for the toxins). This would be expected since production of toxins by cyanobacteria cells has been suggested to be linked to possible chemical defenses (i.e. feeding deterrency) against potential grazer, and evidence (see below) does, in fact, suggest that toxins may deter potential phytoplanktivorous grazers. As a corollary of this, it is suggested by this avoidance that potential grazers are capable of "detecting" the presence of toxins in algal cells. On the other hand, little or no evidence exists to suggest that toxin subsequent present in animal tissues can be so detected, and thus it is generally assumed that selection further "up the chain" is not a factor in higher trophic transfer. That said, other aspects of feeding behavior, including both general feeding preferences/strategies (e.g. herbivory versus carnivory), and more specific behaviors, particularly including selection of certain tissues by predators (e.g. preference of human consumers toward fish muscle versus other organs/tissues), might be argued to contribute to selection, and consequently the potential for trophic transfer.

A preponderance of evidence, in fact, supports a possible avoidance of toxigenic cyanobacteria by phytoplanktivores. In particular, selectivity with regards to trophic transfer is perhaps best demonstrated by numerous studies that have investigated feeding by zooplankton, and particularly *Daphnia* spp., as a widespread cladoceran micrograzer, in relation to the MCs. Microcystins have been shown to be toxic to *Daphnia* and other micrograzers, and toxicity has been shown to specifically correlate with rate of ingestion of the toxin. However, subsequent studies – specifically using "knock-out"non-toxic strains of *Microcystis* – have also, in contrast, indicated that *Daphnia* may not have the ability to distinguish toxic versus non-toxic algal cells (Rohrlack et al., 2001). Moreover, it has been generally found that interaction between grazers and their cyanobacterial prey are dependent on class of grazer (e.g. micro- versus mesozooplankton), species and even inter-specific genetic differences (Kurmayer and Jüttner, 1999; Davis and Gobler, 2011). More recently, it has been proposed (e.g. Wilson et al., 2005 and 2006; Lemaire et al., 2012) that differences in the observed feeding deterrence, relative to toxin content, may be explained by so-called "genotype x genotype interactions" whereby effects on feeding behavior are determined by the combination of grazer genotype (e.g. tolerance or susceptibility to toxin) and algal genotype (i.e. toxic or non-toxic). Finally, studies have suggested (e.g. Kurmayer and Jüttner, 1999; Reinikainen et al., 2001) that avoidance of potentially toxic cyanobacterial cells may be related to currently unknown, and particularly lipophilic, metabolites rather than recognized toxins (e.g. MCs). Understanding of the role of selection in trophic transfer, therefore, will rely on our increasing knowledge of genetic and chemical variability of both cyanobacteria and their grazers.

Even if toxin-containing items are selected for ingestion, however, several lines of evidence suggest both rather limited uptake of diet-derived toxin, as well as active and passive mechanisms for detoxification and/or elimination of these toxins, which together would be expected to limit the potential for trophic transfer. Understanding the contribution of these factors to trophic transfer, requires knowledge of – and/or means to investigate - the physiological, cellular and possible molecular processes involved in both uptake and potential detoxification/elimination. In the cases of MCs, for example, it has been suggested by multiple studies that the gastrointestinal tract, and particularly mid-gut wall, of fish may be an important site for toxin absorption (Chen et al., 2007; Dyble et al., 2011). Given the assumption that bioaccumulation is generally limited to lower trophic levels, it is not perhaps surprising, however, that most insight in this regard has been, likewise, largely limited to phytoplanktivore models. In order, for example, to evaluate the uptake (and subsequent elimination) of MC-LR by fish, in relation to possible human exposure, specifically using the juvenile yellow perch (*Perca flavescens*) model, Dyble et al. (2011) fed known doses of the toxin to fish orally via diet (i.e. "toxin-doped" pellets), and determined concentration and distribution within relevant tissues (i.e. muscle and liver) over time. Consistent with active transport of MCs to (for subsequent detoxification in) hepatocytes, higher levels were found in fish livers, and kinetically speaking, achieved a maximum level in liver cells (8-10 hours following dosing) prior to a subsequent peak in muscle tissue (12-16 hours post-dosing). Moreover, the concentrations measured represented orders of magnitude lower levels than those expected if the entire dose was assimilated. Moreover, roughly equivalent concentrations were observed for two doses used (5 and 20 μg), suggesting a possible maximum capacity for uptake. Furthermore, studies showed a rapid increase in the toxin concentration (dependent in magnitude on dose) following peak levels measured in the fish tissues (after approximately 10 hours), implying a rather rapid elimination of the toxin by excretion (i.e. urine, feces). These finding support both rather limited uptake, and rapid elimination of the toxin, however, it should be noted that these data also correspond to a single dosing of the fish, whereas in aquatic habitats (i.e. during blooms, or through persistent occurrence of toxic cyanobacteria) it would be expected that possible grazers (and even other higher trophic levels) would be exposed more continuously to toxins, such that the effective "window" of time for trophic transfer would be considerably longer.

As pointed-out, the initial step for trophic transfer (from cyanobacterial cell to grazer) might be expected to represent, in terms of selectivity, uptake and detoxification/elimination, a rather distinct process compared to subsequent uptake by higher trophic levels. To understand this higher-level transfer, therefore, it is necessary to evaluate the role of toxin derived from primary consumer with respect to secondary (and subsequent) consumers. In a particularly elegant example, Karjalainen et al. (2005) experimentally demonstrated uptake of NOD by planktivorous fish larvae (i.e. Northern Pike) and invertebrate (i.e. mysid shrimp, *Neomysis integer*) via pre-exposure of relevant zooplankton prey to the toxin both in pure form, and as cell-free extracts of *N. spumigens* (as would be representative of the toxin released by decaying blooms). Prior studies had shown that zooplankton accumulate NOD directly from water (Karjalainen et al., 2003). In these subsequent studies, equal amounts of NOD (approximately 0.20 ng produced by an individual per 24 h) were detected in fecal pellets of pike larvae - suggesting diet derived uptake and passage of the toxin - fed zooplankton exposed to both pure toxin and NOD-containing extracts. Moreover, the authors of the study utilized radiolabeled NOD (i.e. ^{3}H-dihydronodularin) to quantify the transfer of the toxin from zooplankton to planktivores. Indeed, radiolabel was detected in both *N. integer* and pike larvae fed zoo-

http://dx.doi.org/10.5772/55111

plankton, previously exposed to ^{3}H-NOD, with a maximum calculated accumulation of the toxin at 12 h (0.31 ng/individual) and 48 h (0.47 ng/individual), respectively, for the two species. Levels of NOD calculated based on these studies, however, were quite low (approximately 0.12% and 0.03%, respectively, for shrimp and fish larvae) compared to the amounts predicted based on measured ingestion rate and concentration of toxin in zooplankton. These results are, therefore, generally consistent with a proposed biodilution, rather than biomagnifications, of this toxin within this food-chain. Furthermore, although ingestion rates were quite different (i.e. more than 5-fold higher) for fish larvae compared to shrimp, both accumulated rather similar levels (i.e. concentration per weight or individual) of the toxin. Accordingly, these studies point to both a difference in the type of potential planktivore vector (i.e. fish versus invertebrate systems), as well as a likely role of uptake and/or detoxification (and subsequent elimination) of the toxin in relation to the observed biodilution.

In addition to understanding physiological, cellular and molecular aspects of potential grazers/predators, uptake and detoxification can also be closely tied to the chemistry of the toxin. Certainly, among the cyanobacterial toxins, the potential for uptake, and subsequent detoxification/elimination, might be expected – due the chemically diverse nature of these compounds – to vary considerably with this chemical variability. This is most obviously exemplified by the distinction of so-called "hepatotoxins" (e.g. CYN, MCs) that, as implied by this classification, and unlike other cyanotoxins (e.g. PSTs, ATX-a, BMAA), are actively transported via characterized organic anion transporter (OAT) proteins to hepatocytes for subsequent detoxification/elimination. However, even with toxin families, variability in uptake and elimination has been reported. For example, in studies on the uptake of MCs, Xie et al. (2004) compared relative distribution following dosing with two common variants, namely MC-LR and MC-RR, in phytoplanktivorous silver carp. Interestingly, dietary exposure to MC-LR and MC-RR (in algal cells) resulted in considerably higher levels of the latter distributed in various tissues, but rather limited tissue concentration/distribution of the former, and more toxic, variant (Xie et al., 2004). Moreover, detection of relative amounts of the two variants in gut and feces specifically supported an apparent barrier to uptake of MC-LR, compared to the less toxic MC-RR (Xie et al, 2004). It should be pointed-out, however, that results in this phytoplanktivorous model differ substantially from similar studies in a generally carnivorous fish model, namely rainbow trout, particularly with respect to apparently rapid uptake of MC-LR by the latter species, and consequently suggest a role of both consumer species, and differential species physiology, relative to the potential for uptake (and subsequent trophic transfer). Finally, uptake (and subsequent trophic transfer) may even be determined, in part, by chemical presentation of the toxin. For example, it has been shown that in a benthic grazer model, namely the snail, *Lymnaea stagnalis,* that MCs are more readily taken-up from ingested cyanobacterial cells compared to dissolved toxin (Lance et al., 2010a). Furthermore, concurrent studies comparing the fate of MC-LR presented in either dissolved or cell-bound form (Lance et al., 2010b) suggested that, whereas no toxin from ambient/dissolved dosings was found covalently bound in tissues, as much as 67% of cell-derived MCs were accumulated via covalent binding (to targed PPase enzymes) representing a potentially considerable reservoir of the toxin for subsequent trophic transfer (as discussed further below).

The potential for trophic transfer is not likely limited to the most studied cyanobacterial hepatotoxins (i.e. MCs). Although relatively few studies have evaluated their bioaccumulation, the transfer of the neurotoxic STX/PSTs, for example, has been studied with respect to its accumulation in marine animals, and specifically in relation to non-cyanobacterially (i.e. marine dinoflagellate) derived toxin. As a particularly important vector for PSTs, several filter-feeding mollusks are recognized to accumulate toxin-containing algal cells, and represent a possible route for both direct exposure (i.e. "shellfish" consumption), as well as possible indirect exposure to these toxins (i.e. trophic transfer to, and consumption of, secondary consumers/vectors, e.g. fish). There is, in fact, emerging (albeit currently limited) evidence to suggest that these neurotoxins may be transferred, to some extent, from filter-feeding invertebrates to higher trophic levels. In particular, however, these studies suggest that biotransformation via metabolism of PSTs – represented, as a group, by as many as fifty variants (Wiese et al., 2010) - may be a critical consideration. In studies by Kwong et al. (2006), black sea bream were exposed to green-lipped mussels, previously exposed to the PST-producing dinoflagellate, *Alexandrium fundyense.* Through these studies, it was generally found that relatively little PST was transferred to the fish, and that the toxins were rapidly depurated after transferring to toxin-free mussels. Mooreover, toxin profiles suggested considerable biotransformation, and particularly conversion of C2 to C1 variants (see *2.2.2. Saxitoxins and "Paralytic Shellfish Toxins,"* above). Likewise, subsequent studies (Costa et al., 2010) using white seabream, similarly exposed to PST-contaminated cockles, confirmed the rather low uptake of the toxin, and additionally reported an apparently selective uptake/elimination and/or biotransformation such that only B1 and dcSTX were found in fish. This conversion and/or selective uptake/elimination during trophic transfer would have clear implications for subsequent bioavailability of this neurotoxin, and associated health concerns, as there is considerable variability in the toxicity of the PST congeners. Most generally, these studies point to the importance of the vectors (e.g. fish versus shellfish) for the toxin.

Before moving on, to consider bioavailability, perhaps the one exception to the observed pattern of biodilution, which consequently bears discussion, appears to be the trophic transfer of BMAA. In the limited studies that have investigated BMAA in marine and freshwater food-webs, it was shown, in fact, that levels of the toxic amino acid were higher for top trophic levels (e.g. predatory fish) compared to lower trophic levels (e.g. Brand et al., 2010; Jonasson et al., 2010). In a recent study, for example, Jonasson et al. (2010) examined BMAA within food webs of the Baltic Sea, and reported a discernible positive correlation between levels of the toxin and trophic level. It seems likely, though, that the pattern is not quite as simple as classic biomagnification. For example, the Jonasson et al. (2010) and other studies (e.g. Brand et al., 2010) also suggest particularly high levels for benthic versus pelagic species (of both vertebrates and invertebrates). These studies also suggest differences in tissue distribution of the toxin with highest levels of BMAA observed in brain compared to, for example, muscle, and, therefore, underscore the importance of feeding ecology within food-webs, as well as the likely important role of subsequent bioavailability (including uptake and metabolism) and tissue distribution of toxins, in regards to trophic transfer.

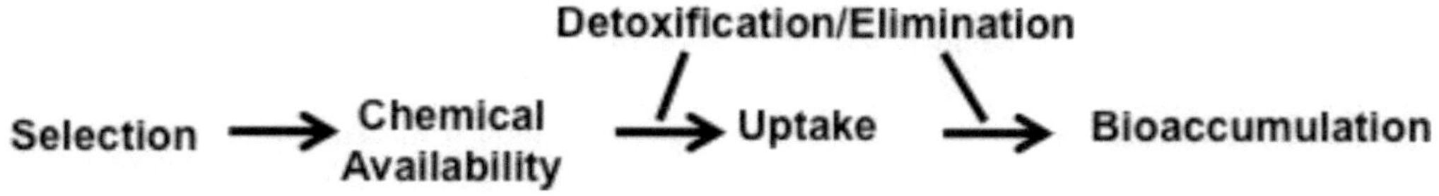

Figure 8. Factors affecting trophic transfer and bioavailabily of cyanobacterial toxins in food webs.

4.2. Bioavailability

Just as selection, chemical availability, uptake and detoxification/elimination would determine trophic transfer of cyanobacterial toxins through food-webs, these factors are, likewise, expected to primarily determine the bioavailability of these toxins to human as would be ostensibly considered – with respect to the current discussion of emerging public health concerns – the "top predator" in this regard. Although not perhaps, strictly speaking, a "bioavailability factor" selectivity with respect to human consumption can certainly contribute to the potential for exposure to food-borne cyanotoxins. In a general sense, several Tiers of selectivity can dictate the likelihood of exposure (in concert with other bioavailability factors) to cyanobacterial toxins in food. As mentioned previously, the generally limited consumption of freshwater fish and shellfish, relative to much more common consumption of fish and other seafood from marine sources, would be expected – given the recognized abundance of cyanobacterial toxins in freshwater systems – to, likewise, generally limit the possible exposure to these toxins. Even within freshwater systems, the relative consumption of fish and shellfish species from lower trophic (i.e. phytoplanktivorous) levels of food webs would similarly contribute to the possible exposure. However, as detailed above (*3. Evidence for bioaccumulation of cyanobacterial toxins in aquatic food-webs)*, there are certainly numerous documented cases of toxin bioaccumulation by phytoplanktivorous species of freshwater fish and invertebrates (e.g. snails, bivalves) which are, indeed, consumed by humans. Finally, even with species, and particularly fish species, selectivity of certain tissues/organs can influence possible exposure scenarios. Most notably, with respect to this latter tier, the general preference for fish flesh (i.e. muscle) versus viscera (e.g. toxin-accumulating liver, etc.) has clear implications for the potential for exposure to these toxins. Selectivity aside, however, the real issue of bioavailability is clearly expected to be most closely linked to those biochemical and physiological processes of digestion (i.e. uptake) and possible detoxification/elimination.

Cyanobacterial toxins, as discussed previously (see *2. Recognized cyanobacterial toxins: chemistry and toxicology*), have been traditionally classified based on their "target" organs. Specifically, the most commonly studied cyanotoxins have been grouped into those targeting either the liver/hepatocytes or brain/CNS, respectively, in the case of the so-called "hepatotoxins" (i.e. MCs, CYN) and "neurotoxins" (i.e. STX/PSTs, ATX-a, BMAA). Based on both evaluation of toxin distribution (e.g. high levels of MC and CYN in livers of exposed animals), and recognized manifestations of toxicity (e.g. neurotoxicity of STX/PSTs and ATX-a), following exposure, effective bioavailability to these organs is largely assumed. In the case of the MCs, however, active transport of the toxin to hepatocytes has actually been shown to be specifically facilitated by a family of organic anion transporter polypeptides (OATPs) that are particularly abundant in these cells (Fischer et al., 2005; Lu et al., 2008; Fischer et al., 2010), and even suggested to play a role in the selective uptake of certain MC congeners by hepatocytes (Fischer et al., 2010). That said, OATPs are, in fact, found in other cell types, and it has been also been suggested, for example, that OATPs in the brain may allow passage of MCs across the blood-brain barrier (Fischer et al., 2005), and they have, accordingly, been linked to oxidative stress in neurons, and subsequent effects on short and long term memory, caused by the toxin in a rat model (Maidana et al., 2006). Although, likewise, considered a hepatotoxin, and found to accumulate primarily in hepatocytes, the mechanism for CYN is not currently known. On the other hand, studies of neurotoxic cyanotoxins have demonstrated the apparent ability of STX/PSTs, ATX-a and BMAA to cross the blood-brain barrier (BBB) as a fundamentally limiting step for all toxins that affect the CNS. For example, STX - as a representative PST - was detected through brain tissues (from sacrificed animals), and consequently suggested to cross the BBB, following both intravenous (Andrinolo et al., 1999) and intraperitoneal (Cervantes Cianca et al., 2007) in mammalian (i.e. cat, rat) models. In support of the implied passage to - as suggested by its purported toxicity, and measured presence in the brain - studies of BMAA, dating back more than twenty years, and well prior to the recent resurgence of interest in this putative neurotoxin, not only have shown that this unusual amino acid is capable of crossing the BBB, but that transport might be specifically facilitated by large neutral amino acid carriers at the blood-brain interface (Smith et al., 1992).

Although the potential for bioavailability of cyanobacterial toxins to target organs is implied by their patterns of bioaccumulation, and observed toxic effects on certain organ systems, as well as limited number of *in vivo* studies, most studies have focused on either exposure to toxins via water ingestion, or in the case of laboratory studies, have examined fate of the toxin, following intraperitoneal injection, or related forms of administering the toxin. The actual bioavailability, with respect to foodborne toxins, is obviously limited by the prior chemical availability (discussed further below), as determined by release (from food), uptake and detoxification/elimination, prior to transport to target organs. To-date, however, studies on uptake and detoxification/elimination of cyanobacterial toxins derived from foods are essentially non-existent.

Rather, as with other aspects of health concerns regarding cyanobacterial toxins, the very few studies that have considered bioavailablity of these toxins – and implicitly uptake and detoxification/elimination as key factors - have generally relied on data, and subsequent inferences, extrapolated from water-borne cyanotoxins, including dissolved or algal cell-derived toxins. Most notably, several authors have considered World Health Organization (WHO) guidelines regarding acceptable concentrations of MCs - as the clearly most widespread cyanobacterial toxin family - in water, and subsequently derived guideline values for total daily intake (TDI) of this toxin. Values of TDI are generally based on observed *no* or *lowest observable adverse effect levels* (NOAELs and LOAELs, respectively) from very a very limited number of oral exposure studies in mouse and pig models (Falconer et al., 1994; Fawell et al., 1999). Accordingly, acceptable values for lifetime, one-time and occasional TDI have been estimated, respectively, as 0.04, 25 and 0.4 μg per kg body weight

http://dx.doi.org/10.5772/55111

(Fromme et al., 1999; Ibelings and Chorus, 2007). In a particular thorough treatment, Ibelings and Chorus (2007) extrapolated this to proposed guideline values that incorporate exposure via both water and food (and particularly "seafood"). Acknowledging a high variability in the amounts of food consumed, as well as other relevant factors (e.g. body weight), the guidelines estimated in this way ranged greatly from 6 μg/kg for daily lifetime exposures to 1900 μg/kg for acute (i.e. "one-time") exposures for adults, with corresponding lower values for children (i.e. 0.08-250 μg/kg body weight). That said, all such values regarding intake (and, implicitly, the necessary consideration of subsequent uptake and detoxification/elimination) are, as mentioned, solely based on (very limited) estimates derived from oral exposure to a single toxin in water, and out of necessity, ignore bioavailability from a more complex "matrix" of animal tissues. Of course, as more information is obtained with respect to the uptake, and subsequent detoxification/elimination, of toxins from animal-based diet, it is hoped that a more realistic understanding of the potential for food-borne exposure will emerge. In particular, a clearer understanding of these toxins in relation to the dietary matrix, and consequently those factors (e.g. digestion, cellular uptake) that determine fate is still needed.

Aside from considerations of uptake and subsequent detoxification/elimination, as it relates to bioavailablity, it has become clear that, in certain cases, the potential (or lack thereof) for human bioavailability may be considerably affected by *chemical* availability. This has been specifically studied, to-date, in two cases: (1) irreversible, covalent binding of MCs to PPases targets; and (2) erroneous translation and consequent incorporation of BMAA into proteins. In the latter case, for example, it has been suggested that BMAA, as a non-essential amino acid, can be potential incorporated (via faulty translation mechanisms) into growing protein chains. Specifically, investigating this possibility, Murch et al. (2004) analyzed BMAA in cyanobacteria, and brains of patients who died of ALS/Parkinsonism dementia complex (along with cycads and flying foxes from Guam as suggested vectors for the toxin), both with and without prior acid hydrolysis. Measured levels of BMAA were on the order of 10- to 240-fold higher following acid hydrolysis, suggesting an apparent release of this amino acid from proteins in these samples. This finding, therefore, not only supported incorporation of BMAA into proteins as a mechanism of toxicity (see *1. Recognized cyanobacterial toxins: chemistry and toxicology*, above), as well as possible limitations in the analytical methodologies applied to this toxin (discussed further below; see *Methodologies for evaluating cyanobacterial toxins in food-webs*), but furthermore, pointed to an "endogenous reservoir" of the toxin. Such a reservoir would specifically provide a means of "slow release," of the toxin as possible mechanism for BMAA bioavailability, and would correlate with the generally late onset of these diseases. It is, of course, implied from these studies that BMAA bound in proteins in this way would, in fact, be readily available following peptidolytic digestion, however, this remains to be confirmed.

As discussed earlier in the chapter (see *1. Recognized cyanobacterial toxins: chemistry and toxicology*), MCs are known to bind to PPases found ubiquitously in cells of all known organisms. In addition, however, to reversible binding to the active site of PPases, it has been shown (MacKintosh et al., 1995; Pereira et al., 2012) that the toxin, once in the active site, will form covalent bonds (via Michael addition) between the Mdha (present in many MCs) and a cysteine (Cys273) found in the active site of Ser/Thr Type 1/2A PPases. Accordingly, it has been suggested that a portion of all Mdha-containing MCs might become bound in this way (Williams et al., 1997a and 1997b; Yuan et al., 2006; Suchy and Berry, 2012), and indeed, estimates - based on specific analysis of the bound toxin (see *5. Methodologies for analysis of cyanobacterial toxins in the food-web*) - suggest a considerable pool of so bound MCs. In classic studies by Williams et al. (1997a and 1997b), for example, analysis of bound MC demonstrated that as little as 24% of MC administered (via i.p. injection) to salmon could be recovered by conventional solvent extraction and analyses, and likewise that as much as 10,000-fold more of the toxin, measured in Dungeness crab larvae, could be detected in the presumptively "bound form" compared to the "free form." More recently, Hilborn et al. (2007) measured both free and bound MCs in dialysis patients exposed (through improperly treated water) to the toxin, and similarly measured significantly higher levels when total (i.e. free and bound) levels were compared to those of the unbound toxin (i.e. measured by solvent extraction and conventional detection, e.g. ELISA), and specifically that only approximately 8-51% of MCs were measured by the latter method, compared to the former.

A preponderance of evidence continues to suggest that bound MCs do, indeed, represent a considerable pool of the toxin, however, very few studies have investigated whether these bound MCs are, in fact, biologically available. To address this question, Smith et al. (2010) recently investigated the potential for digestive enzymes to release covalently bound MC from PPases. Whereas digestive proteases (e.g. trypsin, chymotrypsin, pepsin) were found, as expected, to effectively hydrolyze a control protein (i.e. angiotensin), they had no effect on the cyclic peptides (i.e. MC-LR and MC-LY). Furthermore, based on the assumption that protein-bound MCs could be partially released by these peptidolytic enzymes, the investigators synthesized four Cys-containing MC-oligopeptide adducts, specifically predicted for hydrolytic digestion of the PPase active site by these enzymes, and subsequently evaluated them for toxicity (i.e. inhibition of protein phosphatase). Although inhibition was reduced (compared to MC-LR alone) to approximately 58% for MC-peptide adducts - composed of the cyclic MC-LR covalently bound, via cysteine, to predicted tetra- and nonomeric peptide fragments - this residual biological activity supports the possible bioavailability of potentially toxic bound MCs following protein hydrolysis in the digestive system. Interestingly, concurrent studies (Zhang et al., 2010) evaluated the effects of cooking as an alternative mechanism for release of covalently bound MCs with respect to potential availability of the toxin. In these studies, it was specifically found that levels of MC-LR in carp (injected intraperitoneally with the toxin) were significantly higher (approximately 4-fold) in both muscle tissue and water following boiling, compared to lyophilization and subsequent solvent extraction only, and it was suggested that elevated levels were due to release of covalently bound toxin from these tissues. Although such studies do point to the possible chemical availability of covalent bound toxins, clearly further studies are needed to fully elucidate the possible bioavailability of these in relation to human exposure.

http://dx.doi.org/10.5772/55111

5. Methodologies for evaluating cyanobacterial toxins in the food-web

Techniques for chemical detection and quantitative analysis of cyanobacterial toxins have evolved alongside recognition of their potential health impacts. The majority of the previously established analytical methods (e.g. HPLC-UV, LC-MS, ELISA) have, therefore, primarily focused on the identification of toxin in algal cells and/or dissolved in water, with water (i.e. contamination of drinking water, recreational exposure) being an established direct route of exposure. As for these applications, analytical techniques applied to measurement of toxins in food webs have, likewise, generally focused on two approaches (Sivonen, 2008; Humpage et al., 2010). The first, and arguably most common - given the complex nature of these biological matrices (discussed further below) - has included a number of so-called "hyphenated methods" in which analytical separation, including liquid chromatography (LC) and capillary electrophoresis (CE), in particular, are coupled to one or more suitable detection/measurement technique, including UV absorbance, fluorescent derivatization/detection (FL), mass spectrometry (MS) and electrochemical detection. Alternatively, with the relatively recent commercial availability of enzyme-linked immunosorbent assay (ELISA) kits for several cyanobacterial toxins, as well as growing understanding of the toxicology of these metabolites - and thus development of several biochemical techniques (e.g. protein phosphatase inhibition assays for MCs) - these bioanalytical techniques have been also applied to the evaluation of cyanobacterial toxin in relation to food-webs and bioaccumulation (e.g. Lance et al., 2006; Berry and Lind, 2010; Berry et al., 2011; Berry et al., 2012). However, unlike detection of several non-cyanobacterial, marine algal toxins as contaminants of fish and seafood for which there are validated analytical techniques, there are presently no validated methods for evaluating cyanobacterial toxins in biological matrices.

Both of the aforementioned approaches present potential limitations, but generally speaking, it would be argued that the two consequently complement one another. In particular, ELISA-based methods have been somewhat criticized (Metcalf et al., 2000; Mountfort et al., 2005) as being potentially susceptible to non-targeted molecules (i.e. matrix components) in samples that may immunologically cross-react with antibodies, or alternatively not being able to distinguish more toxic variants among co-occurring congeners within toxin groups. As antibodies used in ELISAs are typically generated in relation to a particular representative variant of these toxins, relying on chemical similarity and cross-reactivity to detect other variants, they do not enable co-occurring congeners to be distinguished from total toxin concentrations. This latter limitation is perhaps best exemplified by the ELISA-based analysis of MCs. Although commercially available ELISAs for MCs exploit the generally conserved Adda moiety found in most variants (Fig. 2), MC variants lacking (or containing modified versions of) Adda have been reported (Namikoshi et al., 1990 and 1992; Sivonen et al., 1992; Oksanen et al., 2004), and would be missed in these analyses leading to some degree of "false negatives," or at least possible underestimation of MC content. Alternatively, studies have shown that improper use of ELISA kits – as well as factors such as organic solvents, salinity and pH - can contribute to the potential for false positives (Metcalf et al., 2005). Additionally, it is recognized that toxicity of MCs varies with congener, and therefore the inability to distinguish particular variants, with respect to this relative toxicity, does not enable what is essentially a proxy of "total MC" to be evaluated in terms of actual relevance to toxicity (Mountfort et al., 2005). As an alternative, enzyme assays - and particularly the various PPase inhibition assays developed for MCs (Mountfort et al., 2005) – are, in fact, capable of assessing cyanobacterial toxins based on relevant biological activity. However, such assays are typically not as sensitive as, for example, ELISA, and likewise may be susceptible to matrix components, as well as being unable to chemically distinguish particular toxin variants. That said, sensitivity of methods such as ELISA are generally higher than for most other methods, and moreover, although coupling analytical separation to detection (e.g. LC-MS) may enable identification of particular chemical variants, this is only applicable to those variant which are specifically targeted. In other words, even though LC coupled to tandem mass spectrometry (MS/MS) can, for example, selectively detect several common MC variants based on characteristic molecular ions, and subsequent "daughter ions," without prior knowledge of the optimal parameters (i.e. parent/daughter ions, ionization energy, etc.) - and/or availability of suitable analytical standards - to use for other for other less common (or perhaps yet uncharacterized) variants, and their metabolic products, these would be generally missed by such an approach (Mountfort et al., 2005). Accordingly, a strategy which incorporates both approaches and their relative benefits (i.e. highly sensitive detection of "total" MC by ELISA, target-based bioassay and selective analytical separation and detection of individual MC variants) might be expect to provide the most comprehensive toxin profile.

In general, the obvious challenge posed in adapting analytical techniques, originally developed for water (and, to a lesser extent, algal) samples, to bioaccumulation in food webs is the relatively more complex matrix of biological specimens (i.e. animal tissues). Other components of these biological matrices can interfere with analyses by specifically requiring a higher degree of selectivity (to discern the analyte from other components of the matrix), and as well as leading to suppression of the detection response (e.g. suppression of ionization in MS). To some extent, these challenges are inherently addressed when coupling detection to optimized analytical separation (e.g. LC-MS) that essentially isolates components (e.g. as chromatographic *peaks* based on retention time, etc.), but has also been generally supplemented by sample preparation steps prior to analysis. In particular, sample preparation steps have included selective extraction (e.g. Metcalf et al., 2002; Msagati et al., 2006), solid-phase extraction (SPE; e.g. James et al., 1998; Metcalf et al., 2002; McElhiney and Lawton, 2005; Scott et al., 2009) and other so-called "clean-up steps" to remove these potential interfering chemical species. Of course, in the case of less stable toxins (e.g. ATX-a; discussed below), extensive sample work-up can chemically jeopardize the analyte leading to underestimation or even complete non-detection of these compounds; generally speaking though, most approaches require some degree of sample preparation prior to analysis, particularly when dealing with complex bio-matrices.

One of the particular challenges of a biological matrix is due to the lack of specificity of certain detection methods. For example, although none of the recognized cyanobacterial toxins discussed have a particularly specific chromophore, as to enable unambiguous detection, HPLC coupled to UV spectrophotometric detection has been successfully used – specifically based on shortwave UV detection and established chromatographic retention time, and in conjunction with analytical standards – to detect and measure several cyanobacterial toxins in water samples (e.g. Harada et al., 1994; Gugger et al., 2005; McElhiney and Lawton, 2005; Berry and Lind, 2010). However, in more complex bio-matrices, this lack of a distinguishing UV chromophore, and potential for co-eluting non-targeted components of the matrix generally limit this approach. Similarly, although fluorescence derivatization – and subsequent fluorescence detection coupled to chromatography or other analytical separation techniques (e.g. CE) - has been used as a highly sensitive means of detection/measurement of cyanobacterial toxins (e.g. Harada et al., 1997; James et al., 1998), the derivatization chemistry frequently employed in these approaches exploit common functional groups (e.g. amines, carboxylic acids, dienes). As such, non-toxin analytes (e.g. peptides) present in biological matrices can be coincidentally derivatized and, by co-elution and/or simply poor resolution, interfere with identification of the analyte of interest. Possible overlap in analytical response is not limited to these analytical separation/detection techniques, and indeed, it has been suggested that for ELISA, antibody cross-reactivity with chemically related components of the matrix might, likewise, lead to non-selective detection, and erroneous results in analyses.

Even in the case of highly selective detection techniques, interference due to the bio-matrix can arise. This is particularly seen with quantitative analyses based on mass spectrometry, including LC-MS, and particularly the most commonly used (at present) method of electrospray ionization (LC-ESI-MS). Components of the sample matrix, including inorganic (e.g. pH, salts/ions) and organic (e.g. proteins and other biomolecules) components, can both interfere with ionization; the former can directly interfere with ionization, whereas the latter can indirectly effect ionization of the analyte, particularly through competitive ionization. In the case of MCs, for example, it has been shown that dissolved organic carbon, pH and ionic strength can suppress signal in LC-MS with the latter being the most significant (Li et al., 2010). More notably in relation to the present discussion, Karlsson et al. (2005) investigated the effect of a biological matrix with respect to the LC-MS detection of MCs and NOD in biological tissues, including aquatic invertebrates (i.e. Blue Mussels, *Mytilus edulis*), fish (i.e. Rainbow Trout, *Onchorhyncus mykiss*) and waterfowl (i.e. Common Eider, *Somateria mollissima*). In these studies, it was found that ion signal varied from 16-134% of the expected signal (from spiked toxin), suggesting a good deal of both ionization suppression and enhancement, which varied with toxin variant (i.e. six MC variants and NOD) and biological matrix. In related studies, investigating the use of an MC oxidation product (discussed below) for LC-MS analysis, Ott and Carmichael (2006) reported losses in signal strength of more than 41% for this analyte. More recently, Li et al. (2012) examined the effects of ionization suppression with respect to quantitative analysis of BMAA, as well as its non-toxic isomer, 2,4,-diaminobutyric acid (DAB), by LC-MS/MS. Although considerable matrix effects were observed for DAB, there appeared to be no contribution to the BMAA signal. Notably, however, this optimized method was used to suggest that BMAA was not seemingly present in several cyanobacterial samples evaluated, and to support the growing indication that this putative toxin is not as widespread as previously suggested. Indeed, although matrix effects represent an analytical challenge, the effects of signal suppression (e.g. ion suppression) can generally be addressed by various strategies, including the use of appropriate *internal standards* and techniques of *standard addition* to assess the extent of this effect on quantitation.

	Limitations	Advantages
Biochemical Methods		
ELISA	Cost (~$400-500/plate) No chemical information, e.g. identification of chemical variants No toxicity information	Highly sensitive (< ppb) Rapid/analyze multiple samples at once Easy/little training required Relatively inexpensive instrumentation (i.e plate readers)
"Target-Based" e.g. PPase inhibition	No chemical information, e.g. identification of chemical variants Somewhat lower sensitivity Low selectivity, e.g. false positives	Provides toxicity information Relatively inexpensive (reagents) Rapid/analyze multiple samples at once Easy/little training required Relatively inexpensive instrumentation (i.e plate readers)
Instrumental Analysis (i.e. analytical separation/detection)		
HPLC/CE-UV	Low sensitivity Low selectivity, e.g. false positives Requires training Limited chemical information, e.g. can't identify unknown variants Moderately expensive instrumentation Relatively slow/can't analyze multiple samples at once Requires sample clean-up	Provides some chemical information, e.g. can identify chemical variants (if standards available) Analysis can be automated
HPLC/CE-FL	Requires derivatization Somewhat low selectivity, e.g. false positives Requires training Limited chemical information, e.g. can't identify unknowns Moderately expensive instrumentation Relatively slow/can't analyze multiple samples at once Requires sample clean-up	Highly sensitive Provides some chemical information, e.g. can identify chemical variants (if standards available) Analysis can be automated
HPLC/CE-MS	Requires training Expensive instrumentation Relatively slow/can't analyze multiple samples at once Requires (some) sample clean-up	Provides chemical information, e.g. can identify chemical variants (if standards available), possible information regarding unknowns Analysis can be automated

Table 2. Limitations and advantages of different analytical techniques used for detection/measurement of cyanobacterial toxins.

Aside from issues specifically related to the complex biological matrices encountered in food webs, some of the same general challenges associated with quantitative analysis of cyanobacterial toxins in water are, likewise, associated with analysis of bioaccumulation. A common consideration, in this regard, includes a requirement of selectively to detect, and discern, isomers and chemically related congeners. Indeed, this is exemplified by all of the recognized cyanobacterial toxins. For example, both PSTs and the MCs belong to rather large families of chemically related, but structurally distinct, variants – specifically represented, at present, by as many as fifty, and more than ninety, reported variants, respectively - with equally variable toxicity for each. In both cases, especially toxic and common variants (i.e. STX and MC-LR) are most frequently considered as a proxies for these toxin families, however, it is known that several other congeners from these groups can, in fact, potentially contribute to toxicity, and moreover, due to differential uptake and bioavailability hold, likewise, variable potential with respect to bioaccumulation. This presents, as discussed above, a clear limitation to ELISA-based analyses of the MCs that is unable to distinguish specific contributions of individual congeners. Likewise, although LC-MS and related methods, which employ analytical separation prior to detection, are able (if sufficiently optimized) to chromatographically resolve/separate congeners, the requirement for established molecular ionization and fragmentation parameters to detect these variants (by mass spectrometry) limits which variants will, and will not, be detected. Although considerably less complex, on the other hand, both CYN and ATX-a, likewise, have structurally related congeners and/or structural isomers, including for homoATX-a and 7-epiCYN, respectively, that are found alongside the "primary" toxins. In both of these cases, the congeners are also associated with toxicity, and evaluation of their contribution with respect to food-borne toxins needs to be included. On the other hand, although only BMAA (among several structural isomers) has been reported as potentially toxic, it has been suggested that natural occurrence of numerous possible isomeric congeners, all sharing the same molecular mass (Fig. 9), may greatly confound mass spectrometric analysis of this toxic amino acid (Banack et al., 2010), and specifically it has been suggested that, due to this, the once considered widespread occurrence of this neurotoxin may, in fact, be considerably over-estimated (Jiang et al., 2012; Li et al., 2012).

Although many of the cyanotoxins are generally considered chemically quite stable, and thus persistent in the environment, stability has, likewise, been suggested to limit quantitative analysis in some cases - and particularly ATX-a as perhaps the most chemically labile of the known toxins from cyanobacteria. Indeed, ATX-a has an estimated (Stevens and Krieger, 1991) half-life of only about 1-2 days – or even as low as 4-10 hours - in solutions emulating relevant biological conditions, including sunlight (i.e. photolysis) and pH (i.e. acidification). Degradation products, moreover, are generally not considered toxic (Stevens and Krieger, 1991). This instability poses obvious challenges, and particularly the potential for this toxin being underestimated or even missed in chemical analyses, and may, in fact, contribute to the absence of any reports on its bioaccumulation in food webs. Accordingly, it is generally advised that appropriate precautions regarding sample collection, transport and storage be taken to minimize recognized factors (i.e. light exposure, pH), and methods have been developed to increase speed of analysis (e.g. Smith and Lewis, 1987), to minimize this factor in assessing the possible role of ATX-a in relation to food-borne health concerns.

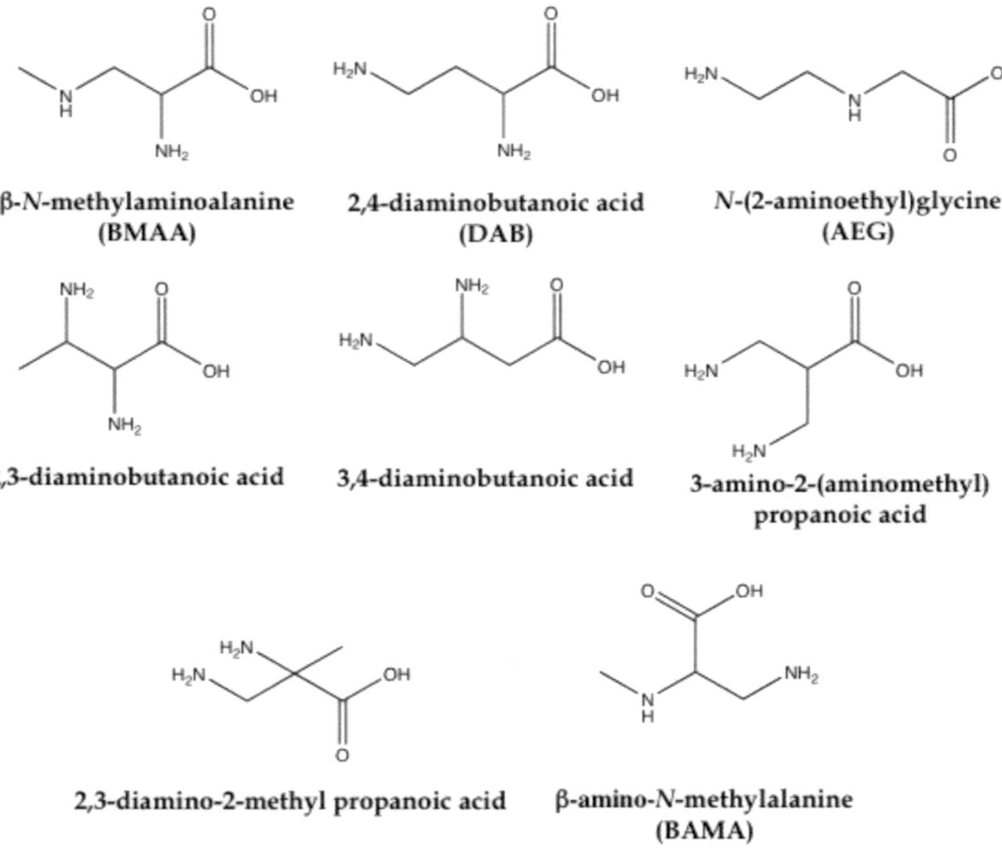

Figure 9. Isomers of the toxic amino acid, BMAA, suggested to potentially confound MS analysis.

As we learn more about the fate of cyanobacterial toxins in food webs, it is becoming increasingly recognized that at least two of the recognized cyanotoxins, namely MCs and BMAA, may present specific analytical challenges due to their specific chemical toxicology. As previously discussed (see *4.2 Bioavailability*), in addition to reversible binding of the MCs to "targeted" PPases, covalent and thus effectively irreversible binding of these toxins, specifically via Mdha (Fig. 10), may lead to considerable underestimation of the total MC content as quantitative chemical analyses based on solvent extraction, and subsequent detection of the non-bound molecule, would generally miss these bound-forms of the toxin. Indeed, it has been estimated that more than 75% of MC-LR (as representative Mdha-containing variant) in exposed fish, and as much as 99.9% in exposed invertebrates (e.g. mussels), is effectively "tied up" by covalent, irreversible binding (Williams et al., 1997a and 1997b). Similarly, as also discussed previously, one of the proposed mechanisms of toxicity for BMAA is erroneous incorporation into proteins, leading to aberrant protein aggregates which are hallmarks of neurodegenerative disease (e.g. ALS, Alzheimers' Disease) linked to this toxic amino acid. Accordingly, this bound pool of the amino acid would not be immediately available to subsequent analyses relying solely on solvent extraction from the biological matrix. Considering this, several recent developments have focused on analytical strategies for including these "bound-forms" of the toxins in the overall assessment of their contribution to food-web bioaccumulation.

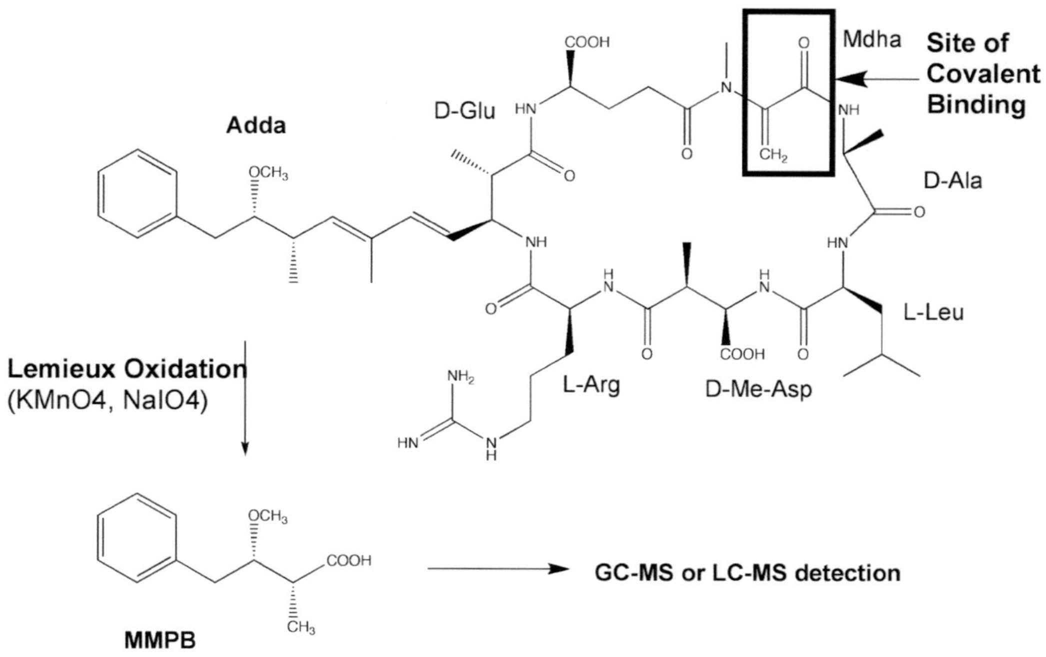

Figure 10. Lemieux oxidation of MC-LR, and detection of product (MMPB) as a surrogate for total MCs.

Perhaps the most elegant of these has been the development of the so-called "MMPB method," based on detection of the Adda oxidative cleavage product, 3-methyl-4-methoxy-phenylbutanoic acid (MMPB), as a proxy for total (i.e. bound and unbound) microcystins. As stated previously, Adda is both a key component of the MCs with respect to their toxicity, and is, indeed, conserved in the vast majority of variants (Fig. 2). Taking advantage of this conserved moiety, Sano et al. (1992) developed an analytical technique, specifically based on *Lemieux oxidation* that utilizes permanganate/periodate oxidation to cleave MMPB from the pendant Adda of microcystins (Fig. 10). This analyte can be subsequently quantified by several techniques, including GC-MS (Sano et al., 1992; Williams et al., 1997a and Williams et al., 1997b; Suchy and Berry, 2012) and LC-MS (e.g. Ott and Carmichael, 2006; Yuan et al., 2006). As Adda is distal to the Mdha, and site of covalent linkage to the PPase active site, the liberated MMPB can be used as a proxy – with no otherwise known naturally occurring counterpart – for both bound and free MCs. In fact, when subsequently applied to a range of fish and invertebrates, it became clear both that a the vast majority of MCs in exposed animals are not detected by analytical methods based on solvent extraction of the free toxin (suggesting a considerable loss of the exposure dose), and that significantly more of the toxin were detectable by the MMPB method (suggesting covalent binding as a likely "sink" for this lost toxin). Williams et al. (1997a and 1997b) most famously applied this method to the analysis of experimentally (i.e. intraperitoneally) exposed salmon, as well as samples of Dungeness crab larvae and mussels (*Mytilus edulis*). In these studies it was found, for example, that while nearly 100% of exposure dose (from *Microcystis* cells) could be recovered by the MMPB method, only approximately 0.1% of MC of the expected levels were detected by MeOH extraction coupled to a PPase inhibition assay (Williams et al., 1997a). Likewise, for i.p.-exposed salmon, approximately 34% recovery of MC by Lemieux oxidation, specifically coupled to GC-MS, was reported, compared to approximately 8% recovery for MeOH extraction and PPase inhibition assay, and similarly more than 10,000-fold higher MC was detected by the MMPB method compared to extraction/PPase inhibition in populations of crab larvae (Williams et al., 1997b). More recently, the modified MMPB method (i.e. SPME-GC-MS detection of MMPB) was applied to evaluation of MCs in several fish species, including those consumed by humans, from various freshwater lake systems, and it was similarly found that this approach measured significantly higher levels of the toxin (5- to 40-fold higher) than those detected by ELISA (Suchy and Berry, 2012). Since initial development of the technique, the MMPB has been further refined to include improvements in the sample preparation steps, including SPE (Ott and Carmichael, 2006) and solid-phase microextraction (SPME; Suchy and Berry, 2012), as well as subsequent detection methods (e.g. LC-MS, and LC-MS/MS, versus GC-MS; Ott and Carmichael, 2006; Yuan et al., 2006; Neffling et al., 2010), and it has been applied to a range of matrices including assessment of human exposure (e.g. Yuan et al., 2006). Accordingly, the MMPB method represents a tremendous advancement to both our understanding of trophic transfer/bioavailability of this toxin, as well as our ability to assess its role in food webs and bioaccumulation with respect to public health.

Similar to the covalent binding of MCs to PPase targets, the possible incorporation of BMAA into proteins, and consequent potential for underestimation, has been addressed in recent – albeit much fewer - studies. Incorporation of BMAA into proteins, with respect to both analytical challenges, and its possible role in bioavailability and trophic transfer of the toxin, was first reported by Murch et al. (2004). In this study, acid hydrolysis (i.e. 24 h boiling in 6 M HCl) – to digest proteins, and release BMAA - coupled to subsequent HPLC-FL analysis measured levels of the toxin in cycad flours exceeding those previously measured, following simple solvent extraction (i.e. presumptively unbound BMAA), by as much as 90-fold. In the same study, BMAA in brain tissues from patients who had died of Alzheimer's Disease were, likewise, analyzed following acid digestion, and similarly showed levels of the toxin that were 60- to 130-fold great than those measured following solvent extraction (i.e. "free BMAA" only). The presence of this bound pool of BMAA in proteins was accordingly suggested to represent a previously unrecognized reservoir of the toxin available for both trophic transfer (i.e. following proteolytic enzyme digestion), and as a slowly released form of the toxin with respect to the recurrent damage and "latency period" observed in the onset of these neurodegenerative diseases (Murch et al., 2004). Moreover, these results point to a limitation in the prior analytical approach, and specifically a likely underestimation of the toxin in food webs. Accordingly, subsequent studies (Rosen and Hellenäs, 2008; Baptista et al., 2011; Cervantes Cianca et al., 2012) have undertaken development and validation – as well as application - of various

http://dx.doi.org/10.5772/55111

analytical techniques (e.g. HPLC-FL, LC-MS/MS and CE-UV) that incorporate acid hydrolysis a means of characterizing "total BMAA" content. As these methods are validated, they will no doubt provide a key tool for evaluating both the ecology (e.g. trophic transfer within food-webs) and toxicology of this cyanobacterial metabolite, and clarify its possible role in human health.

6. Other cyanobacterial toxins and their bioaccumulation

A rather limited number of secondary metabolites produced by cyanobacteria – as discussed throughout this chapter (i.e. MCs, CYN, STX/PSTs, ATX-a and BMAA) – are generally considered, specifically based on association with documented intoxication events, as "toxins." However, the blue-green algae are, in fact, widely recognized to produce a myriad of biologically active metabolites (Gerwick et al., 2001; Tan, 2007; Tan, 2010). Rather than toxins though, the majority of these chemically diverse, bioactive compounds have been identified as part of "drug discovery" efforts (Tan, 2007). That said, many of the biological systems used to prospect for potential pharmaceuticals – most notably perhaps including cytotoxicity as a means of identifying anticancer drugs – could clearly be extended to include those compounds (i.e. "cytotoxins") which may have negative impacts on human health, as toxins, rather than, or in addition to, their intended therapeutic targets. Indeed, it has been argued (e.g. Berry et al., 2008) that many (or perhaps even most) of the bioactive secondary metabolites from cyanobacteria – including several investigated as drug leads - are likely produced as *allelelochemicals*, serving a role as chemical agents for deterrence, specifically through their "toxicity," toward other organisms.

Although limited to no literature exists, due to the nature of their discovery (as drug candidates), on either the potential for either toxicity or bioaccumulation of these many previously identified bioactive metabolites, indirect evidence suggests that as-of-yet unidentified metabolites do, indeed, contribute to toxicity of the cyanobacteria. Specifically, several studies (e.g. Pietsch et al., 2001; Kurmayer and Jüttner, 2009) have compared relative toxicity of pure cyanobacterial toxins to crude extracts, and consistently found higher degrees of biological activity for the latter suggesting an additive or even synergistic role of congeners in these mixtures, including both chemically related (i.e. variants within a toxin family) and/or potentially unrelated, and likely uncharacterized, metabolites. These finding, therefore, generally point to the higher toxicity of metabolic mixtures, and specifically suggest the possibility of unknown toxins which might be relevant to bioaccumulation – and, thus, consequent health concerns - within food-webs. Identification of these additional toxic metabolites will, therefore, be essential to a holistic understanding of the health effects of cyanobacterial toxins, including their potential contribution to food-borne toxicity.

Due, perhaps in part, to the nature of the biological assays used (e.g. cytotoxicity assays, enzyme inhibition assays) that rely on water-solubility of test compounds, the majority of the bioactive metabolites identified from blue-green algae as potential drug candidates have typically focused on rather water-soluble or polar compounds, and particularly the diverse non-ribosomal peptides (NRPs) characteristic of the cyanobacteria (Welker and Von Döhren, 2006). Indeed, a few such NRPs have, in fact, been identified alongside recognized toxins, specifically based on potential relevance to chemical ecology. A particularly notable example is the identification of several chemically related, and apparently quite widespread, peptides – isolated, alongside MCs, from *Microcystis* - as protease inhibitors (e.g. microviridin J, aeruginosin) with demonstrated ability to serve as feeding deterrents to the zooplankton, *Daphnia* (Harada et al., 1993; Martin et al., 1993; Okino et al., 1993; Tsukamoto et al., 1993; Rohrlack et al., 2004; von Elert et al., 2005). As for MCs, very recent studies suggest a genotype x genotype interaction between toxin and grazer, and consequent development of tolerance to these protease inhibitors (Schwarzenberger et al., 2012; von Elert et al., 2012). Accordingly, these latter findings would open up the door to possible bioaccumulation, and possible human exposure, although to-date there have not been any studies to investigate this aspect within freshwater food-webs.

In marine environments, a particularly salient example is lyngbyatoxin, and severally chemically related cyclic peptides (e.g. aplysiatoxin, debromoaplysiatoxin), isolated from marine species of the genus, *Lyngbya,* a well known producer of several known cyanobacterial toxins (i.e. MCs, CYN, STX/PSTs). Although these former peptide toxins, specifically acting as activators of protein kinase C, have been associated with direct human exposure (i.e. dermatotoxins) – as well as being investigated with respect to possible pharmacological potential – the toxins, found in filamentous cyanobacteria in marine shallows, have also been reported to be incidentally grazed by marine animals, including invertebrates – and particularly various species of gastropods that accumulate the toxin (Capper et al., 2005) - and vertebrates, most notably including sea turtles (Yasumoto et al., 1998; Arthur et al., 2008). Given the recognized toxicity to mammals (e.g. Ito et al., 2002), it is suggested that possible bioaccumulation, and subsequent consumption, could represent a route of human exposure and toxicity. In fact, as one of the few examples of acute toxicosis possibly associated with foodborne cyanotoxins, the presence of these toxins in turtle meat has been linked (Yasumoto et al., 1998) to several cases of human intoxication in the South Pacific and Madagascar (Hashimoto et al., 1967; Champetier et al., 1998) specifically characterized by ulceration of mucosal membranes, as well as apparent neurotoxic effects. It is also worth noting that these toxins have been hypothesized (Arthur et al., 2008) to explain chronic health effects – and specifically promotion of tumors associated with fibropapillomatosis – in exposed turtles, and these results, therefore, underscore the largely unstudied, possible contribution of these toxins to similar human health concerns associated with long-term, food-borne exposure.

Although the vast majority of bioactive secondary metabolites identified have, for reasons stated above, particularly included a number of peptides and other hydrophilic compounds, the cyanobacteria are known to produce a variety of lipophilic metabolites as well. In support of a possible role of these metabolites in relation to food webs, when evaluating the effects of toxic metabolites from the recognized toxigenic cyanobacterial species, *Planktothrix rubescens,* Kurmayer and Jüttner (1999) observed that lipophilic extraction reduced feeding deterrence of the cyanobacterial cells with respect to zooplankton grazers, and pointed to an uncharacterized lipophilic metabolite in this species. In more recent

http://dx.doi.org/10.5772/55111

studies, Berry et al. (2009) evaluated non-polar extracts of the CYN-producing species, *Aphanizomenon ovalisporum* and *Cylindrospermopsis raciborskii*, specifically using the zebrafish embryo model, and identified apparent lipophilic toxins, chemically unrelated to CYN or other water-soluble toxins produced by these species. It is not, therefore, surprising that considerable research in this area has identified numerous lipophilic metabolites ranging from alkaloids to lipopeptides (Orjala et al., 1995; Wu et al., 2000; Li et al., 2001; Edwards et al., 2004) to fatty acids (e.g. polyunsaturated fatty acid [PUFAs], Reinikainen et al., 2001) and seemingly simple hydrocarbons (Jaja-Chimedza et al., 2012).

Although much of the chemistry behind these observations remains to be characterized, one particularly well-studied group of lipophilic metabolites is a diverse family of indole alkaloids produced by members of the relatively widespread, but otherwise understudied, Stigonemataceae (e.g. Raveh and Carmeli, 2007; Mo et al., 2010; Kim et al., 2012; and many more). Although this chemically diverse, and taxonomically restricted, group of metabolites have been generally identified based on antimicrobial activity (e.g. Raveh and Carmeli, 2007; Mo et al., 2012), and in fact, have been linked to possible allelopathy (i.e. inhibition of photosynthetic microbial competitors) in their natural environment, several biological activities supporting animal toxicity have also been reported (e.g. inhibition of RNA polymerase; Doan et al., 2001). This finding, and their seemingly widespread occurrence, raises the question as to whether these quite lipophilic metabolites may contribution to toxicity within food webs, including perhaps human health concerns.

Similarly, considerable work over the past 15 years or more has identified a diversity of lipopeptides, particularly isolated from the widespread marine cyanobacterial species, *Lyngbya majuscula* (Orjala et al., 1995; Orjala et al., 1996; Li et al., 2001; Nogle et al., 2001; Edwards et al., 2004; Choi et al., 2010) and others (e.g. *Anabaena;* Kaya et al., 2002). Although bioactivity associated with these metabolites runs the gamut from inhibition of specific enzymes to cytotoxicity in mammalian cells to toxicity in a range of organisms (e.g. antifungal, molluscicidal, ichthyotoxicity), potent neurotoxicity has, in particular, been associated with a number of these (e.g. Li et al., 2001; Nogle et al., 2001; Edwards et al., 2004; Choi et al., 2010). However, although a wealth of information regarding toxicity has emerged alongside their chemical discovery, essentially no insight as to possible bioaccumulation – despite the global abundance of these taxa, e.g. *Lyngbya,* in marine and freshwater habitats – currently exists.

More recently – following-up on prior studies (Berry et al., 2009; as discussed briefly above) – an apparently widespread group of toxic, lipophilic metabolites have been identified from several species of otherwise toxigenic cyanobacteria. Utilizing the zebrafish (*Danio rerio*) embryo as a vertebrate model of so-called developmental toxicity, and specifically as a means of *bioassay-guided fractionation,* Jaja-Chimedza et al. (2012), in very recent studies, identified a family of isotactic polymethoxy-1-alkenes (PMAs) from *Aphanizomenon ovalisporum*, specifically as lipophilic inhibitors of developmental pathways in this model system. Both this species, and the genus (i.e. *Aphanizomenon),* more generally, are recognized producers of CYN (genus/species; e.g. Preussel et al., 2006), as well as the neurotoxic STX/PSTs and ATX-a (species; e.g. Mahmood and Carmichael, 1986 and Ballot et al, 2010, respectively). The identification of PMAs as lipophilic metabolites in this species, including CYN-producing strains (Berry et al., 2009), suggests that they may contribute to the overall toxicity of this widely distributed species, as well as - given the highly lipid-soluble nature of these compounds - the potential for their bioaccumulation, and even biomagnfication, within food-webs. Moreover, prior studies have identified the same or similar PMAs from a wide range of cyanobacteria (e.g. Mynderse and Moore, 1979; Mori et al., 1991), although previous studies did not originally link their presence to potential toxicity (but rather identified them based on chemical characterization), and subsequent studies (Jaja-Chimedza et al., forthcoming), using the same toxicity, have identified them in otherwise recognized toxigenic species (e.g. *C. raciborkskii*, *M. aeruginosa*). These emerging findings suggest that this group of metabolites may be widespread, and further underscore the potential role in food-derived toxicity. In fact, identification of closely related metabolites in marine sponges (Rama and Faulkner, 2002) has been attributed to a cyanobacterial biosynthetic origin/source (likely via filter-feeding of algal cells), and further support the potential for their uptake and accumulation in higher trophic levels. To-date, however, studies on their bioaccumulation (beyond this example) in food-webs remains to be addressed.

7. Implications for ecosystem health

Finally, although beyond the scope of this chapter (and volume), it is worthwhile to consider – before concluding our discussion with respect to public health implications of cyanobacterial toxins in food webs – the apparent contribution of cyanobacterial toxins in food webs with respect to animal and ecosystem health. Obviously, understanding the impacts of these toxins on animal health with respect to ecosystems is essential to understanding the potential for trophic transfer of these toxins. Moreover, insights regarding the potential for human health concerns of food-borne toxins – especially as contaminants of shared food-webs - can be often studied indirectly, and to some extent extrapolated, by understanding the role of these toxins in non-human animals. Indeed, with regards to the toxicity of cyanobacterial metabolites, the first reported case of intoxication by a cyanobacterial bloom was made based on animal health, and specifically reported livestock poisonings associated with pond scums (later identified as cyanobacteria) in a so-called "poisonous lake," famously detailed in the pioneering works by George Francis in the late 19th century (Francis, 1878).

Given that current evidence generally suggests limited trophic transfer of most of the known cyanobacterial toxins, and consequent restriction of foodborne cyanobacterial toxins to lower trophic levels in food-webs, it is not surprising that toxicity to animals has particularly focused on those vertebrate (i.e. fish) and invertebrates which are exposed either directly (through phytoplanktivory), or through "single vector" (e.g. zooplanktivory), transfer. For example, the previously discussed studies of Karjalainen et al. (2005), not only demonstrated that pre-exposure of zooplankton to cell-free, NOD-containing extracts of *N. spumigens* – representative of the toxin released during blooms –resulted in subsequent bioaccumulation of this toxin in zooplanktivorous, larval fish predators, but also decreased (compared to unexposed controls) ingestion, growth rate and fecal production of the experimentally fed zooplanktivorous larvae of Northern Pike (*Esox lucius*), suggesting a possible toxic effect to these predators without direct exposure to the toxin-containing water or algal cells. Interestingly enough, no such statistically significant effects was observed for larvae fed zooplankton which were pre-exposed to pure NOD, suggesting a possible contribution of other, currently unknown, toxins (Karjalainen et al., 2005).

Numerous studies, encompassing essentially all of the other known cyanotoxins, as well as yet uncharacterized, but apparently toxic, metabolites, likewise, have demonstrated the potential toxic effects to various aquatic species exposed at this lower end of the trophic scale. At the level of zooplanktivorous grazers, numerous studies have documented the apparent toxic effects of, not only MCs (as discussed above), but also other cyanobacterial toxins, including CYN (Nogueira et al., 2004), STX/PSTs (Filho et al., 2008) and ATX-a (Sieroslawska et al., 2010) - as well as perhaps other unidentified metabolites (present in extracts) - on *Daphnia,* and various other species. Likewise, biochemical and histopathologic analyses of both benthic grazers, particularly including snail species (Lance et al., 2010), and filter-feeding bivalves (Puerto et al., 2011; Sabatini et al., 2011), exposed to cell-bound toxins, including MCs and CYN, as well as unidentified toxic metabolites, demonstrate toxicity – along with apparent bioaccumulation – corresponding to uptake and transport pathways from the digestive system. Similarly, toxicity of several cyanobacterial metabolites to fish – and particularly several, representative phytoplanktivorous species (e.g. carp, tilapia) - exposed to dietary sources of these toxins has been well documented (e.g. Jos et al., 2005; Osswald et al., 2007; El Ghazali et al., 2010; Qiao et al., 2012).

On the other hand, relatively fewer studies to-date have clearly documented toxic effects of subsequent predation on toxin-laden invertebrates (e.g. zooplankton, benthic invertebrates), or phytoplanktivorous fish. However, the limited studies that have do generally point to the potential for toxicity – along with toxin transfer – to higher trophic levels. In one particularly notable study, Qiu et al. (2007) examined – using biochemical and histopathological approaches - four trophic levels, comprised of a phytoplanktivorous, omnivorous and carnivorous fish species in a Chinese lake in relation to a MC-producing bloom. Surprisingly in this case, the most pronounced histopathological signs of toxicity were observed for carnivorous fish, whereas the largest biochemical response (i.e. particularly the production of several antioxidant enzymes/pathway, e.g. superoxide disumutase, catalase, glutathione, glutathione peroxidase), were measured for phytoplanktivorous species. These results suggest not only that carnivores can be exposed to cyanobacterial metabolites, and toxic effects via food webs, but that grazers of cyanobacteria (i.e. phytoplanktivores) may, as such, be specifically adapted to the direct exposure to these toxins.

The toxic effects of cyanobacterial metabolites on higher trophic levels, aside from fish, in aquatic food webs remain quite scarce, despite the fact that numerous taxa, including bird and mammalian species, are recognized as frequent "top consumers" in these systems. However, examples are beginning to emerge in the literature. In an especially insightful example, Miller et al. (2010) recently reported on the apparent toxic effects - including several animal deaths among - among southern sea otters, along the Pacific coast of the U.S., exposed to MCs bioaccumulated by bivalves (i.e. clams, mussels and oysters) consumed by these carnivorous predators. Following an unusually high number of sea otters deaths in the Monterey Bay, and surrounding coastal areas, particularly during the period of 2005-2008, necropsy on these stranded animals was performed. Based on the detection of relatively high levels (up to 348 ppb) of several variants of microcystins, including MC-RR, -LR and -desmethyl LR, in livers of sea otters, along with gross and microscopic pathological indications - particularly in livers of the animals - consistent with MC intoxication, it was concluded that animals had, indeed, died from exposure to this cyanobacterial toxin. The source of the toxin was ultimately traced to outflow from the nearby Pinto Lake into the marine waters of Monterey Bay, and subsequent bioaccumulation of the toxin by mollusks, consumed by sea otters, in the Bay. Characterized as a "super-bloom" of cyanobacteria, levels of MC in Pinto Lake, during this time, were measured as high as 2,100 ppm (more than six orders of magnitude higher than the WHO limit of 1 ppb), and use of Solid Phase Adsorption Toxin Tracking (SPATT) samples enabled tracking of the toxin from the lake toward the Bay. Subsequent laboratory studies confirmed the bioaccumulation of MC - at levels as high 1,324 ppb - by various bivalve (i.e. clam, mussel, oyster) species that make up a primary component of the sea otters' diet. Indeed, this case is particularly revealing as it not only supports hypothesis that higher trophic levels – including mammalian carnivores - can, in fact, be exposed to toxic (and even lethal) levels of cyanobacterial toxins through food-webs, but also that toxins can transfer not only within ecocystems, but between (in this case, freshwater and marine) systems. Moroever, although levels of MCs, in this case, were exceptionally high, this study further provides – through quantificationof the toxin in (livers of) exposed animals – a first estimation of relevant (i.e. lethal) exposure doses for mammalian consumers in relation to environmental concentration both in water, and vectors (i.e. bioaccumulation in bivalves) of the toxin.

8. Conclusions

Cyanobacteria are prolific producers of toxic, and otherwise biologically (i.e. pharmacologically) active, metabolites. Although ubiquitous in the environment, the cyanobacteria are arguably most conspicuous, and generally more abundant, in aquatic systems, particularly in association with so-called "harmful algal blooms." As such, exposure to several cyanobacterial toxins through contamination of drinking water, and related routes, has been clearly linked to both acute toxicoses, including human and animal mortalities, as well as being increasingly tied to several long-term health effects (e.g. cancer, neurodegenerative disease). Consequently, waterborne cyanotoxins are widely acknowledged as a global health concern.

Given this particularly widespread occurrence of the "blue-green algae" in marine and freshwater ecosystems, it is not, therefore, surprising, that bioaccumulation of nearly all of the "recognized" cyanobacterial toxins within relevant species of aquatic food webs has been reported. In light of the enormous human reliance on the world's oceans and freshwater systems, particularly as a source of food (i.e. fish, seafood), as well as culminating evidence to suggest that global climate change is fueling an apparently rapid increase in cyanobacterial abundance, bloom frequency and perhaps even toxigenicity in aquatic systems, cyanobacterial toxins in food webs, likewise, represent a clearly important human health issue.

http://dx.doi.org/10.5772/55111

As an emerging concern, however, clearly more questions than answers remain, at present, regarding the potential role of cyanobacterial toxins in food webs, particularly in terms of possible human and environmental health concerns. Although a preponderance of evidence indicates that diverse taxa of aquatic animal species do, in fact, accumulate cyanotoxins, the biochemical, physiological and ecological processes that control trophic transfer within food-webs remains to be clarified. Likewise, although trophic transfer of the largely water-soluble "known" cyanobacterial toxins appears to follow a pattern of biodilution, rather than biomagnification to top consumers, a growing number cases indicate that species, known to be consumed as part of human diets, do bioaccumulate significant quantities of these toxins, yet the potential implications for human health remains to be elucidated. This, it is argued is due, in part, to the lack of information regarding bioavailability, as well as limitations and challenges in current analytical methodologies used to assess this contribution.

Although the scientific evidence that does exist strongly suggests a potential (and, in fact, high probability) for human exposure to, and consequent health concerns associated with, food-borne cyanobacterial toxins, the implications with respect to public health policy remains almost entirely to be addressed. Indeed, while our scientific understanding of the bioaccumulation of cyanobacterial toxins in relation to human health currently remains rather limited - particularly relative to many other environmental health concerns – the public health implications, including relevance to policy makers and stakeholders, lags even more so. And, in fact, it is asserted that it is many of the same gaps in knowledge that limit our scientific understanding which, likewise, limit public health policy with regards to food-borne cyanotoxins, and thus addressing these gaps will be critical in this regard. First, and perhaps foremost, is the preeminent need to understand the toxicology of food-borne cyanotoxins, including both laboratory and (currently non-existent) epidemiological studies to elucidate what (if any) health effects exist, and which groups are most likely affected. Similarly, clarifying the actual health effects, including relevant doses, mechanisms of action, bioavailability, etc., will be fudnamental to developing effective regulatory guidelines. Although, as described above, attempts have been made (e.g. Ibelings and Chorus, 2007) to extrapolate current (albeit limited) toxicological knowledge in this regard to possible acceptable levels for food-borne cyanotoxins, these are based entirely on data from water-borne toxins, and are not likely to be accurate in terms of exposure through food. Furthermore, even the provisional guidelines that exist for cyanobacterial toxins in water are only recommendations, and policy will not only need to clarify acceptable levels, but also address monitoring and enforcement of these guidelines. As such, improvements, validation and standardization of methods for chemical analysis of cyanobacterial toxins – toward effective monitoring and enforcement - in food will be key. Continued investigations in these areas will, therefore be of the crucial toward developing a comprehensive picture of this emerging public health concern.

Author details

John Berry*

Department of Chemistry and Biochemistry, Florida International University, U.S.A.

References

[1] Andrinolo, D, Michea, L. F, & Lago, N. (1999). Toxic effects, pharmacokinetics and clearance of saxitoxin, a component of paralytic shellfish poison (PSP) in cats. *Toxicon*, , 37, 447-464.

[2] Aráoz, R, & Molgó, J. Tandeau de Marsac, N. ((2010). Neurotoxic cyanobacterial toxins. *Toxicon*, , 56, 813-828.

[3] Arthur, K, Limpus, C, Balazs, G, Capper, A, Udy, J, Shaw, G, Keuper-bennet, U, & Bennet, P. (2008). The exposure of green turtles (*Chelonia mydas*) to tumour promoting compounds produced by the cyanobacterium *Lyngbya majuscula* and their potential role in the aetiology of fibropapillomatosis. *Harmful Algae*, , 7, 114-125.

[4] Ballot, A, Fastner, J, Lentz, M, & Weidner, C. (2010). First report of anatoxin-a-producing cyanobacterium *Aphanizomenon issatschenkoi* in northeastern Germany. *Toxicon*, , 56, 964-971.

[5] Banack, S. A, Downing, T. G, Spacil, Z, Purdie, E. L, Metcalf, J. S, Downing, S, Esterhulzen, M, Codd, G. A, & Cox, P. A. (2010). Distinguishing the cyanobacterial neurotoxin beta=N-methylamino alanine (BMAA) from its structural isomer 2,4-diaminobutyric acid (DAB). *Toxicon*, 56, 868-879., 2(4)

[6] Banker, R. S, Carmeli, O, Hadas, B, Teltsch, R, Porat, R, & Sukenik, A. (1997). Identification of cylindrospermopsin in *Aphanizomenon ovalisporum* isolated from Lake Kinneret, Israel. *Journal of Phycology*, , 35, 613-616.

[7] Banker, R. S, Carmeli, S, Werman, M, Teltsch, B, Porat, R, & Sukenik, A. (2001). Uracil moiety is required for toxicity of the cyanobacterial hepatotoxin cylindrospermopsin. *Journal of Toxicology and Environmental Health, Part A*, , 62, 281-288.

[8] Baptista, M. S, Cianca, R. C, Lopes, V. R, Almeida, C. M, & Vasconcelos, V. M. (2011). Determination of the non protein amino acid β-N-methylamino-L-alanine in estuarine caynobacteria by capillary electrophoresis. *Toxicon*, , 58, 410-414.

[9] Bazin, E, Huet, S, & Jarry, G. Le Hegarat, L.; Munday, J. S.; Humpage, A. R. & Fessard, Cytotoxic and genotoxic effects of cylindrospermopsin in mice treated by gavage or intraperitoneal injection. *Environmental Toxicology*, 27, 277-284., 2012

[10] Beltran, E. C, & Neilan, B. A. (2000). Geographical separation of the neurotoxin-producing cyanobacterium *Anabaena circinalis*. *Applied Environmental Microbiology*, , 66, 4468-4474.

[11] Berry, J. P, Gantar, M, Perez, M. H, Berry, G, & Noriega, F. G. (2008). Cyanobacterial toxins as allelochemicals with potential applications as algaecides, herbicides and insecticides. *Marine Drugs*, , 6, 117-146.

[12] Berry, J. P, Gibbs, P. D, Schmale, M. C, & Saker, M. L. (2009). Toxicity of cylindrospermopsin, and other apparent metabolites from *Cylindrospermopsis raciborskii* and *Aphanizomenon ovalisporum*, to the zebrafish (*Danio rerio*) embryo. *Toxicon*, , 52, 289-299.

[13] Berry, J. P, & Lind, O. (2010). First evidence of "paralytic shellfish toxins" and cylindrospermopsin in a Mexican freshwater system, Lago Catemaco, and apparent bioaccumulation of the toxins in "tegogolo" snails (*Pomacaee patula catemacensis*). *Toxicon*, , 55, 930-938.

[14] Berry, J. P, Lee, E, Walton, K, Wilson, A. E, & Bernal-brooks, F. (2011). Bioaccumulation of microcystins by fish associated with a persistent cyanobacterial bloom in Lago de Patzcuaro (Michoacan, Mexico). *Environmental Toxicology and Chemistry*, , 30, 1621-1628.

[15] Berry, J. P, Jaja-chimedza, A, Davalos-lind, L, & Lind, O. (2012). Apparent bioaccumulation of cylindrospermopsin and paralytic shellfish toxins by finfish in Lake Catemaco (Veracruz, Mexico). *Food Additives and Contaminants Part A*, , 29, 314-321.

[16] Bourke, A. T. C, Hawes, R. B, Neilson, A, & Stallman, N. D. (1983). An outbreak of hepato-enteritis (the Palm Island mystery disease) possibly caused by algal intoxication. *Toxicon*, , 3, 45-48.

[17] Brand, L. E, Pablo, J, Compton, A, Hammerschlag, N, & Mash, D. (2010). Cyanobacterial blooms and the occurrence of the neurotoxin beta-N-methylamino-L-alanine (BMAA) in South Florida aquatic food webs. *Harmful Algae*, , 9, 620-635.

[18] CallerT. A; Doolin, J. W.; Haney, J. F.; Murby, A. J.; West, K. G.; Farrar, H. E.; Ball, A.; Harris, B. T. & Stommel, E. W. ((2009). A cluster of amyotrophic lateral sclerosis in New Hampshire: a possible role for toxic cyanobacteria blooms. *Amyotrophic Lateral Sclerosis*, 10 Suppl. , 2, 101-108.

[19] Capper, A, Tibbets, I. R, Neil, O, & Shaw, J. M. G. R. ((2005). The fate of *Lyngbya majuscula* toxins in three potential consumers. *Journal of Chemical Ecology*, , 31, 1595-1606.

[20] Carmichael, W. W, Evans, W. R, Yin, Q. Q, Bell, P, & Mosczydlowski, E. (1997). Evidence for paralytic shellfish poisons in the freshwater cyanobacterium *Lyngbya wollei*. *Applied Environmental Microbiology*, , 63, 3104-3110.

[21] Carpenter, E. J, & Romans, K. (1991). Major role of the cyanobacterium *Trichodesmium* in nutrient cycling in the North-Atlantic Ocean. *Science*, , 254, 1356-1358.

[22] Cervantes CiancaR. C.; Pallares, M. A.; Barbosa, D. R.; Adan, V. L.; J. M. L. Martins; Gago-Martinez, A. ((2007). Application of precolumn oxidation HPLC method with fluorescence detection to evaluate saxitoxin levels in discrete brain regions of the brain. *Toxicon*, , 49, 89-99.

[23] Cervantes Cianca., R. C.; Baptista, M. S.; Pinto da Silva, L.; Lopes, V. R. & Vasconcelos, V. M. ((2012). Reversed-phase HPLC/FD method for the quantitative analysis of the neurotoxin BMAA (β-N-methylamino-L-alanine) in cyanobacteria. *Toxicon*, , 59, 379-384.

[24] ChampetierR. G; Ranaivoson, G.; Ravaonindrina, N.; Rakotonjabelo, A. L.; Rasolofonirina, N.; Roux, J. F. & Yasumoto, T. ((1998). Un probléma de santé publique réémergent á Madagascar: les intoxications collectives par consommation d'animaux marins. *Arch. Inst. Pasteur Madagascar*, , 64, 71-76.

[25] Chen, J, Xie, P, Zhang, D, & Lei, H. (2007). In situ studies on the distribution patterns and dynamics of microcystins in a biomanipulation fish- bighead carp (*Aristichthys nobilis*). *Environmental Pollution*, , 147, 150-157.

[26] Choi, H, Pereira, A. R, Cao, Z, Shuman, C. F, Engene, N, Byrum, T, Matainaho, T, Murray, T. F, Mangoni, A, & Gerwick, W. H. (2010). The holamides, structurally intriguing neurotoxic lipopeptides from Papua New Guinea marine cyanobacteria. *Journal of Natural Products*, , 73, 1411-1421.

[27] Costa, P. R, Lage, S, Barata, M, & Pousão-ferreira, P. (2011). Uptake, transformation, and elimination kinetics of paralytic shellfish toxins in white seabream (*Diplodus sargus*). *Marine Biology*, , 158, 2805-2811.

[28] Cox, P. A, Banack, S. A, & Murch, S. J. (2003). Biomagnification of cyanobacterial neurotoxins and neurodegenerative disease among the Chamorro people of Guam. *Proceedings of the National Academy of Sciences U.S.A.*, , 100, 13380-13383.

[29] Cox, P. A, Banack, S. A, Murch, S. J, Rasmussen, U, Tien, G, Bidigaire, R. R, & Metcalf, J. S. (2005). Diverse taxa of cyanobacteria produce beta-N-methylamino-L-alanine, a neurotoxic amino acid. *Proceedings of the National Academy of Sciences U.S.A.*, , 102, 5074-5078.

[30] Cox, P. A, Richer, R, Metcalf, J. S, Banack, S. A, Codd, G. A, & Bradley, W. G. (2009). Cyanobacteria and BMAA exposure from desert dust: a possible link to sporadic ALS among Gulf War veterans. *Amyotrophic Lateral Sclerosis*, 10 Suppl. , 2, 109-117.

[31] Craig, M, Luu, H. A, Mccready, T. L, Williams, D, Andersen, R. J, & Holmes, C. F. (1997). Molecular mechanisms underlying the interaction of motuporin and microcystins with type-1 and type-2A protein phosphatases. *Biochemical and Cellular Biology*, , 74, 569-578.

[32] Cucchiaroni, M. L, Viscomi, M. T, Bernardi, G, Molinari, M, Guatteo, E, & Mercuri, N. B. (2010). Metabotropic glutamate receptor 1 mediates electrophysiological and

toxic actions of the cycad derivative beta-N-methylamino-L-alanine on substantia nigra pars compacta dopinergic neurons. *The Journal of Neuroscience*, , 30, 5176-5188.

[33] Davis, T. W, & Gobler, C. J. (2011). Grazing by mesozooplankton and microzoolankton on toxic and non-toxic strains of *Microcystis* in the Transquaking River, a tributary of Chesapeake Bay. *Journal of Plankton Research, 33*, 415-430.

[34] Doan, N. T, Stewart, P. R, & Smith, G. D. (2001). Inhibition of bacterial RNA polymerase by the cyanobacterial metabolites 12-epi-hapalindole E isonitrile and calothrixin A. *FEMS Microbiology Letters*, , 196, 135-139.

[35] Dyble, J, Gossiaux, D, Landrum, P, Kashian, D. R, & Pothoven, S. (2011). A kinetic study of accumulation and elimination of microcystin-LR in Yellow Perch (*Perca flavescens*) tissue and implications for human fish consumption. *Marine Drugs*, , 9, 2553-2571.

[36] Edwards, D. J, Marquez, B. L, Nogle, L. M, Mcphail, K, Goeger, D. E, Roberts, M. A, & Gerwick, W. H. (2004). Structure and biosynthesis of the jamaicamides, new mixed polyketide-peptide neurotoxins from the marine cyanobacterium *Lyngbya majuscula*. *Chemical Biology*, , 11, 817-833.

[37] El Ghazali, I, Sagrane, S, & Carvalho, A. P. Ouahid, Y; Del Campo, F. F.; Vasconcelos, V & Oudra, B. ((2010). Effects of mirocystin profile of a cyanobacterial bloom on growth and toxin accumulation in common carp *Cyprinus carpio* larvae. *Journal of Fish Biology*, , 76, 1415-1430.

[38] Etheridge, S. M. (2010). Paralytic shellfish poisoning: seafood safety and human health perspectives. *Toxicon*, , 56, 108-122.

[39] Eriksson, J, Jonasson, S, Papaefthimiou, D, Rasmussen, U, & Bergman, B. (2009). Improving deriviatization efficiency of BMAA utilizing AccQ-taq in a complex cyanobacterial matrix. *Amino Acids*, , 36, 43-48.

[40] Falconer, I. R, Burch, M. D, Steffensen, D. A, Choice, M, & Coverdale, O. R. (1994). Toxicity of the blue-green alga (cyanobacterium) *Microcystis aeruginosa* in drinking water to growing pigs, as an animal model for human injury and risk assessment. *Environmental Toxicology and Water Quality*, , 9, 131-139.

[41] FAO Fisheries and Aquaculture Department ((2010). The state of world fisheries and aquaculture 2010United Nations Food and Agriculture Organization, Rome, 2010.

[42] Fawell, J. K, Mitchell, R. E, Everett, D. J, & Hill, R. E. (1999). The toxicity of cyanobacterial toxins in the mouse. I: Microcystin-LR. *Human and Experimental Toxicology*, , 18, 162-167.

[43] Ferrao-filho, A. S, & Kozlowsky-suzuki, B. (2011). Cyanotoxins: bioaccumulation and effects on aquatic organisms. *Marine Drugs*, , 9, 2729-2772.

[44] Filho, A. S. da Costa, S. M.; Ribeiro, M. G. & Azevedo, S. M. ((2008). Effects of a saxitoxin-producer strain of *Cylindrospermopsis raciborskii* (cyanobacteria) on the swimming movements of cladocerans. *Environmental Toxicology*, , 23, 161-168.

[45] Fischer, W. J, Altheimer, S, Cattori, V, Meier, P. J, Dietrich, D. R, & Hagenbuch, B. (2005). Organic anion transporting polypeptides in liver and brain mediate uptake of microcystin. *Toxicology and Applied Pharmacology*, , 203, 257-263.

[46] Fischer, A, Hoeger, S. J, Stemmer, K, Feurstein, D. J, Knobeloch, D, Nussler, A, & Dietrich, D. R. (2010). The role of organic anion transporting polypeptides (OATP/SLCOs) in the toxicity of different microcystin congeners *in vitro*: a comparison of primary human hepatocytes and OATP-transfected HEK293 cells. *Toxicology and Applied Pharmacology*, , 245, 9-20.

[47] Francis, G. (1878). Poisonous Australian lake. *Nature*, , 18, 11-12.

[48] Fromme, H, Kohler, A, Krause, R, & Fuhrling, D. (2000). Occurrence of cyanobacterial toxins- microcystins and anatoxin-a- in Berlin water bodies with implications to human health and regulations. *Environmental Toxicology*, , 15, 120-130.

[49] Froscio, S. M, Humpage, A. R, Burcham, P. C, & Falconer, I. R. (2001). Cell-free protein sysnthesis inhibition assay for cyanobacterial toxin cylindrospermopsin. *Environmental Toxicology*, , 16, 408-412.

[50] Funari, E, & Testai, E. (2008). Human health risk assessment related to cyanotoxins exposure. *Critical Reviews in Toxicology*, , 38, 97-135.

[51] Gerwick, W. H, Tan, L. T, & Sitachitta, N. (2001). Nitrogen-containing metabolites from marine cyanobacteria. *The Alkaloids: Chemistry and Biology*, , 57, 75-184.

[52] Griffiths, D. J, & Saker, M. L. (2003). The Palm Island Mystery Disease 20 years on: a review of research on the cyanotoxin cylindrospermopsin. *Environmental Toxicology*, , 18, 78-93.

[53] Gulledge, B. M, Aggen, J. B, Eng, H, Sweimeh, K, & Chamberlin, A. R. (2003). Microcystin analogues comprised of only Adda and a single additional amino acid retain moderate activity as PP2A inhibitors. *Biorganic and Medicinal Chemistry Letters*, 13, 2907-2911., 1.

[54] Gugger, M, Lenoir, S, Berger, C, Ledreux, A, Druart, J. C, Humbert, J. F, Guette, C, & Bernard, C. (2005). First report in a river in France of the benthic cyanobacterium *Phormidium favosum* producing anatoxin-a associated with dog neurotoxicosis. *Toxicon*, , 45, 919-928.

[55] Harada, K. I, Ohtani, I, Iwamoto, K, Suzuki, M, Watanabe, M. F, Watanabe, M, & Terao, K. (1994). Isolation of cylindrospermopsin from a cyanobacterium *Umezakia natans* and its screening method. *Toxicon*, , 32, 73-84.

[56] Harada, K, Oshikata, M, Shimada, T, Nagata, A, Ishikawa, N, Suzuki, M, Kondo, F, Shimizu, M, & Yamada, S. (1997). High-performance liquid chromatographic separa-

tion of microcystins derivatized with a highly fluorescent dienophile. *Natural Toxins*, , 5, 201-207.

[57] Hashimoto, Y, Ko-nosu, S, & Yasumoto, T. (1967). Epidemiological research of poisoining caused by sea turtles in Okinawa.

[58] Hawkins, P. R, Runnegar, M. T. C, Jackson, A. R. B, & Falconer, I. R. (1985). Severe hepatotoxicity caused by the tropical cyanobacterium *Cylindrospermopsis raciborskii* isolated from a domestic water supply reservoir. *Applied and Environmental Microbiology*, , 50, 1291-1295.

[59] Heintzelman, G, Fang, W, Keen, K, Wallace, S. P, & Weinreb, G. A. S. M. ((2001). Stereoselective total synthesis of the cyanobacterial hepatotoxin 7-epicylindrospermopsin: revision of the stereochemistry of cylindrospermopsin. *Journal of the American Chemical Society*, , 123, 8851-8853.

[60] Hilborn, E. D, Carmichael, W. W, Soares, R. M, Yuan, M, Servaites, J. C, Barton, H. A, & Azevedo, S. M. (2007). Serologic evaluation of human microcystin exposure. *Environmental Toxicology*, , 22, 459-463.

[61] Holcombe, G. W, Benoit, D. A, Leonard, E. N, & Mckim, J. M. (1976). Long-term effects of lead exposure on three generations of Brook Trout (*Salvenius fontinalis*). *Journal of Fisheries Research Board of Canada*, , 33, 1731-1741.

[62] Humpage, A. R, Rositano, J, Bretag, A. H, Brown, R, Baker, P. D, Nicholson, B. C, & Steffensen, D. A. (1994). Paralytic shellfish poisons from Australian cyanobacterial blooms. *Australian Journal of Marine and Freshwater Research*, , 45, 761-771.

[63] Humpage, A. R, & Falconer, I. R. (2003). Oral toxicity of the cyanobacterial toxin cylindrospermopsin in male Swiss albino mice: determination of no observed adverse effect level for deriving drinking water guideline value. *Environmental Toxicology*, , 18, 94-103.

[64] Humpage, A. R, Fontaine, F, Froscio, S, Burcham, P, & Falconer, I. R. (2005). Cylindrospermopsin genotoxicity and cytotoxicity: role of cytochrome and oxidative stress. *Journal of Toxicology and Environmental Health A*, 68, 739-753., 450.

[65] Humpage, A. R, Magalhaes, V. F, & Froscio, S. M. (2010). Comparison of analytical tools and biological assays for detection of paralytic shellfish poisoning toxins. *Analytical and Bioanalytical Chemistry*, , 397, 1655-1671.

[66] Ibelings, B. W, Bruning, K, De Jonge, J, Wolfstein, K, Pires, L. M, Postma, J, & Burger, T. (2005). Distribution of microcystins in a lake foodweb: no evidence for biomagnification. *Microbial Ecology*, , 49, 487-500.

[67] Ibelings, B. W, & Chorus, I. (2007). Accumulation of cyanobacterial toxins in freshwater "seafood" and its consequences for public health: a review. *Environmental Pollution*, , 150, 177-192.

[68] Jackim, E, & Gentile, J. (1968). Toxins of a blue-green alga: similarity to saxitoxin. *Science*, , 162, 915-916.

[69] Jaja-chimedza, A, Gantar, M, Gibbs, P. D. L, Schmale, M. C, & Berry, J. P. (2012). Polymethoxy-1-alkenes from *Aphanizomenon ovalisporum* inhibit vertebrate development in the zebrafish (*Danio rerio*) embryo model. *Marine Drugs*, , 10, 2322-2336.

[70] James, K. J, Furey, A, Sherlock, I. R, Stack, M. A, Twohig, M, Caudwell, F. B, & Skulberg, O. M. (1998). Sensitive determination of anatoxin-a, homoanatoxin-a and their degradation products by liquid chromatography with fluorometric detection. *Journal of Chromatography*, , 798, 147-157.

[71] Jiang, L, Aigret, B, De Borggraeve, W. M, Spacil, Z, & Ilag, L. L. MS method for the identification of BMAA from its isomers in biological samples. *Analytical and Bioanalytical Chemistry*, , 403, 1719-1730.

[72] Jonasson, S, Eriksson, J, Berntzon, L, Spacil, Z, Ilag, L. L, Ronnevi, L. O, Rasmussen, U, & Bergman, B. (2010). Transfer of a cyanobacterial neurotoxin within a temperate aquatic ecosytem suggests a pathway for human exposure. *Proceedings of the National Academy of Science U. S. A.*, , 107, 9252-9257.

[73] Jos, A, Pichardo, S, Prieto, A, Repetto, G, Vazquez, C. M, Moreno, I, & Camean, A. M. (2005). Toxic cyanobacterial cells containing microcystins induce oxidative stress in exposed tilapia fish (*Oreochromis* sp.) under laboratory conditions. *Aquatic Toxicology*, , 72, 261-271.

[74] Karjalainen, M, Reinkainen, M, Lindvall, F, Spoof, L, & Meriluoto, J. A. (2003). Uptake and accumulation of dissolved, radiolabeled nodularin in Baltic Sea zooplankton. *Environmental Toxicology*, , 18, 52-60.

[75] Karjalainen, M, Reinikainen, M, Spoof, L, Meriluoto, J. A, Sivonen, K, & Viitasalo, M. (2005). Trophic transfer of cyanobacterial toxins from zooplankton to planktivores: consequences for pike larvae and mysid shrimps. *Environmental Toxicology*, , 20, 354-362.

[76] Karlsson, K. M, Spoof, L. E, & Meriluoto, J. A. (2005). Quantitative LC-ESI-MS analyses of microcystins and nodularin-R in animal tissue- matrix effects and method validation. *Environmental Toxicology*, , 20, 381-390.

[77] Kaya, K, & Mahakhant, A. Keovara, L; Sano, T.; Kubo, T. & Takagi, H. ((2002). Spiroidesin, a novel lipopeptide from the cyanobacterium *Anabaena spiroides* that inhibits cell growth of the cyanobacterium *Microcystis aeruginosa*. *Journal of Natural Products*, , 65, 920-921.

[78] Kim, H, Lantvit, D, Hwang, C. H, Kroll, D. J, Swanson, S. M, Franzblau, S. G, & Orjala, J. (2012). Indole alkaloids from two cultured cyanobacteria, *Westiellopsis* sp. and *Fischerella muscicola*. *Bioorganic and Medicinal Chemistry*, , 20, 5290-5295.

[79] Kinnear, S. (2010). Cylindrospermopsin: a decade of progress on bioaccumulation research. *Marine Drugs*, , 8, 542-564.

[80] Kittler, K, Schreiner, M, Krumbein, A, Manzei, S, Matthias, K, Sascha, R, & Maul, R. (2012). Uptake of the cyanobacterial toxin cylindrospermopsin in *Brassica* vegetables. *Food Chemistry*, , 133, 875-879.

[81] Kozlowsky-suzuki, B, Wilson, A. E, & Ferrao-filho, A. (2012). Biomagnification or biodilution of microcystins in aquatic food-webs? Meta-analyses of laboratory and field studies. *Harmful Algae*, , 18, 47-55.

[82] Kurmayer, R, & Jüttner, F. (1999). Strategies for co-existence of zooplankton with the toxic cyanobacterium *Planktothrix rubescens* in Lake Zürich. *Journal of Plankton Research*, , 21, 659-683.

[83] Kwong, R. W. M, Wang, W, Lam, X, & Yu, P. K. S. P. K. N. ((2006). The uptake, distribution and elimination of paralytic shellfish toxins in mussels and fish exposed to toxic dinoflagellates. *Aquatic Toxicology*, , 80, 82-91.

[84] Lagos, N, Onodera, H, Zagatto, P. A, Andrinolo, D, Azevedo, M. F. Q, & Oshima, Y. (1999). The first evidence of paralytic shellfish toxins in the freshwater cyanobacterium *Cylindrospermopsis raciborskii* isolated from Brazil. *Toxicon*, , 37, 1359-1373.

[85] Lance, E, Neffling, M. R, Gerard, C, Meriluto, J, & Bormans, M. (2010a). Accumulation of free and covalently bound microcystins in tissues of *Lymnaea stagnalis* following toxic cyanobacteria or dissolved microcystin-LR exposure. *Environmental Pollution*, , 158, 674-680.

[86] Lance, E, Josso, C, Dietrich, D, Ernst, B, Paty, C, Senger, F, Bormans, M, & Gerard, C. and microcystin distribution in *Lymnaea stagnalis* following toxic cyanobacterial or dissolved microcysti-LR exposure. *Aquatic Toxicology*, , 98, 211-220.

[87] Landsberg, J. H, Hall, S, Johannessen, J. N, White, K. D, Conrad, S. M, Abbott, J. P, Flewelling, L. J, Richardson, R. W, Dickey, R. W, Jester, E. L, Etheridge, S. M, Deeds, J. R, Van Dolah, F. M, Leighfield, T. A, Zou, Y, Beaudry, C. G, Benner, R. A, Rogers, P. L, Scott, P. S, Kawabata, K, Wolny, J. L, & Steidinger, K. A. (2006). Saxitoxin puffer fish poisoning in the United States, with the first report of *Pyrodinium bahamense* as the putative toxin source. *Environmental Health Perspectives*, , 114, 1502-1507.

[88] Lemaire, V, Brusciotti, S, Van Gremberghe, I, Vyverman, W, Vanoverbeke, J, & De Meester, L. (2012). Genotype x genotype interactions between the toxic cyanobacterium *Microcystis* and its grazer, the waterflea *Daphnia*. *Evolutionary Applications*, , 5, 168-182.

[89] Li, A, Fan, H, Ma, F, Mccarron, P, Thomas, K, Tan, X, & Quilliam, M. A. (2012). Elucidation of matrix effects and performance of solid-phase extraction for LC-MS/MS analysis of β-*N*-methylamino-L-alanine (BMAA) and diaminobutyric acid (DAB) neurotoxins in cyanobacteria. *Analyst*, 137, 1210-1219., 2(4)

[90] Li, W, Duan, J, Niu, C, Qiang, N, & Mulcahy, D. (2010). Determination of microcystin-LR in drinking water using UPLC tandem mass spectrometry- matrix effects and measurement. *Journal of Chromatographic Science*, , 49, 665-670.

[91] Li, W. I, Berman, F. W, Okino, T, Yokokawa, F, Shioiri, T, Gerwick, W. H, & Murray, T. F. (2001). Antillatoxin is a marine cyanobacterial toxin that potently activates voltage-gated sodium channels. *Proceedings of the National Academy of Sciences U.S.A.* , 98, 7599-7604.

[92] Lobner, D, Piana, P. M, Salous, A. K, & Peoples, R. W. (2007). Beta-N-methylamino-L-alanine enhances neurotoxicity through multiple mechanisms. *Neurobiological Disease*, , 25, 360-366.

[93] Lu, H, Choudhuri, S, Ogura, K, Csanaky, I. L, Lei, X, Cheng, X, Song, P. Z, & Klaassen, C. D. (2008). Characterization of organic anion transporting polypeptide 1b2-null mice: essential role in hepatic uptake/toxicity of phalloidin and microcystin-LR. *Toxicological Science*, , 103, 35-45.

[94] MacKintoshR. W.; Dalby, K. N.; Campbell, D. G.; Cohen, P. T.; Cohen, P. & MacKintosh, C. ((1995). The cyanobacterial toxin microcystin binds covalently to cystein-273 on protein phosphatase 1. *FEBS Letters*, , 371, 236-240.

[95] Mahmood, N. A, & Carmichael, W. W. (1986). Paralytic shellfish poisons produced by the freshwater cyanobacterium *Aphanizomenon flos-aquae*). *Toxicon*, , 24, 175-186.

[96] Maidana, M, Carlis, V, Galhardi, F. G, Yunes, J. S, Geracitano, L. A, Monserrat, J. M, & Barros, D. M. (2006). Effects of microcystins over short- and long-term memory and oxidative stress generation in hippocampus of rats. *Chemico-Biological Interactions*, , 159, 223-234.

[97] Martin, C, Oberer, L, Ino, T, König, W. A, Busch, M, & Weckesser, J. (1993). Cyanopeptolins, new depsipeptides from the cyanobacterium *Microcystis* sp. PCC 7806. *Journal of Antibiotics* (Tokyo), , 46, 1550-1556.

[98] Mcelhiney, J, & Lawton, L. A. (2005). Detection of the cyanobacterial hepatotoxins microcystins. *Toxicology and Applied Pharmacology*, , 203, 219-230.

[99] Mejean, A, Peyraud-thomas, C, Kerbrat, A. S, Golubic, S, Pauillac, S, Chinain, M, & Laurent, D. (2010). First identification of the neurotoxin homoanatoxin-a from mats of *Hydrocoleum lyngbyaceum* (marine cyanobacterium) possibly linked to giant clam poisoning in New Caledonia. *Toxicon*, , 56, 829-835.

[100] Metcalf, J. S, Hyenstrand, P, Beattie, K. A, & Codd, G. A. (2000). Effects of physiochemical variables and cyanobacterial extracts on the immunoassay of microcystin-LR by two ELISA kits. *Journal of Applied Microbiology*, , 89, 532-538.

[101] Metcalf, J. S, Beattie, K. A, Saker, M. L, & Codd, G. A. (2002). Effects of organic solvents on the high performance liquid chromatographic analysis of the cyanobacterial

toxin cylindrospermopsin, and its recovery from environmental eutrophic waters by solid-phase extraction. *FEMS Microbiology Letters*, , 216, 159-164.

[102] Miller, M. A, Kudela, R. M, Mekebri, A, Crane, D, Oates, S. C, Tinker, M. T, Staedler, M, Miller, W. A, Toy-choutka, S, Dominik, C, Hardin, D, Langlois, G, Murray, M, Ward, K, & Jessup, D. A. (2010). Evidence for a novel marine harmful algal bloom: cyanotoxin (microcystin) transfer from land to sea otters. *PLoS One*, 5, e12576.

[103] Mo, S, Krunic, A, Chlipala, G, & Orjala, J. (2009). Antimicrobial ambiguine isonitriles from the cyanobacterium *Fischerella ambigua*. *Journal of Natural Products*, , 72, 894-899.

[104] Mondo, K, Hammerschlag, N, Basile, M, Pablo, J, Banack, S. A, & Mash, D. C. (2012). Cyanobacterial neurotoxin beta-N-methylamino-L-alanine (BMAA) in shark fins. *Marine Drugs*, , 10, 509-520.

[105] Mori, Y, Kohchi, Y, Suzuki, M, Carmeli, S, Moore, R. E, & Patterson, G. M. L. (1991). Isotactic polymethoxy 1-alkenes from the blue-green algae. Synthesis and absolute stereochemistry. *Journal of Organic Chemistry*, , 56, 631-637.

[106] Mountfort, D. O, Holland, P, & Sprosen, J. (2005). Method for detecting classes of microcystins by combination of protein phosphatase inhibition assay and ELISA: comparison with LC-MS. *Toxicon*, , 45, 199-206.

[107] Msagati, T. A, Siame, B. A, & Shushu, D. D. (2006). Evaluation of methods for the isolation, detection and quantification of caynobacterial hepatotoxins. *Aquatic Toxicology*, , 78, 382-397.

[108] Murch, S. J, Cox, P. A, & Banack, S. A. (2004). A mechanism for slow release of biomagnified cyanobacterial neurotoxins and neurodegenerative disease in Guam. *Proceedings of the National Academy of Science U.S.A.*, , 101, 12228-12231.

[109] Mynderse, J. S, & Moore, R. E. (1979). Isotactic polymethoxy-1-alkene from the blue-green alga *Tolypothrix conglutinata* var. *Chlorata*. *Phytochemistry*, , 18, 1181-1183.

[110] Namikoshi, M, Rinehart, K. L, Sakai, R, Sivonen, K, & Carmichael, W. W. (1990). Structures of three new cyclic hepatotoxins produced by the cyanobacterium (blue-green alga) *Nostoc* sp. strain 152. *Journal of Organic Chemistry*, , 55, 6135-6139.

[111] Namikoshi, M, Rinehart, K. L, Sakai, R, Stotts, R. R, Dahlem, A. M, Beasley, C. R, Carmichael, W. W, & Evans, A. M. (1992). Identification of 12 hepatotoxins from Homer lake bloom of the cyanobacterium *Microcystis aeruginosa*, *Microcystis viridis*, and *Microcystis wesenbergii*: nine new microcystins. *Journal of Organic Chemistry*, , 57, 866-872.

[112] Nakamura, M, Oshima, Y, & Yasumoto, T. (1984). Occurrence of saxitoxin in puffer fish. *Toxicon*, , 22, 381-385.

[113] Negri, A. P, Jones, G. J, & Hindmarsh, M. (1995). Sheep mortality associated with paralytic shellfish poisons from the cyanobacterium *Anabaena circinalis*. *Toxicon*, , 33, 1321-1329.

[114] Nishiwaki-matsushima, R, Nishiwaki, S, Ohta, T, Yoshizawa, S, Suganuma, M, Harada, K, Watanabe, M. F, & Fujiki, H. (1991). Structure-function relationships of microcystins, liver tumor promoters, in interaction with protein phosphatases. *Japanese Journal of Cancer Research,* , 82, 993-996.

[115] Nogle, L. M, Okino, T, & Gerwick, W. H. a neurotoxic lipopeptide from the marine cyanobacterium *Lyngbya majuscula. Journal of Natural Products,* , 65, 983-985.

[116] Nogueira, I. C, Saker, M. L, Pflugmacher, S, Wiegand, C, & Vasconcelos, V. M. (2004). Toxicity of the cyanobacterium *Cylindrospermopsis raciborskii* to *Daphnia magna. Environmental Toxicology,* , 19, 453-459.

[117] Norris, R. L, Seawright, A. A, Shaw, G. R, Smith, M. J, Chiswell, R. K, & Moore, M. R. (2001). Distribution of 14C cylindrospermopsin in vivo in the mouse. *Environmental Toxicology,* , 16, 498-505.

[118] Ohtani, I, Moore, R. E, & Runnegar, M. T. C. (1992). Cylindrospermopsin: a potent hepatotoxin from the blue-green alga *Cylindrospermopsis raciborskii. Journal of the American Chemical Society,* , 114, 7942-7944.

[119] Okino, T, Murakami, M, Haraguchi, R, Munetata, H, Matsuda, H, & Yamaguchi, K. and trypsin inhibitors from the blue-gren alga *Microcystis aeruginosa. Tetrahedron Letters,* , 34, 8131-8134.

[120] Oksanen, I, Jokela, J, Fewer, D. P, Wahlsten, M, Rikkinen, J, & Sivonen, K. (2004). Discovery of rare and highly toxic microcystins from lichen-associated cyanobacterium *Nostoc* sp strain IO-102-I. *Applied and Environmental Microbiology,* , 70, 5756-5763.

[121] Orjala, J, Nagle, D. G, Hsu, V, & Gerwick, W. H. (1995). Antillatoxin: an exceptionally ichthyotoxic cyclic lipopeptide from the tropical cyanobacterium *Lyngbya majuscula. Journal of the American Chemical Society,* , 117, 8281-8282.

[122] Osborne, N. J, & Shaw, G. R. (2008). Dermatitis associated with exposure to a marine cyanobacterum during recreational water exposure. *BMC Dermatology,* 8, 5.

[123] Osswald, J, Rellan, S, Carvalho, A. P, Gago, A, & Vasconcelos, V. (2007). Acute effects of an anatoxin-a producing cyanobacterium on juvenile fish- *Cyprinus carpio. Toxicon,* , 49, 693-698.

[124] Osswald, J. A, Vasconcelos, V, & Guilhermino, L. (2011). Experimental determination of bioconcentration factors for anatoxin-a in juvenile rainbow trout (*Oncorhynchus mykiss*). *Proceedings of the International Academy of Ecology and Environmental Sciences,* 1, 77-86.

[125] Osswald, J, Rellan, S, Gago, A, & Vasconcelos, V. (2008). Uptake and depuration of anatoxin-a by the mussel *Mytilus galloprovincialis* under laboratory conditions. *Chemosphere,* , 72, 1235-1241.

[126] Ott, J. L, & Carmichael, W. W. MS method development for the analysis of hepatotoxic cyclic peptide microcystin in animal tissues. *Toxicon*, , 47, 734-741.

[127] Pablo, J, Banack, S. A, Cox, P. A, Johnson, T. E, Papapetropoulos, S, Bradley, W. G, Buck, A, & Mash, D. C. (2009). Cyanobacterial neurotoxin BMAA in ALS and Alzheimer's disease. *Acta Neurological Scandinavica*, , 120, 216-225.

[128] Paerl, H, & Huisman, J. (2009). Climate change: a catalyst for global expansion of harmful cyanobacterial blooms. *Environmental Microbiology Reports*, , 1, 27-37.

[129] Pereira, P, Dias, E, Franca, S, Pereira, E, Carolino, M, & Vasconcelos, V. (2004). Accumulation and depuration of cyanobacterial paralytic shellfish toxins by the freshwater mussel *Anodonta cygnea*. *Aquatic Toxicology*, , 68, 339-350.

[130] Pereira, S. R, Vasconcelos, V. M, & Antunes, A. (2012). Computational study of the covalent bonding of microcystins to cystein residues- a reaction involved in the inhibition of the PPP family of protein phosphatases. *FEBS Journal*, in press.

[131] Peuthert, A, Chakrabarti, S, & Pflugmacher, S. (2007). Uptake of microcystins-LR and-LF (cyanobacterial toxins) in seedlings of several important agricultural plant species and the correlation with cellular damage (lipid peroxidation). *Environmental Toxicology*, , 22, 436-442.

[132] Pflugmacher, S, Wiegand, C, Beattie, K. A, Krause, E, Steinberg, C. E, & Codd, G. A. (2001). Uptake, effects, and metabolism of cyanobacterial toxins in the emergent reed plant *Phragmites australis*, *Environmental Toxicology and Chemistry*, , 20, 846-852.

[133] Pietsch, C, Wiegand, C, Ame, M. V, Nicklisch, A, Wunderlin, D, & Pflugmacher, S. (2001). The effects of cyanobacterial crude extract on different aquatic organisms: evidence for cyanobacterial toxin modulating factors. *Environmental Toxicology*, , 16, 535-542.

[134] Pomati, F, Sacchi, S, Rossetti, C, Giovannardi, S, Onodera, H, Oshima, Y, & Neilan, B. A. (2000). The freshwater cyanobacterium *Planktothrix* sp. FP1: molecular identification and detection of paralytic shellfish poisoning toxins. *Journal of Phycology*, , 36, 553-562.

[135] Preu, K, Stüken, A, Wiedner, C, Chorus, I, & Fastner, J. (2006). First report on cylindrospermopsin producing *Aphanizomenon flos-aquae* (Cyanobacteria) isolated from two German Lakes. *Toxicon*, , 47, 156-162.

[136] Proksh, P, Edrada, R. A, & Ebel, R. (2002). Drugs from the seas- current status and microbiological implications. *Applied Microbiology and Technology*, , 59, 125-134.

[137] Puerto, M, Campos, A, Prieto, A, & Camean, A. da Almeida, A. M.; Coelho, A. V. & Vasconcelos, Differential protein expression in two bivalve species: *Mytilus galloprovincalis* and *Corbicula fluminea*, exposed to *Cylindrospermopsis raciborskii* cells. *Aquatic Toxicology*, 101, 109-116., 2011

[138] Qiao, Q, Liang, H, & Zhang, X. (2012). Effect of cyanobacteria on immune function of crucian carp (*Carassius auratus*) via chronic exposure in diet. *Chemosphere,* in press.

[139] Qiu, T, Xie, P, Ke, Z, & Guo, L. (2007). In situ studies on physiological and biochemical respones in four fishes with different trophic levels to toxic cyanobacterial blooms in a large Chinese lake. *Toxicon,* , 50, 365-376.

[140] Rama, R. M, & Faulkner, D. J. (2002). Isotactic polymethoxydienes from the Philippines sponge *Myriastra clavosa. Journal of Natural Products,* , 65, 1201-1203.

[141] Rao, P. V, Gupta, N, Bhaskar, A. S, & Jayaraj, R. (2002). Toxins and bioactive compounds from cyanobacteria and their implications on human health. *Journal of Environmental Biology,* , 23, 215-224.

[142] Rao, S. D, Banack, S. A, Cox, P. A, & Weiss, J. H. (2006). BMAA selectively injures motor neurons via AMPA/kainite receptor activation. *Experimental Neurology,* , 201, 244-252.

[143] Raveh, A, & Carmeli, S. (2007). Antimicrobial ambigues from the cyanobacterium *Fischerella* sp. collected in Israel. *Journal of Natural Product,* , 70, 196-201.

[144] Reinikainen, M, Meriluoto, J. A. O, Spoof, L, & Harada, K. (2001). The toxicities of a polyunsaturated fatty acid and a microcystin to *Daphnia magna. Environmental Toxicology,* , 16, 444-448.

[145] Ricciardi, A, & Bourget, E. (1998). Weight-to-weight conversion factors for marine benthic macroinvertebrates. *Marine Ecology Progress Series,* , 163, 245-251.

[146] Rogers, E. H, Zehr, R. D, Gage, M. I, Humpage, A. R, Falconer, I. R, Marr, M, & Chernoff, N. (2007). The cyanobacterial toxin, cylindrospermopsin, induces fetal toxicity in the mouse after exposure late in gestation. *Toxicon,* , 49, 855-864.

[147] Rohrlack, T, Dittman, E, Börner, T, & Christoffersen, K. (2001). Effects of cell-bound microcystins on survival and feeding of *Daphnia* spp. *Applied and Environmental Microbiology,* , 67, 3523-3529.

[148] Rohrlack, T, Christoffersen, K, Kaebernick, M, & Neilan, B. A. (2004). Cyanobacterial protease inhibitor microviridin J causes lethal molting disruption in *Daphnia pulicaria. Applied Environmental Microbiology,* , 70, 5047-5050.

[149] Rosen, J, & Hellenäs, K. E. Determination of the neurotoxin BMAA (beta-N-methylamino-L-alanine) in cycad seed and cyanobacteria by LC-MS/MS (liquid chromatography tandem mass spectrometry). *Analyst,* , 133, 1785-1789.

[150] Runnegar, M. T. C, Kong, S. M, Zhong, Y. Z, Ge, J. L, & Lu, S. C. (1994). The role of glutathione in the toxicity of a novel cyanobacterial alkaloid cylindrospermopsin in cultured rat hepatocytes. *Biochemistry and Biophysics Research Communication,* , 201, 235-241.

[151] Runnegar, M. T. C, Kong, C. M, Zhong, Y. Z, & Lu, S. (1995). Inhbition of reduced glutathione synthesis by cyanobacterial alkaloid cylindrospermopsin in cultured rat hepatocytes. *Biochemical Pharmacology*, , 49, 219-225.

[152] Sabitini, S. E, Brena, B. M, & Luquet, C. M. San Julian, M.; Pirez, M. & Carmen Rios de Molina, M. D. ((2011). Microcystin accumulation and antioxidant responses in the freshwater clam *Diplodon chilensis patagonicus* upon subchronic exposure to toxic *Microcystis aeruginosa*. *Ecotoxicology and Environmental Safety*, , 74, 1188-1194.

[153] Saker, M. L, & Eaglesham, G. K. (1999). The accumulation of cylindrospermopsin from the cyanobacterium *Cylindrospermopsis raciborskii* in tissues of the Redclaw crayfish (*Cherax quadricarinatus*). *Toxicon*, , 37, 1065-1077.

[154] Sano, T, Nohara, K, Shiraishi, F, & Kaya, K. (1992). A method for micro-determination of total microcystin content in waterblooms of cyanobacteria (blue-green algae). *International Journal of Environmental Analytical Chemistry*, , 49, 163-170.

[155] Schwarzenberger, A, Kuster, C. J, & Von Elert, E. (2012). Molecular mechanisms of tolerance to cyanobacterial protease inhibitors revealed by clonal differences in *Daphnia magna*. *Molecular Ecology*, in press.

[156] Scott, P. M, Niedzwladek, B, Rawn, D. F, & Lau, B. P. (2009). Liquid chromatographic determination of the cyanobacterial toxin beta-n-methylamino-L-alanine in algae food supplements, freshwater fish, and bottled water. *Journal of Food Protection*, , 72, 1769-1773.

[157] Seifert, M. (2007). The ecological effects of the cyanobacterial toxin cylindrospermopsin. Dissertation, The University of Queensland, Brisbane, Australia.

[158] Shaw, G. R, Seawright, A. A, Moore, M. R, & Lam, P. K. S. (2000). Cylindrospermopsin, a cyanobacterial alkaloid: evaluation of its toxicological activity. *Therapeutic Drug Monitoring*, , 22, 89-92.

[159] Shen, X, Lam, P. K. S, Shaw, G. R, & Wikramsinghe, W. (2002). Genotoxicity investigation of a cyanobacterial toxin, cylindrospermopsin. *Toxicon*, , 40, 1499-1501.

[160] Sieroslawska, A, Rymuszka, A, Kalinowska, R, Skowronski, T, Bownik, A, & Pawlik-skowronska, B. (2010). Toxicity of cyanobacterial bloom in the eutrophic dam reservoir (Southeast Poland). *Environmental and Toxicological Chemistry*, , 29, 556-560.

[161] Simmons, T. L, Coates, R. C, Clark, B. R, Engene, N, Gonzalez, D, Esquenazi, E, Correstein, P. C, & Gerwick, W. H. (2008). Biosynthetic origin of natural products isolated from marine microorganism-invertebrate assemblages. *Proceedings of the National Academy of Sciences*, , 105, 4587-4594.

[162] Sivonen, K, Namikoshi, M, Evans, W. R, Fardig, M, Carmichael, W. W, & Rinehart, K. L. (1992). Three new microcystins, cyclic heptapeptide hepatotoxins, from *Nostoc* sp. strain 152. *Chemical Research in Toxicology*, , 5, 464-469.

[163] Sivonen, K. (2008). Emerging high throughput analyses of cyanobacterial toxins and toxic cyanobacteria. *Advances in Experimental Medicine and Biology,* , 619, 539-557.

[164] Smith, F. M, Wood, S. A, Van Ginkel, R, Broady, P. A, & Gaw, S. (2011). First report of saxitoxin production by a species of the freshwater benthic cyanobacterium, *Scytonema. Toxicon,* , 57, 566-573.

[165] Smith, J. L, Schulz, K. L, Zimba, P. V, & Boyer, G. L. (2010). Possible mechanism for the foodweb transfer of covalently bound microcystins. *Ecotoxicology and Environmental Safety,* , 73, 757-761.

[166] Smith, Q. R, Nagura, H, Takada, Y, & Duncan, M. W. (1992). Facilitated transport of the neurotoxin, beta-N-methylamino-L-alanine, across the blood brain barrier. *Journal of Neurochemistry,* , 58, 1330-1337.

[167] Smith, R. A, & Lewis, D. (1987). A rapid analysis of water for anatoxin a, the unstable toxic alkaloid from *Anabaena flos-aquae,* the stable non-toxic alkaloids left after bioreduction and a related amine which may be nature's precursor to anatoxin a. *Veterinary and Human Toxicology,* , 29, 153-154.

[168] Spencer, P. S, Nunn, P. B, Hugon, J, Ludolph, A. C, Ross, S. M, Roy, D. N, & Robertson, R. C. (1987). Guam amyotrophic lateral sclerosis-parkinsonism-dementia linked to a plant excitant neurotoxin. *Science,* , 237, 517-522.

[169] SpoofL; Berg, K. A.; Rapala, J.; Lahti, K.; Lepistö, L.; Metcalf, J. S.; Codd, G. A. & Meriluoto, J. ((2006). First observation of cylindrospermopsin in *Anabaena lapponica* isolated from the boreal environment (Finland). *Environmental Toxicology, 21,* 552-560.

[170] Staton, P. C, & Bristow, D. R. (1997). The dietary excitotoxins beta-N-methylamino-L-alanine and beta-N-oxalylamino-L-alanin induce necrotic and apoptotic-like cell death of rat cerebellar granule cells. *Journal of Neurochemistry,* , 69, 1508-1518.

[171] Stevens, D. K, & Krieger, R. I. (1991). Stability studies on the cyanobacterial nicotinic alkaloid anatoxin-a. *Toxicon,* , 29, 167-179.

[172] Stevens, M, Peigneur, S, & Tytgat, J. (2011). Neurotoxins and their binding areas on voltage-gated sodium channels. *Frontiers in Pharmacology,* 2, 71.

[173] Stewart, I, Webb, P. M, Schluter, P. J, & Shaw, G. R. (2006). Recreational and occupational field exposure to freshwater cyanobacteria- a review of anecdotal and case reports, epidemiological studies and the challenges for epidemiologic assessment. *Environmental Health,* 5, 6.

[174] Suchy, P, & Berry, J. (2012). Detection of total microcystin in fish tissues based on lemieux oxidation and recovery of 2-methyl-3-methoxy-4-phenylbutanoic acid (MMPB) by solid-phase microextraction gas chromatography-mass spectrometry (SPME-GC/MS). *International Journal of Environmental Analytical Chemistry,* , 92, 1443-1456.

[175] Sukenik, A, Reisner, M, Carmeli, S, & Werman, M. (2006). Oral toxicity of the cyanobacterial toxin cylindrospermopsin in mice: long-term exposure to low doses. *Environmental Toxicology*, , 21, 575-582.

[176] Tan, L. T. (2007). Bioactive natural products from marine cyanobacteria for drug discovery. *Phytochemistry*, , 68, 954-979.

[177] Tan, L. T. (2010). Filamentous tropical marine cyanobacteria: a rich source of natural products for anticancer drug discovery. *Journal of Applied Phycology*, , 22, 659-676.

[178] Terao, K, Ohmori, S, Igarashi, K, Ohtani, I, Watanabe, M. F, Harada, K. I, Ito, E, & Watanabe, M. (1994). Electron microscopic studies on experimental poisoning in mice induced by cylindrospermopsin isolated from blue-green alga *Uzmekia natans*. *Toxicon*, , 32, 833-843.

[179] Ting, C. S, Rocap, G, King, J, & Chisholm, S. W. (2002). Cyanobacterial photosynthesis in the oceans: the origins and significance of divergent light-harvesting strategies. *Trends in Microbiology*, , 10, 134-142.

[180] Tsukamoto, S, Painuly, P, Young, K. A, Yang, X, Shimizu, Y, & Cornell, L. a novel cell differentiation-promoting depsipeptide from *Microcystis aeruginosa Journal of the American Chemical Society*, , 115(15-1840), 11046-11047.

[181] Ueno, Y, Nagata, S, Tsutsumi, T, Hasegawa, A, Watanabe, M. F, Park, H, Chen, D, Chen, G. -C, & Yu, G. S.-Z. ((1996). Detection of microcystsins, a blue-green algal hepatotoxin, in drinking water sampled in Haimen and Fusui, endemic areas of primary liver cancer in China, by highly sensitive immunoassay. *Carcinogenesis*, , 17, 1317-1321.

[182] Van Dolah, F. M. (2000). Marine algal toxins: origins, health effects, and their increased occurrence. *Environmental Health Perspectives*, , 108, 133-141.

[183] Vega, A, & Bell, E. A. (1967). amino-β-methylaminopropionic acid, a new amino acid from seeds of *Cycas circinalis*. *Phytochemistry*, , 6, 759-762.

[184] Von Elert, E, Oberer, L, Merkel, P, Huhn, T, & Blom, J. F. (2005). Cyanopeptolin 954, a chlorine-containing chymotrypsin inhibitor of *Microcystis aeruginosa* NIVA Cya 43. *Journal of Natural Products*, , 68, 1324-1327.

[185] Von Elert, E, & Zitt, A. Schwarzenberger ((2012). Inducible tolerance to dietary protease inhibitors in *Daphnia magna*. *Journal of Experimental Biology*, , 215, 2051-2059.

[186] Xie, L, Xie, P, Ozawa, K, Honma, T, Yokoyama, A, & Park, H. D. (2004). Dynamics of microcystins-LR and-RR in the phytoplanktivorous silver carp in a sub-chronic toxicity experiment. *Environmental Pollution*, , 127, 431-439.

[187] Welker, M, & Von Döhren, H. (2006). Cyanobacterial peptides- nature's own combinatorial biosynthesis. *FEMS Microbiology Reviews*, , 30, 530-563.

[188] White, S. H, Duivenvoorden, L. J, Fabbro, L. D, & Eaglesham, G. K. (2006). Influence of intracellular toxin concentrations on cylindrospermopsin bioaccumulation in a freshwater gastropod (*Melanoides tuberculata*). *Toxicon*, , 47, 497-509.

[189] White, S. H, Duivenvoorden, L. J, Fabbro, L. D, & Eaglesham, G. K. (2007). Mortality and toxin bioaccumulation in *Bufo marinus* following exposure to *Cylindrospermopsis raciborskii* cell extracts and live cultures. *Environmental Pollution*, , 147, 158-167.

[190] Williams, D. E, Dawe, S. C, Kent, M. L, Andersen, R. J, Craig, M, & Holmes, C. F. and clearance of microcystins from salt water mussels, *Mytilus edulis*, and in vivo evidence for covalently bound microcystins in mussel tissues. *Toxicon*, , 35, 1617-1625.

[191] Williams, D. E, & Craig, M. McCready; Dawe, S. C.; Kent, M. L.; Holmes, C. F. & Andersen, R. J. ((1997b). Evidence for covalently bound form of microcystin-LR in salmon liver and Dungeness crab larvae. *Chemical Research in Toxicology*, , 10, 463-469.

[192] Wilson, A. E, Sarnelle, O, Neilan, B. A, Salmon, T. P, Gehringer, M. M, & Hay, M. E. (2005). Genetic variation of the bloom-forming cyanobacterium *Microcystis aeruginosa* within and among lakes: implications for harmful algal blooms. *Applied and Environmental Microbiology*, , 71, 6126-6133.

[193] Wilson, A. E, Wilson, W. A, & Hay, M. E. (2006). Interspecific variation in growth and morphology of the bloom-forming cyanobacterium *Microcystis aeruginosa*. *Applied and Environmental Microbiology*, , 72, 7386-7389.

[194] Wu, M, Okino, T, Nogle, L. M, Marquez, B. L, Williamson, R. T, Sitachitta, N, Berman, F. W, Murray, T. F, Mcgough, K, Jacobs, R, Colsen, K, Asano, T, Yokokawa, F, Shioiri, T, & Gerwick, W. H. (2000). Structure, synthesis, and biological properties of Kalkitoxin, a novel neurotoxin from the marine cyanobacterium *Lyngbya majuscula*. *Journal of the American Chemical Society*, , 122, 12041-12042.

[195] Yasumoto, T. (1998). Fish poisonings due to toxins due to microalgal origins in the Pacific. *Toxicon*, , 36, 1515-1518.

[196] Yu, S. Z. ((1995). Primary prevention of hepatocellular carcinoma. *Journal of Gastroenterology and Hepatology*, , 10, 674-682.

[197] Yu, S, Zhao, N, & Zi, X. (2001). The relationship between cyanotoxin (microcystin, MC) in pond-ditch water and primary liver cancer in China. *Zhonghua Zhong Liu Za Zhi*, , 23, 96-99.

[198] Yuan, M, Carmichael, W. W, & Hilborn, E. D. (2006). Microcystin analysis in human sera and liver from human fatalities in Caruaru, Brazil 1996. *Toxicon*, , 48, 627-640.

[199] Zhang, D, Xie, P, & Chen, J. (2010). Effects of temperature on the stability of microcystins in muscle of fish and its consequences for food safety. *Bulletin of Environmental Contamination and Toxicology*, , 84, 202-207.

http://dx.doi.org/10.5772/55111

[200] Zurawell, R. W, Chen, H, Burke, J. M, & Prepas, E. E. (2005). Hepatotoxic cyanobacteria: a review of the biological importance of microcystins in freshwater environments. *Journal of Toxicology and Environmental Health B Critical Reviews*, , 8, 1-37.

Section 7

Pharmacoepidemiology and Pharmacosurveillance in Public Health

Chapter 25

Epidemiology of Patients Diagnosed with Prescription and Non-Prescription Drug Overdose at the Riyadh Security Forces Hospital Between January 2007 and December 2011

Naser Al-Jaser, M. Cli. Epi and Niyi Awofeso

Additional information is available at the end of the chapter

http://dx.doi.org/10.5772/52879

1. Introduction

There is global concern concerning the higher rate of drug overdose morbidity and mortality, particularly from opioid medicines.[1] Drug overdose is one of the leading causes of death in many countries.[2] In the US, prescription drug mortality rate is higher than the death rate from illicit drugs, and drug overdose mortality currently exceeds mortality from motor vehicle accidents.[3] Moreover, there has been a tenfold increase in painkiller prescriptions in the US over the past 15 years.[4] In Saudi Arabia, there has been a significant increase in the use of prescription drugs compared with the previous decade, as the Ministry of Health stated in its 2009 annual report.[5] A number of studies have been conducted that investigate the epidemiology of drug overdose in Saudi Arabia. However, most of these studies were conducted in the late twentieth century.[6,7]

The purpose of this research is to investigate prescription and non-prescription overdose cases admitted to the emergency department of the Security Forces Hospital, Riyadh, from 2007 to 2011. The study sought to identify demographic characteristics of patients who were admitted to the emergency department with drug overdose, including age, gender, income and occupation.

The findings of this study have a number of implications for the Security Forces Hospital and drug overdoses in Saudi Arabia, particularly for elderly patients who take Warfarin continuously. Further, it appears that parents leave their medications unsecured and unprotected from children; thus, preventive and awareness programs are needed to address these issues.

2. Literature review

An Adverse Drug Event (ADE) is defined as an injury resulting from medical intervention related to a drug.[8] It is considered a major problem in medicine because it results in hospital admissions. ADEs include harm caused by the drug, such as adverse drug reactions and overdoses, and harm resulting from using the drug, such as dose reductions and discontinuation of drug therapies.[9] Previous studies have found that ADEs account for 3.9–6.2 per cent of hospital admissions. Further, drug overdoses account for a higher hospital admission rate of ADEs.[10,11]

Drug overdose can be defined as intentionally or unintentionally administering a higher dose of prescription or non-prescription drugs than recommended.[12] Drug overdose is considered a major health problem, particularly in developed countries. In the United States (US), the Centers for Disease Control and Prevention (CDC) recently reported that fatal overdoses from opiate painkillers currently exceed those from cocaine and heroin combined.[12] The rate of prescription drug use is increasing globally.[13] In Saudi Arabia, there has been a significant increase in prescription drug use since 2000 compared with the previous decades; however, there is a dearth of information relating to drug use and overdoses.[5]

In many Asian countries, drug overdose mortality is considered a major problem. For example, a study in northern Thailand which investigated the overdose mortality rate of injecting drug users between 1999 and 2002 found a death rate of 8.97 per 1,000 people among 861 drug users who were Human Immunodeficiency Virus (HIV)-negative.[14] A study in Xichang City, China, found a heroin overdose mortality rate of 4.7 per 100 people among 379 people who injected drugs during 2002 to 2003.[15] Further, in a review conducted in several central Asian countries, emergency medical services stated that there were 21 drug overdose deaths in Tajikistan and 57 in Kyrgyzstan in 2006.[1]

Many European countries also consider drug overdose a major concern, and it is considered one of the leading causes of death. The average mortality rate is 21 deaths per 1 million people aged 15–64.[16] Drug overdose in Europeans aged 15–39 accounted for 4 per cent of all deaths. Males were at a greater risk than females in all countries, with males accounting for 81 per cent of all drug-related deaths reported in European countries. The male to female ratio varied across countries, with the lowest rate in Poland (4:1) and the highest rate in Romania (31:1). The most common drugs used in almost all countries were opioids, which accounted for 90 per cent of drugs used in five countries and 80–90 per cent in 12 countries.[16]

Drug overdose is also considered a major public health threat in the US. There, the drug overdose mortality rate among adults increased from 4 per 100,000 people in 1999 to 8.8 per 100,000 in 2006. Moreover, deaths from drug overdose increased from 11,155 in 1999 to

22,448 in 2005, which can be attributed mainly to prescription drugs rather than illicit drugs. [3] Drug overdose is the second leading cause of death among all unintentional deaths in the US. The most common drugs that caused death by overdose were heroin, cocaine and painkillers. The use of prescription medicines has increased, thus contributing to the death rate. [4] According to the CDC, from 2005 to 2007, prescription drugs such as benzodiazepine, anti-depressants and opioid medicines were found in 79 per cent (2,165 cases) of all substance overdoses.[17]

In Australia, there appears to be a lower risk of drug overdose than in other countries. For instance, the rate of death from opioids was 101.9 per 1 million people in 1999 and 31.3 deaths per 1 million in 2004.[18] Moreover, in 2005, the Illicit Drug Reporting System distributed a survey among intravenous drug users and found that 46 per cent had experienced an overdose.[18] It was also found that 357 deaths were caused by opioid overdose and 40 per cent of deaths occurred in New South Wales. Males accounted for 75 per cent of overdose deaths, and those aged 25–34 were most at risk, accounting for 40 per cent of deaths.[19] Recently released Australian prisoners are at significantly increased risks of illicit drug overdose and deaths.[20]

In Saudi Arabia, studies have noted an increase in drug overdoses in localised cohorts over the past several decades. However, there are no significant statistics for drug overdose morbidity and mortality in Saudi Arabia as a whole.[6,21] Several studies have been undertaken in Saudi Arabia to investigate the drug overdose in hospitals. Moazzam's and Aljahdali's studies found that paracetamol accounted for 24.1 per cent of 170 drug overdose cases and 30 per cent of 79 cases, respectively.[21,22] Ahmed's study found that mefenamic acid accounted for 20 per cent of 50 cases investigated.[6] The rate of death amongst drug overdose was investigated in some studies in Saudi Arabia. Ahmed stated that there was one death among 106 drug overdoses admitted between 1992 and 1994.[6] Elfawal investigated 249 deaths from substance overdose between 1990 and 1997, and found 20 per cent of cases related to medically prescribed drugs.[7] Aljahdali and Ahmed found females accounted for a higher percentage of drug overdose cases.[6,22] Moazzam and Elfawal found males were represented in a higher percentage of cases.[7,21]

Drug overdoses could result from non-prescription substances such as herbal medicines.[23] The problem with herbal remedies relates to limited control and regulation among stores that provide them.[24] Many people believe that herbal substances are harmless and that it is safe to administer excessive amounts because they come from natural sources.[25] Although the rate of usage has increased, fewer than half of patients consult their physicians before administrating herbal remedies.[26] Further, the accurate dosage of herbal medicines is variable, and there are no guidelines to determine correct dosage.[25]

Drug overdoses could result from administering illicit drugs such as heroin and hashish. [27,28] As Saudi Arabia is a strict Islamic country, and Islam prohibits the use of illicit drugs, overdose cases involving illicit drugs are rare.[22] However, according to a world drug report, Saudi Arabia is considered a major market of phenethylline (Captagon) in the Middle East. The Saudi government confiscated more than 10 million pills in one seizure in 2010. However, the prevalence of amphetamines in Saudi Arabia is low compared with other western countries: in 2006, the prevalence of amphetamines in Saudi Arabia was 0.4 per 100,000 people, whereas in Australia and the US, the prevalence was 2.7 and 1.5 per 100,000 people respectively. Further, the prevalence of opioids and cannabis was 0.06 and 0.3 per 100,000 respectively in Saudi Arabia, 0.4 and 10.6 per 100,000 respectively in Australia and 5.9 and 13.7 per 100,000 respectively in the US. Therefore, the prevalence of opioids and cannabis are markedly lower in Saudi Arabia than in Australia and the US.[13]

Suicide is one of the major motivations and outcomes of intentional drug overdose.[29] Suicide accounts for 2 per cent of all deaths in the world. In 2005, there were about 800,000 deaths from suicide, and about 56 million deaths globally.[30] Drugs cause 11 per cent of suicides in Australia.[30] A study found that suicide is a greater risk among people who had a history of drug overdoses compared with people who did not.[31] Another study found a positive correlation between suicide and drug overdose.[32] Moreover, research has found that committing suicide by administering drugs is common among adolescents.[33] One study found suicide was associated with both prescription and non-prescription drugs, with a strong association between opiates and suicide, and opioid users were 14 times more likely to attempt suicide compared with non-opioid users.[34]

The excessive availability of medicines in households is due to the relative affordability of drugs, which can be bought from a range of places including markets, internet pharmacies and cosmetic stores. For instance, patients can purchase prescription drugs from an internet pharmacy without a prescription.[35] One survey investigated how easy it was for adolescents to acquire prescription medications. The question asked was 'which is easiest for someone your age to buy: cigarettes, beer, marijuana or prescription drugs without prescription?' Nineteen per cent of respondents said it was easier to buy prescription drugs compared to 13 per cent in the previous year.[36]

Two main factors contribute to the excessive availability of medicines: physicians and patients. Physicians appear to prescribe more medicines than in the past. For example, there was a 300 per cent increase in the prescription of painkillers in the US in 1999.[35,37] According to the National Institute on Drug Abuse (NIDA), the number of potentially addictive drug prescriptions for pain rose to 200 million in 2011.[38] There is also an association between patient death and physicians who frequently prescribe painkillers. Dhalla published a study in Ontario in 2011 that investigated the opioid prescription rate in family physicians and their relation to opioid-related deaths. He found that 20 per cent of physicians have a prescription rate that is 55 times higher than the 20 per cent of physicians who prescribed the lowest. The top 20 per cent of physicians were responsible for 64 per cent of patient deaths caused by painkillers.[39] In addition, many people falsely reporting symptoms in order to obtain a prescription and this is defined as drug seeking behaviour. The most drugs associated with drug seeking behaviour are benzodiazepine and opioids.[40]

Alcoholism is considered a major risk factor for intentional overdoses. Several studies state that the risk of drug overdose from prescription medicines is higher among people who drink alcohol.[41-43] A study by Li in 2011 investigated trends of paracetamol overdose in US emergency departments from 1993 to 2007 using data from physicians' diagnoses codes and cause of injury codes. The author found those who drank alcohol were 5.48 times more

http://dx.doi.org/10.5772/52879

likely to overdose compared to people who did not drink alcohol, and the p-values were statistically significant.[41]

A study published by Wazaify in 2005 examined OTC drugs and prescription drug overdoses for three months, as well as the potential risk factors. The study investigated 247 overdose cases, excluding alcohol intoxication and spiked drinks. He found alcohol was a major risk factor for overdoses of both OTC and prescription drugs, and that alcohol contributed more to OTC drug overdoses (32.2 per cent) than prescription drugs combined with OTC drugs (24.7 per cent).[42] Moreover, the prescription drug overdose death rate increased with alcohol consumption. West Virginia found 32.9 per cent of overdose deaths were associated with alcohol consumption.[43] Another study on paracetamol overdose found more than one-third of drug overdoses were associated with alcohol consumption at the time of overdose, and it was slightly higher in males (12 per cent) than females (11 per cent).[44] In addition, people who consumed alcohol could overdose on lower doses of paracetamol compared with those who did not consume alcohol.[45] Paulozzi conducted a study on methadone overdose and found that the concentration of methadone was lower when alcohol was involved.[28] Mixing drugs with alcohol is therefore considered a risk factor for drug overdose.[46]

Violence involving sex and family could also be associated to intentional drug overdose.[33,47] A study by Budnitz investigated the pattern of acetaminophen overdoses in the emergency department from two components of the National Electronic Injury Surveillance System. Of the 2,717 annual acetaminophen overdose cases, 69.8 per cent were related to self-directed violence. Further, females had a greater rate of self-directed violence (27.2 per 100,000) compared with males (14.4 per 100,000).[33] Violence and strife have also contributed to the increased rate of illicit drug use in the US.[47]

Drug overdoses can be associated with people who take drugs for recreational purposes. According to the Centers for Disease Control and Prevention (CDC), opioids are involved in more overdose deaths than heroin and cocaine combined, and they are often associated with recreational use.[4] Further, several studies found that recreational use contributed to many of the drug overdoses presenting to emergency departments. For example, a study found that 15.4 per cent of 500 overdose cases presented to emergency departments resulted from recreational use.[48] Further, a survey of 975 students found that 16 per cent abused medicine for recreational purposes.[49]

Buykx found that many people overdose on drugs after they experience interpersonal conflicts.[31] Britton's 2010 study investigated the risk factors of non-fatal overdoses over 12 months. The author recruited 2,966 participants and found that 23.5 per cent of all overdose cases had experienced sexual abuse. Moreover, victims of sexual abuse were 2.02 times more likely to overdose, and the result was statistically significant.[50] Other forms of physical abuse were also addressed in the study: 33.4 per cent of all overdose cases had experienced physical abuse, and they were 1.91 times more likely to overdose, which was statistically significant.[50]

The level of a medicine's purity could lead to a drug overdose, particularly for people using non-prescription medicines. Previous studies have found the fluctuation of heroin purity contributed to the overdose rate.[51] Moreover, in a survey of healthcare providers that asked about risk factors for opioid overdose, approximately 90 per cent mentioned the fluctuation of opioid purity.[52] Of 855 heroin users, 29 per cent split the tablets in half when the purity was unknown.[53] In addition, a study stated that many heroin users believed that purity fluctuation contributed to drug overdose.[54] Conversely, several studies on heroin (e.g. Toprak and Risser) found no association between drug overdose and purity.[55,56]

Other factors that contribute to intentional drug overdose include psychiatric illness, marital problems and family size.[6] Ahmed found that psychiatric illness was a greater risk among males than females, and it was a risk factor in 10 of the 50 cases he investigated. Further, five cases had experienced marital problems.[6] Family size could be a major factor in drug overdose. Large families are common in Saudi culture. A 2011 study by Bani found that 43 per cent of participants had six to eight family members.[57] A study by TNS Middle East of demographic characteristics in Saudi Arabia in 2006 found that 40 per cent of Saudi families are considered large, with six or more members.[58] Aljahdali found that large family size was a risk factor in drug overdoses: 59 per cent of the 79 cases in his study had more than five family members This could indicate that because large families have more children, parental supervision amongst the children is lowered, potentially increasing the chance of the unsupervised ingestion of drugs.[22]

A previous drug overdose might also be a risk factor for another drug overdose, as many studies have attested.[59],[60],[46] For example, Kinner's study in 2012 investigated the risk factors of non-fatal overdoses among illicit drug users, recruiting 2,515 illicit drug users in Vancouver, Canada. The author found an association between drug overdoses and previous drug experiences; people with previous overdoses were four times more likely to overdose compared with people who had no previous experience.[59] This finding is similar to that of a study by Hall in 2008, which investigated the pattern of unintentional drug overdose caused by prescription drugs, recruiting 295 participants. The author found that people who had experienced a previous overdose had a 30.2 per cent chance of overdose compared with 14.4 per cent of people who had not.[60] In addition, a New York study that investigated the risk factors of heroin users found that participants who had overdosed were 28 times more likely to overdose than those who had not experienced a previous overdose.[46] In contrast, some previous studies found no associations between drug overdose and previous overdose experience.[59]

Doctor shopping is considered the most common method of obtaining prescription drugs for legal and illegal use.[61-64] It is defined as patients visiting several doctors to obtain prescription medicines without medical need, and it is considered one of the major mechanisms of diversion.[35] Several studies have found that doctor shopping contributes to drug overdose. For example, the author Hall found that doctor shopping contributed to 21.4 per cent of 259 overdose cases.[65] Further, it found that 19 per cent of participants who overdosed acquired their medicines through doctor shopping.[49] Moreover, doctor shopping is attrib-

http://dx.doi.org/10.5772/52879

uted to a higher rate of drug overdose death.[65,66] Several studies have stated that controlling doctor shopping would assist in preventing drug overdoses.[35,67]

The consumption of prescription drugs, especially opioids, has increased due to their euphoric and energising effects.[4] For example, methamphetamine and alprazolam users tend to redose every three-to-eight hours to maintain the euphoric effect.[46] Further, drug users tend to abuse cocaine to feel euphoric and increase a feeling of sexual desirability.[68] Some medicines do not enhance euphoria until taken in higher doses. For example, drug users take higher doses of benzodiazepine to experience the euphoria effect.[24] Many fatal overdoses occur when larger doses of medicines have been taken to achieve the euphoric effect.[37]

Long-term therapy could be related to overdoses, especially in patients suffering from chronic pain. Further, such patients have easy access to painkillers in the home, which increases the chance of a fatal overdose.[69] Previously, long-term therapy was restricted to cancer patients; however, currently, it is commonly used for chronic pain in non-cancer patients. Unfortunately, the latter have been associated with higher overdose rates.[70] One of the reasons for drug overdose in chronic patients is inadequate pain management.[69,70] The critical issue with chronic pain is pain management, and inadequate pain management could lead to increased doses of painkillers and consequently, an increased rate of drug overdoses.[71]

Calculating the dose is an important factor, and miscalculated doses could lead to unintentional overdoses.[72] Many parents have difficulty measuring and calculating the appropriate dose of paracetamol for their children.[73] One survey asked 100 caregivers if they were able to determine the appropriate dose for their children; only 30 per cent were able to do so.[73] Hixson conducted a study in 2010 to compare the ability of parents to calculate the appropriate dose of acetaminophen using product information leaflets or the Parental Analgesia Slide. Participants were divided into two groups, and a questionnaire was distributed to each group. The author found that caregivers using the Parental Analgesia Slide had fewer dosing errors than caregivers using product information leaflets, but the difference was not statistically significant.[74] Limited literacy and numeracy skills are also associated with poor clinical outcomes and overdoses. Many people with limited numeracy skills are confused with dosing instructions and warning labels. Moreover, people could be confused with the information on the labels of prescription medicines.[75]

Mental states could be a major risk factor of drug overdose, as patients with mental disorders and drug addictions are more vulnerable.[76] For example, Hasin's study found that 15–20 per cent of patients with mental disorders overdosed on drugs at least once in their lives, and patients with depressive disorders were 3.7 times more likely to overdose.[76] Fischer's study found that people with mental problems were 1.51 times more likely to overdose than people without mental problems, but this result was not statistically significant.[77]

Children are considered at greater risk of drug overdose for several reasons. Inappropriate storage and disposal of medicines can contribute to this risk.[78] For example, according to the CDC and Prevention, one of the main causes of drug overdose reported to emergency departments is the unsupervised ingestion of OTC and prescription medicines. Further, the CDC stated that of the 72,000 overdose cases presented to emergency departments in 2004, more than 26,000 were caused by OTC drugs.[79] Additionally, Li's study found that children under the age of five accounted for a higher percentage of drug overdose cases in emergency departments,[41] while another study which investigated 3,034 overdose cases among children found 97 per cent of the cases resulted from the unsupervised ingestion of drugs.[80]

Older age is associated with a higher drug overdose rate for several reasons. First, elderly people aged 65 years and over tend to have more medical problems; thus, they may take many medicines that might interact with each other and cause an overdose.[79] Second, many elderly people live independently and might find it difficult to calculate the correct dose. In addition, they may not recognise the symptoms of drug overdose when it occurs.[81] Suicide attempts are common among elderly people by taking an excessive amount of a drug. Several factors contribute to suicide attempts, such as old age, failing physical and mental health, reduced income and social support.[82]

Maintaining a dose is an important factor in preventing intentional overdoses among chronic patients.[83,84] When medicines such as Warfarin have a narrow therapeutic index, it is critical to adjust the appropriate dose.[83] Physicians prefer not to dispense Warfarin because of the uncertainty of patient compliance with monitoring, dietary implications and the fear of haemorrhagic complications.[85] The initial dose is challengeable, which could result in bleeding, and many patients might overdose at the beginning because they might have Warfarin sensitivity or a poor metabolism, thus requiring reduced dose. The maintenance of the dose depends on several factors, such as weight, diet, disease state and concomitant use of other medications, as well as genetic factors.[84] Genetic variability is considered a major factor in determining Warfarin overdose. There are two genes which are cytochrome P450, family 2, subfamily C, polypeptide 9 (CYP2C9), and vitamin K epoxide reductase complex, subunit 1 (VKORC1) contributing significantly to the variability among patients in dose requirements for Warfarin.[84],[86]

Misunderstanding and misreading the abbreviation of prescriptions can lead to medication errors and overdoses. One report demonstrated that a woman had a severe digoxin overdose because her nurse misread the pharmacist's instructions. The pharmacist had used the abbreviation (=), which was unclear because the pen had trailed ink.[87] Maged conducted a study in Saudi Arabia in 2010 to investigate medication errors in prescription medicines. Of the 529 dosing errors, the author found that 46 per cent caused overdoses. The two main errors were the route and frequency of the medicines.[88] Further, many parents have difficulty understanding the instructions to administer appropriate doses for their children. A study in 2008 examined caregivers' understandings of the age indication of OTC drugs and cough medications. Of the 182 participants whose misunderstood dose instruction, the author found that more than 80 per cent had given medicine to their infants when they should have consulted a physician first.[75]

http://dx.doi.org/10.5772/52879

Many people believe that using excessive amounts of OTC medicines is safe and effective. Some people believe that if a medicine is OTC, it is safe to consume in large quantities.[33], [44] For example, paracetamol is considered a safe medication. However, it has a narrow therapeutic index, so the dangerous dose is close to the recommended dose, and an excessive dose could lead to liver toxicity.[33] Simkin's study found that 20 per cent of the 60 participants did not know the dose that could cause death, and 15 per cent believed that 100 tablets or more would cause death.[44] Advertising and media could contribute to the excessive amounts of OTC drugs administered; for example, advertisements could suggest that the consumption of large amounts is effective before seeing a doctor.[89] Wazaify claims that there is aggressive marketing and advertising for OTC medicines.[42]

There is a higher risk of drug-related deaths among recently released prisoners,[20,90] who are associated with overdoses in the first few weeks after release.[90,91] Many studies state that the leading cause of death for recently released prisoners is accidental drug overdose.[92] For example, a study found that recently released prisoners have an overdose rate that is 12 times higher than the general population.[91] In addition, another study found that the overdose mortality rate is three-to-eight times higher in the first two weeks after release compared to the subsequent 10 weeks.[20] The reasons for higher overdose rates are not understood; however, previous studies have suggested that possible reasons include poor housing, unemployment, psychosocial problems and barriers to health care.[93-95]

Another major factor related to the increase in drug overdose rates is the lack of education, which includes the education of healthcare providers, miscalculation of doses, and limited literacy and numeracy.[35,45,67] Manchikant states that many healthcare providers, such as physicians and pharmacists, do not have adequate education regarding drug misuse.[35] In 2012, Taylor investigated the pattern of acetaminophen overdose in the military and found that a lack of education was a risk factor.[45] The CDC stated that the majority of healthcare providers have the minimum education background regarding prescription drug misuse, and they could prescribe addictive medicines without being aware of the risks involved.[67] Wallace demonstrated that physicians have limited knowledge in detecting, investigating and managing acetaminophen overdoses. Further, Wallace's study proved that the management of overdoses improved when physicians had more knowledge. A management flowchart for paracetamol poisoning was introduced to help physicians treat overdose cases.[96]

Income could be a major factor in drug overdose. People with low incomes could have lower education and numeracy levels compared to those with higher incomes. This is supported by Lokker's study of parental misinterpretations of OTC medication labels, which found that 42 per cent of parents who misinterpreted the labels had an income of less than $20,000 per annum.[75] Further, people with low incomes had more motivation to misuse prescription medicines compared to those with higher incomes.[97] In addition, low-income people were six times more likely to overdose on prescription painkillers, and a US study found that low-income people accounted for 45 per cent of prescription overdose deaths.[37] The CDC also noted that low-income people are at a greater risk of drug overdose.[67]

In contrast, Yu's study in 2005 investigated drug misuse admissions to the emergency department in a large metropolitan teaching hospital in Taipei, Taiwan. The author found that those on high-incomes were more likely to misuse drugs than low and medium income people, and the result was statistically significant.[98] Another study by Hall, which examined the pattern of unintentional drug overdoses, categorised participants' incomes into four quartiles. He found that the higher-quartile income had a greater risk of drug overdose (24.7 per 100,000 people) than the other quartiles. Further, doctor shopping is related to the higher quartile; 58 per cent of doctor shoppers were represented by the higher-quartile income. [60] Paulozzi's study also categorised income into four quartiles and found that the higher-quartile income was at a greater risk of death from methadone overdose (29.9 per cent) and other opioid analgesics (33.1 per cent).[28]

Adverse Drug Reaction (ADR) consider as the fifth leading cause of death and illness in the developed world with direct medical costs estimated to be US$30–130 billion annually in the US and claiming 100,000-218,000 lives annually.[99] Despite this, health-related associations estimate that 95 per cent of all ADRs in Canada and the US are not reported.[100] Many drugs have caused adverse drug reactions after there have been proved, and this were attributed to the drug safety issue. For example in Canada, 3–4 per cent of drugs approved will eventually be withdrawn from the market because of safety issues, Faster approval of new drugs has the potential to produce more safety problems once drugs are on the market. Many agencies have launched post marketing surveillance and pharmacosurveillance systems, and these are aimed to generate safety signals for marketed drugs.[101]

Identifying patterns of drug overdose will help to implement evidence-based policies. In a study in the UK on the effects of the withdrawal of Distalgesic (a prescription-only analgesic compound) from the market, the author found an 84 per cent reduction in intentional drug overdoses presenting to emergency departments in hospitals compared with the three years before the drug was withdrawn. Further, there was a marked reduction in tablet sales after the medicine was withdrawn, from 40 million in 2005 to 500,000 in 2006. Thus, identifying drugs that are commonly involved in overdoses will help in reducing the overdose rate.[102]

3. Methodology

An emergency department visit for drug overdose was the primary outcome measure, including unintentional and intentional overdoses. Drug overdoses are identified by physicians in the emergency department using the terms overdose, poisoning and drug relayed problem. Secondary measures include the patient's age, gender, interior personal occupation, Length of Stay (LOS) in the emergency department, patient type, drug level, previous admission, previous overdose and measurement outcome.

In this research, participants are categorised into three groups. First, interior personnel are identified as people who work in the Ministry of Interior. The second group is interior personnel relatives, where each employee has the right to have his family treated in the hospital. The third group is called exceptional people; many people do not belong to the Ministry of Interior, but they seek treatment in the hospital because they have acquired an exceptional letter, as they require special health intervention.

Overdose cases obtained in the study are divided according to prescription and non- prescription drugs in order to test the hypothesis of the study. Moreover, the number of medicines involved in the cases is addressed and the drugs are categorised into three groups: single, double and triple. In addition, drug level is addressed in the study and it is standardised to moderate or severe according to the level of drug in the body. The LOS of patients was determined by calculating the period between the time of admission and the time of discharge from the emergency department, or the time when admitted to the inpatient management is included in the study and all cases are divided into two categories: discharged from the emergency department and admitted to the inpatient department.

Descriptive statistics such as frequencies and cross-tabulations were obtained to describe the various motives reported by the sample. All drugs involved in overdoses were obtained, as well as their frequency, to identify the medicine that accounted for the highest percentage. Further, the medicines used in overdoses were tabulated according to their medical indication of use and then each medicine was categorised according to their medical indication group. Fisher and chi-square tests were conducted to test the differences between categorical variables. As the chi-square prefers two-by-two tables and each cell must have at least five cells, the patients' type needed to be re-categorised into two groups: interior and non-interior. Although the patients' type was allocated to two groups, one of the cells had less than five, so a Fisher exact test was used.

The data was obtained from medical records, which raises the issue of confidentiality. However, the anonymity of participants will be protected, and only de-identified data was accessed. A letter was obtained from the hospital to ensure the anonymity of the research. The data was obtained only from files that were considered essential for the research. No patient was contacted as part of this study. Each participant will have a unique three-digit code. The data collection complies with the National Health and Medical Research Council's National Statement on Ethical Conduct in Human Research. Further, the study has been approved by the Security Forces Hospital's Research Committee. In addition, the UWA's Human Research Ethics Committee has approved this study.

4. Results

4.1. Demographic characteristics

One hundred and forty drug overdose cases were admitted to the emergency department of the Riyadh Security Forces Hospital between 1 January 2007 and 31 December 2011. Table 1 describes the demographic characteristics of patients associated with drug overdose, and the findings are discussed below. Females accounted for 57.90 per cent of cases and males accounted for 42.10 per cent. In this study, there is a variety in age distribution, with patients aged between 11 months and 86 years. The patients' ages were divided into seven groups:

(0.01–1.12), (2.00–9.12), (10.00–19.12), (20.00–29.12), (30.00–44.12), (45.00–59.12) and (over 60 years). This study demonstrates that groups (2.00–9.12 years) and (over 60 years) accounted for the highest percentage of drug overdose cases (22.9 per cent).

Characteristics	Number	Per cent
Gender:		
Male	59	42.1
Female	81	57.9
Age groups:		
0.01–1.12 years	8	5.7
2.00–9.12 years	32	22.9
10.00–19.12 years	9	6.4
20.00–29.12 years	25	17.9
30.00–44.12 years	19	13.6
45.00–59.12 years	15	10.7
Over 60 years	32	22.9
Type:		
Interior Personnel	30	21.4
Relatives	105	75.0
Exceptional people	5	3.60
Income groups:		
Less than 22,000 USD	37	27.4
22,001–45,000USD	69	51.1
45,001–67,001USD	18	13.3
More than 67,001 USD	11	8.1

Table 1. Socio-demographic characteristics of drug overdose cases.

The interior personnel relatives group accounted for the highest percentage of cases (n=105, 75 per cent), and interior personnel and exceptional people accounted for 21.4 and 3.60 per cent respectively. Income was divided into four groups that were represented by United State Dollar (USD) per annum: (less than 22,000 USD), (22,001–45,000USD), 3 (45,001–

http://dx.doi.org/10.5772/52879

67,001USD) and (more than 67,001 USD). The study showed that (22,001–45,000USD) group represents the highest percentage of participants.

According to Table 2, 96.4 per cent of all drug overdose cases reported to the emergency department between January 2007 and December 2011 were caused by prescription medicines. Previous overdoses were addressed in the study, and only eight patients were found to have previous overdose experiences. Further, the study found that 53.6 per cent of cases were associated with previous admission, and patients with one previous admission represented 20 per cent of all participants who had been admitted previously. In the study, some patients used more than one drug to overdose. It found that 91.4 per cent of patients were taking one drug, while double and triple drugs accounted for 7.9 per cent and 0.7 per cent respectively. In addition, 67.5 per cent of the cases were found to have moderate drug levels, while severe drug levels accounted for 26.4 per cent of cases.

LOS groups were categorised into the following: (less than five hours), (5.01–10.01 hours), (10.01–15.00 hours), (15.01–20.00 hours), (20.01–35.00 hours) and (over 40 hours). It found that 50.0 per cent of all cases reported to the emergency department stayed for less than five hours, and these cases were either discharged or transferred to the inpatient admission department. The study found that 106 drug overdose cases were referred to the inpatient admission department.

Interior relatives accounted for 75 per cent of all overdose cases in the study. It found that 28.6 per cent of the cases were aged 2–9.12 years. Further, 54 per cent of the participants' income was between (22,001–45,000USD) per annum. Eight cases were associated with previous overdose cases, and seven of them were relatives. Moreover, 49.5 per cent of cases stayed in the emergency department for less than five hours. Further, there were 34 discharged cases in the study, 28 of which were relative cases.

The outcome of a drug overdose is statistically different between patients' type (one-sided p-value = 0.007). It found that the inpatient admission department accounted for 93.3 per cent for all interior personnel cases, while non-interior people who were relatives and exceptional people accounted for 78 per cent of the cases, and the difference of outcome management among patient type is significant. By using the Fisher exact test, previous admission is statistically relevant to patient type (one-sided p-value = 0.033). It found that 70 and 50.1 per cent of interior and non interior cases were associated with previous admission; thus, the difference is significant. The difference between drug level and outcome management was tested using a chi-square test, and a significant difference was found. It found that 72.6 per cent of moderate-level cases were admitted to the inpatient department and 91.9 per cent of severe-level cases were admitted to the inpatient department. The management outcome from admission is statistically relevant to the level of drug (one-sided p-value = 0.008). The difference between gender and patients' type was tested using the Fisher exact test; thus, gender is statistically relevant to patients' type (one-sided p-value = 0.000).

Characteristics	Number	Per cent
Previous overdose:		
Yes	8	5.7
No	132	94.3
Previous admission:		
Yes	75	53.6
No	65	46.4
Number of previous admissions:		
0	65	46.4
1	28	20.0
2	21	15.0
3	8	5.7
4	6	4.3
5	4	2.9
7 and more	8	5.6
Drug kind:		
Prescription	135	96.4
Non-prescription	5	3.6
Drug combination:		
Single drug	128	91.4
Double drugs	11	7.9
Triple drugs	1	0.7
Drug level:		
Moderate	95	67.9
Severe	37	26.4
LOS groups:		
Less than five hours	70	50.0
5.01–10.01 hours	24	17.1
10.01–15.00 hours	12	8.6
15.01–20.00 hours	13	9.3
20.01–35.00 hours	10	7.1
Over 40 hours	11	7.9
Outcome management:		
Discharge	34	24.3
Inpatient admission	106	75.7

Table 2. Characteristics of drug overdose cases

4.2. Drug overdose percentages and rates

The means of LOS age and income per annum of patients in the emergency department are addressed, and it was found that the average LOS was around 11 hours, average age was 33 years and four months, and average income was around 35,951 USD.

The number of drug overdose cases was calculated for each year of the study. The annual number of emergency admissions was requested from the medical records department to identify the rate of drug overdose cases among all emergency cases. All results are shown in Table 3. According to the results, the rate of drug overdose reduced between 2007 and 2011.

Year	Number of cases	Number of emergency cases	Rate
2007	33	9576	3.45 per 1,000
2008	30	9131	3.26 per 1,000
2009	26	8707	2.99 per 1,000
2010	26	8209	3.17 per 1,000
2011	25	7883	3.17 per 1,000

Table 3. Number and rate of drug overdose for each year in the study

Most patients overdosed on one drug. Fifty-eight prescription and non-prescription medicines were included in the study. These medicines were categorised in terms of medical indication purpose. Seven drug categories were found in the study, and each one involved more than seven cases. Further, anti-coagulants and analgesics accounted for 35.3 per cent of drug overdose cases. These categories were investigated in terms of age groups. The findings show that 55 per cent of anti-coagulant overdose cases occurred in patients aged over 60 years, while 41 per cent of analgesic overdose cases occurred in patients aged 20–30 years. According to the findings, Warfarin accounted for the highest percentage of drug overdoses. Warfarin accounted for 85 per cent of overdoses in patients aged over 50 years, while two cases occurred in children and middle-aged people respectively. Further, people in lower and middle-income groups accounted for 85.7 per cent of anti-coagulant cases.

The results show that four patients from age (20.00–29.12 years), had a previous overdose, and this age group represented 50 per cent of patients associated with previous overdoses. Moreover, two patients overdosed on OTC medicines twice, and one patient overdosed twice on Warfarin. Two deaths occurred from drug overdoses: one death was a patient who overdosed on paracetamol twice, and the other was attributed to amphetamine. In addition, there were 18 overdose cases aged from 15 to 25 years. It found that analgesics and antipsychotics accounted for 38.8 and 22.2 per cent of the cases respectively. Cholesterol-lowering and diabetic medicines were involved in two cases and antihistamine and antiepileptic drugs were involved in one case each.

As the hospital belongs to the Ministry of Interior, it is important to identify the occupations that are more involved in drug overdoses. There were 30 interior personnel cases, and eleven positions represented all interior personnel drug overdose cases. The system of occupation in the Ministry of Interior has two major categories: officer and non-officer. Non-officer personnel presented at a higher rate in drug overdoses than non-officer personnel. In this study, five of 30 cases belong to officers and the rest belong to non-officers.

Position name	Frequency
Soldier	7
First soldier	5
Captain	4
First Sargent	3
Sargent	2
Staff-Sargent	2
Unknown	2
Colonel	1
Corporal	1
Chief-Sargent	1
Porter	1
Senior-Sargent	1

Table 4. Occupations of interior personnel cases and their frequency

5. Discussion

We found that females accounted for a higher percentage of drug overdose cases than males, which is similar to findings in previous studies.[6,22,103,104] In contrast, Alfawal's study found that males accounted for 88 per cent of the cases.[7] Further, it found that (2.00–9.12 years) and (over 60 years) patients accounted for the highest percentage, at 22.9 per cent of cases. Previous studies associated the elderly with a higher percentage of drug overdoses, and this study had a similar result.[79,82] Further, the CDC found that the highest risk group of drug overdose among children was amongst those aged two years.[80] This research reached the same conclusion. Thus, most cases might have occurred unintentionally because previous studies demonstrated that children and the elderly are at a higher risk of unintentional overdose.[80]

The finding stated that 75.7 per cent of cases were referred to the inpatients admission department. According to the medical records department supervisor, this high percentage is not because most cases were severe; rather, many cases that were presented and discharged from the emergency department were missing and did not register to the medical files. There are two possible reasons for missing drug overdose cases. First, there is a higher load on emergency physicians; so many diagnostic forms are not fully completed. Second, many cases present to the emergency department have not been registered in the patients' medical records, so some overdose cases may have been missed and not caught by the ICD-9-CM. This explains why there were only 140 drug overdose cases in the five-year period. A study conducted in the National Guard Hospital in Riyadh, which is considered larger than the

Security Force Hospital, found nine drug overdose cases per month,[105] compared to this study, which found around three cases per month. This is further evidence that there might be missing cases.

Fifty-eight medicines were involved in the drug overdose cases, and the most common drug was Warfarin, which caused 29 overdose cases. This finding differs from previous studies conducted in Saudi Arabia, which found that OTC medicines accounted for a large percentage of drug overdoses. Moazzam's and Aljahdali's studies found that paracetamol accounted for 24.1 per cent of 170 drug overdose cases and 30 per cent of 79 cases, respectively. [21,22]Ahmed's study found that mefenamic acid accounted for 20 per cent of 50 cases investigated.[6] Moreover, Malik's study found that the most common drugs used were analgesics and non-steroid anti- inflammatory drugs.[104] AbuMadini's study found that 80 per cent of cases were caused by paracetamol,[103] which was the second most common medicine in this study (12 cases).

According to the findings, children aged 2–9 years accounted for 22.4 per cent of drug overdose cases. This might indicate that many parents leave medicines unprotected from children, so children might administer excessive amounts of drugs accidentally. Education and awareness campaigns should be conducted to educate people about the risk of leaving medicines unprotected, as well as how to store their medicines correctly.[1,75,106, 107] Further, leaving medicines unsecured from children can contribute to an increase in the rate of drug overdose.[78,108,109] According to the American Association of Poison Control Centers, in 2009, prescription and OTC drugs caused more than 30 per cent of children's death in the US.[110]

Many policy and prevention measures can be implemented to protect children from drug overdoses, such as child-resistant packaging (CRP), product reformulations and heightened parental awareness. CRP reduced the drug overdose mortality rate of children by 45 per cent between 1974 and 1992.[22,80] Medication packaging will not protect children from overdose, and it becomes ineffective if the medication is not re-secured correctly.[109] Further, packaging has not proved to be effective, as young children have the dexterity to open these containers.[111] Some prevention programs have been conducted to educate parents about storing medicine in safe places. The Preventing Overdoses and Treatment Exposures Task Force (PROTECT) launched a program called 'Up and Away', which aims to educate parents about effectively storing medicines, and it emphasises the need to return medicines to a safe storage location immediately after every use to prevent children from reaching them.[109]

Other strategies might be helpful in preventing drug overdoses in children. For example, the use of adaptors on bottles of liquid medication so that the medication can be accessed only with a needleless syringe; parents should not allow children to drink medicine directly from the bottle; and using unit dose packaging might reduce the amount of accidental drug ingestion. These strategies are highly recommended for common medicines such as OTC drugs.[80]

As children account for a higher percentage of drug overdose cases, parents' misunderstanding and miscalculation of doses can contribute to a higher percentage of overdoses. Contributing factors include limited literacy and numeracy, particularly in age indication. This problem is emphasised in terms of OTC medicines, as no instructions are provided directly by healthcare providers.[28,112] Applying simple language instructions and warning labels in the leaflets of medicines might be helpful in terms of calculating correct doses.[75] Further, healthcare providers should request that parents with low literacy levels use one product for all children in the family, which might help to prevent dose miscalculation.[73]

Another major factor contributing to drug overdoses in children is the availability of unused drugs in homes.[113] The solution for this problem is medication disposal. Campaigns for the disposal of medications have been used in many countries, which would help to reduce accidental drug overdoses in children, intentional drug abuse and the accumulation of drugs by elderly people, as well as protect the physical environment and eliminate waste in the healthcare system.[113,114] The government of Ireland launched a campaign called Dispose of Unused Medicines Properly (DUMP), which encouraged the public to return unused or expired medicines to community pharmacies. The project was launched in 2005, and 9,608 items were returned in the first year and 2,951 kilograms were returned in 2006. The most common medicine group returned was the nervous system class, which accounted for 26.3 per cent.[115]

A study conducted in Saudi Arabia in 2003 identified the issue of unused and expired medicines in Saudi dwellings. The study recruited 1,641 households in 22 cities. The study found that more than 80 per cent of Saudi families had more than five medicines, with an average of more than two medicines that were expired or unused. The most common drugs found in the participants' houses were respiratory drugs (16.8 per cent), followed by central nervous system (CNS) agents (16.4 per cent) and antibiotics (14.3 per cent). Of the 2,050 CNS medications, OTC analgesics (including non-steroidal anti-inflammatory agents) constituted 49.9 per cent of the total (n = 1,023). Further, 51 per cent of all medicines found were not currently used and, of these, 40 per cent were expired. So medication wastage can provide greater opportunity to access prescription drugs in Saudi Arabia. The study recommended disposal medication campaigns to reduce the danger of available unused and expired medicines.[116]

According to the results a large number of medicines were involved in drug overdose, and thus might indicated that many patients have excessive amount of medicines in there dwelling. One reason might contribute to the excessive amount of medicines is drug seeking behaviour. Warfarin accounted for the highest percentage of drug overdoses. Eighty-five per cent of all Warfarin overdoses occurred in patients aged over 50 years, while two cases occurred in children and the middle-aged, respectively. This might indicate that the overdoses occurred unintentionally. One of major reasons for Warfarin overdoses is that it has a narrow therapeutic index; thus, administrating a larger dose would easily lead to overdoses.[117] Further, Warfarin is associated with complex pharmacology and inherent risk of outcome. As it is used continuously, maintaining the dose is critical to ensure safe and effective therapy.[117]

According to the results, females accounted for a higher percentage of drug overdoses. Several factors might contribute to this. First, family conflict was stated as a higher-risk factor of drug overdoses in women. Aljahdali's study found that 80 per cent of the 79 overdose cases investigated were female, and 60 per cent had family conflicts.[22] Further, a study was conducted in the King Fahd Hospital of the University (KFHU) to investigate cases of deliberate self-harm presented to the emergency department of the hospital. The study recruited 362 cases, and the female to male ratio was 1.8:1. The study found that 71 per cent of cases were drug overdoses, of which 50.3 per cent were caused by family problems.[103] Moreover, a study was conducted in Saudi Arabia in KFHU to investigate non-fatal, deliberate self-harm cases. There were 55 cases investigated over nine months, and 80 per cent of them were female. The most common method used was self-poisoning (drug and chemical). The study found that family conflict was the main factor, contributing to 50.9 per cent of cases.[118]

The rate of drug overdose for each year of the study period was reduced from 3.45 to 3.17 per 1,000. However, the number of emergency admissions also reduced annually. This result contrasts with previous studies. For example, Moazzam found an increased rate of drug poisoning in the alQassim region in Saudi Arabia, from 6.6 per 100,000 in 1999 to 10.7 per 100,000.[21] Further, Malik found that the number of drug overdose cases presented in Asir Center Hospital increased from two cases in 1989 to 22 cases in 1993.[104] This indicates that there were perhaps more preventive and awareness programs in Saudi Arabia in the previous years.

There are several pharmacyosurveillance implications; one of them is collecting data regarding motivations and causes of drug overdose. According to the finding most of the cases occurred in elderly and children, so targeting these groups of people would help in reducing the rate of drug overdose cases.[119] Further, another implication would be the use of Electronic prescription. It is defined as a tool for prescribers to electronically prepare and send an accurate, error-free and understandable prescription directly to a pharmacy. Previous study found that electronic prescription system reduced medical errors by 55 per cent - from 10.7 to 4.9 per 1000 patient-days.[120] According to the results the rate of drug overdose cases in the emergency department decreased between 2007 and 2011, and this was attributed for using electronic prescription system in the hospital.

Drug related problems account for large amount of money in hospital cost. For example, in US a probability model in 2002 estimated that morbidity and mortality associated with DRPs account for $76.6 billion in hospital cost. Further, a study conducted in Saudi Arabia in 2008 found that the estimate cost of one day admission for drug related problem is 666$. So Implementing preventable measures such as pharmacosurveillance system would be a cost effective.[105]

Some policies might be implemented to reduce the risk of drug overdose cases. As Warfarin accounted for the highest percentage of drug overdoses, particularly in elderly people, further dose instruction should be given to elderly patients to ensure they have understood the instructions correctly.[85] Further, patients acquired Warfarin from hospital; thus, if the quantity of medicine dispensed is reduced, drug overdose cases might be prevented. In addition, children accounted for the highest percentage of drug overdose cases, so policymakers should implement awareness courses to educate parents to secure and protect medicines from children.[80] There was a wide range of medicines involved in drug overdose cases, so further dose instruction is needed. Moreover, patients must be educated regarding the dangers of overdosing.

6. Conclusion

Despite religious, cultural and legal deterrents, occasional cases of drug overdoses occur in the Saudi population.

The main limitations of this study mainly in relate to the quality of data available in patients' medical records, as many files might not be fully documented, and some variables related to research are not found in the medical records (e.g. education level). Moreover, as the income level is identified based on the household occupation, a number of files did not document the household occupation; thus, some patients' incomes were not available. The sample size is considered small, as there are few statistically significant associations between variables. Thus, the findings relating to associations between variables might not represent the actual validity of the associations between the independent and outcome variables. In addition, the data in this study was collected from a single institution, and the patients of drug overdoses have special characteristics that might not be similar to the general Saudi population. For example, all people treated in the hospital obtain medicines from the pharmacy without any charge. Further, One of the limitations of this study is that it does not state the reasons for drug overdoses, and it does not identify if overdoses occurred intentionally or accidentally.

Some significant findings were made, such as Warfarin causing 29 overdose cases, and patients aged over 50 accounting for 85 per cent of all Warfarin cases. This finding signifies a problem with Warfarin in elderly patients, and further research is needed to identify the major cause of this high percentage and to assist in implementing preventive measures to protect the elderly from the risk of overdosing. Further, children accounted for a high percentage of drug overdoses, and the study stated that 66.6 of anti-hypertensive overdoses were children. Thus, further research should be conducted to identify the reasons why children overdose so they can be protected from drug overdoses.

These findings could help the hospital to implement preventive strategies and policies. As many cases occur accidentally, education and awareness programs are required regarding dose instructions and the storage and disposal of medicines. Further, many patients keep excessive amounts of medicines in their dwellings, so reducing the amount of medicines provided to chronic patients would help to reduce drug overdose cases. Education of physicians on drug-seeking behaviour of patients is important. Further, special courses in dose instructions could be implemented for elderly patients, as well as programs that target parents regarding dose calculations for their children and the safe storage of medicines. In addition, clinical guidelines for overdose management need to be standardised, and the surveillance and recording of overdose information should be improved. Lastly, improved edu-

http://dx.doi.org/10.5772/52879

cation is required for the public and for health workers in order to prevent drug interactions that might precipitate overdoses.

Author details

Naser Al-Jaser, M. Cli. Epi and Niyi Awofeso

School of Population Health, University of Western Australia, Australia

References

[1] Coffin P. Overdose: A Major Cause of Preventable Death in Central and Eastern Europe in Central Asia:Vilnius; 2008 [cited 17/5/2012]. Available from: http://www.harm-reduction.org/images/stories/library/od_report_2008_en.pdf

[2] Warner M, Chen LH, Makuc DM. Increase in fatal poisonings involving opioid analgesics in the United States, 1999-2006. NCHS data brief. 2009 (22):1.

[3] CDC. Prescription Drug Overdose: State Health Agencies Respond. 2008. Available from: http://www.cdc.gov/HomeandRecreationalSafety/pubs/RXReport_web-a.pdf

[4] CDC. Unintentional Drug Poisoning in the United States.; 2006 [cited 11/5/2012]. Available from: http://www.cdc.gov/HomeandRecreationalSafety/pdf/poison-issue-brief.pdf

[5] statistics dgo. Health statistics year book, new outpatient and inpatients in Mental Health Departments. Riyadh: MOH; 2009. Available from: http://www.moh.gov.sa/en/Ministry/Statistics/book/flash/1430/MOH_Report_1430.html

[6] Ahmed M. Drug-associated admissions to a district hospital in Saudi Arabia. Journal of clinical pharmacy and therapeutics. 1997;22(1):61-66.

[7] Elfawal M. Trends in fatal substance overdose in eastern Saudi Arabia. Journal of Clinical Forensic Medicine. 1999;6(1):30-34.

[8] Jha AK, Kuperman GJ, Teich JM, Leape L, Shea B, Rittenberg E, et al. Identifying adverse drug events development of a computer-based monitor and comparison with chart review and stimulated voluntary report. Journal of the American Medical Informatics Association. 1998;5(3):305-314.

[9] Lazarou J, Pomeranz BH, Corey PN. Incidence of adverse drug reactions in hospitalized patients. JAMA: the journal of the American Medical Association. 1998;279(15): 1200-1205.

[10] Moore TJ, Cohen MR, Furberg CD. Serious adverse drug events reported to the Food and Drug Administration, 1998-2005. Archives of internal medicine. 2007;167(16): 1752.

[11] Budnitz DS, Pollock DA, Mendelsohn AB, Weidenbach KN, McDonald AK, Annest JL. Emergency department visits for outpatient adverse drug events: demonstration for a national surveillance system. Annals of emergency medicine. 2005;45(2): 197-206.

[12] CDC. Overdoses of Prescription Opioid Pain Relievers --- United States, 1999--2008. Prevention CfDC; 2011. Available from: http://www.cdc.gov/mmwr/preview/mmwrhtml/mm6043a4.htm

[13] Santiago L, Altamirano P, Torreblanco M, Ruiz S. WORLD DRUG REPORT 2011. Vinne: (UNODC) UNOoDaC; 2011. Available from: http://www.unodc.org/documents/data-and-analysis/WDR2011/World_Drug_Report_2011_ebook.pdf

[14] Quan VM, Vongchak T, Jittiwutikarn J, Kawichai S, Srirak N, Wiboonnatakul K, et al. Predictors of mortality among injecting and non-injecting HIV-negative drug users in northern Thailand. Addiction. 2007;102(3):441-446.

[15] Zhang L, Ruan Y, Jiang Z, Yang Z, Liu S, Zhou F, et al. An 1-year prospective cohort study on mortality of injecting drug users]. Zhonghua liu xing bing xue za zhi= Zhonghua liuxingbingxue zazhi. 2005;26(3):190.

[16] EMCDDA. THE STATE OF THE DRUGS PROBLEM IN EUROPE. Portugal: [cited 1/6/2012]. Available from: http://www.emcdda.europa.eu/publications/annual-report/2011

[17] CDC. Suicides Due to Alcohol and/or Drug Overdose. NVDRS; 2011 [cited 15/5/2012]. Available from: http://www.cdc.gov/ViolencePrevention/pdf/NVDRS_Data_Brief-a.pdf

[18] Health AIo, Welfare. Statistics on Drug Use in Australia 2006. 2007 [cited 7/5/2012]. Report No.: 9781740246606. Available from: http://www.aihw.gov.au/publication-detail/?id=6442467962

[19] Degenhardt L, Roxburgh A. Accidental drug-induced deaths due to opioids in Australia. 2005 [cited 20/5/2012]. Available from: http://ndarc.med.unsw.edu.au/resource/accidental-drug-induced-deaths-australia-1997-2001

[20] Merrall ELC, Kariminia A, Binswanger IA, Hobbs MS, Farrell M, Marsden J, et al. Meta-analysis of drug-related deaths soon after release from prison.Addiction. 2010;105(9):1545-1554.

[21] Moazzam M, Al-Saigul A, Naguib M, Al Alfi M. Pattern of acute poisoning in Al-Qassim region: a surveillance report from Saudi Arabia, 1999-2003. Eastern Mediterranean Health Journal. 2009;15(4):1005-1010.

[22] Al Jahdali, Antipsychotics SG. Pattern and risk factors for intentional drug overdose in Saudi Arabia. Canadian journal of psychiatry. 2004;49:331-334.

[23] WHO, Zhang X. WHO guidelines on safety monitoring of herbal medicines in pharmacovigilance systems. 2004 [cited 10/7/2012]. Report No.: 9241592214. Available from: http://apps.who.int/medicinedocs/documents/s7148e/s7148e.pdf

[24] Lessenger JE, Feinberg SD. Abuse of prescription and over-the-counter medications. The Journal of the American Board of Family Medicine. 2008;21(1):45-54.

[25] Saad B, Azaizeh H, Abu-Hijleh G, Said O. Safety of traditional Arab herbal medicine. Evidence Based Complementary and Alternative Medicine. 2006;3(4):433-440.

[26] Alkharfy K. Community pharmacists' knowledge, attitudes and practices towards herbal remedies in Riyadh, Saudi Arabia. East Mediterr Health J. 2010;16(9):988-993.

[27] Jane B, Trevor S, Andrew T, Bilal W, Alex W, Sunny M. The context of illicit drug overdose deaths in British Columbia, 2006. Harm Reduction Journal. 2009;6.

[28] Paulozzi LJ, Logan JE, Hall AJ, McKinstry E, Kaplan JA, Crosby AE. A comparison of drug overdose deaths involving methadone and other opioid analgesics in West Virginia. Addiction. 2009;104(9):1541-1548.

[29] De Leo D, Evans R. International suicide rates: recent trends and implications for Australia. 2006 [cited 25/5/2012]. Available from: http://www.health.gov.au/internet/main/publishing.nsf/content/1D2B4E895BCD429ECA2572290027094D/$File/intsui.pdf

[30] Suicides, Australia, 1994 to 2004. Canberra,; 2006 [cited 12/4/2012]. Available from: http://www.ausstats.abs.gov.au/ausstats/subscriber.nsf/0/FF573FA817DC3C84CA25713000705C19/$File/33090_1994 to 2004.pdf

[31] Buykx P, Ritter A, Loxley W, Dietze P. Patients Who Attend the Emergency Department Following Medication Overdose: Self-reported Mental Health History and Intended Outcomes of Overdose. International Journal of Mental Health and Addiction. 2011:1-11.

[32] Bohnert ASB, Roeder KM, Ilgen MA. Suicide attempts and overdoses among adults entering addictions treatment: Comparing correlates in a US national study. Drug and alcohol dependence. 2011;119(1-2):106-12.

[33] Budnitz DS, Lovegrove MC, Crosby AE. Emergency department visits for overdoses of acetaminophen-containing products. American Journal of Preventive Medicine. 2011;40(6):585-592.

[34] Darke S, Ross J. The relationship between suicide and heroin overdose among methadone maintenance patients in Sydney, Australia. Addiction. 2001;96(10):1443-1453.

[35] Manchikanti L. Prescription drug abuse: what is being done to address this new drug epidemic? Testimony before the Subcommittee on Criminal Justice, Drug Policy and Human Resources. Pain Physician. 2006;9(4):287.

[36] Leary E, Poisson M. prescription and over the counter drug abuse, Orange County Comprehensive Report. Santa Ana, california; 2010 [cited 2/5/2012]. Available from: http://www.duila.org/Assets/StreetTrends/Prescription and OTC Drug Abuse/prescription-over-the-counter-drug-abuse-report.pdf

[37] CDC. Policy Impact: Prescription Painkiller Overdoses. 2011 [cited 9/5/2012]. Available from: http://www.cdc.gov/HomeandRecreationalSafety/pdf/PolicyImpact-PrescriptionPainkillerOD.pdf

[38] Devi S. USA homes in on prescription drug abuse. The Lancet. 2011;378(9790): 473-474.

[39] Dhalla IA, Mamdani MM, Gomes T, Juurlink DN. Clustering of opioid prescribing and opioid-related mortality among family physicians in Ontario. Canadian Family Physician. 2011;57(3):e92-e96.

[40] White J, Taverner D. Drug-seeking behaviour. Australian prescriber 1997 (20):68-70.

[41] Li C, Martin BC. Trends in emergency department visits attributable to acetaminophen overdoses in the United States: 1993,Äì2007. Pharmacoepidemiology and drug safety. 2011;20(8):810-818.

[42] Wazaify M, Kennedy S, Hughes CM, McElnay JC. Prevalence of over-the-counter drug-related overdoses at Accident and Emergency departments in Northern Ireland--a retrospective evaluation. Journal of clinical pharmacy and therapeutics. 2005;30(1):39-44.

[43] Toblin RL, Paulozzi LJ, Logan JE, Hall AJ, Kaplan JA. Mental illness and psychotropic drug use among prescription drug overdose deaths: a medical examiner chart review. The Journal of clinical psychiatry. 2010;71(4):491-496.

[44] Simkin S, Hawton K, Kapur N, Gunnell D. What can be done to reduce mortality from paracetamol overdoses? A patient interview study. QJM. 2012;105(1):41-51.

[45] Taylor LG, Xie S, Meyer TE, Coster TS. Acetaminophen overdose in the Military Health System. Pharmacoepidemiology and drug safety. 2012.

[46] Curtis M, Guterman L. Overdose Prevention and Response. 2009 [cited 6/5/2012]. Available from: http://harm.live.radicaldesigns.org/downloads/Overdose Prevention and Response Guide.pdf

[47] Shah N. Unintentional Illicit and Prescription Drug Overdose Death Trends, 2008. New Mexico Journal NME; 2009 [cited 7/5/2012]. Available from: http://nmhealth.org/erd/pdf/ER prescription drug overdose 112009.pdf

[48] Craig DGN, Bates CM, Davidson JS, Martin KG, Hayes PC, Simpson KJ. Overdose pattern and outcome in paracetamol-induced acute severe hepatotoxicity. British journal of clinical pharmacology. 2011;71(2):273-282.

[49] Buykx P, Loxley W, Dietze P, Ritter A. Medications used in overdose and how they are acquired- an investigation of cases attending an inner Melbourne emergency department. Australian and New Zealand journal of public health. 2010;34(4):401-404.

[50] Britton PC, Wines JD, Conner KR. Non-fatal overdose in the 12 months following treatment for substance use disorders. Drug and alcohol dependence. 2010;107(1): 51-55.

[51] Darke S, Duflou J, Torok M. A reduction in blood morphine concentrations amongst heroin overdose fatalities associated with a sustained reduction in street heroin purity. Forensic science international. 2010;198(1-3):118-120.

[52] Mayet S, Manning V, Williams A, Loaring J, Strang J. Impact of training for healthcare professionals on how to manage an opioid overdose with naloxone: Effective, but dissemination is challenging. International Journal of Drug Policy. 2011;22(1): 9-15.

[53] HORYNIAK D, HIGGS P, LEWIS J, WINTER R, DIETZE P, AITKEN C. An evaluation of a heroin overdose prevention and education campaign. Drug and alcohol review. 2010;29(1):5-11.

[54] Maher L, Ho HT. Overdose beliefs and management practices among ethnic Vietnamese heroin users in Sydney, Australia. Harm Reduction Journal. 2009;6(1):6.

[55] Toprak S, Cetin I. Heroin Overdose Deaths and Heroin Purity Between 1990 and 2000 in Istanbul, Turkey*. Journal of forensic sciences. 2009;54(5):1185-1188.

[56] Risser D, Uhl A, Oberndorfer F, Stichenwirth M, Hirz R, Sebald D. Is there a relationship between street heroin purity and drug-related emergencies and/or drug-related deaths? An analysis from Vienna, Austria. Journal of forensic sciences. 2007;52(5): 1171-1176.

[57] Bani I. Prevalence and related risk factors of Essential Hypertension in Jazan region, Saudi Arabia. Sudanese Journal of Public Health 2011;6(2):45-50.

[58] East TM. Saudi Arabia's demographics - the winds of change. [cited 16/5/2012]. Available from: http://www.ameinfo.com/96723.html

[59] Kinner SA, Milloy M, Wood E, Qi J, Zhang R, Kerr T. Incidence and risk factors for non-fatal overdose among a cohort of recently incarcerated illicit drug users. Addictive Behaviors. 2012.

[60] Hall AJ, Logan JE, Toblin RL, Kaplan JA, Kraner JC, Bixler D, et al. Patterns of abuse among unintentional pharmaceutical overdose fatalities. JAMA: the journal of the American Medical Association. 2008;300(22):2613-2620.

[61] Trescot AM, Boswell MV, Atluri SL, Hansen HC, Deer TR, Abdi S, et al. Opioid guidelines in the management of chronic non-cancer pain. Pain Physician. 2006;9(1): 1.

[62] Reporting KASPE. A Comprehensive Report on Kentucky Prescription Monitoring Program Prepared by the Cabinet for Health and Family Services Office of the Inspector General. 2006 [cited 22/5/2012]. Available from: http://chfs.ky.gov/nr/rdonlyres/7057e43d-e1fd-4552-a902-2793f9b226fc/0/kaspersummaryreportversion2.pdf

[63] Manchikanti L, Damron K, Pampati V, McManus C. Prospective evaluation of patients with increasing opiate needs: prescription opiate abuse and illicit drug use. Pain Physician. 2004;7(3):339.

[64] Manchikanti L, Fellows B, Damron K, Pampati V, McManus C. Prevalence of illicit drug use among individuals with chronic pain in the Commonwealth of Kentucky: an evaluation of patterns and trends. The Journal of the Kentucky Medical Association. 2005;103(2):55.

[65] Hall AJ, Logan JE, Toblin RL, Kaplan JA, Kraner JC, Bixler D, et al. Patterns of abuse among unintentional pharmaceutical overdose fatalities. JAMA: the journal of the American Medical Association. 2008;300(22):2613.

[66] Hempstead K. Manner of death and circumstances in fatal poisonings: evidence from New Jersey. Injury Prevention. 2006;12(suppl 2):ii44-ii48.

[67] Strategies P. CDC Grand Rounds: Prescription Drug Overdoses — a U.S. Epidemic. [cited 13/5/2012]. Available from: http://www.cdc.gov/mmwr/preview/mmwrhtml/mm6101a3.htm

[68] Meehan TJ, Bryant SM, Aks SE. Drugs of Abuse: The Highs and Lows of Altered Mental States in the Emergency Department. Emergency medicine clinics of North America. 2010;28(3):663-682.

[69] Von Korff M, Kolodny A, Deyo RA, Chou R. Long-term opioid therapy reconsidered. Annals of internal medicine. 2011;155(5):325-328.

[70] Reidenberg M, Willis O. Prosecution of physicians for prescribing opioids to patients. Clinical Pharmacology & Therapeutics. 2007;81(6):903-906.

[71] Baehren DF, Marco CA, Droz DE, Sinha S, Callan EM, Akpunonu P. A statewide prescription monitoring program affects emergency department prescribing behaviors. Annals of emergency medicine. 2010;56(1):19-23. e3.

[72] Miles FK, Kamath R, Dorney SFA, Gaskin KJ, O'Loughlin EV. Accidental paracetamol overdosing and fulminant hepatic failure in children. Medical Journal of Australia. 1999;171:472-475.

[73] Buck M. Preventing Acetaminophen Overdosage. The Annals of Pharmacotherapy. 2000;34(32-4).

[74] HIXSON R, Franke U, Mittal R, Hamilton M. Parental calculation of pediatric paracetamol dose: a randomized trial comparing the Parental Analgesia Slide with product information leaflets. Pediatric Anesthesia. 2010;20(7):612-619.

[75] Lokker N, Sanders L, Perrin EM, Kumar D, Finkle J, Franco V, et al. Parental misinterpretations of over-the-counter pediatric cough and cold medication labels. Pediatrics. 2009;123(6):1464-1471.

[76] Hasin DS, Goodwin RD, Stinson FS, Grant BF. Epidemiology of major depressive disorder: results from the National Epidemiologic Survey on Alcoholism and Related Conditions. Archives of General Psychiatry. 2005;62(10):1097.

[77] Fischer B, Brissette S, Brochu S, Bruneau J, El-Guebaly N, Rehm J, et al. Determinants of overdose incidents among illicit opioid users in 5 Canadian cities. Canadian Medical Association Journal. 2004;171(3):235-239.

[78] Ozanne-Smith J, Centre MUAR, NPHPG. Pharmaceutical Poisoning to 0-19 Year Olds: National Public Health Partnership Public Health Planning and Practice Framework Trial. 2002 [cited 23/5/2012]. Report No.: 9780732614928. Available from: http://www.monash.edu.au/miri/research/reports/muarc193.pdf

[79] ACPM. Over The Counter Medications: Use In General and Special Population, Therapeutic Errors, Misuse, Storage and Disposal. Washington; 2011 [cited 28/4/2012]. Available from: http://www.acpm.org/resource/resmgr/timetools-files/otcmedstimetool.pdf

[80] Schillie SF, Shehab N, Thomas KE, Budnitz DS. Medication overdoses leading to emergency department visits among children. American Journal of Preventive Medicine. 2009;37(3):181-187.

[81] Conca AJ, Worthen DR. Nonprescription Drug Abuse. Journal of Pharmacy Practice. 2012 February 1, 2012;25(1):13-21.

[82] Gavrielatos G, Komitopoulos N, Kanellos P, Varsamis E, Kogeorgos J. Suicidal attempts by prescription drug overdose in the elderly: a study of 44 cases. Neuropsychiatric disease and treatment. 2006;2(3):359.

[83] Yin T, Miyata T. Warfarin dose and the pharmacogenomics of CYP2C9 and VKORC1--Rationale and perspectives. Thrombosis research. 2007;120(1):1-10.

[84] Klein T, Altman R, Eriksson N, Gage B, Kimmel S, Lee M, et al. Estimation of the warfarin dose with clinical and pharmacogenetic data. The New England journal of medicine. 2009;360(8):753.

[85] Nasser S, Mullan J, Bajorek B. Challenges of Older Patients' Knowledge About Warfarin Therapy. Journal of Primary Care & Community Health. 2012;3(1):65-74.

[86] AMA. Personalized health care report 2008: warfarin and genetic testing. 2008 [cited 15/7/2012]. Available from: http://www.ama-assn.org/ama1/pub/upload/mm/464/warfarin-brochure.pdf

[87] A misread abbreviation that led to a digoxin overdose. Prescriber. 2007;18(12):57-59.

[88] Majed AJ, Menyfah A, Mostafa A. Medication prescribing errors in a pediatric inpatient tertiary care setting in Saudi Arabia. BMC Research Notes. 2011;4(294):1-6.

[89] Awofisayo S, Uwanta E. Colorimetric Detection and Measurement of Paracetamol Exposure in Patients Prior Dispensing at a Pharmaceutical Care Centre. Int J Cur Biomed Phar Res. 2012;2(1):249-251.

[90] Bird SM, Hutchinson SJ. Male drugs-related deaths in the fortnight after release from prison: Scotland, 1996-99. Addiction. 2003;98(2):185-190.

[91] Binswanger IA, Stern MF, Deyo RA, Heagerty PJ, Cheadle A, Elmore JG, et al. Release from prison--a high risk of death for former inmates. New England Journal of Medicine. 2007;356(2):157-165.

[92] Binswanger IA, Blatchford PJ, Lindsay RG, Stern MF. Risk factors for all-cause, overdose and early deaths after release from prison in Washington state. Drug and alcohol dependence. 2011;117(1):1-6.

[93] Iguchi MY, Bell J, Ramchand RN, Fain T. How criminal system racial disparities may translate into health disparities. Journal of health care for the poor and underserved. 2005;16(4 Suppl B):48-56.

[94] Iguchi MY, London JA, Forge NG, Hickman L, Fain T, Riehman K. Elements of well-being affected by criminalizing the drug user. Public Health Reports. 2002;117(Suppl 1):S146.

[95] Fontana L, Beckerman A. Recently released with HIV/AIDS: primary care treatment needs and experiences. Journal of health care for the poor and underserved. 2007;18(3):699.

[96] Wallace C, Dargan P, Jones A. Paracetamol overdose: an evidence based flowchart to guide management. Emergency medicine journal: EMJ. 2002;19(3):202.

[97] Rigg KK, Iba≈Üez GE. Motivations for non-medical prescription drug use: A mixed methods analysis. Journal of substance abuse treatment. 2010;39(3):236-247.

[98] Yu MC, Tang LH, Chang KS, Narayan K, Chen KT. Risk factors associated with emergency room drug abuse admissions in urban Taiwan, 1998-1999. Journal of Addictions Nursing. 2005;16(4):195-198.

[99] Ernst FR, Grizzle AJ. Drug-related morbidity and mortality: updating the cost-of-illness model. JAPHA-WASHINGTON-. 2001;41(2):192-199.

[100] Mittmann N, Knowles SR, Gomez M, Fish JS, Cartotto R, Shear NH. Evaluation of the extent of under-reporting of serious adverse drug reactions: the case of toxic epidermal necrolysis. Drug safety. 2004;27(7):477-487.

[101] Lexchin J. Drug safety and Health Canada. The International Journal of Risk and Safety in Medicine. 2010;22(1):41-53.

[102] Corcoran P, Reulbach U, Keeley H, Perry I, Hawton K, Arensman E. Use of analgesics in intentional drug overdose presentations to hospital before and after the withdrawal of distalgesic from the Irish market. BMC clinical pharmacology. 2010;10(1):6.

[103] AbuMadini M, Abdel Rahim S. Deliberate self-harm in a Saudi university hospital: A case series over six years (1994-2000). Arab Journal of Psychiatry. 2001;12(2):22-35.

[104] Malik G, Bilal A, Mekki T, Al-Kinany H. Drug overdose in the Asir region of Saudi Arabia. Annals of Saudi Medicine. 1996;16(1):33.

[105] Al-Olah YH, Al Thiab KM. Admissions through the emergency department due to drug-related problems. Ann Saudi Med. 2008;28(6):426-9.

[106] Johnson EM, Porucznik CA, Anderson JW, Rolfs RT. State-Level Strategies for Reducing Prescription Drug Overdose Deaths: Utah's Prescription Safety Program. Pain Medicine. 2011;12:S66-S72.

[107] Alliance DP. Preventing Overdose, Saving Lives: Strategies for Combating a National Crisis. 2009 [cited 17/5/2012]. Available from: http://www.drugpolicy.org/docUploads/OverdoseReportMarch2009.pdf

[108] Medical JWGotNPFS, Committee SA, Staff NPF, Scotland SES, Executive SS, Medical S, et al. Prevention and Treatment of Substance Misuse: Delivering the Right Medicine: A Strategy for Pharmaceutical Care in Scotland: A Report of a Joint Working Group of the National Pharmaceutical Forum/Scottish Medical and Scientific Advisory Committee. 2005 [cited 23/5/2012]. Report No.: 9780755946938. Available from: http://www.scotland.gov.uk/Resource/Doc/57346/0017002.pdf

[109] Budnitz DS, Salis S. Preventing medication overdoses in young children: an opportunity for harm elimination. Pediatrics. 2011;127(6):e1597-e1599.

[110] Tucker C. Drug Takebacks Aim to Prevent Abuse, Protect Environment. Nations Health. 2011;41(2):1-3.

[111] Maklad AI, Emara AM, El-Maddah EI, El-Refai MAAM. PEDIATRIC POISONING IN EGYPT. Journal of Applied Pharmaceutical Science. 2012;2(02):01-06.

[112] Shah NG, Lathrop SL, Reichard RR, Landen MG. Unintentional drug overdose death trends in New Mexico, USA, 1990-2005: combinations of heroin, cocaine, prescription opioids and alcohol. Addiction. 2008;103(1):126-136.

[113] Smolen A. Role of the Pharmacist in Proper Medication Disposal. US Pharm. 2011;36(7):52-55.

[114] DHW. Prescription Drug Overdoses in Nova Scotia Working Group recommendations submitted to the Minister of Health and Wellness, the honourable Maureen MacDonald. [Nova Scotia Department of Health and Wellness]: Wellness DoHa; 2011 [cited 27/5/2012]. Available from: http://www.gov.ns.ca/DHW/Working-Group-Recommendations-Prescription-Drug-Overdoses.pdf

[115] HENMAN MC. The DUMP campaign. 2009 [cited 19/5/2012]. Available from: http://www.tara.tcd.ie/bitstream/2262/56870/1/IPJUN09DUMPCAMPAIGN.PDF

[116] Abou-Auda HS. An economic assessment of the extent of medication use and wastage among families in Saudi Arabia and Arabian Gulf countries. Clinical therapeutics. 2003;25(4):1276-1292.

[117] Grice G, Milligan P, Eby C, Gage B. Pharmacogenetic dose refinement prevents warfarin overdose in a patient who is highly warfarin-sensitive. Journal of Thrombosis and Haemostasis. 2008;6(1):207-209.

[118] Osman A, Ibrahim I. Deliberate Non-Fatal Self Harm in Patients Attending a General Hospital in Saudi Arabia. Arab J. Psychiatr.1997;8(1):31-41.

[119] Dart RC. Monitoring risk: post marketing surveillance and signal detection. Drug and alcohol dependence. 2009;105:S26-S32.

[120] Puspitasari IM, Soegijoko S. e-Prescription: An e-Health System for Preventing Adverse Drug Events in Community Healthcare. [cited 15/7/2012] Available from: http://www.ijljecp.or.id/files/IJCP_2012_1_1_5-11.pdf

Section 8

Research, Ethics, Social and Teaching Issues in Public Health

Chapter 26

Contribution of Biomedical Research Ethics in Public Health Advances

CN Fokunang, EA Tembe-Fokunang,
M. Djuidje Ngounoue, P.C. Chi, J Ateudjieu,
Awah Pascal, G. Magne, N.M. Ndje, O.M.T. Abena,
D. Sprumont and Kaptue Lazare

Additional information is available at the end of the chapter

http://dx.doi.org/10.5772/53695

1. Introduction

The term research refers to a class of activities designed to develop or contribute to generalizable knowledge. Generalizable knowledge consists of theories, principles or relationships, or the accumulation of information on which they are based, that can be corroborated by accepted scientific methods of observation and inference [1]. In the present context "research" includes both medical and behavioral studies pertaining to human health. Generally "research" is usually modified by the adjective "biomedical" to indicate that the reference is to health-related research [1, 2].

Progress in medical care and disease prevention depends upon an understanding of physiological and pathological processes or epidemiological findings, and requires at some time research involving human subjects. The collection, analysis and interpretation of information obtained from research involving human beings contribute significantly to the improvement of human health [3].

Research involving human subjects includes patient care (clinical research) and that undertaken on patients or other subjects, or with data pertaining to them, solely to contribute to generalizable knowledge (non-clinical biomedical research) [4]. Research is defined as "clinical" if one or more of its components is designed to be diagnostic, prophylactic or therapeutic for the individual subject of the research. Invariably, in clinical research, there are also components designed not to be diagnostic, prophylactic or therapeutic for the subject;

examples include the administration of placebos and the performance of laboratory tests in addition to those required to serve the purposes of medical care [5].

Advances in biomedical science and technology, and their application in the practice of medicine, are provoking some anxiety among the public and confronting society with new ethical problems. Society is expressing concern about what it fears would be abuses in scientific investigation and biomedical technology [1, 5]. This is understandable in view of the methodology of biomedical experimental research. Investigation begins with the construction of hypotheses and these are then tested in laboratories and with experimental animals. For the findings to be clinically useful, experiments must be performed on human subjects, and, even though carefully designed, such research entails some risk to the subjects [6]. This risk is justified not by any personal benefit to the researcher or the research institution, but rather by its benefit to the human subjects involved, and its potential contribution to human knowledge, to the relief of suffering or to the prolongation of life [7].

Society devises measures to protect against possible abuses. The first international code of ethics for research involving human subjects — the Nuremberg Code — was a response to the atrocities committed by Nazi research physicians, revealed at the Nuremberg War Crimes Trials [8]. Thus it was to prevent any repetition by physicians of such attacks on the rights and welfare of human beings that human-research ethics came into being. The Nuremberg Code, issued in 1947, laid down the standards for carrying out human experimentation, emphasizing the subject's voluntary consent. In 1964 the World Medical Association took an important step further to reassure society: it adopted the Declaration of Helsinki, most recently revised in 1989, which lays down ethical guidelines for research involving human subjects. In 1966 the United Nations General Assembly adopted the International Covenant on Civil and Political Rights, which entered into force in 1976, and which states (Article 7): *"No one shall be subjected to torture or to cruel, inhuman or degrading treatment or punishment. In particular, no one shall be subjected without his free consent to medical or scientific experimentation* ". It is through this statement that society expresses the fundamental, human value that is held to govern all research involving human subjects — the protection of the rights and welfare of all human subjects of scientific experimentation.

In the late 1970s, in view of the special circumstances of developing countries in regard to the applicability of the Nuremberg Code and the Declaration of Helsinki, the Council for International Organizations of Medical Sciences (CIOMS) and the World Health Organization (WHO) undertook a further examination of these matters, and in 1982 issued *Proposed International Guidelines for Biomedical Research Involving Human Subjects.* The purpose of the *Proposed Guidelines* was to indicate how the ethical principles that should guide the conduct of biomedical research involving human subjects, as set forth in the Declaration of Helsinki, could be effectively applied, particularly in developing countries, given their socioeconomic circumstances, laws and regulations, and executive and administrative arrangements [9].

Certain areas of research do not receive special mention in the guidelines; they include human genetic research, embryo and fetal research, and fetal tissue research. These represent research areas in rapid evolution and in various respects controversial.

The mere formulation of ethical guidelines for biomedical research involving human subjects will hardly resolve all the moral doubts that can arise in association with such research, but the guidelines can at least draw the attention of investigators, sponsors and ethical review committees to the need to consider carefully the ethical implications of research protocols and the conduct of research, and thus conduce to high scientific and ethical standards of research.

Given the different perceptions and priority views in the debate over the value and role of biomedical research, it is believed that the biomedical community must take stock and recommit its efforts to diseases that have a major effect on the population. This requires a re-evaluation of funding priorities, open interactions among researchers, and creating a more effective relations among stakeholders, government, foundations and institutions of higher learning. There is also the need for a shift in paradigm in biomedical research towards poverty related diseases and emerging diseases to reduce the 90/10 gap [6, 30].

2. International declarations and guidelines for ethical framework

The first international document on the ethics of research, the Nuremberg Code, was promulgated in 1947 as a consequence of the trial of physicians who had conducted atrocious experiments on unconsenting prisoners and detainees during the Second World War. The Code, designed to protect the integrity of the research subject, sets out conditions for the ethical conduct of research involving human subjects, emphasizing the human subject's "voluntary consent" to research.

To give the Universal Declaration of Human Rights, adopted by the United Nations General Assembly in 1948, legal as well as moral force, the General Assembly of the United Nations adopted in 1966 the International Covenant on Civil and Political Rights, of which Article 7 states " *No one shall be subjected to torture or to cruel, inhuman or degrading treatment or punishment. In particular, no one shall be subjected without his free consent to medical or scientific experimentation.* "

The Declaration of Helsinki, promulgated in 1964 by the World Medical Association, is the fundamental document in the field of ethics in biomedical research and has had considerable influence on the formulation of international, regional and national legislation and codes of conduct. The Declaration, revised in Tokyo in 1975, in Venice in 1983, and again in Hong Kong in 1989, is a comprehensive international statement of the ethics of research involving human subjects. It sets out ethical guidelines for physicians engaged in both clinical and non- clinical biomedical research, and provides among its rules for informed consent of subjects and ethical review of the research protocol [10].

The publication in 1982 of *Proposed International Guidelines for Biomedical Research Involving Human Subjects* was a logical development of the Declaration of Helsinki. As stated in the Introduction of that publication, the Guidelines were intended to indicate how the ethical principles embodied in the Declaration could be effectively applied in developing countries. The text explained the application of established ethical principles to biomedical research involving human subjects and drew attention to new ethical issues arising in the period that preceded its publication. The present publication, *International Ethical Guidelines for Biomedical Research Involving Human Subjects,* supersedes the 1982 *Proposed International Guidelines.*

CIOMS and WHO have continued to work together to provide ethical guidance for research involving human subjects. One important outcome of this cooperation has been *International Guidelines for Ethical Review of Epidemiological Studies,* published by CIOMS in 1991, intended to assist investigators and institutions as well as regional and national authorities in setting and maintaining standards for the ethical review of epidemiological studies [10].

2.1. Fundamental ethical principles

All research involving human subjects should be conducted in accordance with three basic ethical principles, namely respect for persons, beneficence and justice. It is generally agreed that these principles, which in the abstract have equal moral force, guide the conscientious preparation of proposals for scientific studies [11]. In varying circumstances they may be expressed differently and given different moral weight, and their application may lead to different decisions or courses of action. The present guidelines are directed at the application of these principles to research involving human subjects.

2.1.1. Respect for persons

Respect for persons incorporates at least two fundamental ethical considerations, namely:

a) respect for autonomy, which requires that those who are capable of deliberation about their personal choices should be treated with respect for their capacity for self-determination; and b) protection of persons with impaired or diminished autonomy, which requires that those who are dependent or vulnerable be afforded security against harm or abuse [12].

2.1.2. Beneficence

Beneficence refers to the ethical obligation to maximize benefits and to minimize harms and wrongs. This principle gives rise to norms requiring that the risks of research be reasonable in the light of the expected benefits, that the research design be sound, and that the investigators be competent both to conduct the research and to safeguard the welfare of the research subjects. Beneficence further proscribes the deliberate infliction of harm on persons; this aspect of beneficence is sometimes expressed as a separate principle, non-maleficience (do no harm).

2.1.3. Justice

Justice refers to the ethical obligation to treat each person in accordance with what is morally right and proper, to give each person what is due to him or her. In the ethics of research involving human subjects the principle refers primarily to distributive justice, which requires the equitable distribution of both the burdens and the benefits of participation in research. Differences in distribution of burdens and benefits are justifiable only if they are based on morally relevant distinctions between persons; one such distinction is vulnerability [13].

"Vulnerability" refers to a substantial incapacity to protect one's own interests owing to such impediments as lack of capability to give informed consent, lack of alternative means of obtaining medical care or other expensive necessities, or being a junior or subordinate member of a hierarchical group. Accordingly, special provisions must be made for the protection of the rights and welfare of vulnerable persons [14].

2.1.4. Research involving human subjects includes the following areas

i. controlled trials of diagnostic, preventive or therapeutic measures in larger groups of persons, designed to demonstrate a specific generalizable response to these measures against a background of individual biological variation

ii. studies designed to determine the consequences for individuals and communities of specific preventive or therapeutic measures; and studies concerning human health-related behaviour in a variety of circumstances and environmentsstudies of a physiological, biochemical or pathological process, or of the response to a specific intervention, whether physical, chemical or psychological- in healthy subjects or patients;

iii. Research involving human subjects may employ either observation or physical, chemical or psychological intervention; it may also either generate records or make use of existing records containing biomedical or other information about individuals who mayor may not be identifiable from the records or information. The use of such records and the protection of the confidentiality of data obtained from those records are discussed in *International Guidelines for Ethical Review of Epidemiological Studies [15].*

Research involving human subjects also includes research in which environmental factors are manipulated in a way that could affect incidentally-exposed individuals. Research is defined in broad terms in order to embrace field studies of pathogenic organisms and toxic chemicals under investigation for health-related purposes.

Research involving human subjects is to be distinguished from the practice of medicine, public health and other forms of health care, which is designed to contribute directly to the health of individuals or communities. Prospective subjects may find it confusing when research and practice are to be conducted simultaneously, as when research is designed to obtain new information about the efficacy of a drug or other therapeutic, diagnostic or preventive modality.

Research involving human subjects need to be conducted only by, or strictly supervised by, suitably qualified and experienced investigators and in accordance with a protocol that clearly states: the aim of the research; the reasons for proposing that it involve human subjects; the nature and degree of any known risks to the subjects; the sources from which it is proposed to recruit subjects; and the means proposed for ensuring that subjects' consent will be adequately informed and voluntary. The protocol should be scientifically and ethically appraised by one or more suitably constituted review bodies, independent of the investigators [16].

3. Consideration of some important ethical guidelines

3.1. Informed consent human participation in clinical research

3.1.1. Guideline 1: Individual informed consent

For all biomedical research involving human subjects, the investigator must obtain the informed consent of the prospective subject or, in the case of an individual who is not capable of giving informed consent, the proxy consent of a properly authorized representative [5, 13].

Informed consent is consent given by a competent individual who has received the necessary information; who has adequately understood the information; and who, after considering the information, has arrived at a decision without having been subjected to coercion, undue influence or inducement, or intimidation.

Informed consent is based on the principle that competent individuals are entitled to choose freely whether to participate in research. Informed consent protects the individual's freedom of choice and respects the individual's autonomy [17].

In itself, informed consent is an imperfect safeguard for the individual, and it must always be complemented by independent ethical review of research proposals. Moreover, many individuals, including young children, many adults with severe mental or behavioural disorders, and many persons who are totally unfamiliar with modern medical concepts, are limited in their capacity to give adequate informed consent [17]. Because their consent could imply passive and uncomprehending participation, investigators must on no account presume that consent given by such vulnerable individuals is valid, without the prior approval of an independent ethical-review body. When an individual is incapable of making an informed decision whether to participate in research, the investigator must obtain the proxy consent of the individual's legal guardian or other duly authorized representative [18].

When the research design involves no more than minimal risk- that is, risk that is no more likely and not greater than that attached to routine medical or psychological examination -and it is not practicable to obtain informed consent from each subject, the ethical review committee may waive some or all of the elements of informed consent [19]. Investigators should never initiate research involving-human subjects without obtaining each subject's informed consent, unless they have received explicit approval to do so from an ethical review committee.

3.1.2. Guideline 2: Essential information for prospective research subjects

Before requesting an individual's consent to participate in research, the investigator must provide the individual with the following information, in language that he or she is capable of understanding:

i. that each individual is invited to participate as a subject in research, and the aims and methods of the research; -the expected duration of the subject's participation; -the benefits that might reasonably be expected to result to the subject or to others as an outcome of the research;

ii. any foreseeable risks or discomfort to the subject, associated with participation in the research;

iii. any alternative procedures or courses of treatment that might be as advantageous to the subject as the procedure or treatment being tested;

iv. the extent to which confidentiality of records in which the subject is identified will be maintained;

v. the extent of the investigator's responsibility, if any, to provide medical services to the subject;

vi. that therapy will be provided free of charge for specified types of research-related injury;

vii. whether the subject or the subject's family or dependants will be compensated for disability or death resulting from such injury; and

viii. that the individual is free to refuse to participate and will be free to withdraw from the research at any time without penalty or loss of benefits to which he or she would otherwise be entitled [20].

3.1.3. Guideline 3: Obligations of investigators regarding informed consent

The investigator has a duty to:

1. communicate to the prospective subject all the information necessary for adequately informed consent;

2. give the prospective subject full opportunity and encourage- ment to ask questions;

3. exclude the possibility of unjustified deception, undue influence and intimidation;

4. seek consent only after the prospective subject has adequate knowledge of the relevant facts and of the consequences of participation, and has had sufficient opportunity to consider whether to participate;

5. as a general rule, obtain from each prospective subject a signed form as evidence of informed consent; and

6. Renew the informed consent of each subject if there are material changes in the conditions or procedures of the research [21].

3.1.4. Guideline 4: Inducement to participate

Subjects may be paid for inconvenience and time spent, and should be reimbursed for expenses incurred, in connection with their participation in research; they may also receive free medical services. However, the payments should not be so large or the medical services so extensive as to induce prospective subjects to consent to participate in the research against their better judgment ("undue inducement"). All payments, reimbursements and medical services to be provided to research subjects should be approved by an ethical review committee [21].

3.1.5. Guideline 5: Research involving children

Before undertaking research involving children, the investigator must ensure that:

i. children will not be involved in research that might equally well be carried out with adults;

ii. the purpose of the research is to obtain knowledge relevant to the health needs of children;

iii. a parent or legal guardian of each child has given proxy consent;

iv. the consent of each child has been obtained to the extent of the child's capabilities;

v. the child's refusal to participate in research must always be respected unless according to the research protocol the child would receive therapy for which there is no medically- acceptable alternative;

vi. the risk presented by interventions not intended to benefit the individual child-subject is low and commensurate with the importance of the knowledge to be gained; and

vii. interventions that are intended to provide therapeutic benefit are likely to be at least as advantageous to the individual child-subject as any available alternative [22]..

3.1.6. Guideline 6: Research involving persons with mental or behavioural disorders

Before undertaking research involving individuals who by reason of mental or behavioural disorders are not capable of giving adequately informed consent, the investigator must ensure that:

i. such persons will not be subjects of research that might equally well be carried out on persons in full possession of their mental faculties;

ii. the purpose of the research is to obtain knowledge relevant to the particular health needs of persons with mental or behavioural disorders;

iii. the consent of each subject has been obtained to the extent of that subject's capabilities, and a prospective subject's refusal to participate in non-clinical research is always respected;

iv. in the case of incompetent subjects, informed consent is obtained from the legal guardian or other duly authorized person;

v. the degree of risk attached to interventions that are not intended to benefit the individual subject is low and commensurate with the importance of the knowledge to be gained; and

vi. interventions that are intended to provide therapeutic benefit are likely to be at least as advantageous to the individual subject as any alternative [23].

3.1.7. Guideline 7: Research involving prisoners

Prisoners with serious illness or at risk of serious illness should not arbitrarily be denied access to investigational drugs, vaccines or other agents that show promise of therapeutic or preventive benefit.

3.1.8. Guideline 8: Research involving subjects in underdeveloped communities

Before undertaking research involving subjects in underdeveloped communities, whether in developed or developing countries, the investigator must ensure that:

i. persons in underdeveloped communities will not ordinarily be involved in research that could be carried out reasonably well in developed communities;

ii. the research is responsive to the health needs and the priorities of the community in which it is to be carried out;

iii. every effort will be made to secure the ethical imperative that the consent of individual subjects be informed; and

iv. the proposals for the research have been reviewed and approved by an ethical review committee that has among its members or consultants persons who are thoroughly familiar with the customs and traditions of the community [24].

3.1.9. Guideline 9: Informed consent in epidemiological studies

For several types of epidemiological research individual informed consent is either impracticable or inadvisable. In such cases the ethical review committee should determine whether it is ethically acceptable to proceed without individual informed consent and whether the investigator's plans to protect the safety and respect the privacy of research subjects and to maintain the confidentiality of the data are adequate [25].

3.1.10. Guideline 10: Equitable distribution of burdens and benefits

Individuals or communities to be invited to be subjects of research should be selected in such a way that the burdens and benefits of the research will be equitably distributed. Special justification is required for inviting vulnerable individuals and, if they are selected, the means of protecting their rights and welfare must be particularly strictly applied [26].

3.1.11. Guideline 11: Selection of pregnant or nursing (breastfeeding) women as research subjects

Pregnant or nursing women should in no circumstances be the subjects of non-clinical research unless the research carries no more than minimal risk to the fetus or nursing infant and the object of the research is to obtain new knowledge about pregnancy or lactation. As a general rule, pregnant or nursing women should not be subjects of any clinical trials except such trials as are designed to protect or advance the health of pregnant or nursing women or fetuses or nursing infants, and for which women who are not pregnant or nursing would not be suitable subjects [27].

3.1.12. Guideline 12: Safeguarding confidentiality

The investigator must establish secure safeguards of the confidentiality of research data. Subjects should be told of the limits to the investigators' ability to safeguard confidentiality and of the anticipated consequences of breaches of confidentiality [28].

3.1.13. Guideline 13: Right of subjects to compensation

Research subjects who suffer physical injury as a result of their participation are entitled to such financial or other assistance as would compensate them equitably for any temporary or permanent impairment or disability. In the case of death, their dependants are entitled to material compensation. The right to compensation may not be waived [29]

3.1.14. Guideline 14: Constitution and responsibilities of ethical review committees

All proposals to conduct research involving human subjects must be submitted for review and approval to one or more independent ethical and scientific review committees. The investigator must obtain such approval of the proposal to conduct research before the research is begun. The provisions for review of research involving human subjects are influenced by political institutions, the organization of medical practice and research, and the degree of autonomy accorded to medical investigators. Whatever the circumstances, however, society has a dual responsibility to ensure that [30]

- **i.** all drugs, devices and vaccines under investigation in human subjects meet adequate standards of safety; and
- **ii.** the provisions of the Declaration of Helsinki are applied in all biomedical research involving human subjects.

3.2. Externally sponsored research

3.2.1. Guideline 15: Obligations of sponsoring and host countries

Externally sponsored research entails two ethical obligations:

- **i.** An external sponsoring agency should submit the research protocol to ethical and scientific review according to the standards of the country of the sponsoring agency, and the ethical standards applied should be no less exacting than they would be in the case of research carried out in that country.
- **ii.** After scientific and ethical approval in the country of the sponsoring agency, the appropriate authorities of the host country, including a national or local ethical review committee or its equivalent, should satisfy themselves that the proposed research meets their own ethical requirements.

3.2.2. Definition

The term "externally sponsored research" refers to research undertaken in a host country but sponsored, financed, and sometimes wholly or partly carried out by an external international or national agency, with the collaboration or agreement of the appropriate authorities, institutions and personnel of the host country.

Ethical and scientific review. Committees in both the country of the sponsoring agency and the host country have responsibility for conducting both scientific and ethical review, as well as the authority to withhold approval of research proposals that fail to meet their scientific or ethical standards. Special responsibilites may be assigned to review committees in the two countries when a sponsor or investigator in a developed country proposes to carry out research in a developing country. When the external sponsor is an international agency the research protocol must be reviewed according to its own independent ethical review procedures and standards [31].

Committees in the external sponsoring country or international agency have a special responsibility to determine whether the scientific methods are sound and suitable for the aims of the research, whether the drugs, vaccines or devices to be studied meet adequate standards of safety, whether there is sound justification for conducting the research in the host country rather than in the country of the external sponsoring agency, and that the proposed research does not in principle violate the ethical standards of the external sponsoring country or international organization [32].

Committees in the host country have the special responsibility to determine whether the goals of the research are responsive to the health needs and priorities of the host country. Moreover, because of their better understanding of the culture in which the research is proposed to be carried out, they have special responsibility for assuring the equitable selection of subjects and the acceptability of plans to obtain informed consent, to respect privacy, to maintain confidentiality, and to offer benefits that will not be considered excessive inducements to consent.

In short, ethical review in the external sponsoring country may be limited to ensuring compliance with broadly stated ethical standards, on the understanding that ethical review committees in the host country will have greater competence in reviewing the detailed plans for compliance in view of their better understanding of the cultural and moral values of the population in which the research is proposed to be conducted [33].

3.2.3. Research designed to develop therapeutic, diagnostic or preventive products

When externally sponsored research is initiated and financed by an industrial sponsor such as a pharmaceutical company, it is in the interest of the host country to require that the research proposal be submitted with the comments of a responsible authority of the initiating country, such as a health administration, research council, or academy of medicine or science.

Externally sponsored research designed to develop a therapeutic, diagnostic or preventive product must be responsive to the health needs of the host country. It should be conducted only in host countries in which the disease or other condition for which the product is indicated is an important problem. As a general rule, the sponsoring agency should agree in advance of the research that any product developed through such research will be made reasonably available to the inhabitants of the host community or country at the completion of successful testing. Exceptions to this general requirement should be justified and agreed to all concerned parties before the research begins. Consideration should be given to whether the sponsoring agency should agree to maintain in the host country, after the research has been completed, health services and facilities established for purposes of the study [34].

3.2.4. Obligations of external sponsors

An important secondary objective of externally sponsored collaborative research is to help develop the host country's capacity to carry out similar research projects independently, including their ethical review. Accordingly, external sponsors are expected to employ and, if necessary, train local individuals to function as investigators, research assistants, or data managers or in other similar capacities. When indicated, sponsors should also provide facilities and personnel to make necessary health-care services available to the population from which research subjects are recruited.[34]. Although sponsors are not obliged to provide health-care facilities or personnel beyond that which is necessary for the conduct of the research, to do so is morally praiseworthy. However, sponsors have an obligation to ensure that subjects who suffer injury as a consequence of research interventions obtain medical treatment free of charge, and that compensation is provided for death or disability occurring as a consequence of such injury. Also, sponsors and investigators should refer for health care services subjects who are found to have diseases unrelated to the research, and should advise prospective subjects who are rejected as research subjects because they do not meet health criteria for admission to the investigation to seek medical care. Sponsors are expected to ensure that research subjects and the communities for which they are recruited are not made worse off as a result of the research (apart from justifiable risks of research interventions) — for example, by the diversion of scarce local resources to research activities. Sponsors may disclose to the proper authorities in the host country information that relates to the health of the country or community, discovered in the course of a study [35].

External sponsors are expected to provide, as necessary, reasonable amounts of financial, educational and other assistance to enable the host country to develop its own capacity for independent ethical review of research proposals and to form independent and competent scientific and ethical review committees. To avoid conflict of interest, and to assure the independence of committees, such assistance should not be provided directly to the committees; rather funds should be made available to the host-country government or to the host research-institution [36].

Obligations of sponsors will vary with the circumstances of particular studies and the needs of host countries. The sponsors' obligations in particular studies should be clarified before research is begun. The research protocol should specify what, if any, resources, facilities, assistance and other goods or services will be made available during and after the research, to the community from which the subjects are drawn and to the host country.The details of these arrangements should be agreed by the sponsor, officials of the host country, other interested parties, and, when relevant, the community from which subjects are to be drawn. The ethical review committee in the host country should determine whether any or all of these details should be made a part of the consent process [36].

4. World medical association declaration of Helsinki

It is the mission of the physician to safeguard the health of the people. His or her knowledge and conscience are dedicated to the fulfillment of this mission. The Declaration of Geneva of the World Medical Association binds the physician with the words, "The health of my patient will be my first consideration," and the International Code of Medical Ethics declares that "A physician shall act only in the patient's interest when providing medical care which might have the effect of weakening the physical and mental condition of the patient."

The purpose of biomedical research involving human subjects must be to improve diagnostic, therapeutic and prophylactic procedures and the understanding of the etiology and pathogenesis of disease.

In current medical practice most diagnostic, therapeutic or prophylactic procedures involve hazards. This applies especially to biomedical research.

Medical progress is based on research which ultimately must rest in part on experimentation involving human subjects.

In the field of biomedical research a fundamental distinction must be recognized between medical research in which the aim is essentially diagnostic or therapeutic for a patient, and medical research, the essential object of which is purely scientific and without implying direct diagnostic or therapeutic value to the person subjected to the research. Special caution must be exercised in the conduct of research which may affect the environment, and the welfare of animals used for research must be respected.

Because it is essential that the results of laboratory experiments be applied to human beings to further scientific knowledge and to help suffering humanity, the World Medical Association has prepared the following recommendations as a guide to every physician in biomedical research involving human subjects. They should be kept under review in the future. It must be stressed that the standards as drafted are only a guide to physicians all over the world. Physicians are not relieved from criminal, civil and ethical responsibilities under the laws of their own countries [37].

4.1. Basic principles

1. Biomedical research involving human subjects must conform to generally accepted scientific principles and should be based on adequately performed laboratory and animal experimentation and a thorough knowledge of the scientific literature.

2. The design and performance of each experimental procedure involving human subjects should be clearly formulated in an experimental protocol which should be transmitted for consideration, comment and guidance to a specially appointed committee independent of the investigator and the sponsor, provided that this independent committee is in conformity with the laws and regulations of the country in which the research experiment is performed.

3. Biomedical research involving human subjects should be conducted only by scientifically qualified persons and under the supervision of a clinically competent medical person. The responsibility for the human subject must always rest with a medically qualified person and never rest on the subject of the research, even though the subject has given his or her consent.

4. Biomedical research involving human subjects cannot legitimately be carried out unless the importance of the objective is in proportion to the inherent risk to the subject.

5. Every biomedical research project involving human subjects should be preceded by careful assessment of predictable risks in comparison with foreseeable benefits to the subject or to others. Concern for the interests of the subject must always prevail over the interests of science and society.

6. The right of the research subject to safeguard his or her integrity must always be respected. Every precaution should be taken to respect the privacy of the subject and to minimize the impact of the study on the subject's physical and mental integrity and on the personality of the subject.

7. Physicians should abstain from engaging in research projects involving human subjects unless they are satisfied that the hazards involved are believed to be predictable. Physicians should cease any investigation if the hazards are found to outweigh the potential benefits.

8. In publication of the results of his or her research, the physician is obliged to preserve the accuracy of the results. Reports of experimentation not in accordance with the principles laid down in this Declaration should not be accepted for publication.

9. In any research on human beings, each potential subject must be adequately informed of the aims, methods, anticipated benefits and potential hazards of the study and the discomfort it may entail. He or she should be informed that he or she is at liberty to abstain from participation in the study and that he or she is free to withdraw his or her consent to participation at any time. The physician should then obtain the subject's freely-given informed consent, preferably in writing.

10. When obtaining informed consent for the research project the physician should be particularly cautious if the subject is in a dependent relationship to him or her or may consent under duress. In that case the informed consent should be obtained by a physician who is not engaged in the investigation and who is completely independent of this official relationship.

11. In case of legal incompetence, informed consent should be obtained from the legal guardian in accordance with national legislation. Where physical or mental incapacity makes it impossible to obtain informed consent, or when the subject is a minor, permission from the responsible relative replaces that of the subject in accordance with national legislation. Whenever the minor child is in fact able to give consent, the minor's consent must be obtained in addition to the consent of the minor's legal guardian.

12. The research protocol should always contain a statement of the ethical considerations involved and should indicate that the principles enunciated in the present Declaration are complied with.

4.2. Medical research combined with professional care (Clinical research)

1. In the treatment of the sick person, the physician must be free to use a new diagnostic and therapeutic measure, if in his or her judgment it offers hope of saving life, reestablishing health or alleviating suffering.
2. The potential benefits, hazards and discomfort of a new method should be weighed against the advantages of the best current diagnostic and therapeutic methods.
3. In any medical study, every patient — including those of a control group, if any — should be assured of the best proven diagnostic and therapeutic method.
4. The refusal of the patient to participate in a study must never interfere with the physician-patient relationship.
5. If the physician considers it essential not to obtain informed consent, the specific reasons for this proposal should be stated in the experimental protocol for transmission to the independent committee.
6. The physician can combine medical research with professional care, the objective being the acquisition of new medical knowledge, only to the extent that medical research is justified by its potential diagnostic or therapeutic value for the patient.

4.3. Non therapeutic research involving human subjects (Non-clinical biomedical research)

1. In the purely scientific application of medical research carried out on a human being, it is the duty of the physician to remain the protector of the life and health of that person on whom biomedical research is being carried out.
2. The subjects should be volunteers, either healthy persons or patients for whom the experimental design is not related to the patient's illness.
3. The investigator or the investigating team should discontinue the research if in his/her or their judgment it may, if continued, be harmful to the individual.
4. In research on man, the interest of science and society should never take precedence over considerations related wellbeing of the subject.

5. The phases of clinical trials of vaccines and drugs

5.1. Vaccine development

Phase I refers to the first introduction of a candidate vaccine into a human population for initial determination of its safety and biological effects, including immunogenicity. This phase may include studies of dose and route of administration, and usually involves fewer than 100 volunteers.

Phase II refers to the initial trials examining effectiveness in a limited number of volunteers (usually between 200 and 500); the focus of this phase is immunogenicity.

Phase III trials are intended for a more complete assessment of safety and effectiveness in the prevention of disease, involving a larger number of volunteers in a multicentre adequately controlled study [5].

5.2. Drug development

5.2.1. Phase I

Phase I refers to the first introduction of a drug into humans. Normal volunteer subjects are usually studied to determine levels of drugs at which toxicity is observed. Such studies are followed by dose-ranging studies in patients for safety and, in some cases, early evidence of effectiveness.

5.2.2. Phase II

Phase II investigation consists of controlled clinical trials designed to demonstrate effectiveness and relative safety. Normally, these are performed on a limited number of closely monitored patients.

5.2.3. Phase III

Phase III trials are performed after a reasonable probability of effectiveness of a drug has been established and are intended to gather additional evidence of effectiveness for specific indications and more precise definition of drug-related adverse effects. This phase includes both controlled and uncontrolled studies.

5.2.4. Phase IV

Phase IV trials are conducted after the national drug registration authority has approved a drug for distribution or marketing. These trials may include research designed to explore a specific pharmacological effect, to establish the incidence of adverse reactions, or to determine the effects of long-term administration of a drug. Phase IV trials may also be designed to evaluate a drug in a population not studied adequately in the premarketing phases (such as children or the elderly) or to establish a new clinical indication for a drug. Such research is to be distinguished from marketing research, sales promotion studies, and routine post-marketing surveillance for adverse drug reactions in that these categories ordinarily need not be reviewed by ethical review committees

In general, Phase I drug trials and Phase I and Phase II vaccine trials should be conducted according to the articles of the Declaration of Helsinki that refer to non-clinical research. However, some exceptions can be justified. For example, it is customary and ethically justifi-

http://dx.doi.org/10.5772/53695

able to conduct Phase I studies of highly toxic chemotherapies of cancer in patients with cancer, rather than in normal volunteers as prescribed in the Declaration of Helsinki, Article III.2. Similarly be ethically it may be ethically justifiable to involve HIV-seropositive individuals as subjects in Phase II trials of candidate vaccines [37].

Phase II and Phase III drug trials should be conducted according to the articles of the Declaration of Helsinki that refer to "medical research, combined with professional care (clinical research)". However, the Declaration does not to provide for controlled clinical trials. Rather, it assures the freedom of the physician "to use a new diagnostic and therapeutic measure, if in his or her judgment it offers hope of saving life reestablishing health or alleviating suffering" (Article II.1). Also in regard to Phase II and Phase III drug trials there are customary and ethically justified exceptions to the requirements of the Declaration of Helsinki. A placebo given to a control group, for example, cannot be justified by its "potential diagnostic or therapeutic value for the patient", as Article II.6 prescribes. Many other interventions and procedures characteristic of late-phase drug development have no possible diagnostic or therapeutic value for the patients and thus must be justified on other grounds; usually such justification consists of a reasonable expectation that they carry little or no risk and that t contribute materially to the achievement of the goals of the research [37].

Phase III trials of vaccines do not use "a new diagnostic and therapeutic measure" that offers "hope of saving life, reestablishing health or alleviating suffering" (clinical research). Yet administration of the vaccine is intended to be a benefit to the subject rather than the purely scientific application of medical research carried out on a being" (non-clinical biomedical research). Thus, Phase III vaccine-trials do not conform to either of the categories defined in the Declaration of Helsinki.

6. Advances in biomedical research in 2012

Biomedical research in the United States is a $100 billion enterprise, with approximately 65% supported by industry, 30% by government (predominately the NIH), and 5% by charities, foundations, or individual donors. Although total sponsorship tripled between the mid-1990s and mid-2000s [15], the rate of increase has fallen since 2003 and declined in real (inflation-adjusted) terms since 2007 [3, 17]. The number of new drugs entering human trials has also fallen during the past two decades, especially for new molecular entities and entirely new classes of drugs. In contrast, the number of approvals of medical devices by the Food and Drug Administration (FDA) has increased steadily each year [23]. Driven by demand, total medical spending on devices has increased at a rate that is several times that for health services and twice that for drugs [5, 30].

Since the mid-1990s, the United States has invested approximately 4.5% of its total health expenditures on biomedical research. In contrast, only 0.1% supports research in health services, comparative effectiveness, new care models, best practices, and quality, outcome, or service innovations [37]. This funding will increase to approximately 0.3% from appropriations in 2010 health legislation.

Misconceptions regarding the scientific process are common. Research is costly, capital-intensive, and collaborative. Researchers in both academic and industrial settings require access to much the same information, samples and tissue, instrumentation, and specialized technical skills. They also depend on one another as a source of new ideas. It is a paradox, during this decade of growing scrutiny of ties between academic institutions and companies, that academic investigators value their nonfinancial company ties (with access to technology or research materials) more than personal compensation or support of their laboratory [4, 19]. Moreover, the notion that "pure" (basic) and "applied" (clinical) research exist as distinct activities is belied by their source of sponsorship and the self-reports of how researchers actually spend their time [27]. Such multimode researchers are more productive, as judged by the number of publications, impact factor, success at winning peer-reviewed NIH funding, and number of patents. This reality was cited by a recent U.S. Federal Court opinion overturning the patentability of several genes that predispose women to breast cancer. The court called for patenting practices that favor openness whenever basic discovery is inhibited [3, 20].

Sponsors have sought to improve their research productivity through the NIH Roadmap initiative (especially Clinical and Translational Science Awards) by encouraging alliances between companies and universities, alternative organizational models, and joint investment in costly facilities, such as imaging or gene sequencing [1, 23]. We reviewed the lessons from 70 such alliances from the mid-1960s through 2000 [5]. Although it is too soon to judge the success of the most recent models, in the main, earlier ones have not accelerated the pace of either discovery or clinical application. The sources of difficulty are idiosyncratic, but recurrent problems are a failure at inception to agree on intellectual-property provisions, excessive secrecy, and disagreements over research aims. In our view, the most salient reason for failure is the centralization of authority within large, inherently cautious bureaucracies in government, universities, foundations, and companies. Collectively, such factors inhibit scientists' creativity by disregarding the pluralism of ideas and the diversity of approaches that are necessary for innovation. Conversely, the most successful collaborations have found a balance between external direction and scientists' curiosity. Many of the most experienced observers from government, industry, and academia concur with this viewpoint [25, 31].

Economic forces are also relevant. In the United States, the gain in life expectancy between 1970 and 1990 added $2.4 trillion per year to the gross domestic product by 2000. Moreover, biomedical research bolsters employment, economic development, balance of trade, and exports. Studies from many countries show that investment in new technology of all types is the primary source of economic growth, especially when such investment is made by the private sector [2, 35]. In contrast, in areas in which public spending on technology is dominant, the rates of productivity and growth are lower. The differences are most marked in medical research [15, 44].

Despite these observations, some federal policymakers express doubt that scientific advance is a prerequisite for improved health. They favor predictable, low-cost public health measures and expanded access to basic care during the current decade of austerity [11, 26]. Other policymakers question whether spending on new devices and high-cost bioengineered drugs produce commensurate clinical value [7], 39. Such criticism is driven by estimates that new technology of marginal benefit (as measured by reduced disease burden or improved longevity) accounts for one half to two thirds of health care inflation in Western countries [31, 46] Even the commercial value of biomedical research is questioned by some companies, as is reflected by their reduced rates of research and development because of unfavorable returns as compared with marketing [1, 17], or mergers and acquisitions [6].

Other observers assert that social, educational, and macroeconomic factors are more important than medicine or public health practice in promoting a population's health [20]. They see technology as a distraction from enlightened social, tax, and regulatory policies. Debate over the goals has already begun [14, 22].

As a consequence, we believe that steps must be taken to reestablish public confidence in researchers and clinicians, along with their institutions. Measures are needed that go beyond those recommended by the Institute of Medicine [3] the Council of Medical Specialty Societies and the National Institute of Health. These reports emphasize remedies that focus primarily on competing interests without dealing with the opportunities. We are concerned that the recommendations overlook the potential for new models to foster productivity[52].

6.1. Seven remedies for consideration

The discontent arising from the current circumstances demands the consideration of sweeping changes in the way we conduct biomedical research. We believe that seven measures should be considered to reconcile competing goals. They require recognition of the multilayered sources of conflict, especially those based on different scientific aims and social values [15].

6.2. Improve data on clinical value

We must develop and apply better objective information about clinical value. This goal implies a higher standard for adopting new devices (including clinical trials similar to those for drugs) and better information on the effectiveness of existing drugs and devices, especially data that are available only from proprietary insurance databases. It is unlikely that provisions for comparative-effectiveness research in the 2010 health care legislation or the changes proposed by the FDA for device approval will be sufficient. New incentives are needed for private and government insurers to disclose clinical data to researchers, along with expanded access to device registries, easier access to data from Medicare and Medicaid, and development of more robust analytical techniques for ascertaining clinical value. Moreover, physicians and surgeons must commit to a new level of objectivity in judging clinical value, while resisting the influence of commercial potential or personal financial interests [13, 48].

6.3. Change the role of teaching hospitals

The roles of academic health centers and teaching hospitals must be modified to improve their ability to conduct early-stage (proof-of-concept) clinical trials. Here, entirely new models for interaction are required, probably involving freestanding independent institutes or autonomous units within academic centers, where patients come specifically for access to such early-stage studies and where the mutual expectations for investigators, companies, and patients are clear and unambiguous. This change will hasten the divergence between institutions that offer routine care (and that are managed to provide low-cost, reproducible high quality) and those with capability for scientific innovation (where early-stage investigations occur). Making these interactions effective and avoiding the shortcomings of past attempts will require new models of intellectual property, patents, and licensing by moving these aspects farther down the chain of discovery [5]. Two very different approaches should be tried: creating patent pools involving multiple companies and universities [19] and a renunciation of patenting in return for more latitude to conduct high-risk laboratory experimentation and initial clinical trials [26]. It is likely that only some of the 130 academic health centers will choose to undertake such changes.

6.4. Develop new models for collaboration and financing

In asserting the need for an increase of total spending on biomedical research and the need to foster the diversity of scientific approaches, consideration should be given to new models of collaboration and cooperation. Such measures would allow the NIH to concentrate on basic biomedical science and large, multi-institutional projects, where its scale can be most valuable, while providing offset to industry's declining investment in research. These models might include the following [6, 52].

6.5. Create a new class of bonds

States and the federal government might issue bonds to support innovation in biomedical science and health services, with preference given to high-risk research and diseases important to public health. Such bonds have long been used to support athletic facilities, airports, and roads. They provide a mechanism for private investment to meet public needs [18].

6.7. Defer patents to later in the discovery chain

In return for new sources of funding and greater latitude to conduct high-risk research, the new entities would forgo claims to patents or other intellectual property and place positive and negative findings immediately in the public domain.

Emphasizing new incentives, creating new entities, and mobilizing additional funding sources avoid the risk of disrupting productive research relationships currently found in universities, established research institutes, and the NIH. The measures also allow new laboratories to attract the best talent, while providing a route to enhance the productivity of research and its early clinical application [25].

6.8. Establish biomedical innovation trusts

The formation of new nonprofit, public–private partnerships, biomedical innovation trusts, could enable individuals and corporations to receive immediate federal tax credits for contributions to support research in high-priority diseases. Such trusts might be administered by decentralized new foundations or new regional public entities and be directed at particular diseases, universities, freestanding laboratories, or small companies. Similar tax incentives have been used historically to preserve land, create parks, and build factories [31, 54].

6.9. Use incentives to promote pluralism

To enhance the diversity of scientific approaches and innovation in its application, preference in funding might be given to new research institutes or entities, rather than existing universities or companies.

6.10. Renew professional commitments

All physicians must renew their commitment to professionalism and their duty to their patients. This will not be easy in an age when commercial values are paramount and the competition of the marketplace drives personal and institutional financial decisions. Yet, without such a recommitment, no safeguards will prevent an inexorable loss of trust in our institutions and us. Professionalism, as interpreted today, means not a return to paternalism, but objectivity in judgment on behalf of the patient, with open communication and an absence of bias [37]. It must be translated into action by a blanket proscription of product promotion in any guise.

6.11. Focus on cost-effective targets

We must recognize that new technology creates value to the general economy and has many clinical benefits but that it also usually spurs new clinical costs. Observers who are the most critical of medicine believe we have failed to recognize that historical compromise. In an era in which many favor public-policy goals to ensure a basic level of care for all citizens and a reduction in the rate of increase of aggregate health care spending, the technological imperative will surely be challenged with greater stridency. This requires incentives for researchers to focus on diseases that are common, cannot currently be prevented or effectively treated, are expensive, and have a major effect on the patients' health [2, 13]. Such choices among diseases are onerous but inescapable [47, 60].

6.12. Adopt realistic research goals

We must embrace a new realism about the difficulty of the scientific process and what can (and cannot) be expected from it. We must not overpromise. Such realism will not be popular with patient advocacy groups, the press, politicians, benefactors, or company investors. Each of these groups has a vested interest in overstating their case. Yet to do otherwise runs the risk of eroding the trust on which so much depends. Paradoxically, a commitment to realism may itself have a positive effect on the scientific process by reducing the pressure to promote findings prematurely and by fostering openness [13, 51].

6.13. Redefine the terms of conflict

Finally, we in medicine must recognize that those who have a public health perspective or who see social and economic factors as paramount will not be sympathetic to increasing the technology-driven momentum of the past 60 years. Inevitably, we face growing conflict over individual choice, access to the latest drug or device, the true cost of technology over a lifetime, perceptions of value, and preferences for competition versus regulation. Such tensions have long been implicit. They are now explicit. Not everyone believes biomedical research is essential [8].

7. Promotion of biomedical research in Sub Saharan Africa (SSA)

7.1. Setting the policies by SSA and stakeholders to prioritize funding for health research

The African heads of state during this decade have embarked on the need for poverty disease control supported by health research. In the Abuja Declaration of 2000, the heads of state pledged their commitments to apply strategies needed to improve on malaria control. They also called for additional resources to stimulate the development of malaria vaccines appropriate for Africa and to provide similar incentives for other anti-malaria technologies [39-41]. In addition the African Union has set a target of allocating 15% of national budget to the health sector, and 2% of health budget to finance health research. The AU countries reportedly agreed to allocate 1% of their countries GDP to research. In its 2008 report, the Global Forum for Health Research only list Liberia to have surpassed the set goal of allocating 15% of its national budget to the health sector by 2003; the report listed Burkina Faso, Central African Republic, Gabon, Gambia, Namibia, Niger and Tanzania to be just over 12%. Before then many of these countries invested very little in health systems. From this report, few low and middle income countries collect and report data on investments in health research [42, 53].

Since the 90s, there are only a few institutions enabling developing country scientists to undertake health research. The situation has since changed significantly, in terms of their allocations. There are currently a number of government agencies that support research, such as World Bank, European Union, World Health Organization (WHO), World Health Organization/Special Programme for Research and Training in Tropical Diseases (WHO/TDR), European Developing Countries Clinical Trials Partnership (EDCTP), Kenya Medical Research Institute (KEMRI), African Malaria Network (AMANET), Drug for neglected Diseases Initiatives (DNDI), National Institute of Health (NIH), Japanese Internatioanl cooperation (JICA), Department for International Development (DFID),), United Nation Development Programme (UNDP), Danish International Development Agency, Dutch Ministry of Foreign Affairs (DGIS), International Development Research Centre (IDRC), Swiss Development Cooperation (SDC), Swedish International Development cooperation agency (SIDA), United State Agency for International Development (USAID) and many other unlisted. Some private philanthropic support to health has been very beneficial in promoting health and reducing the 10/90 gap in sub-Saharan Africa. These include the Bill and Melinda Gates Foundation, EXXON Mobil, Rockefeller Foundation, Wellcome Trust, BH Billiton to name but a few. There are other self financing bodies supporting health research such as the Medical Research Council (MRC) of UK, National Institute of Health (NIH), GlaxoSmithKline (GSK), Pfizer, Norvatis and the United States Department of Defence (DOD) [58-60]

7.2. Major agencies promoting biomedical research and capacity building in Sub-Saharan Africa (SSA)

7.2.1. European Developing Countries Clinical Trials Partnership (EDCTP)

The European Developing Countries Clinical Trials Partnership (EDCTP) was created in 2003, as a European response to the global health crisis caused by malaria. HIV/AIDs and tuberculosis, three poverty-related diseases. EDCTP involves 15 members of the European Union, plus Norway, and Switzerland in partnership with the scientific community and policy makers from sub-Saharan Afica (SSA). The EDCTP started off with a five-year budget of €200 million; member states and the private sector were expected to each contribute a similar sum. EDCTP aims at accelerating the development of new or improved drugs, vaccines and microbicides, against HIV/AIDs tuberculosis and malaria, with a focus on phases II and III clinical trials in SSA. In its work, EDCTP supports clinical trials that combine capacity building and networking, in such a way that the developed human and infrastructure capacity is utilized to conduct multicenter trials, often spanning different SSA countries [52].

The impressive performance of EDCTP is reflected in is 2008 annual report when 21 projects were approved for funding, 27 project contracts worth €54 million were signed. The founding of CANTAM (Central Africa Network of Tuberculosis, HIV/AIDs and Malaria) with EDCTP support, in a research neglected area of Africa is worth mention www.edctp.org. With regard to promoting research and capacity building of researchers and research institutions in SSA, there is no doubt that none compares any closer to WHO/TDR, (the special Programme for Research and Training on Tropical Diseases) which is an independent global programme of scientific collaboration that helps to coordinate support of global efforts to combat major diseases of the poor and the disadvantaged [30].

7.2.2. World Health Organization/special programme for research and training in Tropical Diseases (WHO/TDR),

WHO/TDR was established in 1975, and therefore preceded by a decade and a half the work of the Commission on Health Research for Development, whose members included the founding Director of WHO/TDR. WHO/TDR is soibsired by UNICEF, UNDP, World Bank and WHO; it also receives funding from other agencies across the globe [61].

At the start WHO/TDR restricted its activities to addressing what were by then major neglected diseases, namely malaria, bancroftian filariasis, onchocerciasis, leprosy, leishmaniasis, and African and American trypanosomiasis. Dengue, intestinal helminthes, sexually transmitted infections and tuberculosis were added later. In its early years WHO/TDR made unequaled contributions not only to research on these diseases, but also contributed immensely to capacity building of research leaders in Africa today benefitted from WHO/TDR sponsorship. WHO/TDR also contributed financially and strategically to the development of many new tools and strategies against diseases of poverty. http://apps.who.int/tdr/.

7.2.3. The Kenya Medical Research Institute (KEMRI)

KEMRI established in 1979, operates 10 research centres across the country and employs over 200 national researches and another 500 technical staff. KEMRI has an annual budget of nearly

USD 40 million (of which one-half is Government of Kenya contribution). Several international research teams contribute another 45% KEMRI carries out national ethics review. Major achievements of KEMRI include; national policy basis for control of malaria, tuberculosis, leprosy and leishmaniasis, established surveillance and rapid response systems for major disease outbreaks, improved diagnostics such as KEMRI Hep-cell kit for Hepatitis, particle Agglutination (PA) kit for HIV, and HLA tissue typing techniques [42]

KEMRI successfully collaborated with the Government of Japan to establish global training centres for control of parasitic and infectious diseases. The KEMRI Institute of Tropical Medicine and Infectious Diseases, founded in collaboration with local Jomo Kenyatta University of Agriculture and Technology offers training at MSc and PhD levels. KEMRI founded the African Health Sciences Congress and African Health Journal. www.kemri.org/ (accessed 01/07/12). the progress made by KEMRI since its inception are attributable TO: (i) effective n-s and s-s collaboration (ii) implementation of innovative planning and initiatives, (iii) focused local capacity development and (iv) commitment of the national authorities to strengthen health research and development[23].

7.2.4. African Malaria Network Trust (AMANET)

AMANET has its origins in the African Malaria Vaccine Testing Network (AMVTN) which was established in 1995 with the primary goal of preparing African malaria research institutions to participate in malaria vaccine trials, in 2002, AMANET was registered as a Trust in Tazania and became the Legal successor of AMVTN. This change enabled AMANET to carry out holistic capacity strengthening of trial sites and Centres, and to take on legal responsibilities including sponsorship of trials. The change also signaled the network's commitment and interest in a wider range of malaria interventions, although malaria vaccine development would remain its main focus [29].

The mission of ANANET s to promote capacity strengthening and networking of malaria R&D in Africa, where it has provided institutions with support for essential infrastructure improvement, short-term training to over one thousand health researchers, and uniquely postgraduate degree training in preparation for participation in malaria vaccine development AMANET is funding over 40 projects across SSA, and is well known in Africa for its networks in vaccine trials, bioethics and the Afro-immunoassay network. AMANET also sponsors several blood stage malaria vaccine trials across Africa and has hosted the multilateral initiative on Malaria (MIM) since January 2006 [23]. AMANET Research Ethics capacity strengthens Grant: supported by the Gates foundation where identification of specific gaps in the ethical review process followed by a capacity building programme tailor-made for the identified gaps. A total of 32 ECs have been surveyed in Africa and benefitted from the capacity strengthening sub grants and training activities (www.amanet-trust.org): The south African Research Training initiative (SARETI); based at the University of Kwazulu-Natal and Pretoria University in South Africa, providing training inEthics to African researchers and ERC members. (www.whsph.up.ac.za/sareti/sareti/sareti.htm): The international Research Ethics Network for Southern Africa (IRENSA); based at the University of cape Town, running short term training programmes for mid-career African scientist and embers of Ethics Committees (www.irensa.org):The Training and Resources in research Ethics Evaluation (TRREE) for Africa, which focuses on development or research ethics educational programmes for e-learning and provision of e-resources [23].

7.2.5. Drugs for Neglected Diseases Initiative (DNDI)

DNDI was established in 2003 is a not-for-profit drug development organization, focused on improving the health and quality of life of people suffering from neglected diseases. DNDI was founded by Médicins Sans Frontières (MSF) with five public sector organizations, viz Kenya Medical Research Institute, Indian Council of Medical Research, Malaysian Ministry of Health, Oswaldo Cruz Fondation, Institute Pasteur France, and WHO/TDR as observer. DNDi support covers basic science, as well as preclinical and clinical research, focusing on human African trypanosomiasis, leishmaniasis, chaga's disease, and malaria. In 2007 DNDi in partnership with Sanofi Aventis, completed trial of a combination of Artesunate with Amo-diaquine (ASAQ), as a patent free drug against malaria. DNDi is also responsible for the HAT Platform which addresses Human African Trypanosomiasis (HAT) which is truly a neglected disease; there is very limited clinical research activity geared to improving its treatment or diagnosis, and it is endemic only in remote areas. The HAT platform was therefore established through a partnership of the five most affected countries (the Sudan, Democratic Republic of Congo, Uganda, Republic of Congo, and Angola) in collaboration with DNDi and the Swiss Tropical Institute, and other partners to build and strengthen clinical trial capacity including the search for appropriate diagnostics for HAT. In 2008, the HAT Platform received a US$68.2 million grant from the Bill & Melinda Gates Foundation for this purpose[23].

7.2.6. The Japanese chemical giant Sumitomo Chemical Company

They undertook R&D that led to production of Olyset Nets which incorporate an insecticide (permethrin) into the actual fibers of the net, and releases it slowly over a number of years. Olyset nets are guaranteed to last at least five years; they never need retreatment, are tear-resistant, ash proof, provide maximum ventilation; they inhibit mosquito (Anopheles spp.) biting, they repel, knockdown and kill mosquitoes. Olyset nets were the first long-lasting insecticidal net (LLIN) to be submitted and fully registered by the WHO Pesticide Evaluation Scheme (WHOPES) www.olyset.net/.[23]

In 2003 through a PPP a royalty-free technology transfer was undertaken under which Sumitomo Chemical Company would further develop Olyset nets, which eventually led to setting up a factory in Arusha, Tanzania, that was officially launched in early 2008; it aimed at producing 51 million units during 2009, employing 6000 people in Arusha alone, and supporting over 20,000 others. The factory in Arusha is now a 50/50 joint venture between Sumitomo Chemical Company and A to Z textile Mills, a Tanzania company. Another factory is being set up in Nigeria that will bring global production to more than 60 million nets annually, www.olyset.net/olysetnet/manurfacturinginafrica/ (accessed 06.07.12).

7.2.7.Medical research council UK

The MRC supports and advances medical research in three main ways: through their research facilities, by funding research centres in partnership with universities, and by providing research grants and career awards to scientists in UK universities and hospitals. Supporting scientists. Around 5,700 research staff are supported by the MRC, either employed directly in our institutes and units or funded through grants and fellowships. It spends about £86m on training awards for postgraduate students and fellows in 2011/12, including those in the MRC's own institutes and units[59].

The MRC expects valuable data arising from MRC-funded research to be made available to the scientific community with as few restrictions as possible so as to maximize the value of the data for research and for eventual patient and public benefit. Such data must be shared in a timely and responsible manner.The MRC believes that data sharers should receive full and appropriate recognition by funders, their academic institutions and new users for promoting secondary research. New studies that result from this data-sharing should meet the high standards of all MRC research regarding scientific quality, ethical requirements and value for money. It should also add recognizable value to the original dataset. Such research is often most fruitful when it is a collaboration between the new user and the original data creators or curators, with the responsibilities and rights of all parties agreed at the outset. Data arising from MRC-funded research must be properly curated throughout its life-cycle and released with the appropriate high-quality metadata. This is the responsibility of the data custodians, who are often those individuals or organisations that received MRC funding to create or collect the data[55].

Research fish (formerly known as MRC e-Val) gathers outputs, outcomes and impacts arising from MRC-funded research. MRC e-Val is an online survey designed to gather feedback from MRC-funded researchers about the results of their work. The aim is to compile accurate information about the outputs of MRC research and to capture impact as it occurs. This information will then be used to communicate the benefits of MRC funding; support evaluations of the economic, social and academic impact of MRC research; and provide evidence for strategy development. Information was sought across the whole MRC portfolio from all MRC researchers that had held MRC support since 2006 (approximately 3000 principal investigators) [60]. A full set of responses was submitted for 2541 Awards. This represents 83% of Awards that were invited to complete MRC e-Val as shown in figure 1.

8. Use of animal in biomedical research

8.1. Using animals in research: Benefits and ethical consideration

In 1780, Jeremy Bentham, an English Philosopher, first initiated the arguments of ethics in the vicinity of protection and treatment against animal by stating that animals should be treated equally as humans and they should not be neglected because they can not speak nor express their emotions [38]. In 1859, Darwin's theory on evolution placed human and animals on the same physical and emotional continuum. From late 19th century till now, a number of animal rights advocates have presented various arguments against animal uses in biomedical research. Using animals in the discovery of scientific knowledge is not only subject to the prosperity of mankind but also that of all species on earth:

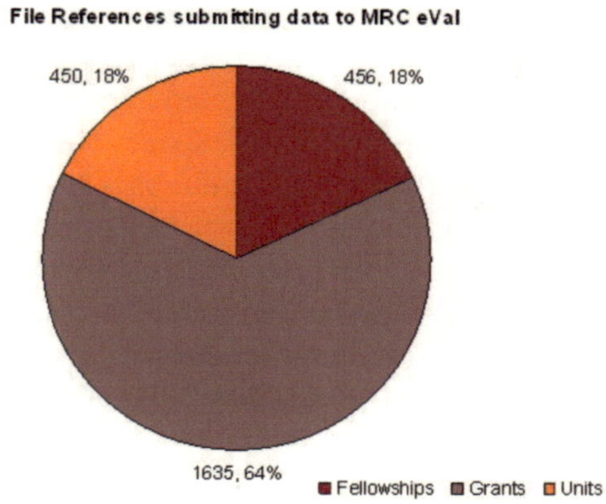

Figure 1. Representation of 83% of Awards that were invited to complete MRC e-Val [51]

The welfare of animals used in research, testing and teaching is affected by a combination of a number of factors. It is the combined effect of biological factors, environmental factors and interactions with the researchers that determine the welfare of animals used for research or teaching purposes [39]. The various factors that affect the welfare of animals used in research have been outlined in table 1.

Biological factors	Environmental factors	Interaction with researchers or teachers
Age if the animals	Ventilation of the room where the animals are kept	Nature of handing (gentle or rough; pain or distress could be caused)
Sex of the animals	Room temperature	Frequency of research procedures could be stressful
Reproductive status of the animals	Relative humidity of the room	Duration of manipulations or procedures (e.g. a class of students using animals in 5-h practical). The same animals may be used by more than one class over a certain period of time
Genetic factors based on the genotype of the animals	Diet during breeding and experimentation	Management practices such as number tags castration, dehorning and tail docking
Stress of the animals	Water availability for the animals	
Physiological/metabolic state of the animals	Light cycle and quality in the room where the animals are kept Noise in the vicinity of the room where the animals are kept Bedding in the cages Size of cages and number of animals per cage Transportation of animal	

Table 1. Types of independent factors that may affect welfare of animals used in research or teaching [46].

One of the strongest grounds of using animals in scientific research is the values of research toward animals and human beings. In the perspective of human health, many diseases such as small pox virus that our forefathers significantly suffered from have now been eradicated or controlled with the aid of biomedical research on animals. The use of animals in research is prevalent because they share at least 200 common illnesses and diseases with humans [38]. Animals are used in research or experimentation in place of human subjects for various reasons. Using animals in research affords the scientist to monitor reactions to stimuli and other variables in complex organs and tissue, while allowing the scientist to minimize environmental variables. Animals are used in scientific research to further science in many arenas. They are used most often in the following cases: Disease Treatment, Prevention, Treatment of Injuries, Basic Medical Testing, and Medical Diagnosis. Animals in research have made possible many scientific breakthroughs that humans benefit from each day such as in; Vaccinations, Anesthesia, Antibiotics, Numerous medical treatments for various diseases. Animals provide the scientist with unique possibilities especially using animals for medical research [39, 40].

When experimenting with new drugs for the treatment of disease it would be virtually impossible to isolate a human the way an animal can be isolated. All mammals share the same systems, there are variants but they are far outweighed by the likeness that humans and animals share. There are just certain testing that can not be accomplished without the use of live organs and tissue. There is no way to duplicate a complex disease in a culture, nor to enable a computer to completely analyze the effects of drugs on a system. Animals play a vital role in medical research [40-42].

8.1.2. Some facts about animal biomedical research

85 % of the animals used in research are rodents - rats and mice that have been bred for laboratory use. Most laboratory tests on animals are simple single type tests - change in diet, drawing a simple blood sample, administering a drug, Animals are given anesthetics if a procedure is going to be invasive in any way. Dogs, cats and non-human primates account for only 3 out of 1000 subjects in experimentation. Humans are still the largest group that is used for research and experimentation and beats out all other lab animals when it comes to testing [44].

A criterion which all scientists must follow is known as the three R's. The three R's in research refer to the following: Refinement, Reduction, and Replacement. Refinement of testing must be arranged so that animal distress is minimal. The scientist must reduce the number of animals used in the experimentation whenever possible and if possible, replace animals with other adequate research methods. There are animal restrictions in place to insure that animals are not used when not necessary[45]. When there are other viable models to conduct research those methods supposed to be used instead of using an animal subject. Only the minimal number of animals is to be used as subjects in an experiment or research project. Unnecessary research and experimentation is considered unethical and use of animals is not supported. The use of animals in research is heavily regulated[46]. The care is mandated through regulatory guidelines and there are heavy damages and fines assessed when these regulations are not followed. The regulations dictate how the animals will be housed and treated to include veterinary care, pain management and other measures to make sure the animals do not suffer throughout the course of the experiment. The scientist needs to get permission from an ethical committee, which have a full description of the project, before starting any research on animals, to ensure for minimum of suffer among the animals [47-49].

8.1.2.1. Replacement

Animals should be replaced in experiments by less sentient alternatives such as invertebrates or in vitro methods whenever possible.

8.1.2.2. Refinement

If animal experiments can not be avoided protocols should be refined to minimize any adverse effects for each individual animal. Appropriate anaesthesia and analgesia should be used for any surgical intervention. Humane endpoints should be used whenever possible. Staff should be well trained, and housing should be of a high standard with appropriate environmental enrichment. Animals should be protected from pathogens[50, 51].

8.1.2.3. Reduction

The number of animals should be reduced to the minimum consistent with achieving the scientific objectives of the study, recognizing that important biological effects may be missed if too few animals are used. Alternatively, methods should be found to obtain more information from each experiment, thus speeding up the pace of research. This can be achieved by careful control of variation and by appropriate experimental design and statistical analysis [52]..

The use of animals in medical research remains essential. However, in accordance with the law, scientists must avoid using animals wherever possible. If applying for funding for studies involving animals, researchers must give sound scientific reasons for using them and explain why there are no realistic alternatives [52, 55] Around 30 per cent of the research we fund involves animals. Some of the key players involved in one way or another in promoting the implementation of the 3 Rs and the dissemination of information about alternatives to animals in research and teaching are illustrated in table 2.

Organization	**Web site address**
European centre for the Validation of Alternative Methods (ECVAM)	http://ecvam.jrc.it/index.htm(Accessed on 04 June 2009).
Interagency Coordinating Committee on Validation of Alternative methods (ICCVAM) in the USA	http://iccvam.niehs.nih.gov/(Accessed on 04 June 2009).
National interagency Center for the Evaluation of Alternative Toxicological methods (NICEATM) which provides support to the ICCVAM	http://ntp.niehs.nih.gov/ntpweb/index.cfm?objectid =7182FF48-BDB7-CEBA-F8980E5DD01A1E2D (accessed on 04 June 2009)
Norwegian Reference Centre for laboratory Animal Science and Alternatives that maintains the NORINA database containing guidelines on use of animals in	

Organization	Web site address
research as well as audiovisual aids and other teaching materials.	
Alternative to Animal Testing Web Site (Alweb) developed by the John Hopkins Centre for Alternatives to Animal Use	Htt://www.altweb.org (accessed on 04 June 2009)
InterNICHE which promotes humane use of animals in education	www.interniche.org (accessed on o4 June, 2009)
The Netherlands Centre for Alternatives to Animal Use	www.nca-nl.org (accessed on 04 June 2009)
Australian and New Zealand Council for the Care of Animals in Research and teaching (ANZCCART)	anzccart@adelaide.edu.au (Accessed on 04 June 2009).

Table 2. some organizations involved in promoting implementation of the 3Rs [53].

9. Conclusion

Ethical consideration in biomedical research has created a great impact in improving clinical trial research initiatives in both low income economies and industrialized nations. However the lack of scientific expertise and the slow response of scientists, sponsors to ethical questions involving some clinical projects has had a negative effect in the promotion of ethics in biomedical research initiatives. These considerations will require decades of reorientation of our biomedical research efforts. The failure to resolve ethical conflicts be it politically motivated, policy-related, or personal (scientist bias), claims of legitimately competing priorities has limited progress in biomedical research and has encouraged new regulatory constraints in new product development. The IRBs should therefore build a solid working framework, advance capacity building strategies and implement a synergy working platform to promote biomedical and clinical research geared to promote science contribution to human development.

It is also of importance to recognize the contribution of animals used in biomedical research to the good health of humans as well as animal, as moral agents, human beings should always make efforts to ensure that animals are treated humanely in research and teaching.

Efforts should be made to uphold the principles of 3Rs, which ensures that researchers should replace animals with other alternatives whenever possible, and if not possible then the number of animals used should be reduced to the minimum possible sample size as regards to the required statistical power, and refine the methodologies in order to minimize any harm that may be caused by the experimental procedures. It is a welcome idea for the creation of animal ethics committee, and the development of credible national ethics and legal framework, capacity building of research on humane treatment of experimental animals and dialogue among the different stakeholders concerned with the welfare of animal implicated in research.

Special effort have been made to identify some key players in the promotion of biomedical research and their responsibilities, and all the guidelines indicated in this study are intended to protect research participants, and uphold the fundamental ethical principles.

http://dx.doi.org/10.5772/53695

Although there are many action put in place to resolve the 10/90 gap and much has been achieved, the gap still persist. There is the need for more investments towards strengthening of capacities in health research and institutions in sub-saharan Africa to bridge the 10/90 gap.There is also the need to find better ways of translating health research results conducted within the framework of fundamental ethical principles into action and policy implementations.

Acknowledgements

The authors wish to thank the Council for International Organizations of Medical Sciences (CIOMS), the World Health Organization (WHO) for the free accessible document that facilitated the preparation of this document. International Ethical Guidelines for Biomedical Research Involving Human Subjects of Geneva 1993 that was very useful for the preparation of this document. The national ethics committee of Cameroon for the technical support in putting together this writes up. The Ministry of Higher Education is also acknowledged for the research allowance that supported processing charge of the manuscript.

Author details

CN Fokunang[1,2,3], EA Tembe-Fokunang[1], M. Djuidje Ngounoue[2], P.C. Chi[2], J Ateudjieu[2], Awah Pascal[4], G. Magne[2], N.M. Ndje[2], O.M.T. Abena[1], D. Sprumont[5] and Kaptue Lazare[2]

*Address all correspondence to: charlesfokunang@yahoo.co.uk

1 Faculty of Medicine and Biomedical Sciences, University of Yaoundé 1, Cameroon

2 Cameroon National Ethics Committee (CNEC), Yaoundé, Cameroon

3 Faculty of Health Sciences, University of Bamenda, Bambili, Cameroon

4 Department of Philosophy, Faculty of Arts and Social Sciences, University of Yaoundé 1, Cameroon

5 Chaire de Droit de la Santé, University of Neuchatel, Switzerland

References

[1] Barrett DH, Bernier RH, Sowell AL .Strengthening public health ethics at the centers for disease control and prevention.; Centers for Disease Control and Prevention Public Health Ethics Committee Steering Group. Journal Public Health Management Practice. 2008; 14(4):348-53.

[2] Beauchamp, T.L., Childress, J.F. Principles of Biomedical Ethics, 5th edition Oxford University Press. 2001.

[3] Beauchamp, T. The concept of paternalism in biomedical ethics. In Beauchamp, T. Standing on principles. New York: Oxford University Press 2010; pp. 101–119).

[4] Beecher, H.K. Ethics and Clinical Research. New England Journal of Medicine. 1966. 274, 1354.

[5] Benatar, S. R. (2002). Reflections and recommendations on research ethics in developing countries. Social Science and Medicine, 54(7), 1131–1141.

[6] Bernheim, R.G., Melnick, A. Principled leadership in public health: integrating ethics into practice and management. Journal Public Health Management Practice.2008; 14(4):358-66.

[7] Beskow, L.M., Namey, E.E., Cadigan, R.J., Brazg, T., Crouch, J., Henderson, G.E., Michie M., Nelson, D.K., Tabor, H.K., Wilfond, B.S. Research participants' perspectives on genotype-driven research recruitment. Journal of Empirical Research for Human Research Ethics.2011; 6(4):3-20.

[8] Bhutta, Z.A., (2002). Ethics in international health research:a perspective from the developing world. Bulletin WHO, 80:114-120.

[9] Buchanan, D. R. Autonomy, paternalism, and justice: Ethical priorities in public health. American Journal of Public Health, 2008; 98(1), 15.

[10] Cadigan, R.J., Michie, M., Henderson, G., Davis, A.M., Beskow, L.M. The meaning of genetic research results: reflections from individuals with and without a known genetic disorder.J Empirical Research and Human Research Ethics. 2011; 6(4):30-40.

[11] Chilengi, R. An ethics perspective on responsibilities of investigators, sponsors and research participants. Acta Tropica, 2009; 112S:S53-S62.

[12] Council for International Organizations of Medical Sciences (CIOMS) .International Guidelines for Biomedical Research Involving Human Subjects. Geneva.CIOMS; 2002; pp.112.

[13] Department of Health. Tackling health inequalities: 10 years on, Publication No. 291444, London: Crown.2009.

[14] Emanuel, E., Wendler, D., Killen, J., and Grady, C. What makes clinical research in developing countries ethical? the benchmarks of ethical research. The Journal of Infectious Diseases,2004; 189(5), 930–937.

[15] Fineberg, H.V.Shattuck Lecture. A successful and sustainable health system--how to get there from here. North England Journal of Medicine. 2012; 15; 366(11):1020-7.

[16] Gitau-Mburu, D. Should public health is exempt from ethical regulations? Intricacies of research versus activity.East Africa Journal of Public Health. 2008; (3):160-2.

[17] Gollust, S.E., Baum, N.M., Jacobson, P.D. Politics and public health ethics in practice: right and left meet right and wrong. Journal of Public Health Management Practice. 2008. 14(4):340-7.

[18] Huddle TS. Honesty is an internal norm of medical practice and the best policy.American Journal of Bioethics.2012; 12(3):15-27.

[19] Hyder, A.A., Merritt, M., Ali, J., Tran, N.T., Subramaniam, K., Akhtar, T. Integrating ethics, health policy and health systems in low- and middle-income countries: case studies from Malaysia and Pakistan. Bulletin World Health Organization.2008; 86 (8): 606-611.

[20] International Conference on Harmonization (ICH) Guidelines for Good Clinical Practice,1996. Available freely on the websites and other sources.

[21] Jefferson, A.L., Carmona, H., Gifford, K.A., Lambe, S., Byerly, L.K., Cantwell, N.G., Tripodis, Y., Karlawish, J. Clinical Research Risk Assessment among Individuals with Mild Cognitive Impairment. American Journal of Geriatrics and Psychiatry. 2012; 30. 12-30.

[22] Joyce, G.F., Carrera, M.P., Goldman, D.P., Sood, N., Physician prescribing behavior and its impact on patient-level outcomes.American Journal of Management Care. 2011; 1;17(12):e462-71.

[23] Kilama, W.L. The 10/90 gap in sub-Saaran Africa: Resolving inequities in health Research. Acta Tropica 2009; 112S:S8-S15.

[24] Kost, R.G., Lee, L.M., Yessis, J., Coller, B.S., Henderson, D.K. Assessing research participants' perceptions of their clinical research experiences; Research Participant Perception Survey Focus Group Subcommittee. Clinical Translational Science.2011; 4(6): 403-13.

[25] Krech R.Working on the social determinants of health is central to public health. Journal Public Health Policy.2012; 33(2):279-84.2012.10.

[26] Lavery, J.V., Harrington, L.C., Scott, T.W. Ethical , Social, and Cultural considerations for the site selection for research with genetically modified mosquitoes. American Journal of Tropical Medicine and Hygiene, 2008; 79 (3), 312-318.

[27] London AJ, Kimmelman J, Carlisle B . Research ethics. Rethinking research ethics: the case of post-marketing trials. Science 2012; 4; 336(6081):544-5.

[28] Nicholas, J. Next steps in clinical trial redesign. Journal of National Cancer Institute. 2012; 18;104(2):90-2.

[29] Nuffield Council on Bioethics. Public health: Ethical issues. Cambridge: Cambridge Publishers, 2007, p212.

[30] Nyika, A., Kilama, W., Chilengi, R., Tangwa, G., Tindana, P., Ndebele, P., Ikingura, J., Composition, training needs and independence of ethics review committees across

Africa: are the gate-keepers rising to the emerging challenges? Journal of Medical Ethics, 2009: 35, 189-193.

[31] Omonzejele, P.FIs the codification of vulnerability in international documents a sufficient mechanism of protection in the clinical research ethics context? Medical Law. 2011: 30(4):497-515.

[32] Reiter-Theil, S., Agich, G.J., Research on clinical ethics and consultation. Introduction to the theme. Medical Health Care Philos. 2008; 11(1):3-5.

[33] Sade, R.M. Why physicians should not lie for their patients. American Journal of Bioethics. 2012:12(3):17-9.

[34] Tangwa, G.B., Ethical principles in health research and review process. Acta Tropica, 2009. 112S:S2-S7.

[35] Thomas, J.C., MacDonald, P.D., Wenink, E., Ethical decision making in a crisis: a case study of ethics in public health emergencies : Journal Public Health Management Practice; 2009. 15, (2):E16-21.

[36] Wikler, D., and Brock, D. W. Population-level bioethics: Mapping a new agenda. In Dawson, A., and Verweij, M, Ethics, prevention, and public health, 2007. p. 78. New York: Oxford University Press.

[37] World Medical Association Declaration of Helsinki, Available at http://www.wma.net/e/policy/17-c-e.html. Ethical principles for Medical Research Involving Human Subjects. 52nd WMA General Assembly, Edinburgh, Scotland. www.dndi.org (accessed 04.08.12).

[38] Blakemore C: Misguided thinking on animals. Nature 1989;339:414.

[39] Bowman P: Institutional animal care and use committee review of wildlife field research. Lab Animal 1989;18:28-30.

[40] Britt D: Ethics, ethical committees and animal experimentation. Nature 1984;311:503-506.

[41] Dawkins MS: From an animal's point of view: Motivation, fitness, and animal welfare. Behav Brain Sci 1990;13:1-61.

[42] Duggan JM: Resource allocation and bioethics. Lancet 1989;1:772-773.

[43] Fox MW: A call for common understanding of animal welfare, animal rights, and animal well-being. J Am Vet Med Assoc 1990;196:832-833.

[44] Good RA: The value of animal research. Science 1990;248:538

[45] Harvard University's Office of Government and Community Affairs: The Animal Rights Movement in the United States: Its Composition, Funding Sources, Goals, Strategies and Potential Impact on Research. Clarks Summit, PA, Society for Animal Rights, Inc., 1982..

[46] Hoff C: Immoral and moral uses of animals. New England Journal of Medicine 1980;302:115-118.

[47] Lutts RH: The Nature Fakers: Wildlife, Science and Sentiment. Golden, CO, Fulcrum Publishing, 1990.

[48] Markell DL: The case for revising our laws on animal experimentation. International Journal for the Study of Animal Problems 1981;2:87-95.

[49] Meischke HRC, Begbie RA: Philosophical and moral aspects of the use of animals in experimentation. Australian Veterinary Association Yearbook 1981;232-237.

[50] Miller HB, Williams WH: Ethics and Animals. Clifton,NJ, Humanic Press, 1983..

[51] National Research Council: Use of Laboratory Animals in Biomedical and Behavioral Research. Washington, D.C., National Academy Press, 1988..

[52] Thelestam M, Gunnarsson A: The ethics of animal experimentation. Proceedings of the second CFN symposium held in Stockholm, Sweden, August 12-14, 1985. Acta Physiologica Scandinavica 1986;128:269pp.

[53] National Commission for the Protection of Human Subjects of Biomedical and Behavioural Research subjects (NCPHSBBRS). Protection of Human Subjects: Institutional Review Boards. Fed Regist; 1978; 43:231-561.

[54] ICH-GCP E6. International Conference on Harmonization Guidance: Good Clinical Practices. Global Medical Education and Development. 1997. Available at http//www.icr-global.org.

[55] Lavery VJ, Grady C, Wahl RE, Emmanuel JE. Ethical issues in International Biomedical Research: A case book, Oxford University Press, 2007.

[56] United Nation. Universal Declaration of Human Rights. Available at http://www.un.org/en/document/udhr/.1948.

[57] World Health Organization. Operational Guidelines for ethics committees that review biomedical research, available at http://apps.who.int/tdr/svc/publications/training-guideline-publications/operational-guidelines-ethics-biomedical-research, 2000.

[58] Shemdoe GS. Introduction to intellectual property rights for investigator in health research and institutional intellectual property policy. Acta Tropica 2009; 112S:S80-S83.

[59] Kilama W. From Research to control: Translating research findings into health policies operational guidelines and health products. Acta Tropica, 2009; 112S:S91-S101.

[60] World Medical Association. Declaration of Helsinki. Ethical principles for research involving human subjects. Adopted by the 52 nd WMA General Assembly, Seoul, South Korea, 2008.

[61] Amir JA. Research and Legal Liability. Acta Tropica, 2009;112S:S71-S75).

Chapter 27

The Role of Ethics in Public Health Clinical Research

C. N. Fokunang, E. A. Tembe-Fokunang, P. Awah,
M. Djuidje Ngounoue, P. C. Chi, J. Ateudjieu,
R. Langsi, Lazare Kaptue and O. M. T. Abena

Additional information is available at the end of the chapter

http://dx.doi.org/10.5772/52478

1. Introduction

The public health ethics look at the moral basis of the health of human as a guiding support put in place to maximize welfare, and therefore health as a component of welfare [1,2]. This view frames the core moral challenge of public health as balancing individual liberties with the advancement of good health outcomes.

An alternative view of public health ethics characterizes the fundamental problematic of public health ethics differently: what lies at the moral foundation of public health is social justice [2]. While balancing individuals' liberties with promoting social goods is one area of concern, it is embedded within a broader commitment to secure a sufficient level of health for all and to narrow unjust inequalities [2, 3]. Another important area of concern is the balancing of this commitment with the injunction to maximize good aggregate or collective health outcomes. Public health ethics has therefore a strong moral connection to broader questions of social justice, poverty, and systematic disadvantage [3,4].

1.1. Historical ethical perspective

Although there have been some manifested concerns about the vulnerability of human subjects implicated in clinical research for over a century, it was the scandals and tragedies of the Nazi doctors during the second World War that gave birth to the discipline of bioethics [4, 5]. Other recent concerns in bioethics are attempting to extend ethical debate beyond the one-to-one physician-patient relationship, to enter the domain of public health where focused is geared towards the health of the entire populations. In the Africa setting, these extended concerns are being driven in part by the persisting iniquities and disparities in the health status of the low income resource countries and the rich countries, the differences in access to health services, the differences in the effort put into solving health problems, whereby the larger health burdens of the South receive scarce research attention, and the fewer problems of the North receive most of the attention in what has been termed the 10/90 gap [6, 35]. More attempts made to redress these inequalities have led to greater research investment and North-South research collaboration with the aim of solving the major health problems affecting the population in the poor countries of the South [7, 35].

1.2. The Ethical fundamental principles

Four fundamental principles of ethics have been universally recognized namely; autonomy, beneficence, non-maleficence and justice. These principles universally deals with the respect for all other humans as moral equals, making sure that all our actions are intended to achieve results with less harm, and treating others with fairness and equity [8, 48].

1.2.1. Beneficence and non maleficence

The principle of beneficence and non-maleficence are best considered together as they are like mirror images of each other. Literally beneficence means doing good and non-maleficence means avoiding evil or harm [9, 38, 42].

1.2.2. The harm principle

It is likely that no classic philosophical work is cited more often in the public health ethics literature than John Stuart Mill's essay "On Liberty" [10]. In that essay, Mill defends what has come to be called the harm principle, in which the only justification for interfering with the liberty of an individual, against her will, is to prevent harm to others. The harm principle is relied upon to justify various infectious disease control interventions including quarantine, isolation, and compulsory treatment. In liberal democracies, the harm principle is often viewed as the most compelling justification for public health policies that interfere with individual liberty [10, 19]. For example, a prominent view in the United States is that it was not until the public became persuaded of the harmful effects of "second hand smoke" that the first significant intrusion into smoking practices—the banning of smoking in public places—became politically possible. Perhaps because of the principle's broad persuasiveness, it is not uncommon to see appeals made about harm to others in less than obvious contexts [11]. Defenders of compulsory motorcycle helmet laws, for example, argued that the serious head injuries sustained by unprotected cyclists diverted emergency room personnel and resources, thus harming other patients[12, 32]. The harm principle has been interpreted to include credible threat of significant economic harm to others as well as physical harm. Regarding smoking policy, various restrictions on the behavior of smokers have been justified by appeal to the financial burden on the health care system of caring for smoking-related illnesses [13].

As with all such principles, questions remain about its specification. How significant must the threat of harm be, with regard to both its likelihood and magnitude of effect? Are physical harms to the health of others to be weighted more than economic harms or other setbacks to interests? Whether interpreted narrowly or broadly, there are limits to the public health cases that can plausibly be placed in the harm principle box [14, 15]. Moreover, in the context of commitments to social justice and general welfare, and the other justifications described above, too exclusive a focus on the harm principle can undermine otherwise justifiable government mandates and regulation. It is undeniable that individuals have much broader and more multidimensional interests than narrowly self-directed physical ones, and in that sense, it is not unreasonable to have a fairly expansive understanding of "harm" in a public health context [16-18]. The summary of the fundamental ethical principles and their applications in public health and biomedical research illustrated by Chilengi [17], is shown in table 1.

PRINCIPLES	DESCRIPTION	APPLICATION
AUTONOMY	Human beings are born as autonomous agents. This autonomy gives them the rights to self determination that must be respected. Autonomy demands that the wishes of all persons must be respected and we do so by asking their opinion or willingness to get involved or not	Informed Consent
NON-MALEFICENCE	*Primun non nocere,* Latin translation for first, do no harm. Research must primarily and actively seek not to do harm regardless of the extent of potential good that may arise from the research.	Evaluate foreseeable risks and minimize harm
BENEFICENCE	While minimizing harm research must be of benefit to individuals and society at large. Beneficence is a group of norms for providing benefits and balancing benefits against risks and costs	Maximize benefits
JUSTICE	A group of norms for distributing benefits risks and costs fairly. The benefits of research must equitably be shared by those who bore the cost and risk of the research.	Fair subject selection and fair distribution of benefits.

Table 1. Summary of fundamental ethical principles and their applications in public health and biomedical research [17].

2. Some challenges related to public health research ethics

There is no standardized method of organizing either the ethics of clinical practice, or the public health and biomedical research. Although these distinctive concerns are often dealt with under the broader term of bioethics, sometimes bioethics is presented as the equivalent of medical ethics. Whichever approach is preferred, a key question remains: what distinguishes public health ethics from medical ethics? The answer lies in the distinctive nature of public health [23,51].

Public health has four characteristics that provide much of the subject matter for public health ethics as follows: (1) its promotion involves a particular focus on prevention; (2) it is a public or collective good; (3) it involves an intrinsic outcome-orientation and (4) its promotion often entails government action; [11, 24-26].

First, in public health the main point of concern is the population, not individuals. Public health is, by its very nature, a public, communal good, where the benefits to one person cannot readily be individuated from those to another, though its burdens and benefits often appear to fall unevenly on different sub-groups of the population [25]. This raises a particular set of challenges the public health ethics has to address. Whose health are we concerned about, and then what sacrifices is it acceptable to ask of individuals in order to achieve it? Is there a difference between public health and population health? And why is public health a good worth promoting? [26]. Any answer to these questions has to take into account the fact that public health measures are often based on the prospect of benefit to individuals, not immediately securable benefits [23, 27].

Second, promoting public health involves a high degree of commitment to the prevention of disease and injury. However, although much of the discussion surrounding public health focuses primarily on this preventive aspect, public health agencies and services also involve diagnosing and treating illnesses, with all the attendant clinical services that those activities require [28, 29].

Achieving good public health results frequently requires government action: many public health measures are coercive or are otherwise backed by the force of law. Public health is focused on regulation and public policy, and relies less often on individual actions and services. In this as in all other areas of official state action, we therefore have to address tensions among justice, security, and the scope of legal restrictions and regulations [19, 30].

2.1. The rationale of public health programs and policies

Public health draws its fundamental legitimacy from the essential and direct role that health plays in human flourishing, whether that role is understood ultimately in terms of maximizing health or promoting health in the context of advancing social justice [31, 38]. This general justification is sometimes too broad, however, to provide sufficient moral warrant for specific public health policies and institutions, especially when, as is so often the case, these policies and institutions are implemented by the state and affect the liberty or privacy of corporate or individual persons (Beauchamp, 2010). This section puts forward six justifications or reasons that can be put forward to defend a particular public health institution or policy [32].

Two observations are worth making at the outset. First, public health policies are rarely defended by only one reason. Usually a mixed set of justifications can be provided. For

http://dx.doi.org/10.5772/52478

example, tax policies intended to decrease cigarette consumption can be defended both by appeal to paternalism and by appeal to reducing the harms of second hand smoke to children in the home and in automobiles[20, 33]. Second, the impact of public health policies is often not uniform across all the individuals affected by the policy, and thus different justifications are sometimes put forward specific to these different people. This complexity is unavoidable, since it results from the nature of public health: The focus of public health is population health, but populations are rarely internally uniform with regard to all features that are morally relevant to any particular policy [28, 34-35]. Some people may stand to benefit from the policy while others may not. Moreover, in line with concerns about democratic legitimacy and state over-reaching, some members of the population may support the aims of the policy while others may object [36].

The first four of the justifications for public health policies- overall benefit, collective efficiency/ action, and fairness- speak specifically to the context in which some members of the affected population are not directly benefited by the policy or object to it [37]. The next two justifications appeal to the significance of harm, both to others and to oneself. They apply more specifically to traditional concerns about balancing respect for liberty with advancing health and are more prevalent in the public health ethics literature than the previous four. In the fifth justification, the argument is from a relatively uncontroversial Millian harm principle, and in the sixth justification, from somewhat more tendentious paternalistic principles [12, 38].

2.2. Some benefits of public health

It is difficult to estimate direct benefits of the majority of public health interventions since some of these interventions target many health problems and many interventions can contribute to reduce the burden of one health problem. Furtherer, it is known that some of health determinants like those associated to environment change naturally. At individual level, it is even more complicated as the efficacy of public health intervention is the absence of a particular health event that is difficult to justify by the intervention [39, 40].

Generally, we all benefit from having public health interventions, and from having trusted regulatory agencies such as the Centers for Disease Control and Prevention (CDC) or the Food and Drug Administration (FDA) make decisions about such interventions and their reach [16, 41]. All things considered, having public health regulation is better than not having it. Having public health decisions made on the basis of overall statistics and demographic trends is ultimately better for each one of us, even if particular interventions may not directly benefit some of us. Thus, the task of public health ethics is not necessarily to justify each particular intervention directly [16, 41]. Rather, public health interventions in general, as long as they stay within certain pre-established parameters, can be justified in the same way a market economy, the institution of private property, or other similarly broad and useful conventions that involve some coercive action but also enable individuals to access greater benefits can be justified: when properly regulated and managed, its existence is by and large better than its absence for everyone [43].

2.3. The public health policy action strategies

A related justification views health as a public good the pursuit of which is not possible without ground rules for coordinated action and near-universal participation. The public health is viewed as having the structure of a coordination or collective efficiency problem. For example, if one person (or a sufficient critical mass of such persons) decides not to abide by a public health regulation because the regulation does not directly benefit he or she otherwise objects, the ramifications will likely be felt by others in her environment and beyond (Daniels, 2008). Everybody has to participate because, failing their involvement, neither they nor anyone else can reap the benefit of a healthy society (Crawford, 2008).

The collective efficiency class of arguments relies on claims about the sheer number and technical complexity of the decisions that need to be made to protect health in the environment and in the market place, as well as the indivisible character of responses to some health threats [15, 21, 46].

2.4. Public health community engagement

The communitarian argument relies on the idea that is good for the whole is necessarily good for its parts [47]. Communitarians view individuals' identities and the meaningfulness of their lives as indelibly tied to the well-being of their community. Clinical research in a developing nation to be deemed ethical requires community engagement, so that the research can contribute to the social value. Thus, on this view, public health interventions are good for individuals simply because they benefit the community as a whole. It thus encourages a cooperative way of thinking about public health interventions. Its main shortcoming, however, is that it assumes too tight a connection between individuals and the communities to which they belong, thereby incurring the potential for abuses of less privileged individuals within certain communities in the name of communal well-being [48]. It is unfortunately not always the case that the interests of individuals and the interests of their communities coincide in this convenient way. Rather, such interests often come apart, and can come into conflict in ways that require us to address yet again the questions: how much can we ask of individuals for the sake of others, of which individuals can we ask sacrifices for the sake of the community, and why? There is a conceptual distance between what is good for particular individuals, what is good for all individual members of a community, and what is good for the community [8, 49]. Thus, there can sometimes be direct trade-offs between what is good for the community and what is good for particular individuals within it. Notwithstanding these difficulties, this is certainly a strategy worth giving serious consideration as a possible avenue for the justification of public health interventions, particularly in some contexts where there is a strong sense of community solidarity [3, 50].

3. Aspect of justice and fairness in public health

Whether social justice is viewed as a side constraint on the beneficence-based foundation of public health, or as foundational in its own right, there is broad agreement that a commitment to improving the health of those who are systematically disadvantaged is as constitutive of public health as is the commitment to promote health generally (Powers and Faden 2006, Institute of Medicine's Committee for the Study of the Future of Public Health [50-52].

In this regard, there is an intimate connection between public health and the field of health and human rights. Many in public health accept that there is a fundamental right to health, as codified in the United Nations Universal Declaration of Human Rights or otherwise, although there is less agreement about the justification for such a right or what precisely the right entails [24]. A key question for public health ethics is on whom the duties generated by a right to health fall. Since so many of these duties require collective action. The governments are obvious candidates, but so, too, are other social institutions in the private sector as well as those global in structure that bear on the right to health [8, 35]. A failure on the part of these institutions to ensure the social conditions necessary to achieve a sufficient level of health is an injustice that on the view of many violates a basic human right. Note that as a basic human right, the claims of the right to health are not in any fundamental respect restricted to national borders but rather fall on the human community [9].

When inequalities in health exist between socially dominant and socially disadvantaged groups, they are all the more important because they occur in conjunction with other disparities in well-being and compound them [1, 15]. Reducing such inequalities are specific priorities in the public health goals of national and international institutions.

One of the most difficult challenges for public health ethics emerges when moral function conflicts with the injunction to improve, if not maximize, aggregate or collective health outcomes [39]. Although the health of the world's most desperately poor can in many cases be improved by extremely cost-efficient interventions like basic childhood immunizations and vitamin supplementation, reducing other unjust inequalities in health can consume significant resources.

Another challenge in social justice for public health ethics emerges when the health needs of systematically disadvantaged groups conflict with other dimensions of well-being as well as with considerations of collective efficiency. Targeting a public health program to poor and minority communities can sometimes both serve social justice concerns and be efficient if, for example, the health problem the intervention targets occurs disproportionately in these groups [7, 42]. At the same time, however, if the health problem is itself associated with stigma or shame, targeting the poor and minorities may reinforce existing invidious stereotypes, thereby undermining another critical concern of social justice, equality of social respect. In such cases, public health authorities must decide whether a commitment to social justice requires foregoing an efficient, targeted program in favor of a relatively inefficient, universal program that also may produce less improvement in health for the disadvantaged group (thus failing to narrow unjust inequalities) in order to avoid exacerbating existing disrespectful social attitudes [19].

Some formal methods, including most notably cost-utility analysis, rely on what are referred to as summary health measures in which mortality and diverse morbidities are combined in a single metric such as a quality-adjusted or disability-adjusted life year. These measures, and the formal methods that employ them, sometimes rely on assessments of what may be only vague individual preferences for trade-offs between different states of health or different kinds of benefits. Moreover, they make morally problematic assumptions including, for example, whether to differentially value years saved in different stages of life and about how to disvalue specific disabilities [34]. Depending on how these and other assumptions are determined and specified, summary health measures have been criticized as being ageist or not ageist enough, as discriminating unfairly against people with disabilities, as failing to capture the moral uniqueness of life-saving, as treating as commensurable qualitatively different losses and benefits, and as failing to take adequate account of the claims of those who are most disadvantaged [14, 50].

3.1. Burden distributions in ethical research

Another appeal that can be used to defend certain public health interventions that impose unequal burdens on different members of a population relies on considerations of fairness. The basic premise of this line or argument would be that burdens have to be roughly equivalent for everyone [23]. The same could be said for certain public health "burdens," understood as both the burdens of disease and disability and the burdens of public health interventions. Based on considerations such as a particular group's likelihood to contract a certain disease, and their overall health status, other parts of the population can legitimately be asked to "contribute," as it were, in order to make the distribution of disease burdens more equitable [9, 50]. For example, part of the rationale for requiring child immunization prior to enrollment in school is that this is a way to ensure that low-income children, who are generally less healthy than other children, have access to the needed vaccines [44]. Another example of public health interventions that appear to be guided by this justification is rubella vaccination of children for the sake of pregnant women and their fetuses [50]. This reasoning can help explain why individuals are sometimes asked to bear public health burdens that do not directly benefit them. However, the question of how far we can go in redistributing health-related burdens will likely continue to plague any proponent of this justificatory strategy. Moreover, questions about the plausibility of viewing health-related burdens as subject to distribution in this manner may also arise [6, 17].

3.2. Paternalism

Paternalism is classically understood as interfering with the liberty of action of a person, against his/her will, to protect or promote his/her welfare is as controversial as the harm principle is uncontroversial (Dworkin 2005). Few public health interventions are justified exclusively or even primarily on unmediated, classic paternalistic grounds, although many more public health programs may have paternalistic effects. By contrast, other classes of arguments that are sometimes described as paternalistic, including soft paternalism, weak paternalism, and libertarian paternalism, are evoked more frequently [19, 21].

Soft and weak paternalism are usually interpreted as interchangeable, though they have sometimes been taken to denote different concepts [14, 46]. A common interpretation defines this kind of paternalism as interferences with choices that are compromised with regard to voluntariness or autonomy. Though a person might voice or hold a preference different from the one that is sought for him, his preference is not entitled to robust respect if it is formed under conditions that significantly compromise its autonomy or voluntariness, such as cognitive disability or immaturity and, in very limited cases, ignorance or false beliefs [20]. Adaptive preferences are also considered compromised with regards to autonomy: sometimes, individuals modify their preferences in order to be able to adapt to difficult, unjust, or undesirable circumstances [32]. Such preferences also do not have the same standing as preferences formed under normal conditions and are therefore viewed as subject to interference [32].

Libertarian paternalism defends interventions by planners (such as public health authorities) in the environmental architecture in which individuals decide and act in order to make it easier for people to behave in ways that are in their best interests (including their health), provided two conditions are satisfied [5, 31]. First, individuals are steered by these interventions in ways that make them better off, as judged by themselves. Thus, in libertarian paternalism there is no attempt to contravene the will of individuals, in contrast to what some hold to be a necessary feature of paternalism. Second, the interventions must not overly burden individuals who want to exercise their freedom in ways that run counter to welfare. In this sense, libertarian paternalism claims to be liberty-preserving, hence libertarian.

A key conceptual question about paternalism is whether the interference with individual liberty must be against the person's will [3]. If this feature is a necessary condition of paternalism, then libertarian paternalism is inappropriately titled. From the standpoint of public health ethics, however, whether libertarian paternalism is appropriately titled is less important than the moral issues it raises and how it is justified [1, 52].

3.3. Mutual benefit

Finally, there is a more pragmatic reason to attend to public health in the developing world. Beyond claims of justice, morality, and common decency, we live in a world where mobility and interaction within and across countries is very high. Diseases such as SARS, H1N1, and drug-resistant TB, as well as less headline-grabbing ailments such as cholera and malaria, are not neatly contained within one national boundary. Citizens of all countries would benefit from improving public health in the developing world. Contributing to the availability and improvement of medical, sanitary, and other health-related resources for those who live in poverty and deprivation is ultimately good for us all, whether we are in the habit of traveling around the world or not [7]. There is also the need for understanding the emerging diseases and those poverty related diseases that is of major economic concerns [36, 52].

4. Research for low income ecomomies

Medical research is sometimes undertaken in the low income economies in order to further the understanding and treatment of diseases, not primarily for the benefit of those in the developing world, but rather for the benefit of citizens of the developed world. In such cases, participants and their communities might well claim that they are entitled to share in the benefits of the research [9, 16]. However, compensation to participants and their communities is often non-existent or not nearly in line with the potential benefits their participation will bring to those fortunate enough to have been born in a different geographical location [6, 36]. Note that this is a different issue from the question of whether researchers working on indigenous diseases in the developing world have a duty to provide medical care or other ancillary services to their research subjects [5, 21].This is less a question of justice as of research ethics more generally.

4.1. Uneven research focus

Much medical research is focused on diseases that affect less than 10% of the world's population, while millions die every year from diseases that potentially could be prevented or more easily treated if only enough research and other medical resources were devoted to them [1, 20]. Given the sheer numbers of people who needlessly die every day from such neglected but widespread diseases, and given that the developed world clearly has the resources to change that state of affairs, justice claims arguably also arise in this context [22, 35].

4.2. The legal compensatory claims

Many poor, underdeveloped countries that are massively underserved when it comes to public health resources continue to suffer from the direct and indirect effects of historical, unjust harms perpetrated by many of the world's wealthiest countries such as colonialism, war, occupation, and other forms of violent economic exploitation [36, 43]. In many cases, harms are more recent or are continuing, for example the diamond wars in Sierra Leone and other African countries as well as the more general on-going exploitation of local natural resources. Both the historical effects and the persistent effects of such violence and exploitation on public health in those countries ground additional justice-based claims against the wealthy nations to reduce the profound inequalities in health that exist between the world's poor and advantaged people [8, 26].

4.2.1. The role of the ethics committee

There are many synonymous for committees that review and approve biomedical research protocols to safeguard the dignity, rights, safety and well being of actual or potential research participants (WHO, 2000; Tedlock, 1983).Terminologies such as Independent Ethics Committee (IEC), Institutional Review Boards (IRB), Institutional Ethics Committee (IEC), National Ethics Committee (NEC) and Ethics Review Boards (ERB) are interchangeably used. The two WHO guidelines have addressed in details the description of what ERB are, or are intended to be, recommended compositions, what ethical review entails, how they should operate, reach decisions and communicate those decisions. Other publications have provided ethical framework for evaluating whether proposed research is ethical (CIOMS, 2008, Emmanuel et al., 2000; Amdur and Elizabeth, 2002. It is important therefore to look at the different roles of stakeholders in ethical research.

Responsibilities of the participants

The greatest role of ERB is to ensure that research that is conducted among the communities is ethical. Also important to this obligation is to ensure that in its basic setup, composition, operations and follow up activities are such that the mandate of protecting research participants is carried out effectively.

Research and legal liability

Legal liability claims against health professionals were traditionally confined to those who engaged in clinical practice. However, in recent years an increasing number of civil claims have emerged in the health research realm. In this regard, three trends have emerged: (1) the types of legal claims have diversified; (2) the number and types of defendants named in such lawsuits have increased beyond researchers; and (3) class action lawsuits are increasingly being lodged on behalf of groups of research subjects (Mello et al., 2003). While the overwhelming number of research-related lawsuits has arisen in affluent countries, the filing of multi-jurisdictional lawsuits against drug maker, Pfizer, in relation to its Trovan drug trial in Nigeria illustrates that developing countries are also becoming battlegrounds from lawsuits against those involved in research. This work outlines the liability risks of researchers, host institutions, research ethics committees, consulting bioethicists, and research sponsors through a review of sample cases involving these parties.

There exist a number of liabilities in the ethical conduct of research involving all the stakeholder that can be outline as follows:

Research liability

This involves civil claims against researchers which in the early days centered around the notion of informed consent If we consider the case of Wess versus Solomon (1989), the heirs of a subject who died while a volunteer in a non therapeutic study successfully sued the investigator and his university-affiliated hospital. The judge found the principal investigator and hospital, through its research ethics committee responsible for not disclosing a rare fatal complication caused by fluorescent dye and not adequately screening the subject who suffered from undisclosed hypertropic cardiomyopathy.

Research ethics committee liability

Research ethics committee (RECs) or Institutional Review Boards (IRBs), are responsible for assessing human research protocols for conformity to ethical principles (Zlotnik Shaul, 2002). RECs liability has been recognized as far back as in the 70s, when the US National Commission for the protection of Human Subjects of Biomedical and Behavioral research published a report captioned *Report and Recommendation: Institutional Review Board* (NCPHSBBR, 1978).The principles state that one who undertakes to protect others must act responsibly. IRB members could be liable if they did not exercise reasonable care in carrying out their review. This may occur if their approval led to a research activity and injuries that would not have occurred if a reasonable person, confronted with the same information would have placed conditions on the research that would have prevented the injury. Therefore an injured can possibly press charges for negligence by the IRB members in assessing the risks and benefits of proposed research, or in approving consent procedures not necessarily likely to assure legally effective consent.

4.2.2. Institutional liability

Institutional liability arises from the Common Law doctrine of vicarious liability, which holds superiors accountable for the wrongs of their subordinates (Amir, 2009). Amir JA. Research and Legal Liability. Acta Tropica, 2009;112S:S71-S75).An illustrated case is that in the US of Berman versus Fred Hutshinson cancer centre (2002) where the husband of a research participant (Hamilton) died in a chemotherapy trail brought filed a law suit against the Fred Hutchinson Cancer Centre alleging that his wife's consent to participate in the study was not informed because the institution failed to disclosed the following:

That the researchers had no idea whether the relevant drugs would have any protective effect against organ damage; Hamilton would not receive the planned dosage of the drug if she were unable to ingest the oral version of the drug; seven prior protocol participants had died, one of whom had suffered serious organ damage; and there were alternative treatments that were less risky and were reporting a significantly higher cure rate. In summary Berman argued that his diseased wife did not give informed consent to participate in the trial as she was not informed that an experimental drug to prevent lethal side effects of chemotherapy was not available was not available in the intravenous form. After trying to swallow the pills, the participant vomited the pills and died. The trial court handling the case ruled that the Fred Hutchinson Cancer Research Centre's failure to disclose the unavailability of the intravenous form of the drug invalidated Hamilton's consent to participate in the trial.

Bioethicist liability

The bioethicist liability case can be exemplified in the Robertson case where the plaintiffs' alleged that the consulting bioethicist in the matter was careless, negligent and reckless for the following: failing to exercise reasonable care under all of the circumstance, in accordance with the accepted bioethical practice; failing to follow and abide by by the guidelines set forth by various governmental agencies and acting negligently.

Sponsor laibility

The most high profile lawsuit filed against a study sponsor are those lodged against the US pharmaceutical firm, Pfizer, y the Nigerian plaintiffs and authorities. The lawsuits arose from a 1996 drug study conducted by Pfizer in the Northern State of Kano during a meningitis epidemic. In the US case of Abdullahi versus Pfizer Inc (2003), the plaintiffs, parents of the child participants in the trial, alleged the use of the drug TROVAN on children with meningitis was done without the parental informed consent and resulted in nearly a dozen dying, and others being left with brain damage, paralysis and slurred speech. In January 2009, the US Court of Appeals for the Second Circuit in New York overturned a lower court's finding that the cases brought by the plaintiffs could not be heard in the United States (Perlroth, 2009). In April 2009, Pfizer reportedly settled the case for $75 million (Howden, 2009).However, the settlement of the US case did not affect other pending cases against Pfizer in Nigeria such as the $7 billion case lodged by the Nigeria Federal Government in June 2007 and a $2 billion case

http://dx.doi.org/10.5772/52478

lodged by the Kano State Government (Sturcke, 2007).The Pfizer case is significant for various reasons. To begin with, it illustrates that research participants in the developing countries are gaining increasing awareness of their rights and are prepared to act accordingly. The second point is that research conducted by US sponsors of research in developing countries is actionable against those sponsors in the US. Thirdly, research liability lawsuits may also be brought by government authorities, even though they were not the affected parties. Lastly, liability suits may be filed concurrently in different countries and a judgment or settlement in one country does not affect pending cases elsewhere. Some countries require sponsors and investigators to obtain insurance coverage for trial participants for trial-related injuries as a prerequisite to trial commencement. The Pfizer case demonstrates that it is important for sponsors and investigators to have insurance cover clinical drug testing trials.

There exist other potential areas of law suit given the increase in multi-country, multi-national collaborations. Potential lawsuits are emerging from legal issue with material transfer agreement, data sharing agreement and intellectual property rights. The use and storage of biological materials/samples, particularly those exported for storage and analysis to institutions in sponsor countries for use such as to determine biomarkers that confer protective immunity where capacity to conduct such analysis is not available in host countries in the developing countries. Solutions to solving such potential problems involve signing contractual agreements, memoranda of understanding such as data sharing agreement (DSA), Material Transfer Agreement (MTA), entered into between the disputing parties. Such agreements should be negotiated between all relevant stakeholders before any clinical research can commence, and that a dispute resolution mechanism are jurisdictional issues are prospectively determined in the case of any foreseeable dispute.

4.3. Contribution of International Research Integrity (IRI) in public health research promotion

National Science Foundation NSF implementation of Section 7009 of the America Creating Opportunities to Meaningfully Promote Excellence in Technology, Education, and Science (COMPETES) Act requires that the Authorized Organizational Representative complete a certification at the time of proposal submission that the institution has a plan to provide appropriate training and oversight in the responsible and ethical conduct of research to undergraduates, graduate students, and postdoctoral researchers who will be supported by NSF to conduct research. Additional information on NSF's responsible conduct of research (RCR) policy is available in the Award and Administration Guide, Chapter IV.B [46]. While training plans are not required to be included in proposals submitted to NSF, institutions are advised that they are subject to review upon request.

With the increasing globalization of science and engineering research and education, and the associated issues related to the responsible conduct of research within a global context, NSF recognizes that projects involving international partners may present special risks and challenges. Maintaining high standards of ethical and scientific integrity helps to maintain public trust in the research enterprise. An increasing number of authors have pointed to the importance of mentoring and education in relation to the responsible conduct of science in preventing transgressions of scientific integrity. Just like in clinical research and biomedicine, epidemiologists and other public health researchers have the responsibility to exhibit and foster the very highest standards of scientific integrity [46]

The following resources are provided to assist in developing training and oversight plans for the responsible and ethical conduct of research in an international context and to understand the codes of conduct in other countries. NSF does not provide content or endorse these sites' content, but provides them as possible resources.

4.4. National institute of health in public health research clinical excellence

The National Institute for Health and Clinical Excellence (NICE) is a special health authority of the English National Health Service (NHS), serving both English NHS and the Welsh NHS. It was set up as the National Institute for Clinical Excellence in 1999, and on 1 April 2005 joined with the Health Development Agency to become the new National Institute for Health and Clinical Excellence (still abbreviated as NICE). NICE carries out assessments of the most appropriate treatment regimes for different diseases. This must take into account both desired medical outcomes (i.e. the best possible result for the patient) and also economic arguments regarding differing treatments. NICE have set up several National Collaborating Centres bringing together expertise from the royal medical colleges, professional bodies and patient/carer organizations which draw up the guidelines [47]. The centres are the National Collaborating Centre for Cancer, the National Clinical Guidelines Centre for Acute and Chronic Conditions, the National Collaborating Centre for Women and Children´s Health, and the National Collaborating Centre for Mental Health. The National Collaborating Centre then appoints a Guideline Development Group whose job it is to work on the development of the clinical guideline. This group consists of medical professionals, representatives of patient and carer groups and technical experts. They work together to assess the evidence for the guideline topic (e.g. clinical trials of competing products) before preparing a draft guideline. There are then two consultation periods in which stakeholder organizations are able to comment on the draft guideline. After the second consultation period, an independent Guideline Review Panel reviews the guideline and stakeholder comments and ensures that these comments have been taken into account. The Guideline Development Group then finalizes the recommendations and the National Collaboration Centre produces the final guideline. This is submitted to NICE who then formally approve the guideline and issues this guidance to the NHS [47].

4.5. Institute of tropical medicine and hygiene in public health research ethics

The London School of Hygiene and Tropical Medicine is an institution promoting research in public health through the introduction of research training courses which aim at equipping students with skills needed to appreciate and analyze public health problems in developing countries, and to design and evaluate actions to improve public health. The course considers issues of global health, development and the provision of health services from a multidisciplinary perspective. All the public health students are expected to have a substantial experience of planning or implementation of public health programmes, of teaching or research, in developing countries. Graduates from this course work in global health, health service management, in health programmes in developing countries, in international and national NGOs, and in research. In addition to MSc Public Health in Developing Countries. By the end of the course students should be able to: demonstrate knowledge and understanding of theory and practice in the core public health disciplines (epidemiology, statistics, social sciences, health policy and health economics; demonstrate specialized knowledge and skills in other areas relevant to public health from a wide range of options (e.g., primary health care, medical anthropology, epidemiology and control of malaria, and population studies); apply these skills to identify and assess public health problems in developing countries and evaluate actions designed to improve public health; formulate public health strategies and approaches to public health problems appropriate to a given culture and environment; and apply appropriate research skills for evaluation and use of research findings.

4.6. World Health Organization (WHO) in public health research ethics

Health ethics has been an integral part of the activities of many units and departments at WHO for many years and is addressed not only within the Department of Ethics and Social Determinants (ESD) and throughout the organization. ESD works collaboratively with staff from all departments and the regional offices to identify, design, and carry out projects addressing the ethics of health care, public health, and biomedical science. This encompasses projects that originate in the department and those on which it provides advice and assistance to activities located in other clusters and in regional offices. In October 2002, the World Health Organization launched its Ethics and Health Initiative to provide a focal point for the examination of the ethical issues raised by activities throughout the organization, including the regional and country offices, and to develop activities regarding a wide range of global bioethics topics, from organ and tissue transplantation to developments in genomics, and from research with human beings to fair access to health services.

Work in ethics and health is now carried out by the Department of Ethics and Social Determinants in the Innovation, Information, Research and Evidence cluster at headquarters. This department is involved in a wide range of ethics activities, both on its own initiative and in response to the needs of other parts of WHO. The specific projects, many of which link different departments and involve experts from outside the organization, evolve in response to changes in the field.

4.7. NEPAD in promoting public health research in Africa

The New Partnership for Africa's Development (NEPAD) is a socio-economic development programme of the African Union (AU) whose express objective is to stimulate Africa's development by bridging existing gaps in Infrastructure (Energy, Water and Sanitation, Transport and ICT); Agriculture and Food Security; Human Resource Development, especially Health/Education, Youth and Training, Social Affairs; Science, Technology and Innovation; Trade, Industry/Market Access and Private Sector Development; Environment/Climate Change and Tourism; Governance/Public Administration, Peace and Security; Capacity

Development, and Gender Development. The implementation of these programmes is based on the AU/NEPAD principles of African leadership and the ownership of the continent's development agenda and process, as well as a commitment to good political, economic and corporate governance. African leaders have explicitly recognized that socio-economic transformation of the continent cannot be achieved without increased investments in science, technology, and innovation. To that end, the leaders have initiated a number of concrete actions geared towards promoting the continent's scientific and technological development. The actions include the creation of the African Ministerial Council on Science and Technology (AMCOST) and its subsidiary bodies -- the NEPAD Office of Science and Technology, and the AU Commission for Human Development, Science and Technology. These institutions have collectively developed a comprehensive strategy and action plan -- Africa's Science and Technology Consolidated Plan of Action -- adopted at the second African Ministerial Conference on Science and Technology in Dakar, Senegal, in September 2005. The main goals of Africa's Science and Technology Consolidated Plan of Action (CPA) are to strengthen Africa's capacities to develop, harness and apply science, technology, and innovation to achieve millennium development goals (MDGs), as well as mobilizing the continent's expertise and institutions to contribute to the global pool of science and technological innovations. Key to these goals is the promotion of transnational Research and Development (R&D) programmes

4.7.1. Technological trends and Innovation systems in public health delivery in Africa

There is need for a common and shared understanding of what can be done in order to tap science, technology and innovation tools to address Africa's current huge burden of disease. First, African countries and institutions have to show the qualities of leadership necessary for generating and utilizing technology and innovations in health in order to address diseases that are peculiar to this continent. It is evident that many of these diseases are not being addressed by the global scientific community for reasons which need no enumerating here. This can only be Africa's responsibility. Secondly, Africa needs to position itself strategically with regard to shaping and driving a new research and innovation agenda necessary for disease treatment and diagnosis. Today, the continent does not have access to relevant health innovation tools that are widely available around the world. Worse still, Africa is not a key player in the public health research and innovation enterprises. Inequality in science, technology and health innovation capacity in Africa is evident in the extent of the disease burden in many countries. Consequently, the current global funding arrangements for public health, including for global pandemics like HIV/AIDS and neglected diseases, must go beyond merely treating the symptoms through the provision of treatment but should also focus on building requisite health research and development [53] infrastructure on the continent. Thirdly, new continental initiatives must focus on shifting the apparent successes in health innovations to product development and product delivery. It is evident that while promising innovations have been developed in Africa and/or for Africa's specific diseases, not many investments are taking place in product development and product delivery. It is therefore important to address this shortcoming in the context of the Africa health strategies for NEPAD and the AU.

Finally, Africa must take advantage of the wide pool of scientific knowledge and technology tools available globally. This means that, on the one hand, individual countries and continental institutions must invest in technology prospecting in order to exploit existing and relevant health technologies and products. On the other hand, Africa must invest in setting up or transforming research institutions that are not only knowledge-based but also oriented towards product development. There is an immediate need to strengthen African institutions, especially universities and schools of medicine, by increasing funding and revising the curricula. Thus the issue of how science, technology and innovation can alleviate Africa's burden of disease.

4.7.2. Ethics in European Union research

Public attitudes towards science and technology are overwhelmingly positive. The confidence generated by messages such as 'scientifically tested' or 'scientifically proven' is testament to society's support of scientific endeavour. It also highlights the social responsibility that accompanies research. As science advances and evolves, and the relationship between science and society gets better explanations, new challenges are created for the scientific community. Nowadays, there are more scientists than ever before. On a regular basis, exciting research opportunities spring into existence. Grant driven projects and non funded projects are larger, more complex, and more expensive. The role that science plays in our lives continues to gain more significance and recognition in importance, and society, in turn, has a stake in science. Consequently, the relationship between science and society continues to change and intensify in the pursuit of progress [54].

Excellence in science means addressing ethical concerns - to improve the quality of the science itself, but also to highlight the importance of its outcomes to the wider community. The EU's commitment to ethics in research is reflected in explicit requirements, and more specifically in the evaluation of project proposals. Ethics may be context-dependent, but any research team's approach to ethical matters is taken as an indication of the honesty and the clarity of its proposal. While there are rarely clear-cut answers when it comes to ethics, some areas are excluded from EU funding by definition. These are human cloning for reproductive purposes, altering the genetic heritage of human beings, and creating human embryos only to conduct research or obtain stem cells [54].

5. Conclusion

The population of low income economies are highly vulnerable in medical research. The fundamental ethical principles need to have its place in the global public health research sectors. With the increase research in finding new investigational products, developing new disease diagnostics techniques puts the human population into a vulnerable position vis a vis participation into clinical research trials. It is therefore imperative for the public health sector to place more emphasis in the implementation of research that is ethical. By so doing the fundamental principle of morality, autonomy and respect for others, beneficence, non-maleficence and justice shall be practicable and sustainable as within the universal declaration of Helsinki. The public health sector in both developing and developed nations has a duty to set up a working platform that may reduce the 10/90 gap that has remained static in the sub-Saharan Africa. Medical research should be undertaken in the low income economies in order to further the understanding and treatment of poverty related diseases, primarily for the benefit of those in the developing world, not rather for the benefit of citizens of the developed world. Ethics is therefore a non negotiable principle and policy in Public Health Clinical Research practice. It is also evident with increasing clinical research that there shall be more potential legal issues. This calls for more scrutiny in the institutions that be in regulating the ethical framework in the conduct of human research. Those implicate in research should ensure that they are fully versed with their legal rights and obligations associated with the research they are engaged in, and also in tuned with the import and export regulations relevant to biological material transfer, data sharing as the shortcoming of these regulation are potential points for legal liability.

Acknowledgements

We wish to acknowledge the special financial grant from the Ministry of Higher Education of Cameroon, the EDCTP Grant award to the National Ethics Committee of Cameroon, and the financial support from the University of Bamenda. All contributed to the research and processing of this invited write-up by INTECH Publishers.

Author details

C. N. Fokunang[1,2], E. A. Tembe-Fokunang[1], P. Awah[3], M. Djuidje Ngounoue[2,4], P. C. Chi[2], J. Ateudjieu[1,5], R. Langsi[6], Lazare Kaptue[2] and O. M. T. Abena[1]

1 Faculty of Medicine and Biomedical Sciences, University of Yaounde 1, Centre Region, Cameroon

2 Cameroon National Ethics Committee (CNEC), Yaoundé, Cameroon

3 Faculty of Arts and Modern Letters, University of Yaoundé 1. Ipas, Chapel Hill, North Carolina, United States

4 Faculty of Sciences, University of Yaoundé 1, Centre Region, Cameroon

5 Faculty of Sciences, University of Dschang; Division of Health Operations Research, Ministry of Public Health Cameroon, Cameroon

6 Health Division, University of Bamenda, Cameroon

References

[1] Barrett DH, Bernier RH, Sowell AL. Strengthening public health ethics at the centers for disease control and prevention.; Centers for Disease Control and Prevention Public Health Ethics Committee Steering Group. Journal Public Health Management Practice. 2008:.14(4):348-53.

[2] Beauchamp, T.L., Childress, J.F. Principles of Biomedical Ethics, 5th edition Oxford University Press.2001 p.133.

[3] Beauchamp, T. The concept of paternalism in biomedical ethics. In Beauchamp, T. Standing on principles. New York: Oxford University Press. 2010: (pp. 101–119).

[4] Beecher, H.K., Ethics and Clinical Research. New England Journal of Medicine.1966: 274, 1354.

[5] Belsky, L., and Richardson, H. S. Medical researchers' ancillary clinical care responsibilities. *British Medical Journal*, 2004: 328(7454), 1494–1496.

[6] Benatar, S. R. Reflections and recommendations on research ethics in developing countries. Social Science and Medicine, 2002: 54(7), 1131–1141.

[7] Bernheim, R.G., Melnick, A. Principled leadership in public health: integrating ethics into practice and management. Journal Public Health Management Practice. 2008: 14(4):358-66.

[8] Bernheim, R.G. Public health ethics: the voices of practitioners.J Law Med Ethics. 2003:31(4 Suppl):104-9.

[9] Beskow, L.M., Namey, E.E., Cadigan, R.J., Brazg, T., Crouch, J., Henderson, G.E., Michie M., Nelson, D.K., Tabor, H.K., Wilfond, B.S. Research participants' perspectives on genotype-driven research recruitment. Journal of Empirical Research for Human Research Ethics.2011: 6(4):3-20.

[10] Bhan, A., Jerome, A., Singh, R., Upshur, E.G., Grand Challenges in global health: engaging civil society organizations in biomedical research in developing countries. PLoS Med, 2007:. 4 (9), e272, www.plosmedicine.org.

[11] Bhutta, Z.A., Ethics in international health research:a perspective from the developing world. Bulletin WHO, 2002: 80:114-120.

[12] Buchanan, D. R. Autonomy, paternalism, and justice: Ethical priorities in public health. American Journal of Public Health, 2008: 98(1), 15.

[13] Büken NO, Büken E.The legal grounds regarding clinical trial in Turkey.Medical Law. 2011: 30 (4) : 591-611.

[14] Cadigan, R.J., Michie, M., Henderson, G., Davis, A.M., Beskow, L.M.. The meaning of genetic research results: reflections from individuals with and without a known genetic disorder.J Empirical Research and Human Research Ethics. 2011: 6(4):30-40.

[15] Cambon-Thomsen, A., Rial-Sebbag, E., Knoppers, B.M..Trends in ethical and legal frameworks for the use of human biobanks.European Respiratory Journal; 2007 : 30(2):373-82.

[16] Childress, J. F., Faden, R. R., Gaare, R. D., Gostin, L. O., Kahn, J., Bonnie B. Public health ethics: Mapping the terrain. *The Journal of Law, Medicine & Ethics*, (2002:. 30(2), 170–178.

[17] Chilengi, R. An ethics perspective on responsibilities of investigators, sponsors and research participants. Acta Tropica, 2009: 112S:S53-S62.

[18] Cohen, J. T., Neumann, P. J., & Weinstein, M. C. Does preventive care save money? Health economics and the presidential candidates. *The New England Journal of Medicine*, 2008: 358(7), 661–663.

[19] Council for International Organizations of Medical Sciences (CIOMS). International Guidelines for Biomedical Research Involving Human Subjects. Geneva. CIOMS. 2002. pp.112.

[20] Emanuel, E., Wendler, D., Killen, J., and Grady, C. What makes clinical research in developing countries ethical? the benchmarks of ethical research. The Journal of Infectious Diseases, 2004. 189(5), 930–937.

[21] Fineberg, H.VShattuck Lecture. A successful and sustainable health system--how to get there from here.North England Journal of Medicine 2012: 366(11):1020-1027.

[22] Gafni, A. Willingness-to-pay as a measure of benefits: Relevant questions in the context of public decisionmaking about health care programs. *Medical Care*. 1991: 29(12), 1246–1252.

[23] Gitau-Mburu, D. Should public health be exempt from ethical regulations? Intricacies of research versus activity.East Africa Journal of Public Health., 2008: (3):160-162.

[24] Gollust, S.E., Baum, N.M., Jacobson, P.D. Politics and public health ethics in practice: right and left meet right and wrong.Journal of Public Health Management Practice. 2008: 14(4):340-347.

[25] Goodman, E. P. (2006). Stealth marketing and editorial integrity. *Texas Law Review*, 85, 83–152.

[26] Harper, I.. Translating ethics: researching public health and medical practices in Nepal., Canadian Journal of Public Health, 2006: 97 (5) : 402-424.

[27] Horstkötter D, Berghmans R, de Ruiter C, Krumeich A, de Wert G. "We are also normal humans, you know?" Views and attitudes of juvenile delinquents on antisocial

behavior, neurobiology and prevention. International Journal of Law and Psychiatry. 2012:.35(4):289-97.

[28] Huddle TS. 2012. Honesty is an internal norm of medical practice and the best policy.American Journal of Bioethics. 12(3):15-27..

[29] Hyder, A. A., and Merritt, M. W. Ancillary care for public health research in developing countries. *Journal of the American Medical Association*, 2009: 302(4), 429.

[30] International Conference on Harmonization (ICH) Guidelines for Good Clinical Practice, 1996. Available freely on the websites and other sources.

[31] Jefferson, A.L., Carmona, H., Gifford, K.A., Lambe, S., Byerly, L.K., Cantwell, N.G., Tripodis, Y., Karlawish, J. Clinical Research Risk Assessment Among Individuals With Mild Cognitive Impairment. American Journal of Geriatrics and Psychiatry. 2012: 30. 12-30

[32] Jones, M. M., & Bayer, R. Paternalism & its discontents: Motorcycle helmet laws, libertarian values, and public health. *American Journal of Public Health*, 2007:. 97(2), 208–217.

[33] Joyce, G.F., Carrera, M.P., Goldman, D.P., Sood, N., Physician prescribing behavior and its impact on patient-level outcomes.American Journal of Management Care. 2011: 17(12):62-71.

[34] Kass, N. E. An ethics framework for public health. *American Journal of Public Health*, 2001:. 91(11), 1776–1782.

[35] Kilama, W.L). The 10/90 gap in sub-Saaran Africa: Resolving inequities in health Research. Acta Tropica., 2009:112S:S8-S15.

[36] Kost, R.G., Lee, L.M., Yessis, J., Coller, B.S., Henderson, D.K. Assessing research participants' perceptions of their clinical research experiences.; Research Participant Perception Survey Focus Group Subcommittee. Clinical Translational Science. 2011:. 4(6):403-413.

[37] Krech R..Working on the social determinants of health is central to public health. Journal Public Health Policy. 2012: 33(2):279-84.

[38] Lavery, J.V., Harrington, L.C., Scott, T.WEthical,social, and cultural considerations for the site selection for research with genetically modified mosquitoes. American Journal of Tropical Medicine and Hygiene. 2008: 79 (3), 312-318.

[39] London AJ, Kimmelman J, Carlisle B. Research ethics. Rethinking research ethics: the case of postmarketing trials.Science 4; 2012: 336(6081):544-555.

[40] Nicholas, J. Next steps in clinical trial redesign. Journal of National Cancer Institute. 2012:. 18;104(2):90-2.

[41] New Partnership for Africa's Development (NEPAD). Science, Technology and Innovation for Public Health in Africa. In : Fetson Kalua, Abolade Awotedu, Leonard Kamwanja and John Saka editions: 2009, pp 213.www.nepadst.org.

[42] Nyika, A., Kilama, W., Chilengi, R., Tangwa, G., Tindana, P., Ndebele, P., Ikingura, J., Composition, training needs and independence of ethics review committees across Africa: are the gate-keepers rising to the emerging challenges? Journal of Medical Ethics, 2009:. 35, 189-193.

[43] Omonzejele, P.FIs the codification of vulnerability in international documents a sufficient mechanism of protection in the clinical research ethics context? Medical Law. 2011: 30(4):497-515.

[44] Reichert, T. A., Sugaya, N., Fedson, D. S., Glezen, W. P., Simonsen, L., & Tashiro, M. (2001). The japanese experience with vaccinating schoolchildren against influenza. *The New England Journal of Medicine*, 344 (12), 889–896.

[45] Sade, R.M. Why physicians should not lie for their patients. American Journal of Bioethics.(2012:.12(3):17-9.

[46] Steven S C, Amyre B, Angus D. Ethics and Scientific Integrity in Public Health, Epidemiological and Clinical Research. Public Health Reviews, 2009, Vol. 34, No 1.

[47] Sorenson, C; Drummond, M; Kanavos, P; McGuire, A. *National Institute for Health and Clinical Excellence (NICE): How does it work and what are the implications for the U.S.?*. National Pharmaceutical Council. Retrieved 2009-09-18.

[48] Tangwa, G.B., Ethical principles in health research and review process. Acta Tropica, 2009:. 112S:S2-S7.

[49] Thomas, J.C., MacDonald, P.D., Wenink, E., Ethical decision making in a crisis: a case study of ethics in public health emergencies. : Journal Public Health Management Practice; 2009. 15 (2):E16-21.

[50] Thomas, J. C., Sage, M., Dillenberg, J., and Guillory, V. J. A code of ethics for public health. *American Journal of Public Health,* 2002: 92(7), 1057–1059.

[51] Wikler, D., and Brock, D. W. Population-level bioethics: Mapping a new agenda. In Dawson, A., and Verweij, M, *Ethics, prevention, and public health,* New York: Oxford University Press. 2007: p 78.

[52] World Medical Association Declaration of Helsinki, Available at http://www.wma.net/e/policy/17-c-e.html. Ethical principles for Medical Research Involving Human Subjects. 52nd WMA General Assembly, Edinburgh, Scotland.

[53] Andanda P, Awah P, Ndebele P, Onigbogi O, Udatinya D and Mwondela M.The ethical and legal regulation of HIV-vaccine research in Africa: lessons from Cameroon, Malawi, Nigeria, Rwanda and Zambia, African Journal of AIDS Research 2011, 10(4): 451–463 ISSN 1608–5906 EISSN 1727–9445

[54] Http://Cordis.europa.eu/fp7/ethics-en.htm/

[55] Abdullahi v Pfizer Inc., 77 Fed.Appx. 48 (2d Cir. 2003.

[56] Anderlik, MR. Legal Liability for Bioethics Involved in Research. Health Law and Policy Institute. http://www.law.uh.edu/healthlaw/perspectives/Research/001002Best.html/>(assessed 03/09/2012.

[57] Berman v Fred Hutchinson Cancer Centre Case No C01-0727L (BJR), August 8, 2002. United States District Court Western District of Washington at Seattle. Accessible: http://biotech.law.Isu.edu/research/wa/Berman_v_Hutchinson.pdf/ (accessed 03/09/2012.

[58] Mello MM., Joffe S. Compact versus contract-industry sponsor's obligations to their research subjects. Ann. Intern. Med; 2003:43:231—561.

[59] Perlroth N. Pfizer's Nigerian Plaintiffs Get Day In Court, January, 2009 http://www.forbes.com/2009/01/pfizer-nigeria-trovan-business-healthcare-0130_trovan.html/ accessed 03/09/2012.

[60] Robertson v McGee. No 01CV00G0H (M) (ND Okla filed January 29, 2001). Sherman, Silverstein, Kohl, Rose and Podolsky Law Offices.http://www.sskrplaw.com/gene/robertson/complaint.html/ (accessed 03/09/2012).

[61] Weiss v Solomon. A.Q.no 312.1989.http://www.commonlaw.uottawa.ca/index.php?option=com_docmans&task=doc_download&gid=1644/ (accessed 03/09/2012)

[62] Zlotnik Shaul R.Reviewing the reviewers: the vague accountability of research ethics committees. Crit. Care; 2002; 6 (2):12-22.

[63] National Commission for the Protection of Human Subjects of Biomedical and Behavioural Research subjects(NCPHSBBRS). Protection of Human Subjects: Institutional Review Boards. Fed Regist; 1978; 43:231-561.

Chapter 28

Mental Health and Social Capital: Social Capital as a Promising Initiative to Improving the Mental Health of Communities

Emma Bassett and Spencer Moore

Additional information is available at the end of the chapter

http://dx.doi.org/10.5772/53501

1. Introduction

Mental illness is a growing public health concern and has been estimated to impact up to 450 million people across the globe [1]. In countries with particularly high prevalence rates, more than a third of the population will meet the criteria for some form of mental illness during their lifetime [2]. Mood and anxiety disorders tend to have the highest prevalence rates and it has been projected that major depressive disorder will be the second leading disease burden worldwide by 2020 [3]. Mental illness often has chronic effects that can last a life-time and negatively impacts individuals' quality of life at home, work, school, and in social settings [4].

The identification of specific factors that improve or worsen one's mental health is beneficial when aiming to understand onset and course of illness and also for preventing declines in mental health that may sequentially lead to clinical-level cases. Recognizing the key contributors to mental health is a crucial step in enhancing the efficiency of health promotion initiatives. Social capital has been identified as an upstream determinant of mental health and may be particularly beneficial when taking a population health approach. Social capital refers to the material, informational and affective resources to which individuals and, potentially, groups have access through their social connections [5]. It has been proposed that high levels of social capital result in improved mental well-being in both individuals and communities and that enhancing the social resources of groups may allow for improvement in overall population mental health.

To determine social factors that contribute to mental health and to identify who is at greatest risk, there is a need to understand how social capital may help or hinder mental well-being and to examine how predictive factors vary between groups. This chapter will begin by describing the development of social capital, the debates that exist within the current social capital literature, and the ways in which social capital may be connected to health related outcomes. Next, the current literature will be examined in greater detail through the conduction of a systematic search of recently published studies. Findings of these studies, limitations in the current literature and suggestions for future research directions will be outlined. Lastly, public health implications and support for incorporating social capital into population-based mental health promotion programs will be discussed.

2. The development of social capital

Social capital is most often associated with concepts such as trust, norms, power, relationships, and networks and although it is relatively new to health and social sciences research as a whole, its separate components have been studied for centuries [6]. At the basis of social capital is the notion that people invest in social relations with expected returns [7]. While theorists tend to agree upon this underlying understanding, the specific definitions and measurements used in the social capital literature are often disputed [7]. In fact, discrepancies in the definition have existed since the very first attempts to define social capital beginning in the late 1980s and early 1990s. Bourdieu, Coleman, and Putnam are often referred to as early theorists of social capital, and their approaches have influenced the ways in which social capital is viewed in the field of health sciences today [7,8]. Bourdieu was interested in the distribution of social capital within society and explained that like economic or cultural capital, social capital was unequally distributed among individuals and groups [7,8]. Coleman's approach to social capital was similar to Bourdieu's in that they both emphasized the importance of examining social networks. Rather than considering structural measures of social networks, as Bourdieu and Coleman suggested, Putnam focused on relational factors including norms of trust and reciprocity [7]. Despite advances in social capital, there has tended to be a divide between those who follow approaches that are more in line with Putnam's work and those who support Bourdieu or Coleman's definitions of social capital. These approaches have led to two somewhat divergent dimensions of social capital. The first dimension can be labelled 'communitarian', and the second 'network'.

2.1. Debates within the literature

2.1.1. Communitarian versus network approaches to social capital

A central debate within social capital research is whether social capital is a communitarian- or network-driven phenomenon. Communitarian approaches to social capital typically include psychosocial or cognitive constructs (e.g.,perceptions of trust or cohesion) as well as indicators of community participation [8]. Putnam's definition, which focuses on community-level communitarian social capital, has been the most dominant in health sciences to date. In his definition, social capital encompasses five main principles: (1) 'community networks'; the number and density of voluntary, state, and personal networks, (2) 'civic engagement';

http://dx.doi.org/10.5772/53501

the amount of participation in civic networks, (3)'local civic identity'; the degree to which there is a sense of belonging, solidarity, and equality between community members, (4)'reciprocity and cooperation norms'; the degree to which there is a sense of obligation to help others, as well as feelings that others will reciprocate in the future, and (5) 'community trust'; the degree of trust held by individuals within the network [6,10]. Although community networks are included in this definition, Putnam and others who follow a communitarian approach typically focus on the latter four components. A network approach, as represented in the work of Bourdieu, defines social capital as resources that are accessed within social networks for the benefit of individuals or groups [11]. Network approaches to social capital measure directly how and to whom individuals are connected within their social structures by investigating the size, range, and diversity of individuals' social connections, and the resources potentially available within those networks. Although researchers typically adhere to one or the other of these two approaches, some recent studies have sought to compare communitarian and network measures within their work to understand better the potential mechanisms linking social capital to health [5,12]. An approach that includes the incorporation of both communitarian and network dimensions of analysis in studies of social capital is supported throughout this chapter. A more comprehensive approach to social capital will provide researchers and health professionals with a greater understanding of how cognitive, participatory, and network-related elements may work together to influence health outcomes. Understanding the range of social capital processes that may influence health is challenging if social capital dimensions are examined separately.

Critiques of the communitarian approach

Although the communitarian approach to social capital is the most visible in health research today, researchers have expressed several concerns about its prominence. First, the predominance of communitarian approaches in public health research has been largely due to the ways in which social capital was initially translated and cited in the field of public health [8]. Early leading papers on social capital focused on communitarian aspects of social capital, which has resulted in less attention to actual network dimensions [8]. Furthermore, network measures have appeared only recently in the social capital literature, whereas cognitive measures of trust and perceived cohesion appeared early on. Ease of measurement may be a second factor contributing to the uptake of the communitarian approach. The inclusion of network measures in research centred on social capital may give a more complete picture of the association of social capital and mental health outcomes than currently found in the literature.

Second, communitarian measures have often been labelled as proxy, or indirect, measures of social capital since they do not directly assess a person's or group's access to resources [5]. Hence, the communitarian approach has often been criticized for measuring concepts that more closely relate to theories of social cohesion than social capital [7,11]. For example, perceptions of trust may be more suited to measure social cohesion than an individual's general access to resources. Network measures may be advantageous in deciphering the types of resources accessible to individuals and groups within social networks.

A third critique of the communitarian approach lies in its supposed inability to address issues of inequality and power [8]. Other forms of capital (i.e., economic and human) have historically addressed these issues and it seems appropriate that social capital should do the same. Although social capital has been criticized for falling short in this regard, it may not be the concept itself that is ill suited to address distributions and inequalities in social capital within and between societies, but the communitarian measures that are often used. Network measures may offer clearer insights into inequality due in part to the measure's capacity to compare and contrast the types of resources accessed by certain individuals and groups.

2.1.2. Dimensions and levels of social capital

Debates within the social capital literature also concern the levels and dimensions of analysis. Dimensions of social capital include the aforementioned approaches of psychosocial, participation, and network. In terms of the levels of analysis, researchers sometimes differ in their opinions as to whether social capital should be measured with individual- or ecological-level measures. Table 1 provides examples of common individual- and ecological-level measures of social capital according to each dimension. At an ecological level, social capital measures are meant to reflect group and neighbourhood levels of connectivity [6, 14]. Ecological measures capture elements of the community that are often not measurable through individual-level data [13] and are often derived from aggregating individual-level measures. It has been suggested that aggregate data is a proxy measure of exogenous characteristics and more direct measures of neighbourhoods must be created to address this issue [15]. Multilevel studies are increasingly used to assess associations between social capital and health outcomes, and have the benefit of being able to disentangle individual- and neighbourhood-level characteristics [14].

Dimension	**Level**	
	Individual	**Ecological (area)**
Cognitive/Psychosocial	Trust, Perceptions	Community trust, Social cohesion
Participation	Participation	Area participation
Network	Ego networks	Network structures

Table 1. Dimensions and levels of analysis in social capital.

Another debate that has arisen from social capital research has been whether social capital is a concept that should be assessed generally or within certain environments, such as within neighbourhoods. General social capital would represent an individual's general levels of trust towards others, their overall participation in associations, and resources obtained from their entire social networks. Others postulate that although social capital may be measured generally, it can also be assessed in more specific contextual environments [16]. For instance, examining social capital both inside and outside individual's neighbourhoods allows for identifying where people are accessing valued resources [12]. Knowledge of whether the

http://dx.doi.org/10.5772/53501

benefits of social capital for health arise from network sources within or outside the neighbourhood may be important for research and health promotion purposes. Neighbourhood social capital may be measured at an individual-level and is most commonly measured through self-report. With regards to each dimension of social capital, psychosocial measures assess perceived neighbourhood cohesion or trust in neighbours; participation measures would assess involvement in neighbourhood associations; and network measures would examine resources accessed within the neighbourhood. Both general- and neighbourhood-specific measures of social capital are being included in health research to gain a more well-rounded understanding of how and where individuals access their resources.

3. General overview: Social capital and health

3.1. Mechanisms linking social capital to health

Research on social capital has examined a range of health outcomes which have included health-related behaviours, as well as physical and mental illnesses. Social capital may influence health outcomes within neighbourhoods through mechanisms that include: (1) rapid promotion and diffusion of health information, (2) ensuring that health behaviours and norms are adopted, and (3) minimizing opportunities for negative health behaviours [17]. These mechanisms more closely relate to the communitarian rather than the network approach to social capital due to their focus on norms and social cohesion. Several broad areas of physical health are associated with social capital in the communitarian sense, and include mortality and life expectancy, self-rated health, cardiovascular disease, cancer, obesity, diabetes, and infectious disease [18].

High levels of social capital at group, neighbourhood, and network levels has been shown to provide individuals with increased resources in terms of finance, care, and transportation which in turn is found to benefit overall health [19]. The measurement of individual resource access via social connections, along with the emotional support received from these connections, are said to reinforce physical and mental health [19]. For example, those with large social networks may have greater access to social support, which in turn leads to better health [16]. Furthermore, those who have access to network members leading healthy lifestyles may turn to these connections for information which may in turn reinforce positive health behaviours [16]. Researchers have highlighted the benefits of network capital by relating those to the potential positive health benefits that may result from a person's or a group's greater access to informational, material, and socially supportive types of resources. Health-related outcomes that have been shown associated with network components of social capital include self-rated health and obesity [5,12,20]. Thus, research indicates important associations between social capital and health outcomes using both communitarian and network measures. As research moves forward, it is important to understand how both dimensions may work together to influence health outcomes.

3.2. Social capital and mental health

A general search of the social capital and mental health literature show that studies of depression occupy a central part of the literature. The high prevalence rates of depression and the ease of measuring depression through short questionnaires likely contribute in part to prominence of research on depression and social capital. Most studies of social capital and depression have used communitarian measures of social capital, such as trust and participation. Several studies have shown individual-level generalized trust to be inversely related to depressive symptoms [13,21-25]. In studies measuring perceived neighbourhood trust, higher trust in neighbours has also been shown to be a protective factor of depression [22,25]. Studies using indicators of community participation and volunteer work to measure social capital have not shown social capital to be related to depression [22]. While individual-level studies have lent some support for the relationship between depression and social capital, the measures of social capital used in these studies are problematic since they tend to include only communitarian measures such as trust and participation.

Less research has examined social capital and mental health using formal social network data. Analyses that have examined social networks and depression have shown that individuals who report being socially isolated within their social networks are more likely to have depression than those who report more network ties [22,25-28]. Using a resource generator to measure access to specific types of resources within individual's neighbourhoods, researchers did not find any association of social capital with depression over a six-month period [25]. Another study found that women with core neighbourhood ties reported fewer depressive symptoms when compared to women with both neighbourhood and non-neighbourhood core ties, demonstrating the importance of examining neighbourhood connectivity and mental health [29]. One research group [30] conducted a particularly comprehensive study which investigated the spread of depression through social networks. Individuals with several core ties and those who were located centrally within their networks had lower rates of depression [30]. It was found that depressive symptoms do spread within social networks and individuals with depression are more likely to have close ties that also suffer from depression [30]. In fact, having close ties with depression doubled the probability that the respondent will develop depressive symptoms themselves [30]. Initial findings thus demonstrate that both network and communitarian components of social capital may be associated with depressive symptoms, and such relationships require further exploration.

Further research on social capital and other forms of mental illness, including major depression, is needed. On an international level, anxiety disorders typically have even higher prevalence rates than mood disorders with lifetime estimates of approximately 16.6% [31-32]. Anxiety disorders include generalized anxiety, post-traumatic stress, specific phobias, obsessive-compulsive, panic, and social anxiety disorders [32]. Almost half of those diagnosed with depression are also diagnosed with an anxiety disorder [31]. Yet, research studies examining social capital as a potential determinant of anxiety disorders (and other forms of mental illness) are largely understudied. Again, research has tended to focus on communitarian dimensions when examining anxiety. Initial studies suggest inverse associations between psychosocial dimensions of social capital with anxiety symptoms and post-traumatic

http://dx.doi.org/10.5772/53501

stress disorder [33-35]. When network and participation items were measured together in one scale, "structural" social capital was also shown to be negatively associated with anxiety symptoms [34]. More research is needed that examines formal network data in relation to various mental illnesses.

4. Systematic review of literature

4.1. Rationale and objectives

Earlier reviews of social capital and mental health have shown inconsistent results in the association between social capital and mental health [6]. Inconsistencies in the measures of social capital make it difficult to compare studies and to draw common conclusions from the literature. To summarize recent findings on social capital and mental health, we performed a systematic literature review. Compiling and comparing results allows for researchers and health professionals to determine which dimensions of social capital may be most important when examining important mental health outcomes. Gaps within the literature may also be discovered through this process. The main research questions underlying our review were (1) how has social capital been measured in recent studies of social capital and mental health (e.g., psychosocial, participation, or network measures)?; (2) what are the main findings from these studies?

4.2. Methods

Search Procedure. The literature review search was conducted in PubMed; a database that includes access to various health-related articles and journals. Search terms included "social capital AND mental health", "social capital AND mental illness", "social capital AND depression", "social capital AND depressive symptoms", "social capital AND anxiety", and "social capital AND schizophrenia". Search criteria specified that terms were included in the titles of research papers and that articles were published within the last 5 years. After abstracts were gathered, studies that did not in fact examine direct associations between social capital and depressive symptoms, and articles that were not obtainable in English were excluded.

4.3. Results

Search Results. PubMed yielded 31 articles. The majority of articles (n = 16) were derived from the "social capital AND mental health" search. No articles were found with "social capital AND mental illness" or "social capital AND anxiety" searches. The search "social capital AND depression" yielded 10 articles, "social capital AND depressive symptoms" resulted in 4 articles found, and "social capital AND schizophrenia" generated 1 article. Of these articles, 3 were not available in English and 7 did not look at direct associations between social capital and mental health. The final article count included in analyses was 21 [16,21-22,25,33-49].

Table Information. Table 2 includes summary information for each of the 21 studies. Information obtained from each study included: citation number, country of study, study design, sample, measures of social capital, dimension/s of social capital measured, mental health outcome, dimension/s of social capital associated with outcome, and main study findings. In order to compare the findings of studies measuring similar dimensions of social capital, "dimension of analysis" and "social capital dimensions associated with outcome" categories were created. Dimensions of analysis include psychosocial, participation, and network dimensions discussed previously. In many instances, researchers did not use these terms, but may have used 'cognitive' instead of 'psychosocial', or 'structural' instead of 'participation'. In these cases, we re-classified the terms to correspond with one of our defined dimensions (ie. 'cognitive' became 'psychosocial'). Terms used in the "measures of social capital" and " study findings" were consistent with those used in the original research articles.

Descriptive Results. Studies took place in 11 countries across the globe. Most studies measured social capital and mental health outcomes in the general adult population. However, three studies examined social capital and mental health in adolescents, and three examined associations in older adults. Although several studies were cross-sectional in design, seven were longitudinal or prospective cohort studies. The majority of studies examined depression or depressive symptoms as a mental health outcome (n = 15). Other mental health outcomes examined included anxiety (n = 2), post-traumatic stress disorder (PTSD) (n = 2), schizophrenia (n = 1), psychological distress (n = 1), and self-rated mental health (n = 4). Various social capital measures were used in study analyses. Consistent with previous literature, psychosocial (n= 17) and participation (n= 9) dimensions were most frequently measured in conjunction with mental health.

Social Capital and Mental Health Findings

Psychosocial dimensions and mental health. Eleven studies examining the direct association between psychosocial dimensions of social capital and depression or depressive symptoms found that social capital was inversely associated with symptoms. Similar inverse associations were found for studies that included PTSD, anxiety, self-rated poor mental health, and psychological distress as mental health outcomes (N = 7).

Participation dimensions and mental health. Studies reported mixed results when examining direct associations between participation dimensions and mental health outcomes. Of the 3 studies examining participation in relation to depression or depressive symptoms, none found participation in local contexts to be associated with decreased risk of experiencing depressive symptoms. On the other hand, participation was associated with self-rated mental health status in three additional studies.

Network dimensions and mental health. Results of studies examining network dimensions of social capital in association with mental health outcomes were inconsistent. Two of the four studies found network capital to be inversely associated with depressive symptoms. Network dimensions were not examined in relation to other mental health outcomes.

http://dx.doi.org/10.5772/53501

Study	Country of Study	Study Design	Sample	Social Capital (constructs measured)	Social Capital Dimension Measured*	Mental Health Outcome (measure)	Dimension Associated with Outcome?*	Main Findings
16.	USA	Cross-sectional, multilevel	N=497, adults.	Structural Network Capital (reach, range and diversity; Resource Network Capital (embedded employment, transportation, and educational resources)	N	Depressive symptoms (CESD-7)	N = yes	Network density (B = -.54), voluntary organization integration (B = -. 34), access to mainstream individuals (B = -. 13) and access to transportation resources (B = -.48) associated with decreased symptoms. Network social capital was mediator between neighbourhood disadvantage and symptoms.
21.	Sweden	Cross-sectional	N=7757, students aged 13-18.	Psychosocial (general trust) and Neighbourhood social capital (neighbourhood cohesion, reciprocity, safety and cleanliness)	PS	Depression (Depression self-rating scale, DSRS)	PS = yes	Neighbourhood social capital (B = -.10) and general social trust (B = -.20) negatively associated with depression.
22.	USA	Prospective study	N=724, adults.	Cognitive (trust in neighbours, sense of belonging, mutual aid); Structural (volunteer work, community participation)	PS & P	Major depression (CIDI-SF)	PS = yes P = no	Those with neighbourhood trust less likely to develop major depression during follow-up (OR=0.43). After excluding participants with depression at baseline, associations became non-significant. Structural dimensions not associated with depression.
25.	England	Longitudinal, six-month prospective cohort study	N=158, adults.	Network resources (Resource Generator-UK: access to 27 resources and skills)	N	Depression (HAD-D)	N = no	Social capital not independently associated with depression.
33.	England	Cross-sectional survey, multilevel	N=232, adults.	Community social capital (SA-SCAT), structural (know individuals holding certain job titles, participation) and cognitive (ie. trust).	PS, N, & P	Post-traumatic stress as indicator of disaster mental health (PTSD	PS = yes P&N = no	High cognitive social capital negatively associated with posttraumatic stress (B=-.36). Structural social capital not directly associated with PTSD.

						Checklist – Civilian version).		
34.	England	Cross-sectional	N=232, adults.	Cognitive (trust, mutual help, reciprocity) Structural (community linkages) (SA-SCAT-15 item questionnaire)	PS & N	PTSD (PTSD Checklist Civilian Version), anxiety and depression (Hopkins Symptom Checklist-25)	PS = yes (mental health) P&N = yes (anxiety)	Cognitive social capital negatively associated with PTSD (B=-.28), anxiety (B=-.13) and depression (B=-.26), and structural social capital was positively associated with anxiety (B=.13).
35.	USA	Cross-sectional	N=205, adult women.	Trust (neighbourhood trust, trust in people) Volunteering	PS & P	Depressive symptoms (Items from PHQ9, K10, CIDI-SF), anxiety symptoms (CIDI-SF, K10)	PS&P = yes	Social capital negatively associated with depression (B=-.41) and anxiety (B=-.41). Social capital mediated the association between acculturation and depression and anxiety symptoms.
36.	Mexico	Longitudinal	N=2611, adults ages 65-74.	Social capital (groups and networks, trust and solidarity, collective action and cooperation, information and communication, social cohesion and inclusion, empowerment and political action)	PS, N & P	Depressive symptoms (Geriatric Depression Scale). Incidence assessed at 11-month follow-up.	PS&P&N = yes	Higher social capital at baseline associated with lower incidence rates of depressive symptoms in women only (OR=.73).
37.	Ireland	Cross-sectional survey	N=5992, adults.	Trust	PS	Self-reported mental health	PS = yes	Those from rural areas more likely to report high trust and poorer mental health.
38.	Finland	Cross-sectional	N=1102, adults ages 65 and older.	Cognitive social capital (social support, trust, help from neighbours)	PS	Self-reported depression (CIDI-SF) and Psychological distress (General Health Questionnaire)	PS = yes	Cognitive social capital (difficult access to help from neighbours) associated with depression. Not having people to count on, lack of concern from others, and mistrust towards others associated with psychological distress.
39.	Sweden, Finland	Cross-sectional	N=6838, adults aged	Psychosocial (trust in friends and neighbours);	PS & N	Depression (Geriatric	PS = yes N = yes	Low structural capital, measured by infrequent

			65, 70, 75, and 80.	structural (frequency of social contact with friends and neighbours)		Depression Scale-4)		contact with friends (OR=1.53) and neighbours (OR=1.33) associated with depression. Mistrust between friends (OR = 2.01), but not neighbours, associated with increased symptoms.
40.	Japan	National cross-sectional survey, multilevel	N=5956, adults.	Cognitive (trust); structural (membership in sports, recreation, hobby or cultural groups).	PS & P	Self-reported mental health (SF-36).	PS = yes P = yes	Social capital associated with mental health at individual and ecological levels. Cognitive (B= 9.56) and structural social capital (B=8.72) at the ecological level associated with better self-rated mental health.
41.	South Korea	Cross-sectional survey, multilevel	N=5934, adults.	Participation (individual-level participation in organizations); cognitive social capital(individual-level perceived helpfulness); contextual social capital (derived from individual measures)	PS & P	Mental health (self-rated 8-item scale).	PS = yes P = yes	Organizational participation (B=0.151) and cognitive social capital (B=.237) positively associated with mental health. Contextual level of social capital not associated.
42.	USA	Cross-sectional, survey	N=155, adults.	Religious social capital (religious involvement/use of spiritual leader for personal problems); group participation(membership in various groups); social trust(general trust, trust in other homeless, trust in service providers, trust in community leaders); bridging social capital(close ties different to themselves)	PS, N & P	Depression (CESD)	PS = yes P = no N = no P&PS=yes	Higher religious social capital (B = - .21) and higher trust (B = -.18) negatively associated with symptoms. Bridging social capital and group participation not associated.
43.	Germany	Cross-sectional, online survey	N=328, adults.	Perceived social capital at work (Social Capital in Organizations Scale:	PS	Depressive symptoms (German	PS = yes	Lower levels of perceived workplace social capital

				cohesion, trust, values, and support)		version of World Health Organization Five-Item Well-Being Index)		associated with depressive symptoms (OR=.76)
44.	England	Cross-sectional, survey	N=16459, adults.	Neighbourhood-level social capital (social cohesion, trust and social disorganization)	PS	Incidence of schizophrenia (ICD-10 F20). Incidence estimated using local data.	PS = yes	Association between social cohesion and trust and schizophrenia was u-shaped. Compared with neighbourhoods with medial levels of social cohesion and trust, incidence rates significantly higher in neighbourhoods with low (IRR 2.0) and high (IRR 2.5) cohesion and trust.
45.	Finland	Prospective cohort study, multilevel	N=33577, adults.	Workplace social capital (trust, norms, cohesion between other employees and employer)	PS	Depression (self-reported physician-diagnosed and recorded antidepressant prescriptions)	PS = yes	Odds for depression 20-50% higher for employees with low compared to high social capital. Aggregate-level social capital not associated with subsequent depression.
46.	Finland	Longitudinal cohort study	N=25763, adults.	Vertical social capital (trust and reciprocity between employee and employer); horizontal social capital (trust, reciprocity and norms among coworkers)	PS	Depression (self-reported physician-diagnosed and recorded antidepressant prescriptions)	PS = yes	Odds for new physician-diagnosed depression and antidepressant treatment were 30-50% higher for employees with low compared to high vertical and horizontal workplace social capital.
47.	England	Longitudinal, multistage	N=15770, adolescents.	Community social capital (parental involvement at school, sociability, involvement in activities outside the home)	P	Mental health (General Health Questionnaire-12)	P = yes	Adolescent sociability associated with decreased psychological distress only in boys (OR=.64).
48.	South Africa	Cross-sectional	N=16800 adults ages 15 and over.	Neighbourhood-level social capital (aggregated: support and reciprocity, association activity, collective norms, safety);	PS & P	Depressive symptoms (CESD-10)	PS = yes P = no	Compared to those with high neighbourhood-level social capital, those with moderate (B = 0.82) and low (B=0.89) social capital more likely to report symptoms. Compared to those with

				Individual-level trust and civic participation				high trust, moderate trust associated with increased symptoms (B=0.83). No associations found for participation.
49.	China	Longitudinal	N=5164, adolescents and their parents.	Family social capital (frequency have dinner with parents, home alone, go out with unfamiliar friends, parents check homework); Community social capital (perceived safety, neighbourhood ties, neighbourhood cohesion)	PS	Depressive symptoms (CESD)	PS = yes	Higher community social capital associated with lower levels of adolescent depressive symptoms (B=-.97). Family social capital mediated effects of contextual factors on adolescent depressive symptoms. Female adolescents reported more depressive symptoms as result of lower availability of family social capital.

*PS = psychosocial, P = participation, N = network.

Table 2. Search findings of social capital and mental health literature. Studies published within last 5 years.

Composite social capital and mental health. Five studies used scale or composite scores which included two or more dimensions of social capital. When measures of participation and network dimensions of social capital were assessed together, social capital was found to be positively associated with anxiety symptoms. On the other hand, these dimensions were not associated with post-traumatic stress disorder or depressive symptoms. Psychosocial and participation dimensions were also used as composite measures of social capital (N = 2). The fusion of both dimensions is consistent with a communitarian approach to social capital. Both studies found communitarian social capital to be inversely associated with depressive symptoms. Communitarian dimensions were also inversely associated with anxiety symptoms. Lastly, when all three dimensions of social capital were included as a social capital composite score, social capital was negatively associated with depressive symptoms in older adults.

4.4. Discussion

In this literature review, the diverse measurement of social capital in recent studies of mental health and social capital was investigated, and key findings of these studies were highlighted. The first objective of this review was to examine how social capital is currently being measured in the mental health literature. Studies of communitarian social capital were dominant. Psychosocial dimensions of social capital were included in most studies, and participation dimensions were second-most common. Network measures were least common. Yet, with network components increasingly recognized as a core construct of social capital in research on social capital and physical health outcomes [5], it is important that researchers and health professionals also consider network capital in studies of mental health.

Measurement of the psychosocial, participation, and network dimensions of social capital were often inconsistent. Psychosocial measures included a broad range of cognitive and socio-relational characteristics. Despite variations within psychosocial measurement, results consistently found psychosocial social capital to be associated with various mental health outcomes including depression, anxiety, PTSD, psychological distress, and self-reported mental health. Such findings speak to the magnitude of impact that psychosocial characteristics likely have on one's mental health. Measures of participation across studies tended to assess similar constructs and may allow for greater cross-comparison between studies. When examined as a separate dimension, participation was not associated with depressive symptoms. Comparing studies on psychosocial and participatory social capital with those that examined network social capital and mental health is difficult. Studies used various network measures and many failed to conduct comprehensive analyses of social networks and resources. For example, some studies investigated social networks as a complementary component to the participation dimension of social capital, but did not exclusively focus on this dimension of social capital as a potential key contributor to mental health. Nevertheless, network dimensions of social capital were inversely associated with depressive symptoms in two studies, lending support to the notion that network capital plays an important role in mental health outcomes. No studies in the current search observed network social capital in relation to health outcomes other than depression. More rigorous measurement of network connections and resources is needed to understand how network dimensions of social capital may be associated with mental health outcomes.

4.5. Limitations and strengths of current literature review

There are a few limitations to the current literature review. First, search terms were limited to titles of studies. This was to ensure that the articles included in the review focused primarily on social capital and mental health outcomes; yet other studies that examined direct associations may have been missed. Second, articles that were not included in the PubMed database may have been left out from the final list of studies. Third, while common mental illnesses were included in search terms in hopes of capturing a larger range of articles than yielded by general 'mental health' and 'mental illness' searches, studies that examined outcomes other than depression, anxiety, schizophrenia, or general mental health in relation to social capital may have been missed. Researchers who conduct future literature reviews may wish to expand search results to include terms in abstracts or key terms, conduct searches in various databases, and expand searches to include a wider range of mental health outcomes.

This literature review has several strengths. To our knowledge, this is the most recent review of the social capital and mental health literature. Mental health research is an ever-growing field and social capital is increasingly examined as a potential contributor to

http://dx.doi.org/10.5772/53501

well-being. Consequentially, reviews are needed to inform researchers of other works being conducted in an accessible and informative manner. This literature review has also worked towards drawing common conclusions from diverse studies that previously seemed incomparable. This was done by grouping social capital measures into the three most common dimensions of analysis and comparing findings across various mental health outcomes. As far as we are aware, this is the first review of the social capital literature to compare studies in such a manner. Previous review works have focused on individual- and ecological- levels of social capital in attempts to tease out measurement debates [13], however there has also been a need to understand how dimension of social capital is portrayed in the public health field. Lastly, another major strength of conducting this literature review lies in the implications that can be drawn from it. Several gaps within the literature have been highlighted throughout this review process and directions for future research and health promoting programs can be inferred from these gaps. These points will be expanded upon in the following sections.

5. Limitations in current research and suggested future directions

Having compiled and evaluated the literature, it is apparent that more research, particularly from a network perspective, is needed to understand how social capital contributes to mental health. With several debates surrounding the definition and measurement of social capital, it is evident that researchers must work towards building a consensus. An all-inclusive approach that considers psychosocial, participation, and network dimensions may be particularly beneficial when examining mental health outcomes, since it will allow for clearer depictions of contributing factors to the illness. Furthermore, discrepancies of measurement within each dimension must also be addressed. This might be achieved by building a consensus on the definition of social capital. Once social capital is uniformly defined, gold-standard measures of each dimension can be developed and standardized.

Furthermore, an overwhelming number of studies derived from the literature search measured depression or depressive symptoms as the primary mental health outcome. There is a need to understand how social capital, and its separate dimensions, relate to other relevant mental health issues. For example, other social determinants, including socioeconomic status and gender, have been outlined as potential contributors to anxiety spectrum disorder, and more research is needed to examine how social capital might impact one's risk for experiencing anxiety [50]. Co-morbid mental and physical illness may also be necessary to investigate in future studies of social capital. Current research suggests that social capital may have differential effects on different mental illnesses; however co-morbid illnesses within individuals are largely unexplored [34].

Another potential limitation to the current literature is that results are typically generalizable only to others experiencing symptoms of mental illness. Most studies have not conducted formal clinical diagnoses of the mental health outcome of interest, but have relied on brief questionnaires to assess symptomatology. Elevated symptoms may sometimes correspond with a diagnosable illness, however it has not yet been proven that current study results are applicable to those with clinical-level syndromes.

Having established some preliminary associations between social capital and mental health, more research is needed to determine how social capital may impact mental illness in different groups. Initial research suggests that social capital is an important predictor of mental illness at many different life stages. For example, social capital has been found to be associated with depressive symptoms in children, middle-aged, and older adults [21,36,49]. Studies on gender, social capital and health should be advanced. Recent studies suggest important differences in social capital and mental health between men and women. For example, although social capital has been found to be associated with depressive symptoms in both women and men, women may be more prone to experiencing negative mental health consequences in response to decreased levels of psychosocial and network dimensions of social capital in some instances [51]. Further research is needed to examine group differences between social capital and mental health outcomes.

Lastly, some lingering uncertainty exists when attempting to understand the causal relation between social capital and mental health. While cross-sectional studies have many advantages in terms of brevity and reduced resource load and are helpful when gaining an initial understanding of associations, longitudinal studies within the current area of research is a logical next step. Of the longitudinal studies conducted to date, there is some support that suggests social capital may in turn influence mental health [36,47,49]. Programs that promote mental health also seem to follow this rationale by first altering social constructs with hopes of in turn improving mental well-being. Such efforts will be discussed shortly. While the current evidence points to social capital as a potential contributor to mental health, there is a need for long-term longitudinal studies to ease existing uncertainties. Longitudinal investigations of the relationships between social capital and mental health may help identify specific causal directions, and will inform health professionals when developing tailored community programs.

6. Public health implications

Understanding the role that social capital may play in mental health has broader public health implications in terms of treatment and prevention programs. Several studies included in the literature review emphasized the practical public health implications of their findings [21,33,3-36,38,48]. As well as benefitting the general population, increasing social capital may also be used to address mental health issues faced by vulnerable groups including post-disaster victims, ethnic minorities, women, adolescents, older adults, homeless individuals, and those living in disadvantaged neighbourhoods [21,33,35,38,42,51]. Enhancing social capital within vulnerable groups may be achieved by increasing social skills and developing networks [52]. With increased social capital, it was expected that sequential improvements in mental health might be observed [52]. Since various groups are found to face differential barriers to achieving positive mental well-being, it has been suggested that intervention programs be tailored to specific groups of interest [53].

http://dx.doi.org/10.5772/53501

Determinants at individual, social, organizational and community levels must be considered when creating programs aimed at improving population-level mental health. While individual-level intervention programs may be beneficial in aiding those who require critical mental health care, population-based approaches may be most effective when prevention of mental illness and promotion of mental well-being in broader populations is the goal. Social capital is advantageous in that it can be applied at individual and group levels. From an organizational standpoint, it has been suggested that increased social capital between fellow co-workers and between employees and employers may be one potential outlet for improving mental health [45]. Social capital may also be used to foster positive mental well-being at the community level. Because social capital can be measured within neighbourhoods, programs have the potential to be designed from a community or group perspective. These programs may foster a sense of trust and cohesion within broader groups, while also developing community resources to maximize social capital within a given area. This may allow for the improvement or maintenance of positive mental health of larger population-level groups.

Countries across the globe have recognized the potential for social capital to be used as a health promoting mechanism. The improvement of social capital in communities (and its cognitive, network, and resource components), has recently been outlined as an important health promotion initiative in countries including Canada, Australia, and the United Kingdom. The Victorian Government suggest that social capital can be fostered by emphasizing community development, which can be improved by defining community-level goals, mobilizing resources, and developing plans to address collective problems [54]. European initiatives to improve the mental health of population include action goals such as promoting mental health in schools and the workplace, supporting mentally healthy aging and reducing disadvantage [55]. Goals such as these can be accomplished by promoting social inclusion, implementing community development programs, and encouraging social, cultural, economic and political contribution of individuals in society [55]. Through the development of social capital within communities, inequality issues in health and well-being and the ways in which groups come together to promote health can be directly addressed [54].

Canadian initiatives do not yet typically include the term 'social capital' within their mental health initiatives, as does the U.K.; however health promoting goals have included several of its key concepts for decades. For example, in 1986, efforts to improve mental well-being in its population, the Ottawa charter for mental health promotion strived to (1) build health public policy, (2) create supportive environments, (3) strengthen community action, (4) develop personal skills, and (5) reorient health services [56]. Each goal incorporates fundamental concepts of social capital by emphasizing the importance of building connections within social networks, developing health promoting resources and behaviours within communities, and fostering cohesion between individuals and groups. As social capital gains increased recognition in research and public health fields, the use of social capital within health initiatives are likely to become more common. Until then, it is promising that countries recognize the value in its individual components when outlining health promotion goals.

7. Concluding thoughts

Previous and recent evidence strongly suggests that social capital is a key contributor to mental health outcomes. Psychosocial components are consistently shown to be associated with symptoms of depression, anxiety, post-traumatic stress, psychological distress and self-rated mental health. Participation dimensions of social capital may be important for self-rated mental health, but do not seem to be associated with depressive symptoms. Network components on the other hand have been shown associated with depressive symptoms in some instances but have not been examined in relation to other forms of mental illness. More research is needed to establish associations between dimensions of social capital and various mental health outcomes. There remains important gaps within the literature that must be addressed. Nevertheless, social capital is a promising tool that can be used for policy and intervention purposes. Enhancing social capital of communities is thought to contribute to improved mental, and potentially physical, well-being of populations across the globe. With further research, the creation of health promoting programs, changes in policy, and increased knowledge translation between these realms, social capital may be a promising mechanism to improving mental well-being and preventing mental illness.

Author details

Emma Bassett[1*] and Spencer Moore[2]

*Address all correspondence to: 5eb29@queensu.ca

1 School of Kinesiology and Health Studies, Queen's University, Kingston Ontario, Canada

2 School of Kinesiology and Health Studies, Queen's University, Kingston Ontario, Canada

References

[1] World Health Organization. Investigating Mental Health. Switzerland: Nove; 2003. www.who.int/mental_health/media/investing_mnh.pdf

[2] Bulletin of the World Health Organization. Cross-national Comparisons of the Prevalences and Correlates of Mental Disorders. WHO International Consortium in Psychiatric Epidemiology 2000;78(4) 413-426.

[3] Moussavi S, Chatterji S, Verdes E, Tandon A, Patel V, Ustun B. Depression, chronic diseases, and decrements in health: results from the world health surveys. The Lancet 2007;370 851-858.

[4] Government of Canada. The human face of mental health and mental illness in Canada. http://www.phac-aspc.gc.ca/publicat/human-humain06/pdf/human_face_e.pdf (accessed 20 August 2012).

[5] Moore S, Daniel M, Paquet C, Dubé L, Gauvin L. Association of individual network social capital with abdominal adiposity, overweight and obesity. Journal of Public Health, 2009;31(1) 175-183.

[6] Whitley R, McKenzie K. Social capital and psychiatry: review of the literature. Harvard Review of Psychiatry 2005;13(2) 71-84.

[7] Lin, N. Building a network theory of social capital. Connections 1999;22(1) 28-51.

[8] Moore S, Shiell A, Hawe P, Haines V. The privileging of communitarian ideas: citation practices and the translation of social capital into public health research. American Journal of Public Health 2005;85(8) 1330-1337.

[9] Portes A. The two meanings of social capital. Sociological Forum 2000;15(1) 1-12.

[10] Putnam R. Making democracy work: civic traditions in modern Italy. Princeton, NJ: Princeton University Press; 1993.

[11] Carpiano RM. Toward a neighbourhood resource-based theory of social capital for health: can Bourdieu and sociology help? Social Science & Medicine 2006;62 165-175.

[12] Moore S, Bockenholt U, Daniel M, Frohlich K, Kestens Y, Richard L. Social capital and core network ties: a validation study of individual-level social capital measures and their association with extra- and intra-neighborhood ties, and self-rated health. Health & Place 2011;17(2) 536-544.

[13] De Silva MJ, McKenzie K, Harpham T, Huttly SR. Social capital and mental illness: a systematic review. Journal of Epidemiology and Community Health 2005;59 619-627.

[14] Poortinga W. Social capital: an individual or collective resource for health? Social Science & Medicine 2005;62 292-302.

[15] Diez-Roux AV. Neighborhoods and health: where are we and were do we go from here? Revue D'Epidemiologie et de Sante Publique 2007;55 13-21.

[16] Haines VA, Beggs JJ, Hurlbert JS. Neighborhood disadvantage, network social capital, and depressive symptoms. Journal of Health and Social Behavior 2011;52(1) 58-73.

[17] Kawachi I, Kennedy BP, Glass R. Social capital and self-rated health: a contextual analysis. American Journal of Public Health 1999;89(8) 1187-1193.

[18] Kawachi I, Subramanian SV, Kim D., editors. Social Capital and Health. New York: Springer; 2008.

[19] Nakhaie R, Arnold R. A four year (1996-2000) analysis of social capital and health status of Canadians: the difference that love makes. Social Science & Medicine 2010;71 1034-1044.

[20] Verhaeghe PP, Pattyn E, Bracke P, Verhaeghe M, Van De Putte B. The association between network social capital and self-rated health: pouring old wine in new bottles? Health & Place 2012;18(2) 358-365.

[21] Aslund C, Starrin B, Nilsson KW. Social capital in relation to depression, muskoskeletal pain, and psychosomatic symptoms: a cross-sectional study of a large population-based cohort of Swedish adolescents. BMC Public Health 2010;10 715-725.

[22] Fujiwara T, Kawachi I. A prospective study of individual-level social capital and major depression in the United States. Journal of Epidemiology and Community Health 2008;62 627-633.

[23] Sund ER, Jorgensen SH, Jones A, Krokstad S, Heggdal M. The influence of social capital on self-rated health and depression – the Nord-Trondelag health study (HUNT). Norwegian Journal of Epidemiology 2007;17(1) 59-69.

[24] Veenstra G. Location, location, location: contextual and compositional health effects of social capital in British Columbia, Canada. Social Science & Medicine 2005;60 2059-2071.

[25] Webber M, Huxley P, Harris T. Social capital and the course of depression: six-month prospective cohort study. Journal of Affective Disorders 2011;129 149-157.

[26] Berkman LF. The role of social relations in health promotion. Psychosomatic Medicine 1995;57 245-254.

[27] Bruce ML, Hoff RA. Social and physical health risk factors for first-onset major depression disorder in a community sample. Social Psychiatry and Psychiatric Epidemiology 1994;29 165-171.

[28] Walters K, Breeze E, Wilkinson P, Price GM, Bulpitt CJ, Fletcher A. Local area deprivation and urban-rural differences in anxiety and depression among people older than 75 years in Britain. American Journal of Public Health 2004;94(10) 1768-1774.

[29] Bassett E, Moore S. Social capital and depressive symptoms: the association of psychosocial and network dimensions of social capital with depressive symptoms in Montreal, Canada. Unpublished manuscript 2012.

[30] Rosenquist JN, Fowler JH, Christakis NA. Social network determinants of depression. Molecular Psychiatry 2011;16 273-281.

[31] Anxiety and Depression Association of America. Facts and Statistics. http://www.adaa.org/about-adaa/press-room/facts-statistics (accessed August 22 2012).

[32] Somers JM, Goldner EM, Waraich P, Hsu L. Prevalence and incidence studies of anxiety disorders: a systematic review of the literature. Canadian Journal of Psychiatry 2006;51(2) 100-113.

[33] Wind TR, Komproe, IH. The mechanisms that associate community social capital with post-disaster mental health: a multilevel model. Social Science & Medicine 2012; http://dx.doi.org/10.1016/j.socscimed.2012.06.032.

[34] Wind TR, Fordham M, Komproe IH. Social capital and post-disaster mental health. Global Health Action 2011;4. Doi: 10.3402/gha.v4i0.6351.

[35] Valencia-Garcia D, Simoni JM Alegria M, Takeuchi DT. Social capital, acculturation, mental health, and perceived stress to services among Mexican American women. Journal of Consulting and Clinical Psychology 2012;80(2) 177-185.

[36] Bojorquez-Chapela I, Manrique-Espinoza BS, Mejia-Arango S, Solis MM, Salinas-Rodriguez A. Effect of social capital and personal autonomy on the incidence of depressive symptoms in the elderly: evidence from a longitudinal study in Mexico. Aging and Mental Health 2012;16(4) 462-471.

[37] Fitzsimon N, Shiely F, Corradino D, Friel S, Kelleher CC. Predictors of self-reported poor mental health at area level in Ireland: a multilevel analysis of deprivation and social capital indicators. The Irish Medical Journal 2007;100(8) suppl 49-52.

[38] Forsman AK, Nyqvist F, Wahlbeck K. Cognitive components of social capital and mental health status among older adults: a population-based cross-sectional study. Scandinavian Journal of Public Health 2011;39(7) 757-765.

[39] Forsman AK, Nyqvist F, Schierenbeck I, Gustafson Y, Wahlbeck K. Structural and cognitive social capital and depression among older adults in two Nordic regions. Aging and Mental Health 2012;16(6) 771-779.

[40] Hamano T, Fujisawa Y, Ishida Y, Subramanian SV, Kawachi I, Shiwaku K. Social capital and mental health in Japan: a multilevel analysis. PLoS One 2010;5(10):e13214.

[41] Han S, Lee HS. Individual, household and administrative area levels of social capital and their associations with mental health: a multilevel analysis of cross-sectional evidence. International Journal of Social Psychiatry 2012; DOI: 10.1177/0020764012453230.

[42] Irwin J, Lagory M, Ritchey F, Fitzpatrick K. Social assets and mental distress among the homeless: exploring the roles of social support and other forms of social capital on depression. Social Science & Medicine 2008;67(12) 1935-1943.

[43] Jung J, Ernstmann N, Nitzsche A, Driller E, Kowalski C, Lehner B, et al. Exploring the association between social capital and depressive symptoms: results of a survey in German information and communication technology companies. Journal of Occupational and Environmental Medicine 2012;54(1) 23-30.

[44] Kirkbride JB, Boydell J, Ploubidis GB, Morgan C, Dazzan P, McKenzie K, et al. Testing the association between the incidence of schizophrenia and social capital in an urban area. Psychological Medicine 2008;38(8) 1083-1094.

[45] Kouvonen A, Oksanen T, Vahtera J, Stafford M, Wilkinson R, Schneider J, et al. Low workplace social capital as a predictor of depression: the Finnish Public Sector Study. American Journal of Epidemiology 2008;167(10) 1143-1151.

[46] Oksanen T, Kouvonen A, Vahtera J, Virtanen M, Kivimaki M. Prospective study of workplace social capital and depression: are vertical and horizontal components equally important? Journal of Epidemiology and Community Health 2010;64(8) 684-689.

[47] Rothon C, Goodwin L, Stansfeld S. Family social support, community "social capital" and adolescents' mental health and educational outcomes: a longitudinal study in England. Social Psychiatry and Psychiatric Epidemiology 2012;47(5) 697-709.

[48] Tomita A, Burns JK. A multilevel analysis of association between neighborhood social capital and depression: evidence from the first South African National Income Dynamics Study. Journal of Affective Disorders 2012; http://dx.doi.org/10.1016/j.jad.2012.05.066

[49] Wu Q, Xie B, Chou CP, Palmer PH, Gallaher PE, Johnson CA. Understanding the effect of social capital on the depression of urban Chinese adolescents: an integrative framework. American Journal of Community Psychology 2010;45(1-2) 1-16.

[50] Averina M, Nilsson O, Brenn T, Brox J, Arkhipovsky V. et al. Social and lifestyle determinants of depression, anxiety, sleeping disorders and self-evaluated quality of life in Russia: a population-based study in Arkhangelsk. Social Psychiatry and Psychiatric Epidemiology 2005;40(7) 511-518.

[51] Bassett E, Moore S. Perceived neighbourhood cohesion mediates the association between neighbourhood disadvantage and depressive symptoms in Montreal women but not men. Unpublished manuscript 2012.

[52] Dutt K, Webber M. Access to social capital and social support among South East Asian women with severe mental health problems: a cross-sectional survey. International Journal of Social Psychiatry 2010;56(6) 593-605.

[53] Berry HL. Social capital elite, excluded participators, busy working parents and aging, participating less: types of community participators and their mental health. Social Psychiatry and Psychiatric Epidemiology 2008;43(7) 527-537.

[54] State government of Victoria. Social capital & community development. Victorian State Government, Department of Health, Australia 2011. http://www.health.vic.gov.au/healthpromotion/what_is/social_cap.htm (accessed 15 August 2012).

http://dx.doi.org/10.5772/53501

[55] Jané-Llopis E, Anderson P. Mental Health Promotion and Mental Disorder Prevention. A policy for Europe. Nijmegen: Radboud University Nijmegen; 2005.

[56] Public Health Agency of Canada. Ottawa Charter for Health Promotion: An International Conference on Health Promotion, 17-21 November 1986, Ottawa, Canada. http://www.phac-aspc.gc.ca/ph-sp/docs/charter-chartre/index-eng.php (accessed 16 August 2012).

Chapter 29

Communicating, Motivating and Teaching the Significance of Public Health

Claudia Marin-Kelso

Additional information is available at the end of the chapter

http://dx.doi.org/10.5772/53722

1. Introduction

Teaching public health represents a challenge for all health educators, as it includes a wide variety of important subjects that can be general, broad or specific and technical. Keeping students' attention is a difficult task when introducing purely theoretical concepts or subjects that for some, can be obvious, but are the building blocks of public health practice. Pretending to create a "hands on effect" is not an easy task for any health educator. More so, if your students come from different backgrounds, as those interested in Public Health. This chapter intends to address aspects of public health, such as skill sets needed, using technology and strategies to teaching public health, as well as, mentoring students to generate action. Each section will include examples and proposed exercises for the teacher to use in the classroom.

2. Significance of teaching public health

When does a health problem become a public health problem? That's the first question I asked myself when I was in the middle of my medical training. And, while everybody else was thinking about how to do well the semiology oral examination, I was thinking, how I could help not just one, but many people.

Theories in health education vary and they support themselves with behavioral change theories that are no less important, however, these theories are not discussed here due to length and the specific topic of this chapter. This section of the chapter emphasizes the importance of public health's applicability to one's practice, communities, governments and life in general.

After years of public health teaching experience I have come to identify that in order for public health students to understand what public health means and what they can do with it, they first have to learn basic definitions of the subject, a little bit of history, view the complexity of individuals and communities and their determinants of health and be up to date with the health priorities of their community and the world. In short, public health is exciting and challenging!

Public Health is one of those areas that appears to many, as a general science that is "out there" but not necessarily considered the way to go when choosing a career. In the medical world, it is way more attractive (financially speaking) to go further in your clinical training than explore fields related to community health. Public Health is all around us, it encompasses so many areas in which varied professionals can serve and contribute.

One of the earliest definitions of Public Health in the modern world was given by Charles-Edward Winslow in 1920, when he defined it as "the science and art of preventing disease, prolonging life and promoting health through the organized efforts and informed choices of society, organizations, public and private, communities and individuals"[1]. From all the definitions found, this one succinctly describes the subject with its dimensions, determinants and participants. Thereafter you can find other definitions that include terms of functionality, and community participation and involvement that you may relate too, helping facilitate your teaching style and syllabus.

In teaching public health it is very important to transfer not only knowledge but experiences to the students that can lead them to take action in their communities and will show them a breadth of possible areas that can be developed working in the public health field. Some of these include: Child and Maternal Health, Biostatistics, Behavioral Medicine, Environmental Health or Environmental Epidemiology, Epidemiology, Global Health, International Health, Health Care Services Delivery, Preventive Medicine, Public Policy, Health Care Organization amongst others.

Academic training requires students to consider all aspects of a topic, from a range of view-points. It also requires students to state general claims and then prove each claim by providing solid evidence from a range of sources. [2] Giving practical examples allows students to grasp the intricacies of public health challenges and how to face them.

Another recommendation in having people interested and involved in Public Health is to teach them some history. The best way to know what something is, is to know where it comes from. I always recommend to begin your public health teaching activities by exploring some of the history of public health, areas or public health, origins in the different civilizations, examples of actions that were public health efforts but were not considered as such until a definition of public health came out, the relationships of public health with other scientific disciplines, the process of emergence of key concepts, the influence on demographic, health, social, cultural and economic context and the role of public health in society. [3]

As a public health educator it is important to use a variety of teaching methods to meet individual preferences of your students. Possible methods to be used are discussed later.

Some of the best results in public health education are achieved by stimulating research the theory and practice of health education; supporting high quality performance standards for the practice of health education and health promotion; advocating policy and legislation affecting health education and health promotion; and developing and promoting standards for professional preparation of health education professionals [4].

Public health differs from clinical medicine by emphasizing prevention and keying interventions to multiple social and environmental determinants of disease; clinical medicine focuses on the treatment of the individual [4]. The best way to approach a health issue is by integrating both clinical assessment with public health perspective. A health professional can no longer treat his patients symptoms of pathology, but he has to view, analyze and treat all the other determinants of health that surround that individual ensuring a better outcome for the patient.

With the creation and updates of the program "Healthy People", by the United States Department of Health and Human Services, a vision was delineated of where public health wants to be, and it changed the way of planning, organizing and acting in public health. Health promotion and disease-prevention goals were set. It also has analyzed and transformed the determinants of health; including areas to fulfill one's needs and describe all the areas that affect individuals' health.

Determinants of health (as seen in figure 1) have evolved, encompassing five dimensions that need to be studied and understood by public health students. There are personal, social, economic, and environmental factors that influence health status, and those can be summarized as follows: Policymaking, Social factors, Health services, Individual Behavior and Biology and Genetics.

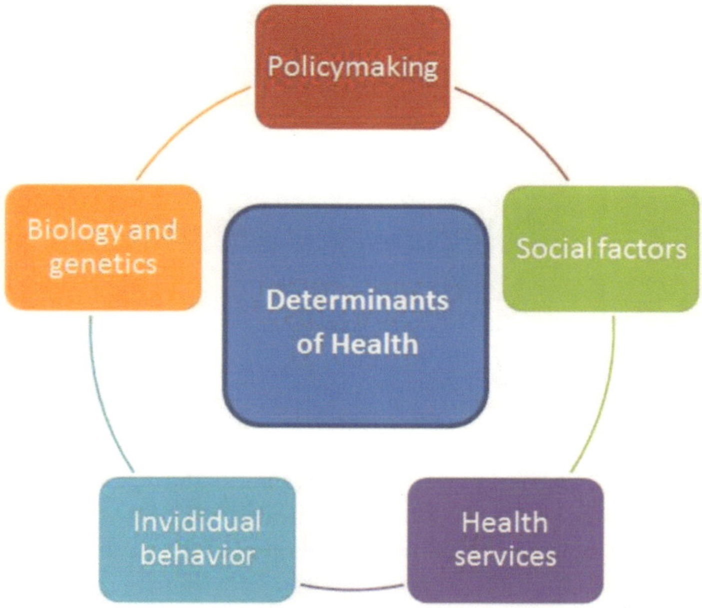

Figure 1. Determinants of Health

As it can be seen in the figure all five determinants are inter-related and each one can be targeted individually or as a group when working out a solution for a health problem.

Example: For the public health problem: "Motor-vehicle crashes among teen agers", one can analyze the problem by using the determinants of health. You can take one or several of the determinants to define what will you target in the intervention (Figure 2).

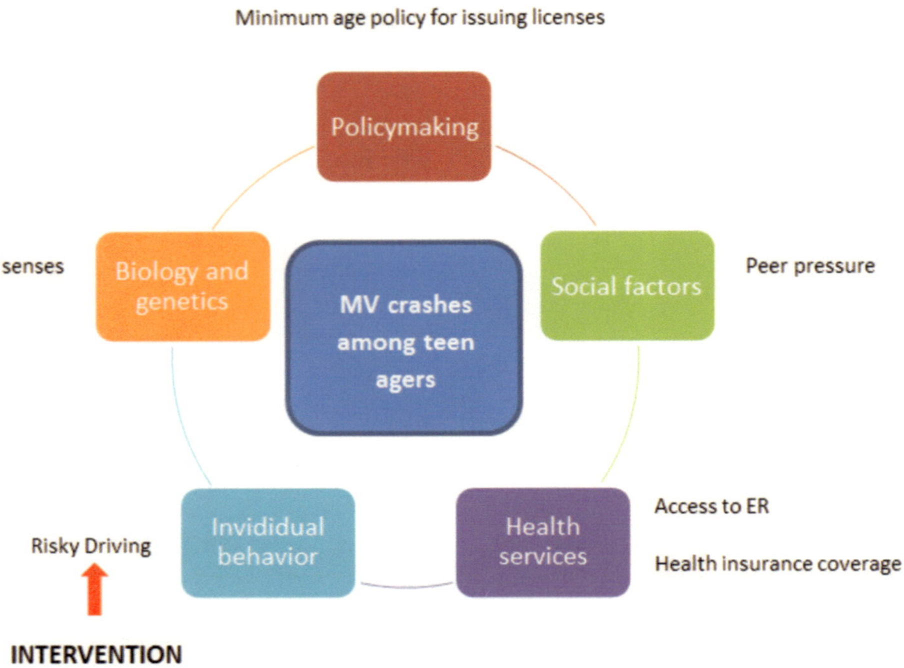

Figure 2. Assessment of Motor-vehicle crashes among teen agers using determinants of health

The world is changing fast. Often unclear is the impact that social, economic, and political change will have on health in general, on health inequities within countries or across the globe in particular. Action on the social determinants of health will be more effective if basic data systems, including vital registration and routine monitoring of health inequity and the social determinants of health are in place and there are mechanisms to ensure that the data can be understood and applied to develop more effective policies, systems, and programs [5]. This being said, education and training in social determinants of health are vital during teaching public health.

http://dx.doi.org/10.5772/53722

In conjunction with Healthy People 2020, we should ask ourselves two questions: "what makes some people healthy and others unhealthy?" and, "how can we create a society in which everyone has a chance to live long healthy lives?". In order to answer these questions, it is recommended to develop objectives that address the relationship between health status and biology, individual behavior, health services, social factors and policies; and emphasize an ecological approach to disease prevention and health promotion. An ecological approach focuses on both individual-level and population-level determinants of health and interventions [6].

Exercise 1	Exercise 1 Characteristics
1. Select a health problem 2. Ask your students to brainstorm and analyze the causes associated to the health problem according to the determinants of health 3. The students can analyze the problem from one or several determinants. 4. Moderate the discussion 5. Write on the board the related causes given by the students 6. Wrap up the discussion	**Type of exercise:** Brainstorming **Setting:** Classroom **Number of students recommended:** From 5 to 30 **Materials:** Bibliography resources, board, markers, eraser. **Duration:** 15 to 20 minutes. **Expected outcome:** Blackboard utilization with a health problem and its possible causes analyzed from each determinant of health.

Figure 3. Exercise 1 - Brainstorming

3. Who is interested in learning about public health?

People interested in public health come from a variety of backgrounds and with different educational levels (Technical, Professional, Masters, PhD). When teaching public health one has to be very well aware of this diversity to use the proper vocabulary, terms and information so it can reach those from non-health and health related backgrounds. Technical jargon should be utilized but only after being thoroughly introduced.

Traditionally, those interested in public health are health practitioners, especially physicians, nurses and social workers. However, I have worked with people from various backgrounds such as finances, administration, anthropology, information technology, biology, etc. actively working on public health. Some of them came into the public health arena by accident and some others because they truly liked it to begin with.

Public Health is a field easy to fall in-love with, challenging different backgrounds seeking the solutions and the outcomes expected for health problems. The recruitment of non-health professionals into public health is not so difficult, but we have an obligation as public health practitioners to promote and communicate that this is an exciting area for many people.

One of my first work experiences at the World Health Organization had me recruiting professionals from non-health backgrounds to work in Public Health specifically from developing countries. In the beginning I thought it was going to be very difficult to motivate these professionals to work in the subject, however, it was highly sought by those who were informed about the job opportunities and areas of work. The main challenge was just to get out there and to deliver the message effectively for public health to be known within some target groups.

The fields of work in Public Health are broad as well. You can work for local, regional, national or world offices, governmental or non-governmental, private and educational institutions. Next is an example of a job description for a non-health professional to work in Public Heath:

Example: Sample Job Description: Performance Improvement Manager
Position Overview: Manages and coordinates organization-wide efforts to ensure that performance management (PM) and quality improvement (QI) programs are developed and managed using a data driven focus that sets priorities for improvements aligned to ongoing strategic imperatives.
Minimum Requirements: Master's degree in public health or MBA and 10 or more years of experience in public health management, planning or public policy development. Experience in Performance Improvement Management and Quality is desired [7].

In the beginning of my public health career, I quickly learned that Public Health needs the work and support of different disciplines and backgrounds. To analyze and act upon a health issue you need the participation of a health professional who knows the theory behind the health issue, people with some knowledge in administration and finances, people that know about policy development, statistics and so on, if you really want to target properly the matter of study and have some impact.

You are able to find all the levels of training in Public Health, while in developing countries, you can mainly find graduate programs such as Masters or PhDs. Perhaps, developing countries are just now entering the world of policy development in public health issues and training programs are just starting to grow.

There are many different degree programs for those interested in studying public health. Some of the programs include:

BA = Bachelor's in public health: Designed to give students a basic grounding in public health issues and methods. [8]

- MPH = Master of Public Health: include coursework in a number of public health disciplines, such as administration, epidemiology, environmental health, and behavioral health. Specialized degrees such as a Master of Health Administration will be more focused on a specific topic.

http://dx.doi.org/10.5772/53722

- MHA = Master of Health Administration: People with experience in public health but often don't have MPH degrees
- MHSA = Master of Health Services Administration: For people interested in administration of Public Health.
- MSPH = Master of Science in Public Health
- DrPH = Doctor of Public Health: It is for people with an interest in public health leadership, or a desire for deeper knowledge than an MPH program can provide.
- PhD = Doctor of Philosophy

The MPH, DrPH, and MHA are example of degrees which are geared towards those who want careers as practitioners of public health in traditional health departments, managed care organizations, community-based organizations, hospitals, consulting firms, international agencies, state and federal agencies, among others.

MS, PhD, and ScD are examples of academic degrees. They are more oriented toward students wishing to seek a career in academics and research rather than public health practice.

However, each school of public health can tailor their degree programs significantly. Students interested in getting a degree in public health should check with individual schools for more information on specific degree programs.

In your classroom, you will have you have an array of backgrounds that represent an opportunity to make your class exciting and fulfilling. Know your students, who they are, what they do, what their expectations are, and more importantly, identify how can they contribute to the public health world.

Exercise 2	Exercise 2 Characteristics
Greet your students and ask them the following information 1. What is your name? 2. What is your background? 3. What do you expect from the class? 4. What previous experiences in public health have you had? 5. Is there a particular career path or job you seek?	**Type of exercise:** Getting acquainted **Setting:** Classroom **Number of students recommended:** From 5 to 30 **Materials:** - **Duration:** 15 to 30 minutes. **Expected outcome:** Knowing your students, identifying what they expect and what they could give to the class.

Figure 4. Exercise 2 – Getting acquainted

Public health is a rewarding field. The field of public health offers great personal fulfillment - working towards improving people's health and well-being is a rewarding day's work. Health status indicators or health outcomes, can tell you whether you've got a clean bill of health or if you and your community are in need of some regular public health attention [9].

4. What skills and competences are needed in a public health practitioner?

An array of skills and competences become the tools of good performance in the field. Those skills and competences need to be developed during public health training. The teacher is directly responsible for assuring that the students get what is needed to execute impeccably the plans and goals delineated for taking action in the community or research fields.

Competency is defined as the ability to apply particular knowledge, skills, attitudes, and values to the standard of performance required in specified contexts. The Core Competencies can serve as a starting point for public health practice and academic organizations as they create workforce development plans, identify training and workforce needs, prepare for accreditation, and more [10]. Generic competencies are the minimum baseline set of competencies that are common to all public health roles across all public health sectors and disciplines and that are necessary for the delivery of essential public health services [11].

The competencies are organized into twelve topic areas. Each topic comprises a set of competency statements as follows (Table 1):

Topic	Generic Competency statement
1. Health systems	• Demonstrates knowledge of the health systems and structures • Demonstrates knowledge of key international agreements.
2. Public Health Science	• Demonstrates knowledge of what constitutes public health and how it relates to public health practice in specific contexts. • Demonstrates knowledge of the determinant factors that affect health and health inequalities. • Demonstrates knowledge of the basic concepts of health. • Demonstrates knowledge of the basic epidemiological concepts.
3. Policy, Legislation and Regulation	• Demonstrates knowledge of the use of policy in a public health context. • Demonstrates knowledge of how legislation and regulations are applied in public health contexts.
4. Research and evaluation	• Demonstrates understanding of the principles of research and its applications in public health. • Demonstrates understanding of the principles of evaluation and its applications in public health.
5. Community health development	• Demonstrates knowledge of community development in a public health context.
6. Public Health Practice	• Demonstrates knowledge and understanding of the intent of public health interventions. • Analyses public health issues.

http://dx.doi.org/10.5772/53722

Topic	Generic Competency statement
	• Uses culturally appropriate values processes and protocols when working in teams.
7. Working across and understanding cultures	• Demonstrates knowledge of the nature of culture. • Demonstrates knowledge of the principles of cultural • safety and takes responsibility for maintaining safety in • regards to cultural values, norms, and practices.
8. Communication	• Listens actively. • Uses different communication styles to facilitate understanding accommodate. • Uses oral communication effectively in a range of contexts. • Communicates clearly in writing for the given context. • Consults with others in a range of settings.
9. Leadership, Teamwork, and professional liaison	• Positively influences the way teams work together. • Demonstrates understanding of the many aspects of leadership. • Instigates, coordinates and facilitates groups. • Establishes and maintains effective professional relationships to improve health outcomes.
10. Advocacy	• Demonstrates the ability to advocate in achieving public health outcomes. • Demonstrates the ability to negotiate to achieve public health outcomes.
11. Professional Development and Self- Management	• Manages self to improve performance and professional development.
12. Planning and Administration	• Accesses a range of organizational information. • Describes how work plan fits with organizational and wider public health priorities. • Completes appropriate administration record keeping and allocated financial responsibilities according to contractual and legal frameworks and organizational policies as they apply. • Demonstrates understanding of the public heath role in an emergency response.

Source: Keating, Gay et al. Generic Competencies for Public Health in Aotearoa-New Zealand. New Zealand: The Public Health Association of New Zealand.

Table 1. Topic areas with their generic competencies in Public Health

A skill is the ability to do something well; to have the expertise. Some of the most important skills for a public health professional to have are: Analytic Assessment Skills, Policy Development/Programa Planning Skills, Communication Skills, Cultural Competency Skills, Community Dimensions of Practice Skills, Basic Public Health Sciences Skills, Financial Planning and Management Skills and Leadership and Systems Thinking Skills [12]

For each domain of skills there are a group of specific competences that apply as shown in table 2.

Skill	Specific Competence
Analytic Assessment Skills	• Defines a problem • Determines appropriate uses and limitations of both quantitative and qualitative data • Selects and defines variables relevant to defined public health problems • Identifies relevant and appropriate data and information sources • Evaluates the integrity and comparability of data and identifies gaps in data sources • Applies ethical principles to the collection, maintenance, use, and dissemination of data and information • Partners with communities to attach meaning to collected quantitative and qualitative data • Makes relevant inferences from quantitative and qualitative data • Obtains and interprets information regarding risks and benefits to the community • Applies data collection processes, information technology applications, and computer systems storage/retrieval strategies • Recognizes how the data illuminates ethical, political, scientific, economic, and overall public health issues
Policy Development/Program Planning Skills	• Collects, summarizes, and interprets information relevant to an issue • States policy options and writes clear and concise policy statements • Identifies, interprets, and implements public health laws, regulations, and policies related to specific programs • Articulates the health, fiscal, administrative, legal, social, and political implications of each policy option • States the feasibility and expected outcomes of each policy option • Utilizes current techniques in decision analysis and health planning • Decides on the appropriate course of action • Develops a plan to implement policy, including goals, outcome and process objectives, and implementation steps • Translates policy into organizational plans, structures, and programs • Prepares and implements emergency response plans • Develops mechanisms to monitor and evaluate programs for their • effectiveness and quality
Communication Skills	• Communicates effectively both in writing and orally, or in other ways • Solicits input from individuals and organizations • Advocates for public health programs and resources • Leads and participates in groups to address specific issues • Uses the media, advanced technologies, and community networks to communicate information • Effectively presents accurate demographic, statistical, programmatic, and scientific information for professional and lay audiences
Cultural Competency Skills	• Utilizes appropriate methods for interacting sensitively, effectively,

http://dx.doi.org/10.5772/53722

Skill	Specific Competence
	• and professionally with persons from diverse cultural, socioeconomic, educational, racial, ethnic and professional • backgrounds, and persons of all ages and lifestyle preferences • Identifies the role of cultural, social, and behavioral factors in • determining the delivery of public health services • Develops and adapts approaches to problems that take into • account cultural differences
Community Dimensions of Practice Skills	• Establishes and maintains linkages with key stakeholders • Utilizes leadership, team building, negotiation, and conflict • resolution skills to build community partnerships • Collaborates with community partners to promote the health of • the population • Identifies how public and private organizations operate within a community • Accomplishes effective community engagements • Identifies community assets and available resources • Develops, implements, and evaluates a community public health assessment, • Describes the role of government in the delivery of community • health services
Basic Public Health Sciences Skills	• Identifies the individual's and organization's responsibilities within the context of the Essential Public Health Services and core functions • Defines, assesses, and understands the health status of populations, determinants of health and illness, factors contributing • to health promotion and disease prevention, and factors influencing the use of health services • Understands the historical development, structure, and interaction of public health and health care systems • Identifies and applies basic research methods used in public health • Applies the basic public health sciences including behavioral and social sciences, biostatistics, epidemiology, environmental public • health, and prevention of chronic and infectious diseases and injuries • Identifies and retrieves current relevant scientific evidence • Identifies the limitations of research and the importance of observations and interrelationships
Financial Planning and Management Skills	• Develops and presents a budget • Manages programs within budget constraints • Applies budget processes • Develops strategies for determining budget priorities • Monitors program performance • Prepares proposals for funding from external sources

Skill	Specific Competence
	• Applies basic human relations skills to the management of organizations, motivation of personnel, and resolution of conflicts • Manages information systems for collection, retrieval, and use of data for decision-making • Negotiates and develops contracts and other documents for • the provision of population-based services • Conducts cost effectiveness, cost benefit, and cost utility analyses
Leadership and Systems Thinking Skills	• Creates a culture of ethical standards within organizations and communities • Helps create key values and shared vision and uses these principles to guide action • Identifies internal and external issues that may impact delivery of • essential public health services (i.e. strategic planning) • Facilitates collaboration with internal and external groups to • ensure participation of key stakeholders • Promotes team and organizational learning • Contributes to development, implementation, and monitoring of organizational performance standards • Uses the legal and political system to effect change • Applies theory of organizational structures to professional practice
Source: PHF. Core Competencies for Public Health Professionals. Washington: Public Health Foundation; 2012.	

Table 2. Skills and specific competences in Public Health.

You can observe in tables 1 and 2, public health professional needs to develop: a series of skills and competences that will make s/he a professional that will be able to perform different duties in several areas and to have a broader understanding of the health problems in his community and the world.

According to the discipline, profiles are outlined to meet the requirement of the tasks as it is presented in the following example:

Example: Sample Job Description: Performance Improvement Manager
Position Overview: Lecturer / Senior Lecturer in Public Health
Essential Factors and Skills: Master's degree or equivalent, Ability to inspire and collaborate, Establishes writing skills, Specialist expertise and experience in public health, Previous experience in coordinating public health research, writing and submitting proposals and bids and mentoring and supervising staff. Excellent verbal and communication skills, presentation skills and IT skills. Organized, with an ability to work methodically, accurately and to deadlines. [13].

http://dx.doi.org/10.5772/53722

Exercise 3	Exercise 3 Characteristics
Invite a guest speaker to your class, who's profile is an experienced Public Health Professional. Ask him to talk about his experience in the field; how he has done it, what skills and competences he has developed. Finish the session with questions and answers from your students.	**Type of exercise:** Guest speaker **Setting:** Classroom or auditorium **Number of students recommended:** From 15 to 100 **Materials:** Audiovisual, video beam, computer **Duration:** 30 to 60 minutes. **Expected outcome:** Students motivated about Public Health

Figure 5. Exercise 3 – Guest speaker

5. Importance of knowing your students and identifying their particular skills

This is a special section with some strategies to identify the potential of your students in the classroom, how to explore and encourage their development and applicability towards public health practice.

It doesn't matter how good a professional can be if s/he doesn't care for who s/he is teaching. A success factor for any one's learning experience is having a teacher that can actively search and find the talents of his/her students.

I always recommend to anyone who works in education, more so in health education, to devote a good amount of time to get to know their students well. I say especially in health education because health sciences tend to depersonalize learning experiences; leaving the themes as just science to be learned no matter the individual makes learning sterile.

From the first encounter with your students take some time getting acquainted, for example, use icebreakers, ask about your student's family, habits, hobbies and why not get into some of the public health subjects you are going to be teaching them utilizing their own health risk factors or determinants of health. That way you will know how much resonance you will have in your lectures. This will also give you the opportunity to select examples that will reach your students in a deeper level that will touch them, that will make them remember!

Learners can be classified according to their learning style or preference as visual, auditory or tactile/kinesthetic [14].

For visual learners it is important to use pictures, diagrams, photographs, graphs, videos, illustrations, flipcharts or any other visual aid that will accompany the main message. Body language it is also important with these types of students. It can become a powerful tool for keeping their interest in the class and the subject.

Auditory learners are those who learn best by listening. Be prepared to use a decisive tone of voice, make changes in volume, intensity, accentuation and speed. Learners get the most out of discussions in small groups, short lectures and interesting subjects. Sometimes you can also use music to emphasize parts of the lecture or discussion.

Tactile or kinesthetic learners learn better by doing, moving or touching. In teaching public health, any type of community work, such as data collection, surveying, prevention activities in the community, education, etc. it is a very used method to motivate and train your students in a particular subject.

Example: Learning Styles	
AUDITORY LEARNERS Like to be read to Like to read at loud Like to use mnemonics to help learn material Like to talk with others about their ideas	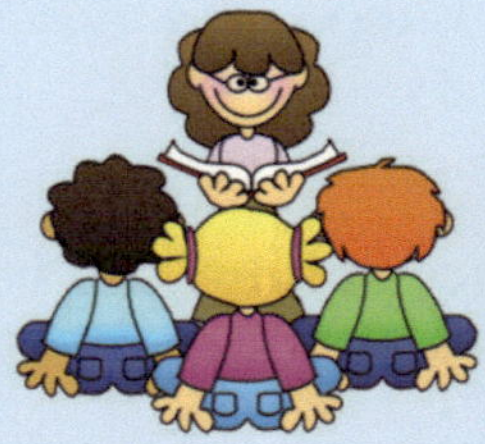
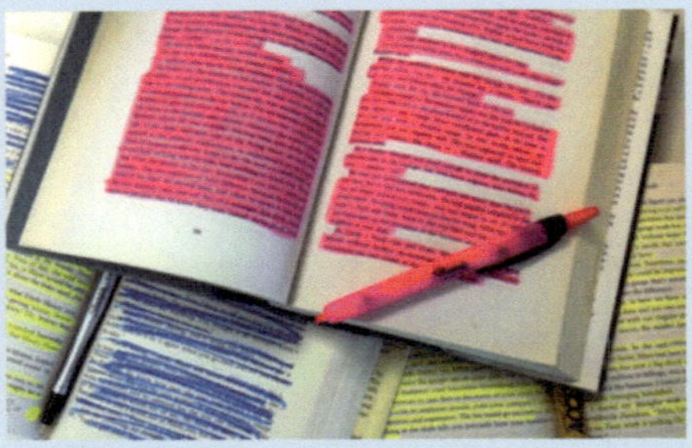	**VISUAL LEARNERS** Like to learn from reading, taking notes, and using worksheets Like to use highlighters to outline important facts Like to see a visual representation of the information Like to use multimedia materials such as computers and transparencies
KINESTHETIC LEARNERS Like to move around to learn new information Like to take frequent breaks Like to use rhythms or music to learn Like to learn in different settings	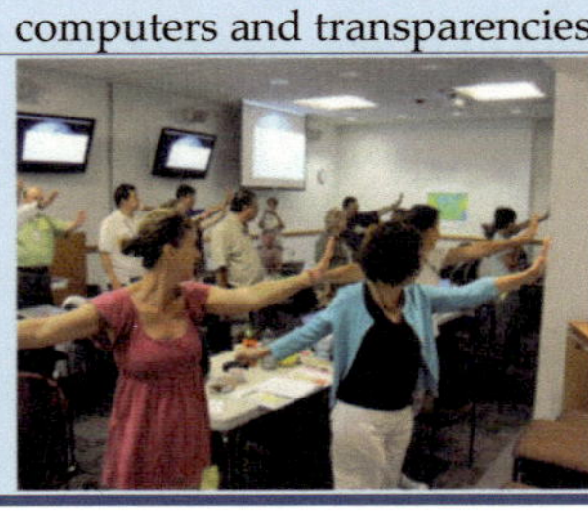

Figure 6. Example of learning styles. Source: BENSLEY, Robert and BROOKINS-FISHER, Jodi. Community Health education and methods. A practical guide. United States: Jones and Barlett Publishers, LLC; 2009.

You can use either or all the methods whenever you feel you need them. Public Health teaching is not limited to the classroom, but can be done in all kinds of settings. Where ever you are, try to use it for your convenience and apply your skills to achieve your main goal: capture your student's interest [15]. You can do this by stimulating research on the theory and practice of health education; supporting high quality performance standards for the practice of health

http://dx.doi.org/10.5772/53722

education and health promotion; and finally, advocating policy and legislation affecting health education.

In the next table there are several methods that can be used in the exercise of teaching public health by developing three types of objectives: cognitive objectives, affective objectives and psychomotor objectives.

Method	Cognitive	Affective	Psychomotor	Time required
Getting acquainted (icebrakers)	X	P	P	15+
Audio	X	P	P	15+
Audiovisual materials	X	P	P	15+
Case studies	X	X		30+
Computer-assisted instruction	X	P		30+
Cooperative learning	P	P	P	30+
Debates	P	P		30+
Educational games	X			20+
Field trips		P		60+
Guest speakers	X	P		30+
Lecture	X			5+
Panels	P	X		30+
Peer education	P	X		120+
Problem solving		X	P	30+
Self-appraisals		X		10+
Service learning	X	X	P	120+
Simulations	X	X	X	30+
Storytelling	P	X		10+

Legend: X = Yes, common use; P = possible

Table 3. Methods for teaching public health and their objectives

Some of the methods described above have been used as examples in this chapter.

Example: Selecting team members
After a getting acquainted section, you noticed you have at least 5 students that know very well SPSS, 3 more that are great speakers, 2 that have field experiences in public health interventions, 4 students with grant writing experiences, and 2 students with managerial and financial skills. You need to put to put together a team of 5 people that can manage and run an intervention in the community. You are able know to select the individuals for your team after knowing the skills your students have.

In order to have a good point of departure in a modern public health course, I recommend choosing an authoritative book on the main concepts of Public Health to be used as course text. Depending on the focus of the class, that book can have only public health theory or more specific information on any of the public health areas.

Prepare your class using at least one of the methods that have been explained or more than one depending on the content of the lecture, number of students, available resources and time.

Create a course syllabus. Schedule topics in advance and inform your students about the materials to be used in the class. Assign some readings so the students have a previous review of the information to be discussed in the class and make sure to make a round of questions (Q&A) about the assigned reading.

This will help you and your students to trace a baseline from which your class will start with generated expectations and a basic knowledge to be developed.

Exercise 4	Exercise 4 Characteristics
Prepare an outline for a lecture using at least 3 methods described in table 3. Input the time dedicated to each activity, materials used and bibliography. Make sure to include exercises for your students.	**Type of exercise:** Lecture **Setting:** Classroom or auditorium **Number of students recommended:** From 5 to 30 **Materials:** Audiovisual, video beam, computer **Duration:** 45 to 90 minutes. **Expected outcome:** Objectives of the lecture met.

Figure 7. Exercise 4 – Lecture

Again, using either one or several of those methods, you should be able to include the students and make them full participant in your class activity. Once you have identified what the student can do and what it that makes her/him special in the classroom, reinforce it and promote it.

6. Guiding your students to generate actions in public health

Public health is a field that offers an abundance of job opportunities to suit a variety of interests and skills. Whether you are more interested in crunching numbers, conducting research, or working with people, there is a place for you. Recent college graduates and those that have been in the field for years have something to offer and to gain in this field. Public health is ideal for those that gain satisfaction knowing that they are working to improve the lives of others.

It is very important for a student to understand the public health priorities that surround her/him, and in that way, should be able to propose solutions that can be taken to actions. Some of the key public health priorities which have become achievements for the world and the United States of America are listed in table 4.

No.	Worldwide 2001-2010	United States 2001-2010
1	Reductions in child mortality	Vaccine-Preventable Diseases
2	Vaccine-Preventable Diseases	Prevention and control of Infectious Diseases
3	Access to Safe Water and Sanitation	Tobacco Control
4	Malaria Prevention and Control	Maternal and Infant Health
5	Prevention and control of HIV/AIDS	Motor Vehicle Safety
6	Tuberculosis Control	Cardiovascular Disease Prevention
7	Control of Neglected Tropical Diseases	Occupational Safety
8	Tobacco Control	Cancer Prevention
9	Increased Awareness and Response for Improving Global Road Safety	Childhood Lead Poisoning Prevention
10	Improved Preparedness and Response to Global Health Threats	Public Health Preparedness and Response

Source: CDC. Ten Great Public Health Achievements

Table 4. Ten great Public Health Achievements

Public Health needs to transcend the assessment of health issues and professionals should be able to propose and deliver interventions in the field that make changes in communities and hopefully in public policies.

Many public health practitioners find the problems, analyze them and give plausible explanations of the causes to health issues. Less come out with ideas for interventions and activities to be made, and even less are able to conjugate the results of those interventions to proposing political exits to public health problems.

Exercise 5	Exercise 5 Characteristics
Take your students on a field trip to visit a vulnerable community to a health problem, example, a community with water problems. Have them talk to the people, look for the water sources, identify the problems, propose solutions and implement intervention activities if already outlined. Wrap up the session with lessons learned. Take pictures and write a field trip report.	**Type of exercise:** **Field trip** **Setting:** Field **Number of students recommended:** 5 to 15 **Materials:** Transportation mean, identifications for students, camera **Duration:** 90 to 180+ minutes. **Expected outcome:** Students motivation, intervention goals reviewed and measured.

Figure 8. Exercise 5 – Field trip

7. Use of technology in the teaching and practicing of public health

Globalization has changed the way in which we work, especially as a scientific community. Networking and technology are quintessential tools for teaching public health now.

Teaching and assessing public health has changed within a century, and now, we face an age in which the Information and communication technologies (ITCs) are the gold standard. ITCs are the integration of telecommunications, computers, audio-visual systems, wired and wireless signals, software, storage and others in order to transmit, store, manipulate and share information efficiently between users.

The ITCs join what used to be telephone networks with computer networks, and has facilitated the delivery of messages to public health practitioners and community.

Dr. Mirta Roses Periago, former Director of the Panamerican Health Organization said in 2003 the following words that I consider relevant: "This century will be the century of networks, connectivity and interdependence, and this will allow us to overcome the barriers of time and space, opening possibilities that we never imagined to improve the life conditions of our people…" [18]

Health services are complex in the way they are built, based upon scientific research and evidence based medicine. In order to do this, it is necessary the collaboration and participation of multiple actors with different profiles, knowledge and skills.

Communication between parties that work in public health has significantly improved through ITCs and social networks. There are other technologies that include digital content and video streaming that also facilitate the interaction of interdisciplinary groups.

The source of knowledge and their spread has evolved as follows (figure 3):

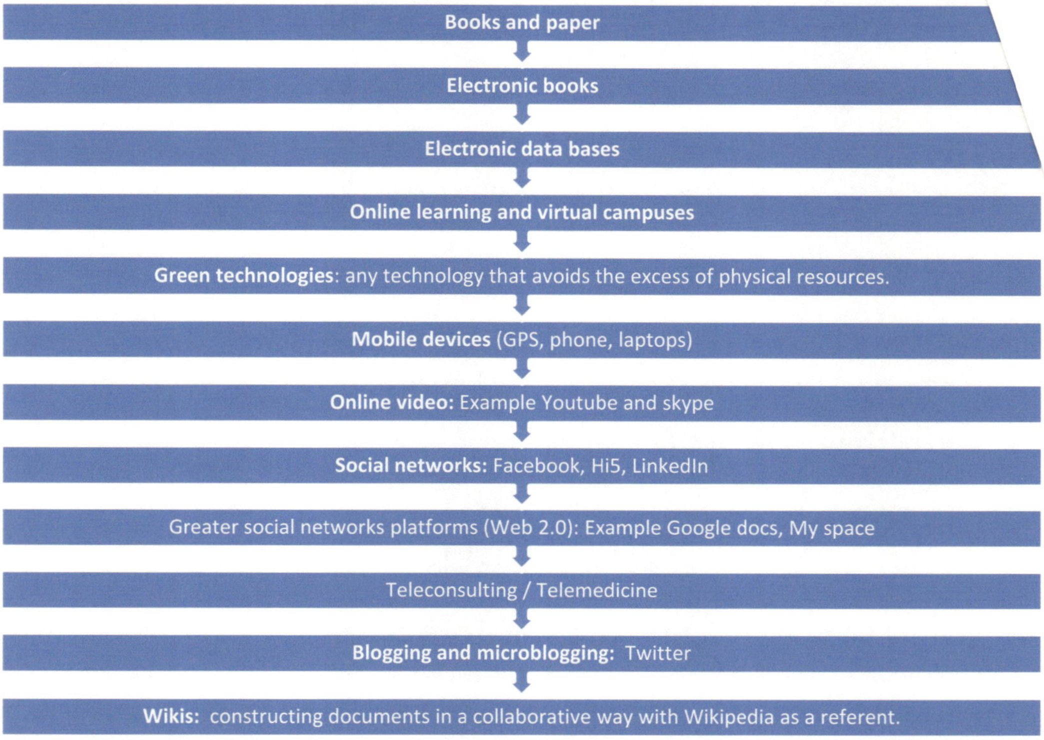

Figure 9. Evolution of knowledge sources and their communication resources

With the use of ITCs you can interact with others, share information and resources efficiently, however, one has to be very cautious when protecting the security and privacy of the health information that is being managed, because of its efficiency and ease of use, sharing this type of knowledge through ITCs can put people at risk.

This is why users, roles and privileges in accessing any type of ITC resource has to be well defined. Computer accounts need to be secure, data storage and back up has to be warranted. [19]

I have personally used all of the tools named in figure 3 for both clinical and public health practice. I believe ITCs and social networking are a powerful tool to access the community and generate highly impacting interventions. However, I also believe the management of the messages being distributed, the discussions created and the rising questions need a careful treatment in order not to allow the transformation or deviation of the core messages that were intended to be delivered.

Example: Blog: U.S Strategy to prevent and respond to gender-based violence globally [20]

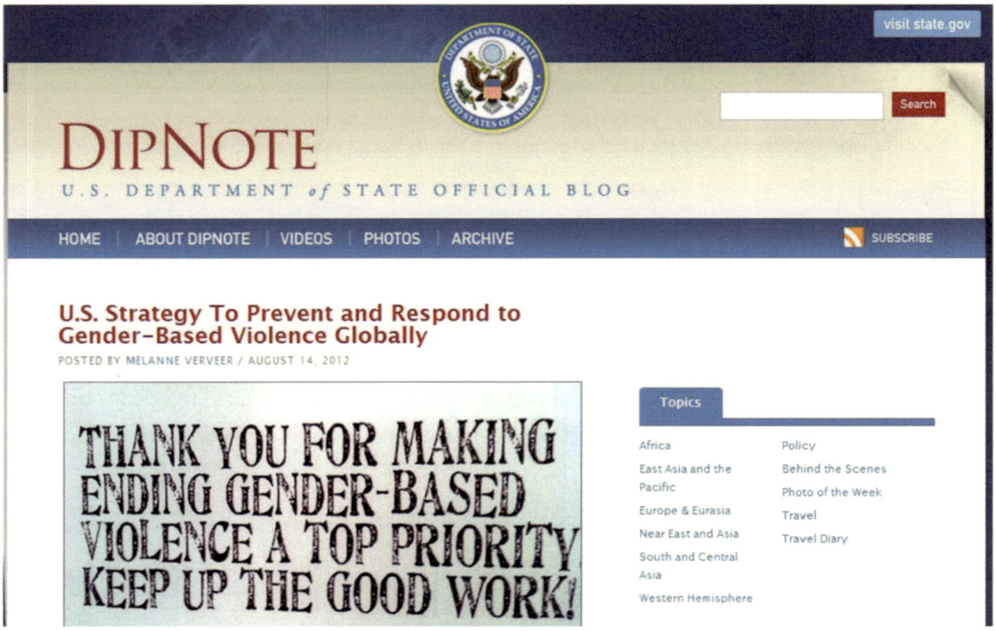

Social networking works especially well in settings where technology is accessible and other communication practices might be more expensive. Some developing countries have good access to internet for instance, and people in the community might be able to participate in activities and discussions, read messages, post queries or getting actively involved in a public health strategy without having to spend a lot or resources.

Exercise 6	Exercise 6 Characteristics
At the computer lab give your students a public health topic to research. Provide them with a list of health databases to be used. Ask them to look for at least 5 scientific articles that discuss the topic selected. Students should write a report and send it to the instructor by e-mail at the end of the class.	**Type of exercise:** Computer-assisted instruction **Setting:** Computer lab **Number of students recommended:** 5 to 30 **Materials:** Computer, video beam **Duration:** 60 to 120 minutes **Expected outcome:** Data bases management

Figure 10. Exercise 6 – Computer-assisted instruction

http://dx.doi.org/10.5772/53722

8. Results expected in the learning process of public health

One of the key messages to be taught is to keep in mind that partnering with the community is the key to success of Public Health practice.

Community diversity and culture must be recognized and respected. Community engagement can only be sustained by identifying and mobilizing community assets, and by developing capacities and resources for community health decisions and action.

The concerns of society are always in the forefront of public health. These concerns keep changing and the methods for addressing keep expanding. New technologies and global, local, and national interventions are becoming a necessary part of public health. [21]

The impact of any public health initiative is proportional to the amount of community involvement and collaboration. They are who, in the end, will acquire long-term commitments with their own health and we as public health practitioners, are the ones who will partner with them and other organizations to make those relationships long lasting and productive.

The final outcome of a public health learning process involves:

- Basic knowledge in public health generalities
- Acute sense of research
- Highly committed and sensible professionals with the community
- Community involvement
- Setting realistic goals that should progress to highly impact the social setting to be applied.
- Setting performance indicators

Goals, objectives, and performance indicators function very much like the elements of an archer and his or her target, in that, they clarify the purpose of the health education intervention.

9. Conclusion

Teaching public health means training individuals to assess effectively health issues, assure the maintenance of health in a community and develop policies, strategies and interventions to improve health.

Public health is an exciting and growing field of study that challenges its professionals to confront complex health issues, such as improving access to health care, controlling infectious disease, and reducing environmental hazards, violence, substance abuse, and injury. The field is dynamic and diverse, and Public Health professionals come from varying educational backgrounds and can specialize in an array of fields. A host of specialists, including teachers, journalists, researchers, administrators, environmentalists, demographers, social workers, laboratory scientists, and attorneys, work to protect the health of the public.

Public health is also a field geared toward serving others. Public health professionals serve local, national, and international communities. They are leaders who meet the many exciting challenges in protecting the public's health today and in the future.

As public health trainers we have the obligation to educate our students develop their skills and make them competent in the areas they select as their preference. A well trained professional should be capable of taking on challenges with confidence, effectiveness and assertiveness.

During training, students need to explore all three dimensions of the core functions of public health: assessment, assurance and policy development. In this way, they would be able to choose which direction to go once they are practicing.

A public health trainer needs to be proficient in the use of ICTs and apply them not only during the academic exercise of teaching public health but during his practice. ICTs facilitate public health intervention outcomes and are an efficient and cost-effective way to promote health.

Author details

Claudia Marin-Kelso[1,2]

Address all correspondence to: claudiamarin@utp.edu.co

1 School of Medicine, Faculty of Health Sciences (Colombian Associated Center for the Iberoamerican Cochrane Network), Universidad Tecnológica de Pereira (UTP), Pereira, Colombia

2 Faculty of Health Sciences (Colombian Associated Center for the Iberoamerican Cochrane Network), Universidad Tecnológica de Pereira (UTP), Pereira, Risaralda, Colombia

References

[1] Winslow, Charles-Edward Amory. The cost of sickness and the price of health. In: Bulletin of the World Health Organization. Geneva: World Health Organization; 2006. Available from http://www.ncbi.nlm.nih.gov/pmc/articles/PMC2626527/pdf/16501735.pdf (accessed August 31, 2012).

[2] Gilbert, Glen; Sawyer, Robin and McNeill, Lisa Beth. Health Education: Creating strategies for school & Community Health. United States: Jones and Barlett Publishers, LLC; 2011.

http://dx.doi.org/10.5772/53722

[3] Saracci, Rodolfo. Introducing the history of epidemiology. In: teaching epidemiology. A guide for teachers in epidemiology, public health and clinical medicine. Third Edition. Oxford: Oxford University Press, 2010.

[4] Novick, Lloyd and Morrow, Cynthia. Defining Public health: Historial and contemporary developments. In: Public Health Administration: Principles for Population-Based Management, Second Edition. Burlington: Jones & Barlett Learning; 2008.

[5] WHO. Closing the gap in a generation. Health equity through action on the social determinants of health. In: commission on social determinants of health. Final Report. Geneva: WHO; 2008. Available from http://whqlibdoc.who.int/hq/2008/WHO_IER_CSDH_08.1_eng.pdf (accessed August 10, 2012).

[6] HSS. Framework. Healthy People 2020. Washington D.C: U.S Department of Health and Human Services (HSS); 2012. Available from http://www.healthypeople.gov/2020/Consortium/HP2020Framework.pdf (accessed August 15, 2012).

[7] CDC. Sample Job Description. Sample Job Description: Performance Improvement Manager. Atlanta: Center for Disease Control and Prevention; 2010. Available from http://www.cdc.gov/stltpublichealth/docs/PHF%20-%20PIM%20Sample%20Job%20Description.pdf (accessed August 1, 2012).

[8] Seltzer, Beth. 101 Careers in Public Health. New York: Springer Publishing Company, LLC; 2011.

[9] Carney, Jan. Public Health in Action: Practicing in the Real world. United States: Jones and Barlett Learning; 2006.

[10] PHF. About the core competencies for public health professionals. Washington: Public Health Foundation; 2012. Available from: http://www.phf.org/programs/corecompetencies/Pages/About_the_Core_Competencies_for_Public_Health_Professionals.aspx (accessed August 25, 2012)

[11] Keating, Gay et al. Generic Competencies for Public Health in Aotearoa-New Zealand. New Zealand: The Public Health Association of New Zealand. Available from http://www.pha.org.nz/documents/GenericCompetenciesforPublicHealth-March2007.pdf (accessed August 28, 2012)

[12] PHF. Core Competencies for Public Health Professionals. Washington: Public Health Foundation; 2012. Available from: https://www.train.org/competencies/corecomp.pdf (accessed August 25, 2012)

[13] WHO. Vacancy: Lecturer / Senior Lecturer in Public Health. Liverpool John Moores University. Liverpool: Collaborating Centre for Violence Prevention, World Health Organization. Available from http://www.nwph.net/JD%20Senior%20Lecturer%20Public%20Health%20IC.pdf (accessed August 20, 2012)

[14] Bensley, Robert and Brookins-Fisher, Jodi. Community Health education and methods. A practical guide. United States: Jones and Barlett Publishers, LLC; 2009.

[15] Barnes, Louis, Roland, Christensen and Hansen, Abby. Teaching and the case method: Text, Cases and Readings. United States: Harvard Business School Press, 1994.

[16] CDC. Ten Great Public Health Achievements – United States, 2001 – 2010. In: Morbidity and Mortality Weekly Report. Vol 19. Atlanta: CDC; 2011. http://www.cdc.gov/mmwr/pdf/wk/mm6019.pdf

[17] CDC. Ten Great Public Health Achievements – Worldwide, 2001 – 2010. In: Morbidity and Mortality Weekly Report. Vol 24. Atlanta: CDC; 2011. http://www.cdc.gov/mmwr/pdf/wk/mm6024.pdf

[18] PAHO. Herramientas y metodologias TIC para mejorar la salud pública en la Región de las Américas. Washington: eSalud OPS. Pan American Health Organization; 2003. Available from http://www.cepal.org/elac/noticias/paginas/7/40837/jorge-walters.pdf (accessed August 30, 2012).

[19] Minelli, Mark and Breckon, Donald. Community Health Education: Settings, Roles, and Skills. 5th edition. United States: Jones and Barlett Publishers; 2009.

[20] USA. U.S. Strategy To Prevent and Respond to Gender-Based Violence Globally. Washingon: U.S Department of State; 2012. Available from http://blogs.state.gov/index.php/site/entry/us_strategy_gbv (accessed August 5, 2012)

[21] Riegelman, Richard. Public Health 101. Healthy people-Healthy populations. United States: Jones and Barlett Publishers, LLC; 2010.